ORTHOPAEDIC PATHOLOGY

Commissioning Editor: Michael Houston
Project Development Manager: Tim Kimber
Project Manager: Nora Naughton
Illustration Manager: Mick Ruddy
Design Manager: Sarah Russell
Illustrator: Paul Banville

ORTHOPAEDIC PATHOLOGY

4th edition

Peter G Bullough MB ChB

Director of Laboratory Medicine, Hospital for Special Surgery, and
Professor of Pathology and Laboratory Medicine, Weill Medical College of Cornell University
New York, NY, USA

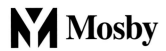 Mosby

Edinburgh London New York Oxford Philadelphia St Louis Sydney Toronto 2004

MOSBY
An imprint of Elsevier Limited

© Gower Medical Publishing Limited 1984
© Gower Medical Publishing Limited 1992
© Times Mirror International Publishers Limited 1997
© 2004, Elsevier Limited. All rights reserved.

The right of Peter Bullough to be identified as author of this work has been asserted by him
in accordance with the Copyright, Designs and Patents Act 1988.

First edition 1984
Second edition 1992
Third edition 1997
Fourth edition 2004

ISBN 0723432244

British Library Cataloguing in Publication Data
A catalogue record for this book is available from the British Library

Library of Congress Cataloging in Publication Data
A catalog record for this book is available from the Library of Congress

Notice
Medical knowledge is constantly changing. Standard safety precautions must be followed, but
as new research and clinical experience broaden our knowledge, changes in treatment and
drug therapy may become necessary or appropriate. Readers are advised to check the most
current product information provided by the manufacturer of each drug to be administered
to verify the recommended dose, the method and duration of administration, and
contraindications. It is the responsibility of the practitioner, relying on experience and
knowledge of the patient, to determine dosages and the best treatment for each individual
patient. Neither the Publisher nor the author assumes any liability for any injury and/or
damage to persons or property arising from this publication.

The Publisher

Printed in China

The
publisher's
policy is to use
**paper manufactured
from sustainable forests**

CONTENTS

LIST OF CONTRIBUTORS

Judith E Adams MBBS, FRCR, FRCP
Professor of Diagnostic Radiology and Academic Group Leader
Imaging Science and Biomedical Engineering
University of Manchester
Manchester, UK

Sarah J Jackson BMed Sci, BMBS, MRCP, FRCR
Consultant Radiologist
Salford Royal Hospitals NHS Trust
Salford, UK

PREFACE

When this text was first published in 1984 it was intended to provide a concise, yet lavishly illustrated and comprehensive introduction to the pathology of bone and joint disorders. The target audience was orthopaedic surgeons, radiologists and pathologists in training. It was one of the first textbooks to be published in full color and this I believe helped to make an understanding of the subject under discussion much more accessible to those whose daily work did not involve the use of the microscope.

When I graduated from medical school in 1956, the standard texts in physiology, pathology and medicine provided little or no information with regard to the pathophysiology of bone and joint disease and even as late as 1970 when I had the temerity to suggest to the chief of the trauma service at a world famous medical school that perhaps we could learn something from studying bone biopsies from old ladies who had fractured their hips; my suggestion was met with incredulity. Today osteoporosis is recognized as one of the most serious problems facing the aging population.

Much of the increasing sophistication in the diagnosis of bone and joint disease I believe we owe to the foundation in 1972 of the International Skeletal Society, which, for the first time, provided a venue for the discussion of bone and joint disease. From its inception, this society was interdisciplinary, drawing its members from the leading exponents of orthopaedics, rheumatology, radiology and pathology in the Americas, Europe, Asia and Australia. As a result of the annual meetings, tremendous progress in diagnostic acumen has been achieved and disseminated through very successful annual refresher courses offered by the society.

Our own interest and understanding depends especially upon our teachers, students, and colleagues.

I was most fortunate in being accepted for a residency in anatomic pathology at the Beth Israel Hospital in Boston. This was followed by a two year fellowship at the Hospital for Joint Disease with Dr Henry Jaffe whose whole life had been dedicated to orthopaedic pathology in that great institution.

Four years spent in the Department of Orthopaedic Surgery at the University of Oxford exposed me to one of the most creative and imaginative orthopaedic surgeons of his generation, Professor Jose Trueta, as well as two of the brightest young minds of orthopaedics at that time, Mr. Michael Freeman and Mr. John Goodfellow. In 1968 at the invitation of Dr Philip Wilson Sr. I came to the Hospital for Special Surgery in New York City.

The foundation in 1988 of a local New York Bone Club whose members have included Dr Lauren Ackerman, Dr Leon Sokoloff, Dr Hubert Sissons, Dr Howard Dorfman, Dr Leonard Kahn, Dr Michael Klein, Dr Gerry Steiner, Dr Aquiles Villacin, Dr Andrew Huvos, Dr Robert Freiberger, Dr Alex Norman and Dr Sam Liu (a veterinary pathologist) has provided a level of intellectual fellowship granted to few. Our monthly meetings over the past 25 years have taught me more of my profession than I would have ever thought possible.

The clinician can observe, using various imaging techniques, the morbid anatomic changes that are associated with musculoskeletal disease. The histologist interpreting tissue sections is helped considerably by clinical and radiologic correlation; without such correlation, serious mistakes are possible. With these thoughts in mind, I have tried to make use of the various imaging techniques now available, and have included a splendid new chapter, written for the nonspecialist by Professor Judith Adams and her colleague Dr Sarah Jackson, on imaging techniques, interpretation, and strategies.

The book uses line drawings to indicate specific features in photographs, and where the three-dimensional or temporal aspects of a structure must be shown, color schematic drawings or anatomic drawings are provided.

The bibliography is arranged by chapter, and subdivided by disease. The references to diseases have been chosen to best amplify the presentations in this book and to provide further access to the literature. Nowadays the easy access to Medline obviates the need for exhaustive bibliographies. Most of the gross photographs and photomicrographs used in the book were taken over the many years of my professional life.

Many of the clinical radiographs are from the Radiology Department at the Hospital for Special Surgery. Additional illustrations have been generously contributed by numerous colleagues throughout the world, mostly members of the International Skeletal Society, to whom I am extremely grateful.

In preparation of the first edition of this book, I was fortunate to have the assistance of Dr Vincent Vigorita, who had just completed his fellowship at Memorial Hospital before joining our staff as assistant pathologist. For the second edition, I had the invaluable help of Dr Rafael Castro. For this as well as the third edition, Dr Philip Rusli, who has been with the pathology department for the past twelve years, has been my amanuensis. With his organizational skills, he has managed the logistics of cataloging illustrations, checking the references, tracking down radiographs, and many, many other tasks that are entailed in such a project as this. I am extremely grateful to him for all his help and support. I am grateful also to Marcia Stone for her reading and helpful suggestions with regard to the sections on Pyogenic Infections and Dr Pierre Mainil-Varlet for his help with Chapter 4.

I am indebted to the professional and technical staff of the Pathology Department at the Hospital for Special Surgery – both past and present and especially Drs. Manjula Bansal and Edward DiCarlo for their never-failing support in this and other projects over the years. We are fortunate at Special Surgery in having an active and vigorous research department; my colleagues there, Dr Adele Boskey, Dr Stephen Doty and Dr Tim Wright have contributed greatly to my understanding of the more basic sciences.

Finally, I thank my friends on the staff of Mosby, especially Michael Houston, Nora Naughton, and Samantha Gear, for the care and hard work that went into the preparation of this book.

Peter G Bullough

To the memory of my Mother and Father,

Any many more, whose names on
Earth and dark,
But whose transmitted effluence can
not die,
So long as fire outlines the
parent spark

Percy Bysshe Shelley (1792–1822)

NORMAL

Chapter 1

NORMAL BONE STRUCTURE AND DEVELOPMENT

The microscopic examination of bone dates back to the earliest days of microscopy (Fig. 1.1). Anton van Leeuwenhoek read a letter to the Royal Society on the topic; soon afterwards, in 1691, Clopton Havers published his *Osteologia Nova*, in which he described the pores in the cortical bone which we now refer to as haversian canals. Since then, major contributions to the study of bone anatomy and histology have been made by many of the most famous names in medicine. Cheselden in 1733 wrote the *Osteographia*, which contained full and accurate descriptions of all human bones gained with the use of the camera obscura. The beautiful and accurate work of Albinus on bone and muscle, in 1754, established a new standard in anatomical illustrations. The experiments of Haller in 1763 contributed greatly to the

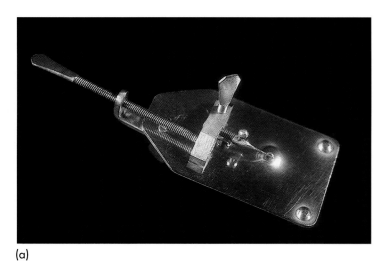

(a)

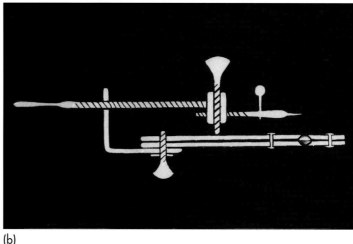

(b)

Figure 1.1   (a and b) Leeuwenhoek's 'microscope' c. 1673. An object attached to the pointed holder was examined by looking through a biconvex lens held between two metal plates. The focus could be adjusted by the screws controlling the pointed rod. Anton van Leeuwenhoek, 1632–1723.

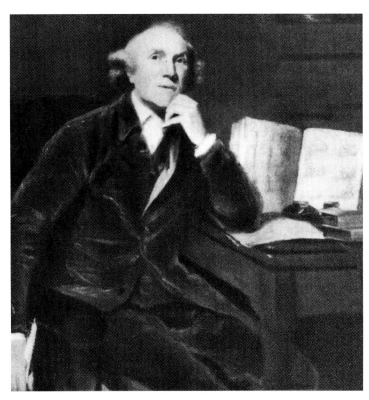

Figure 1.2 John Hunter, 1728–1793. 'To know the effects of disease is to know very little; to know the cause of the effects is the important thing'.

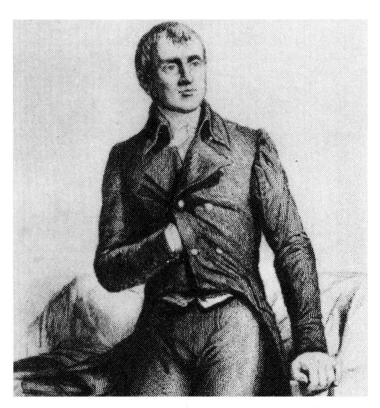

Figure 1.3 Marie Francois Xavier Bichat died in 1802, aged 31 years, of tuberculosis contracted in the autopsy room. During the turbulent years of the Revolution and the Reign of Terror, he effectively reformed the prevailing view of pathology, and brought the autopsy back to a central position. Bichat stressed the importance of the membranes binding together the various organs – the connective tissue.

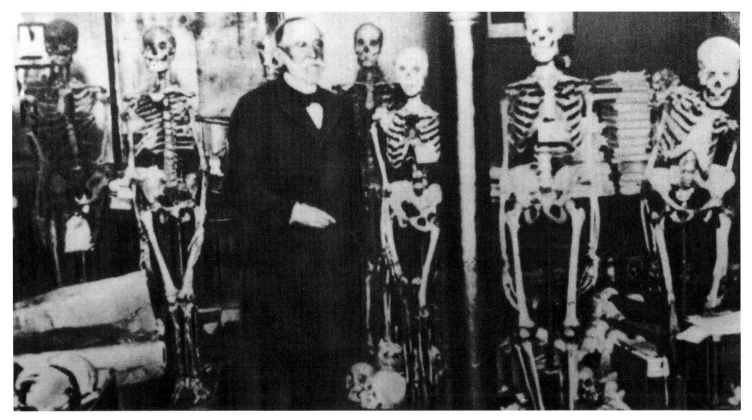

Figure 1.4 Rudolf Virchow, 1821–1902. In defining disease as the cells' reaction to an altered environment, Virchow set the stage for modern medicine. He was not only a great doctor but also a great liberal politician and philosopher. Virchow is seen here with part of his collection.

understanding of bone formation. Hunter, in 1772, did much to elucidate the mechanism of bone growth, particularly the appositional mechanism rather than that of interstitial growth such as occurs in other organ systems. Winslow's *Anatomical Exposition*, in 1776, systematized the approach to bone anatomy. Bichat, in the early 1800s, stressed the importance of the tissue elements shared among the different organ systems (hence histology) and, in particular, described the synovial membrane. Virchow, in the latter half of the nineteenth century, wrote classic descriptions of several bone tumors and metabolic disturbances (Figs 1.2–1.4).

Bone, cartilage, ligaments, and tendons have primarily a mechanical function: providing movement, stability, and protection. Unlike the parenchymal organs, e.g. the liver or kidneys, which are composed mainly of cellular elements with a metabolic function, the connective tissues are mostly formed of an extracellular material (or matrix) made up of substances to resist the tensile and compressive forces.

BONES

GROSS STRUCTURE AND FUNCTION

Each bone has a limiting surface shell: the cortex. Enclosed by the cortical shell are plates and rods of bone tissue variously known as spongy, cancellous, or trabecular bone (Figs 1.5 and 1.6).

Cortical thickness varies considerably, both within a single bone and among different bones. For example, in normal adult vertebral bodies the cortex is very thin, whereas in long bones,

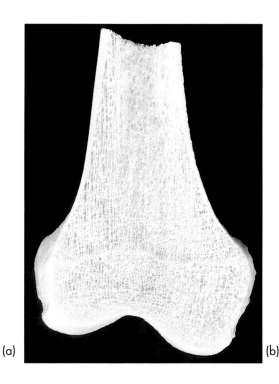

(a)

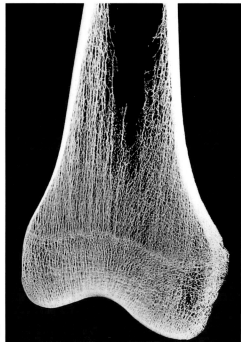

(b)

Figure 1.5 (a) Cleaned and macerated specimen of a lower femur demonstrates the decrease in cancellous bone and the thickening of the cortex as one approaches the diaphysis. (b) Radiograph of the same specimen. Note the arrangement of the trabecular bone as well as the horizontal plate of bone which marks the site of the cartilage growth plate – the 'epiphyseal scar'.

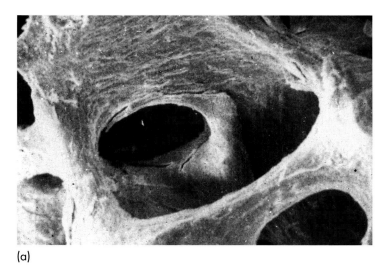

(a)

Figure 1.6 (a) Scanning electron micrograph (× 400), and (b) schematic representation of the perforated plates and the connecting rods of bone in the cancellous bone. Note the packed collagen fibers of the matrix.

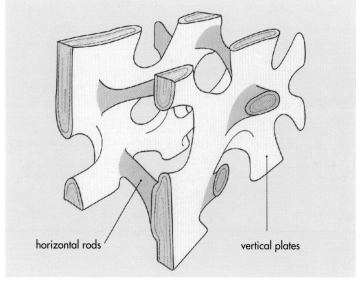

horizontal rods   vertical plates

(b)

such as the adult femur and the tibia, the cortex in the mid-diaphysis may reach more than a quarter inch in thickness. Even in the long bones there is great variation in thickness between the ends of the bone (in which the cortex is thin) and the midshaft of the bone (in which the cortex is thick).

A moment's reflection will make the reason for these differences obvious. The thick cortical bone is well constructed to resist bending, and it is in the middle of the long bones that this force is maximal. In contrast, the cancellous bone is concentrated where compressive forces predominate, i.e. in the vertebral bodies and expanded ends of long bones. Thus, the architecture of the bone reflects its function. This concept is summarized in Wolff's law, which can be simply stated as: 'Every change in the functional loading of a bone is followed by certain definite changes in internal architecture and external conformation in accordance with mathematical laws' (Fig. 1.7). It will be shown later that the microscopic arrangement of the constituents of the extracellular matrix, in the bone and all other connective tissues – e.g. cartilage, tendon, meniscus, intervertebral disc – are no less precisely organized to fulfill their mechanical function.

Bones are often compartmentalized by the morphologist into three indistinct zones: the epiphysis – the region between the articular end of the bone and the growth plate (in adults, the epiphyseal scar); the metaphysis – the region immediately below the growth plate (in the growing animal, the area of growth and most active modeling); and the diaphysis – the region between the metaphyses (i.e. the shaft of the long bones). Epiphysis, metaphysis, and diaphysis are useful descriptive terms, because many diseases predilect one or other of these compartments (Fig. 1.8).

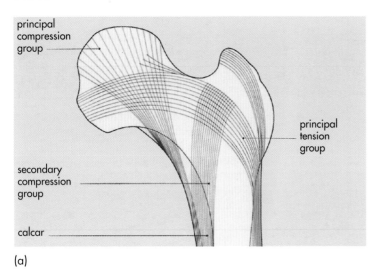
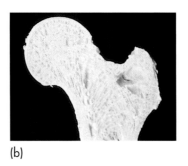
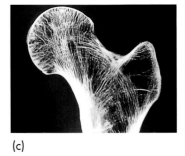

(a)   (b)   (c)

Figure 1.7   (a) Wolff's law is well demonstrated in the head and neck of the femur. In this area, the bone trabeculae radiate from the articular surface down onto the medial cortex of the femoral neck (the calcar), which is much thicker than the cortex on the lateral side of the femoral neck. (b) In this slice through the upper end of the femur, the marrow fat has been washed out of the specimen to demonstrate the distribution of the cancellous bone. (c) Perhaps the best way to demonstrate clearly the arrangement of the bone trabeculae is by radiography of the specimen.

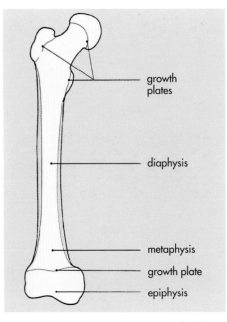

Figure 1.8   Bone compartments in the femur.

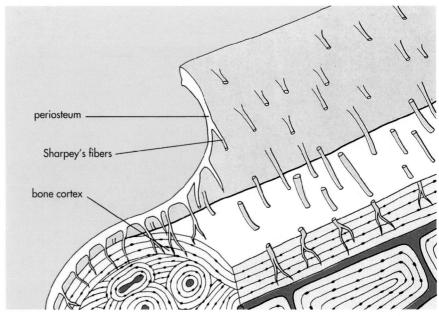

Figure 1.9   The fibers of Sharpey are direct continuations of periosteal collagen fibers around which the circumferential lamellae of the cortical bone have grown, thus firmly anchoring the periosteum.

Periosteum

Except at the musculotendinous insertions and at their articular ends, the bones are covered by a firmly attached thin but tough fibrous membrane, the periosteum. At the articular margins and tendinous insertions the periosteum blends imperceptibly with the surface fibers of the articular cartilage, tendon or ligament.

The periosteum is attached to the surface of the bone cortex by collagen fibers (the fibers of Sharpey), which are direct continuations of the collagen fibers of the periosteum. Where these fibers enter the bone, they are encrusted with mineral (hydroxyapatite), which cements them into the bone (Fig. 1.9). For this rea-

son, any attempt at separation of the periosteum from the bone requires physical tearing of these fibers.

On microscopic examination, the periosteum is seen to have two layers: an outer fibrous layer and an inner cambium layer, which has the potential to form bone. In children the cambium layer provides for the increasing diameter of the bone with growth (Fig. 1.10). In adults, the bone-forming potential of the periosteum is reactivated by trauma, infection, and growing tumors. In children, the periosteum is only loosely attached to the underlying bone, whereas in adults it is firmly attached. Thus the clinical extent of a periosteal reaction is much greater in children than in adults (Fig. 1.11).

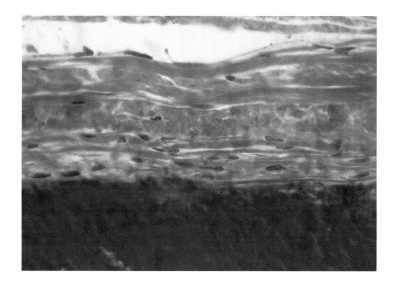

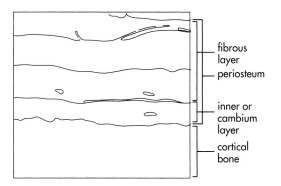

Figure 1.10 Photomicrograph of the periosteum and underlying cortical bone. Note the more cellular inner or cambium layer, which is the more active in producing bone (H&E, × 25 obj.).

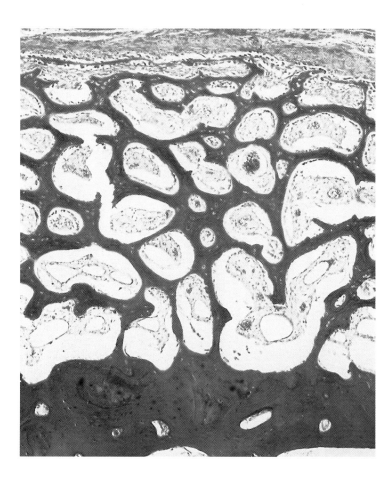

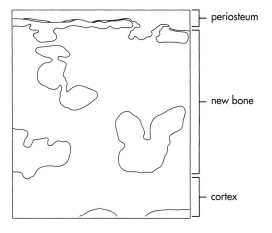

Figure 1.11 Photomicrograph of periosteal new bone layer produced by the cambium of the periosteum following trauma in a child (H&E, × 4 obj.). In a child the periosteal new bone formation following trauma is abundant, because of the weak attachment of the periosteum.

Blood supply

The blood supply of the bone has been studied in cadaveric specimens by injection of latex or other substances into the arteries and/or veins, and the results have been published in several atlases. These studies have shown that many capillaries enter the bone through the periosteum. This periosteal blood supply augments the principal nutrient arteries, which enter the medullary cavity by penetrating the cortex (usually at about the middle of the diaphysis), and the epiphyseal and metaphyseal vessels at the ends of the bone (Figs 1.12 and 1.13).

The intraosseous veins are distinctly different from the arteries in being much more tortuous and having a significantly wider caliber.

MATRIX

A knowledge of the matrix components is essential to the understanding of connective-tissue diseases. The collagens are the principal extracellular components of connective tissues accounting for 70% of all body proteins. Type I collagen is the most common form of collagen and the major collagen found in skin, fascia, tendon and bone. Type I collagen is made up of bundles of fibrils, which in turn are composed of stacked molecules formed from polypeptide chains arranged in a triple helical pattern (Figs 1.14 and 1.15). At least 17 distinct types of collagen composed of at least 31 genetically distinct chains are now known and these vary both in size and configuration. Some contain interrupted helical structures aligned in a staggered array to form fibrils (Table 1.1). There are also nonfiber-forming collagens which

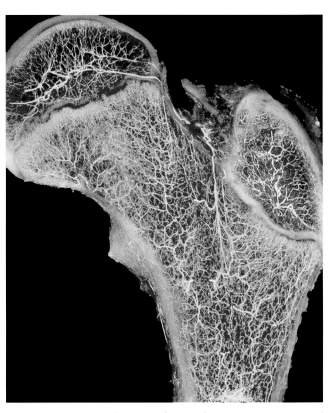

Figure 1.13 Coronal section of upper femur in an immature subject, showing blood supply. Note separate vascular supply to metaphysis, femoral epiphysis, and trochanteric apophysis. (Courtesy of H.V. Crock.)

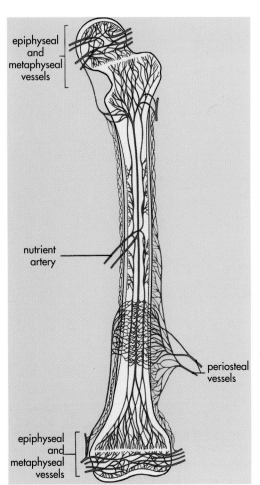

Figure 1.12 Diagram of the several sources of blood supply to the bone.

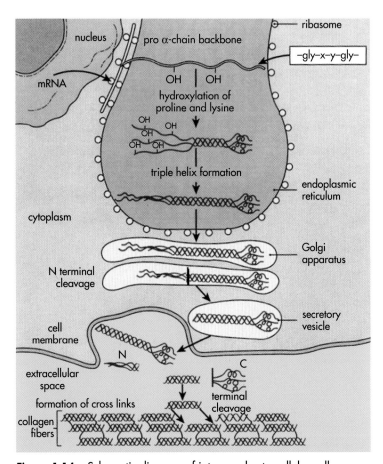

Figure 1.14 Schematic diagram of intra- and extracellular collagen synthesis. In the pro-α-chain, glycine occupies every third position. Commonly, –x– and –y– are lysine and proline. Cleavage of the N and C terminal fragments is an essential step in collagen fiber formation.

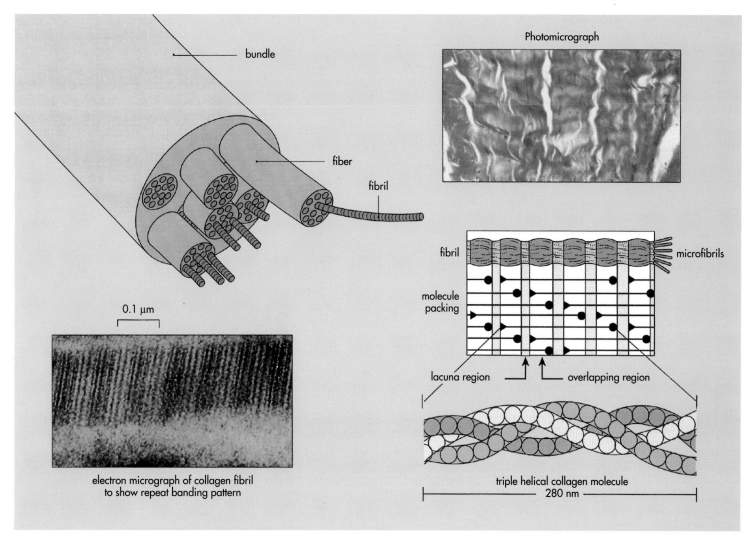

Figure 1.15 Microscopic examination of ligamentous tissue stained with H&E. The wavy homogenous strands of pink material represent bundles of type I collagen fibers. The collagen molecule is a triple helix formed of polypeptide chains, which in turn are formed of repeating tripeptide sequences of glycine-x-y-glycine-x-y etc., in which x and y are frequently proline and lysine. Visualized by transmission electron microscopy, the individual collagen fibrils are seen to have regular light and dark bands. As can be seen from the drawing, the bands result from the gaps between the individual molecules of collagen, which then overlap the adjacent molecules.

Table 1.1 Fiber-forming collagens.

Type	Molecules	Representative tissues
I	$[\alpha 1(I)]_2 \alpha 2(I)$	skin, bone, tendon, dentin etc.
	$[\alpha 1(I)]_3$	dentin, skin (minor form)
II	$[\alpha 1(II)]_3$	hyaline cartilage, vitreous body
III	$[\alpha 1(III)]_3$	skin, vessels
V	$[\alpha 1(V)]_3$	hamster lung cell cultures
	$[\alpha 1(V)]_2 \alpha 2(V)$	fetal membranes, skin, bone
	$[\alpha 1(V)] \alpha 2(V) \alpha 3(V)$	placenta, synovial membranes
XI	$[\alpha 1(XI)] \alpha 2(XI) \alpha 3(XI)$	hyaline cartilage

have varying functions, such as binding sites for other matrix components (type IX) or regulation of vascularization (type X) or fiber size (type XI) (Table 1.2 and Figure 1.16).

Hyaline cartilage has a unique type of collagen, type II, which is structurally characterized by three identical triple helical α-1(II) chains. The type II fibrillar network, which will be discussed in more detail later, is essential both for maintaining the tissue volume and shape as well as providing articular cartilage with its tensile strength when subjected to compressive loads.

Collagen synthesis includes both cellular and extracellular events and is complex. During the processes of transcription and translation of the collagen genes, it is necessary that numbers of

Table 1.2 Nonfiber-forming collagens.

Type	Molecules	Representative tissues
IV	$[\alpha1(IV)]_2\alpha2(IV)$	basement membranes
VI	$\alpha1(VI)]\alpha2(VI)\alpha3(VI)$	vessels, skin, invertebral disc
VII	$[\alpha1(VII)]_3$	dermo-epidermal junction
VIII	(?)	Descemet's membrane, endothelial cells
IX	$\alpha1(IX)]\alpha2(IX)\alpha3(IX)$	hyaline cartilage, vitreous humour
X	$[\alpha1(X)]_3$	growth plate (hypertrophic cartilage)
XII	$[\alpha1(XII)]_3$	embryonic skin and tendon, periodontal ligament
XIII	(?)	endothelial cells
XIV	$[\alpha1(XIV)]_3$	fetal skin and tendon

intervening sequences (known as introns) are spliced out. Defects in this processing of bone (type I collagen) lead to defective collagen chains or reduced amounts of collagen and the disease of osteogenesis imperfecta (OI).

The protein α-chains formed first are made up of sequences of amino acids of which glycine occupies every third position; the intervening positions are frequently occupied by either proline or lysine, which are later hydroxylated in preparation for the formation of the triple helix. (Proline and lysine hydroxylases require the presence of ascorbic acid, α-ketoglutarate, Fe^{++} and O_2.)

The fiber-forming collagens are well suited to resist the effect of pulling, i.e. tension and the principal component of the matrix of tendons and ligaments is type I collagen. However, the fiber-forming collagens do not resist bending or compression, and because the matrices of both bone (mainly type I collagen) and cartilage (mainly types II and IX collagen) are subjected to these latter types of forces, they also contain stiffening substances. In bone, the stiffening substance takes the form of a microcrystalline analog of geologic hydroxyapatite: $Ca_{10}(PO_4)_6(OH)_2$ (Fig. 1.17). The crystals in mineralized tissue are too small to be seen by light microscopy, being approximately only $2 \times 2 \times 25$ nm in size, but they can be visualized by electron microscopy. The apatite crystals provide strength in compression, although, as would be expected, they are weak in bending and tension. During development, the relative mineral content of the bone increases, whereas the water content decreases. The perfection and size of the hydroxyapatite crystals in the bone also increase with age. [It should be remembered that besides its mechanical functions the mineral also has a primary role to play in calcium homeostasis (see Chapter 8, p. 200).]

In articular cartilage, the filler between the collagen fibers is composed of large, negatively charged macromolecules, the proteoglycans (PGs) (Fig. 1.18). These are a group of heterogenous molecules consisting of protein chains and attached carbohydrates, which have a sticky gel-like quality. The major PG in cartilage is aggrecan, which contains a protein core molecular weight (Mr) of approximately 215,000 to which carbohydrate side chains (keratan and chondroitin sulfate) are attached. The aggrecan molecules interact with hyaluronan and this interaction is stabilized by link protein (Fig. 1.19). As many as 200

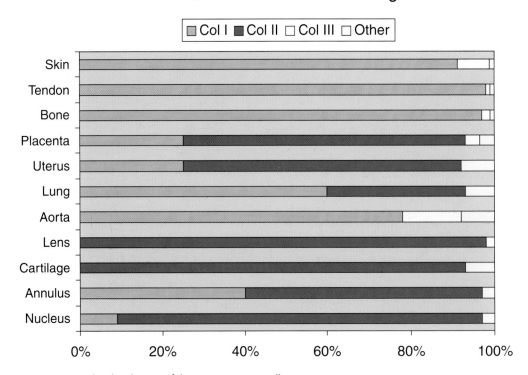

Distribution of Collagen Types in Connective Tissue Matrices as % of Total Collagen

☐ Col I ■ Col II ☐ Col III ☐ Other

Skin · Tendon · Bone · Placenta · Uterus · Lung · Aorta · Lens · Cartilage · Annulus · Nucleus

0%   20%   40%   60%   80%   100%

Figure 1.16 The distribution of the most common collagens in various tissues.

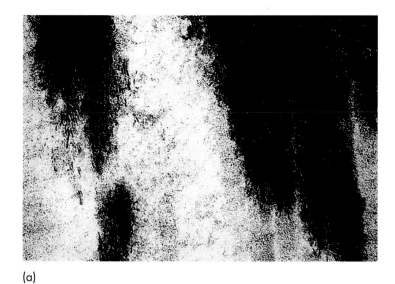

(a)

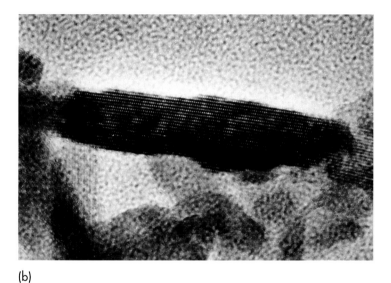

(b)

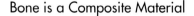

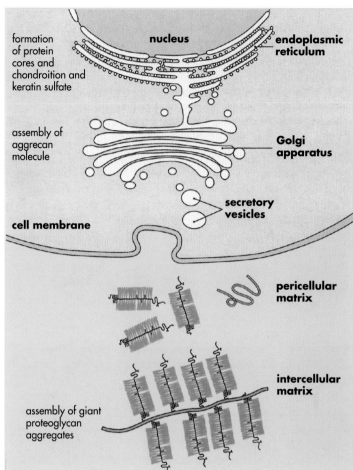

Figure 1.18 Schematic representation of PG synthesis.

Bone is a Composite Material

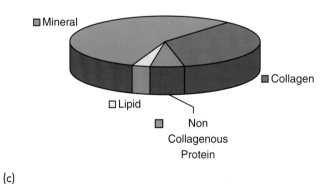

(c)

Figure 1.17 Electron micrographs of bone mineral crystals. (**a**) At a magnification factor of × 101,500, the crystal structure can be clearly seen. (**b**) At higher magnification, × 2,110,000, the lattice formation of the crystals can also be appreciated. (The various stains for demonstrating calcium salts in undecalcified sections are described in Chapter 2, p. 47.) (**c**) The solid matter of bone is distributed as shown in this pie chart. About 10–11% of total bone mass is attributable to water.

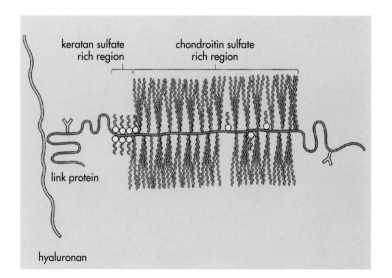

Figure 1.19 Structure of aggrecan. The PG aggrecan is made up of a polypeptide chain interspersed with extended regions, to which are attached sulfated glycosaminoglycan side chains (keratan sulfate and chondroitin sulfate). The PG aggrecan associates with hyaluronic acid in association with link protein. Up to 200 aggrecan molecules can associate with hyaluronic acid to form a large molecular aggregate that is highly charged, and pulls water into the tissue.

individual aggrecan molecules (subunits) bind to one hyaluronic acid chain (Mr $1-2 \times 10^6$) to form a giant aggregate (Mr 5×10^7 to 5×10^8).

PGs are highly charged molecules which bind water and this water accounts for approximately 70% of the wet cartilage tissue mass. PGs in solution can expand to 50% of their volume. However, within hydrated cartilage the expansion of the PGs is restricted by the collagen network to approximately 20% of the maximum possible. The swelling pressure thus created within the cartilage resists applied compressive loads (Fig. 1.20).

When cartilage is loaded, some water is extruded; removal of the load permits the imbibing into the tissue of more water, together with essential nutrients, until the swelling pressure of the PGs is again balanced by the resistance of the collagen network.

The aggrecan shows an age-related decrease in size and enrichment in keratan sulfate relative to chondroitin sulfate. Associated with these changes is cartilage dehydration.

In addition to aggrecan, cartilage contains other smaller PGs which contain dermatan sulfate (biglycan, decorin, fibromodulin, lumican). These PGs are present in lower concentrations than aggrecan and may have a role in preventing joint adhesions. In older individuals they show increasing concentration, especially in the superficial layers.

Articular cartilage also contains other extracellular noncollagenous proteins. Anchorin is a protein on the surface of chondrocytes involved in binding of these cells to extracellular matrix components, possibly transmitting altered stress on type II fibers to chondrocytes. Fibronectin, thrombomodulin, cartilage oligomeric matrix protein, cartilage-associated protein (CASP) etc. are all found in cartilage but their precise functions are not yet known. The possible arrangement of all these components within the cartilage matrix is shown schematically in Figure 1.21.

Cell synthesis and breakdown

The matrix components of the connective tissues are manufactured as well as regulated by cells which themselves occupy only a small volume of the tissues. Nevertheless, these cells, i.e. fibroblasts (cells that produce fibrous tissue, including ligaments and tendons), osteoblasts (cells that produce bone), and chondroblasts (cells that produce cartilage), are essential to the production and maintenance of a healthy matrix. Disturbances in cell function may lead to an alteration in the rate of synthesis or to the production of abnormal matrix constituents or, on the other hand, to altered breakdown. The breakdown of matrix constituents, either as a result of normal turnover or to pathologic state, occurs through the action of enzymes which may derive either, from the connective-tissue cells themselves, from synoviocytes, or from blood-borne inflammatory cells.

The bone matrix is synthesized by a layer of cells on the bone surface (Figs 1.22 and 1.23). These cells, the osteoblasts, are mesenchymal in origin and are characterized by their abundant endoplasmic reticulum, and the enzyme alkaline phosphatase. Although there is an incomplete correlation between actual bone matrix formation, including its mineralization, and the morphologic features of the osteoblasts, nevertheless, the rate of matrix production at the time of biopsy can be approximated by the size

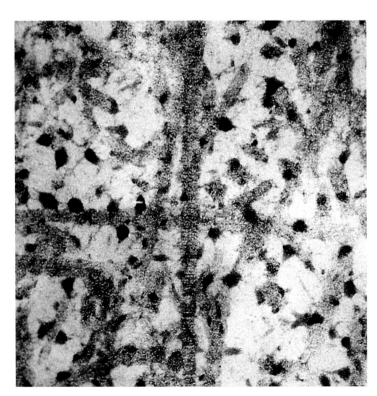

Figure 1.20   Electron microscopic examination of cartilage demonstrates amorphous electron-dense deposits of PG between collagen fibers (× 102,900).

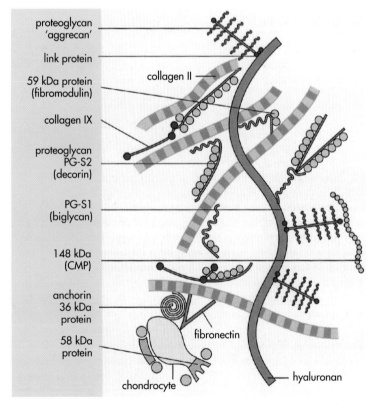

Figure 1.21   Schematic illustration of the possible arrangement of collagen matrix constituents.

of the osteoblasts. 'Active' osteoblasts are plump, whereas cells that line the bone surface and are flat can be considered quiescent or 'inactive' at least with regard to matrix production (Fig. 1.24). However, matrix synthesis should not be considered their sole function vide infra. Because there is a gradual increase in the size of bone-forming cells, the point at which an 'inactive' cell becomes an 'active' cell is necessarily a subjective determination.

As the osteoblasts produce bone matrix and the matrix miner-

alizes, they become surrounded by the mineralized matrix formed, and are thus buried within the substance of the bone. By this process the osteoblasts become osteocytes (Figs 1.25 and 1.26). [Since the spacing of the osteocytes is so obviously different from the closely packed osteoblasts on the surface, it is evident that not all osteoblasts on the surface are buried to become osteocytes. Some die via programmed cell death (apoptosis).] Osteocytes are connected with each other and with some of the

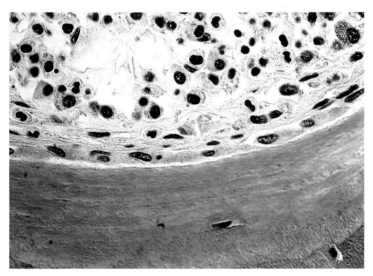

Figure 1.22 Photomicrograph of an actively forming bone surface. A layer of flattened active osteoblasts with abundant basophilic cytoplasm lines the smooth formative surface. (Compare with Figure 1.24.) (H&E, × 25 obj.)

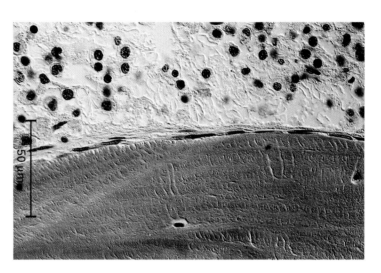

Figure 1.24 Photomicrograph shows a layer of 'inactive', flat osteoblasts at the bone surface (H&E, × 10 obj.).

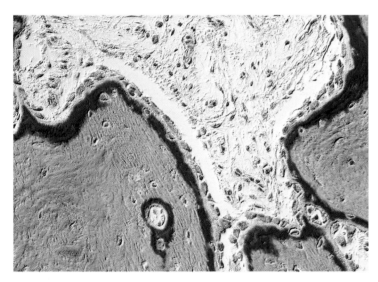

Figure 1.23 Photomicrograph of an undecalcified specimen showing a layer of active, plump osteoblasts at a bone surface. The layer of red-stained tissue beneath the osteoblastic layer represents unmineralized matrix or osteoid. The green-staining material represents calcified matrix. (Goldner Stain, × 10 obj.)

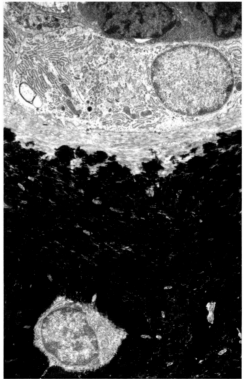

Figure 1.25 Transmission electron photomicrograph to demonstrate an active osteoblast. The cytoplasm is rich in rough endoplasmic reticulum. Underlying the cell is a layer of nonmineralized collagenous matrix (osteoid), which, in H&E sections, is seen as a smooth, pink layer on the bone surface. Directly under the osteoid seam is a layer of mineralized bone containing an osteocyte (× 10,000).

osteoblasts on the surface of the bone by a series of cell processes which run through canals permeating the bone tissue (Figs 1.27–1.30). These canals are called the osteocytic canaliculi. The syncytium of osteocytes that permeate the bone probably plays an important role in physiologic calcium homeostasis, and may also act as a sensing device to regulate skeletal homeostasis in accordance with Wolff's law. The osteocytic canaliculi do not cross the cement lines (see Fig. 1.39 for a description of cement lines).

Associated with the cells that are actively forming bone matrix, a thin layer of nonmineralized bone matrix (osteoid), normally approximately 10 µm thick, separates the cellular layer

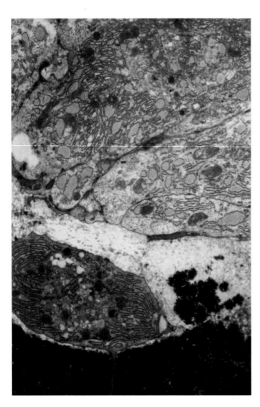

Figure 1.26 Transmission electron photomicrograph demonstrating portions of the cytoplasm of two active osteoblasts lying upon a mineralizing osteoid seam. Within the osteoid seam (lower right) is a newly formed osteocyte (× 10,000).

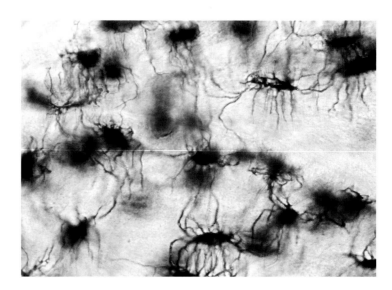

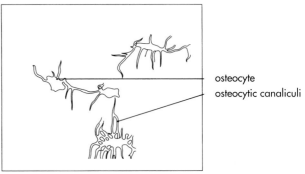

Figure 1.28   Photomicrograph of osteocytes and osteocytic canaliculi seen by transmitted light in ground bone section (× 10 obj.).

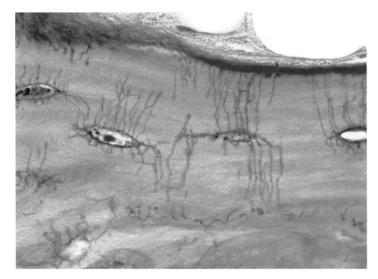

Figure 1.27   Photomicrograph to demonstrate the general disposition of the osteocytic canaliculi through which run the osteocytic processes. These processes join the osteocytes into a network which has attachments to the cells at the bone surface (H&E, × 10 obj.).

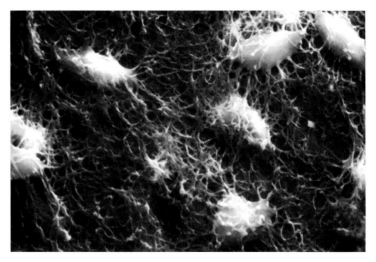

Figure 1.29   Scanning electron photomicrograph demonstrating the osteocytes and their connecting canaliculi (× 750).

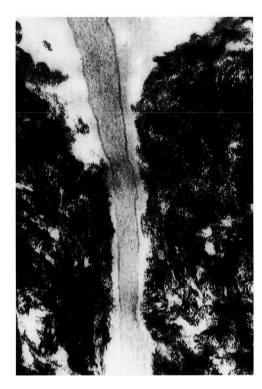

Figure 1.30
Electron
photomicrograph
of a portion of an
osteocytic process
in an osteocytic
canaliculus in
mineralized bone
(× 50,000).

from the mineralized matrix (Fig. 1.31). The time between the deposition and subsequent mineralization of the organic matrix, called the 'mineralization lag time', is about 10 days. (The identification of this nonmineralized bone matrix is a key factor in the diagnosis of certain metabolic disturbances of bone, however its recognition depends on the preparation of undecalcified sections.)

On microscopic examination the actively forming bone surfaces, as well as the inactive formed surfaces, are smooth. However, some bone surfaces have an irregular or 'gnawed out' appearance, and these surfaces either have been resorbed or are actively resorbing (Fig. 1.32). The cells concerned with resorption are the osteoclasts – large, often multinucleated cells with abundant cytoplasm. Osteoclasts frequently lie in cavities (Howship's lacunae) on the bone surface (Figs 1.33 and 1.34). While the osteoclast is usually a multinucleate cell, mononuclear forms of resorbing cells may also be seen.

Electron microscopy reveals that the osteoclast has a ruffled border adjacent to the bone and contains many lysosomal bodies, mitochondria, and vesicular inclusions (Fig. 1.35). The osteoclast is derived from blood-borne monocytes.

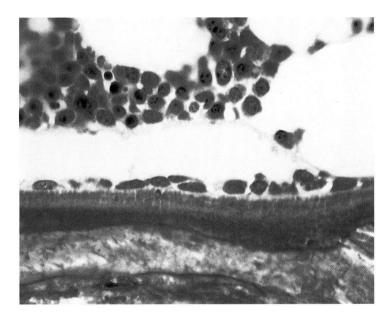

Figure 1.31 Photomicrograph of a section of undecalcified bone showing a prominent layer of active osteoblasts lying on an osteoid seam, with underlying mineralized bone. The calcification front is seen as a deeply staining basophilic line (H&E, × 25 obj.).

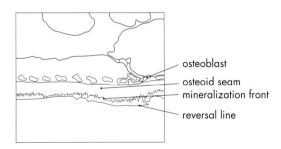

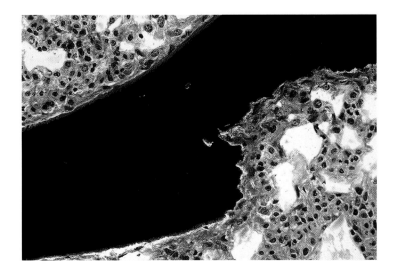

Figure 1.32 Photomicrograph showing contrast of the bone-forming surface (upper left) with an osteoid seam with a resorbing surface (lower right) (Von Kossa, × 10 obj.).

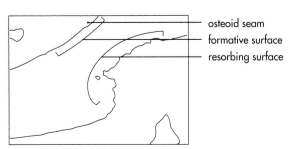

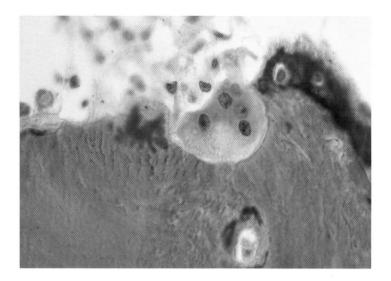

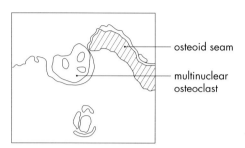

Figure 1.33 Photomicrograph showing an osteoclast in a Howship's lacuna. Osteoclasts are identified by their abundant cytoplasm and multiple nuclei (Goldner stain, × 25 obj.).

osteoid seam

multinuclear osteoclast

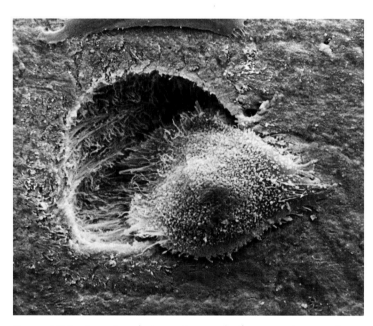

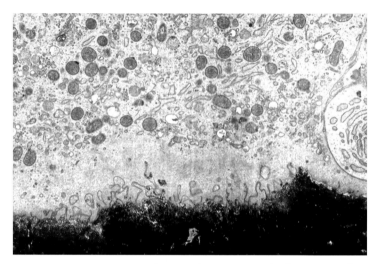

Figure 1.34 Scanning electron micrograph of an osteoclast on a bone slice. Adjacent and partially obscured by the osteoclast is a surface excavation of the bone slice, which was produced by the osteoclast during an 18-hour incubation period (× 1,500). (Courtesy of T.J. Chambers.)

Figure 1.35 Transmission electron photomicrograph of a portion of an osteoclast and its ruffled border in intimate contact with the mineralized surface of the bone. Within the cytoplasm there is abundant mitochondria with interspersed Golgi apparatus (× 15,000).

Bone remodeling, the coordinated balance of bone formation and bone resorption, is regulated both by systemic hormones (Table 1.3), blood-derived factors and local mediators (Table 1.4). In addition to their direct effect, hormones may also regulate the synthesis, as well as the effects, of the local mediators. These complex interactions are actively being investigated.

The established biochemical markers of bone turnover include serum alkaline phosphatase, serum osteocalcin (bone Gla protein), collagen N-telopeptides, and the urinary excretion of calcium and collagen breakdown products, such as hydroxyproline or cross-linked collagen peptides. These cross-linked peptides are

the most specific as they are only formed after synthesis is complete. Further discussion of the biochemical control of bone turnover and of calcification will be found in Chapters 7, p. 173 and 8, p. 200.

HISTOLOGY

Mature bone

In mature bone tissue the collagen fibers of the matrix are arranged in layers or leaves (hence the term 'lamellar bone'), and

Table 1.3 Systemic mediators in cell synthesis and breakdown.

Systemic mediators (hormones)	Site of action	Mode of action
Polypeptide hormones		
Parathyroid hormone (PTH)	Osteoblast	Anabolic effect with ↑ rate of bone formation
	? Pre-osteoblast	Anabolic effect with ↑ rate of bone formation
	Osteoclast (indirect)	Resorption via ↑ osteoclastic activity effected by secondary messenger
Calcitonin (CT)	Osteoclast	Inhibitory ↓ resorption
Insulin	Osteoblast	Stimulates matrix synthesis
	Chondroblast	Stimulates matrix synthesis
	? Osteoclast	Regulates bone resorption
Growth hormone (GH)	—	May have an effect secondarily by stimulating the production of insulin-like growth factor by skeletal cells
Steroid hormones		
1,25-Dihydroxyvitamin-D3 [1,25(OH)$_2$D3]	Osteoblast	Stimulates the synthesis of osteocalcin leads to ↑ bone resorption
		Inhibits bone collagen synthesis
Glucocorticoids	Pre-osteoblast	Increased bone resorption, possibly indirect effect via ↑ PTH
		Decreased matrix synthesis
Sex steroids	Indirect action. Mediated by other hormones?	Important in skeletal maturation and in preventing bone loss during ageing process
Thyroid hormones	Chondroblasts?	Necessary to normal growth and development, especially cartilage
		In adult ↑ thyroid causes increased bone resorption

Table 1.4 Local mediators in cell synthesis and breakdown.

Local mediators	Site of action	Mode of action
Growth factor polypeptides synthesized by bone cells		
Insulin-like growth factor 1 (IGF-1) (somatomedin)	Pre-osteoblast	Increased cell replication
	Osteoblast	Increased matrix synthesis
Transforming growth factor β (TGFβ)	Pre-osteoblast	Increased cell replication
	Osteoblast	Increased matrix synthesis
Fibroblast growth factors (FGF)	Pre-osteoblast	Increased cell replication
Platelet-derived growth factor (PDGF)	Pre-osteoblast	Bone cell replication and bone resorption
Blood cell derived factors		
Interleukin-1 (IL-1)	Pre-osteoblast	Stimulates bone cell replication. In low doses may also stimulate matrix
	Osteoblast	production directly. Also stimulates bone resorption indirectly
Tumor necrosis factor (TNF)	Pre-osteoblast	Increased cell replication. Stimulates bone resorption, possibly indirectly

in each of these layers the collagen bundles lie parallel to each other (Fig. 1.36). However, the orientation of the collagen bundles changes from one layer to the next, in a similar way to the layers in plywood (Fig. 1.37). In this manner, bone tissue gains much of its strength.

In cortical bone the layers are formed concentrically around a vascular core (haversian canal) to form an osteon (Fig. 1.38). On microscopic examination it becomes apparent with hematoxylin and eosin staining, that surrounding each osteon, and irregularly distributed throughout the trabecular bone, there are distinct deep blue lines. These lines are the cement lines (Fig. 1.39). When histologic sections are examined microscopically using polarized light, a discontinuity of the collagen is seen on either side of the cement line. From this observation it can be inferred that the bone is constructed of myriads of separate pieces like a three-dimensional jigsaw puzzle. (It has been demonstrated experimentally that fracture propagation tends to occur along the cement lines.)

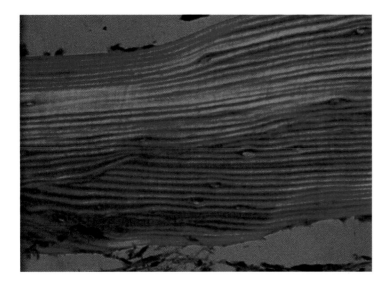

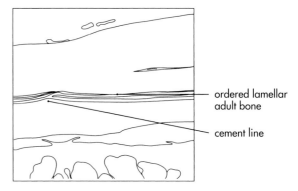

ordered lamellar adult bone

cement line

Figure 1.36   Segment of trabecular bone microscopically examined with polarized light (× 10 obj.). Although at first sight the bone tissue appears as a seamless structure, it is made up of individual fragments which are joined at the cement lines.

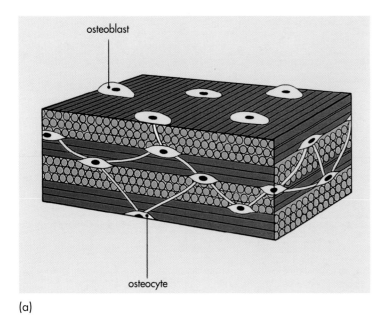

osteoblast

osteocyte

(a)

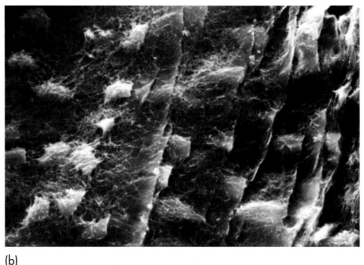

(b)

Figure 1.37   (a) Diagrammatic representation of the layered (lamellar) appearance of bone shows how the alternating dark and light layers seen in Figure 1.36 are explained by the change in direction of the collagen fibers in each layer. (b) Scanning electron photomicrograph demonstrating collagenous lamellae (layers) of the bone with the osteocytes between the lamellae (× 500).

Primary osteons are formed in the infant by the ingrowth of periosteal blood vessels following a 'cutting cone' of osteoclasts which tunnel through the existing cortex. The tunnel thus formed then becomes partially filled in by layers of bone matrix, the most recently formed layer being that adjacent to the vessel. Secondary and subsequent osteons are formed during the process of bone modeling by the outgrowth of vessels from existing haversian systems, each of which are preceded by a cluster of osteoclasts (Fig. 1.40).

Immature bone

In addition to mature lamellar bone, another form of mineralized tissue exists in which the collagen matrix is irregularly arranged in a woven pattern resembling the warp and woof threads in a

fabric (Figs 1.41 and 1.42). The cells within this matrix are larger, more rounded, and closer together than those seen in lamellar bone. This type of mineralized tissue, which has been variously called woven bone, primitive bone, fiber bone, and immature bone, is seen during development, in fracture callus, in bone-forming tumors, and in conditions characterized by a highly accelerated rate of bone formation (e.g. in Paget's disease and other hypermetabolic states). Its recognition by the pathologist is important because it usually indicates the presence of a disease process.

Marrow

The limited tissue space in the haversian canals of the cortical bone is occupied by fat, and neurovascular tissue; in the much

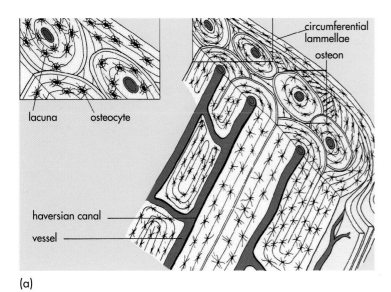

(a)

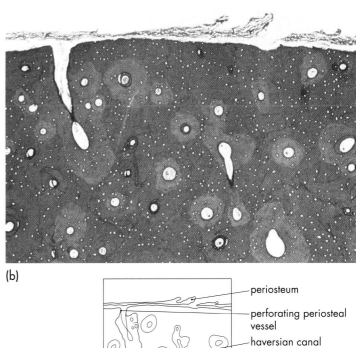

(b)

Figure 1.38 (**a**) Schematic diagram of some of the main features of the microstructure of mature bone. Note the general construction of the osteons, the distribution of the osteocytic lacunae, the haversian canals and their contents. (**b**) Photomicrograph of cortical bone shows lamellae surrounding haversian canals to form osteons. In addition it shows the periosteal surface with a penetrating periosteal vessel (H&E, × 4 obj.).

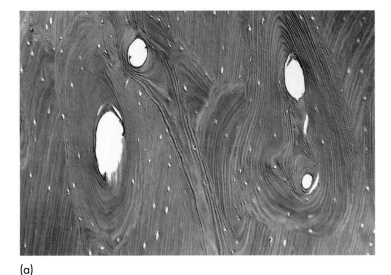

(a)

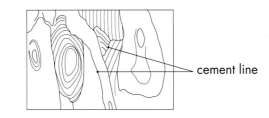

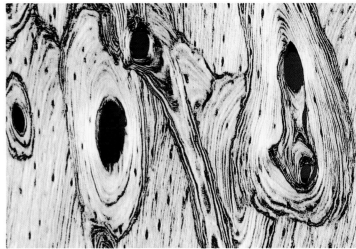

(b)

Figure 1.39 (**a**) Photomicrograph of a portion of the cortical bone in a cross-section. The cement lines are not easy to see, however, the changes in direction of the bone lamellae give some indication of the cement lines (H&E, Nomarski optics, × 10 obj.). (**b**) The same histologic field photographed using polarized light. The structural discontinuity between the various osteons is now seen clearly as dark lines which correspond to cement lines. (Cement lines may stain blue on H&E sections but are often difficult to see.)

ampler tissue space of the cancellous bone in addition there is often hematopoietic tissue. Although hematopoietic tissue is found in all the bones at birth, with maturation it becomes largely confined to the axial skeleton, i.e. the skull, ribs, vertebral column, sternum, and pelvic girdle. The appearance of cellular marrow at other sites during adult life is abnormal and warrants investigation. In areas where hematopoietic tissue is normally present, the ratio of fat to hematopoietic tissue is about equal (Fig. 1.43). An increase or decrease in this ratio may indicate hematologic disease. (Interestingly, although in older individuals

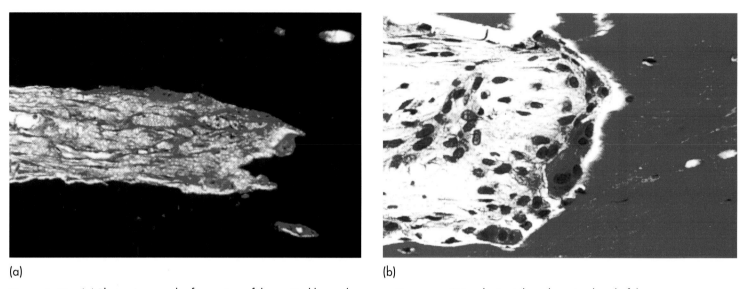

(a)   (b)

Figure 1.40 (a) Photomicrograph of a portion of the cortical bone shows a cutting cone. Osteoclasts at the advancing head of the cone are followed by active osteoblastic activity behind (von Kossa, × 10 obj.). (b) In this photomicrograph obtained at a higher magnification the osteoclastic resorption can be more clearly appreciated (H&E, × 25 obj.).

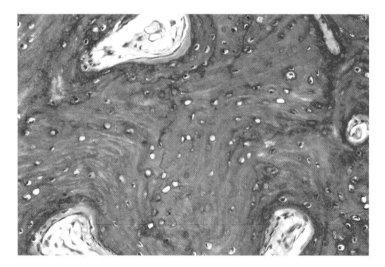

Figure 1.41 Photomicrograph of immature bone from a patient with OI. Note the crowded, oval to round osteocytes (H&E, × 10 obj.).

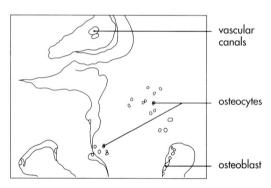

vascular canals

osteocytes

osteoblast

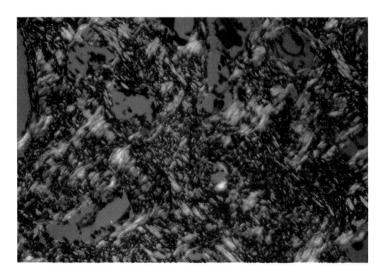

Figure 1.42 Photomicrograph of immature bone taken with polarized light demonstrates the irregular woven appearance of the collagenous matrix (H&E, × 10 obj.).

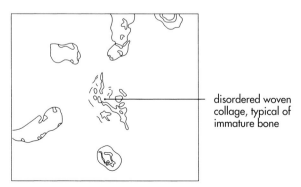

disordered woven collage, typical of immature bone

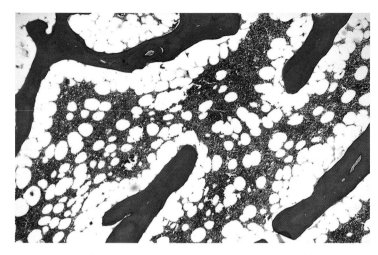

Figure 1.43 Photomicrograph showing the relationship of bone tissue to bone marrow. Normally the ratio of fat to hematopoietic tissue, in bones containing hematopoietic tissue, is 1:1. As clearly shown in this photograph, the marrow immediately around the bone trabeculae is usually devoid of hematopoietic tissue (H&E, × 1.25 obj.).

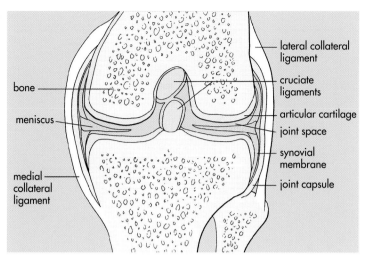

Figure 1.44 Diagram of the knee joint. The radiologic joint space consists of the radiolucent articular cartilage plus the joint cavity.

as well as certain disease states hyperplastic marrow may reappear in the long bones, it is often arrested at the site of the closed epiphyseal plate.)

JOINTS

GROSS STRUCTURE

The ends of contiguous bones, together with their soft-tissue components, articular cartilage, ligaments, and synovium, constitute a functioning unit: the joint. Of the three types of joints, the most common is the diarthrodial joint, which has a cavity to form a freely movable connecting unit between two bones (Figs 1.44 and 1.45). Hyaline cartilage (articular cartilage) covers the articulating surfaces of the diarthrodial joints, with the exception of the sternoclavicular and temporomandibular joints, which are covered by fibrocartilage.

The normal function of a diarthrodial joint has three characteristics. These are: the freedom of the articulating surfaces to move over each other, the ability of the joint to maintain stability during use, and lastly a proper distribution of stress through the tissues which comprise the joint so that these tissues are not damaged. These aspects of joint function depend upon the shape of the articulating surfaces of the joint (Fig. 1.46); the integrity of the ligaments, muscles, and tendons that support the limb; and the cellular control of the mechanical properties of the matrices of the bone, cartilage and the other tissues that together comprise the joint.

The second type of joint is the amphiarthrodial joint or symphysis, which is characterized by limited mobility, and exemplified by the intervertebral disc and symphysis pubis (Fig. 1.47). The intervertebral disc is a fibrocartilaginous complex which forms the articulation between the vertebral bodies. It contributes to the mobility and stability of the spine as well as to the transmission of load through it. It should be noted that disc height is not the same in all segments of the spine; the cervical and thoracic

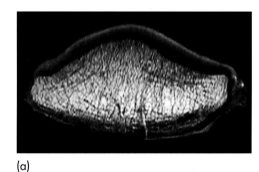

(a)

(b)

Figure 1.45 MRI facilitates visualization of the cartilage. The lamellated appearance shown in (a) reflects the varying water content, the zone of calcification and possibly the collagen orientation at the surface. (b) A clinical MRI shows cartilage thinning and fibrillation in the lateral compartment when compared with the medial compartment.

discs are flatter than those of the lumbar region. Disc height also varies from front to back, relative to the curvature of the spine. In older individuals the disc becomes dehydrated and gets thinner.

The intervertebral disc can be divided into two components: the outermost fibrous ring (annulus fibrosus) and the innermost

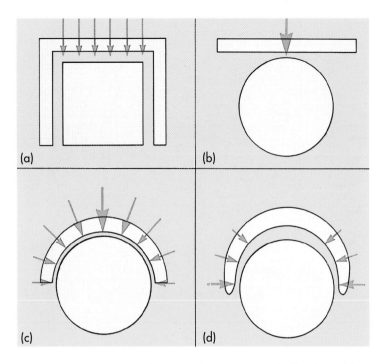

Figure 1.46 The shape of the joint determines: (1) The freedom of the joint surfaces to articulate; (2) The stability of the joint; and (3) The distribution of stress on the tissues. (**a**) Does not allow acceptable freedom of movement. (**b**) Permits total freedom of movement, but is unstable. (**c**) Allows freedom of movement and is stable. However, the shape is not optimal because it is completely congruent and does not provide space between the articulating surfaces for lubrication or nutrition. When the joint is loaded, the stress is not equally distributed over the joint surfaces. (**d**) Is the optimal shape for a joint because it is stable, it articulates easily, and there is some space between the joint surfaces, so that the synovial fluid can move into the joint space to provide for the nutrition of the cartilage cells and the lubrication of the surfaces. This shape also distributes an increasing load equally, because the deformability of cartilage and bone enables the tissues to respond and conform to the stresses imposed on them.

gelatinous core (nucleus pulposus). The annulus, if viewed from above, can be seen to contain fibrous tissue layers arranged in concentric circles. Each layer extends obliquely from vertebral body to vertebral body, with the fibers of one layer running in a direction opposite to that of the adjacent layer. These alternating layers provide for motion that is universal in direction, i.e. flexion–extension–lateral bending and rotation, but restricted in degree (Figs 1.48 and 1.49). The fibers of the annulus are attached by Sharpey's fibers into the bony end-plates of the adja-

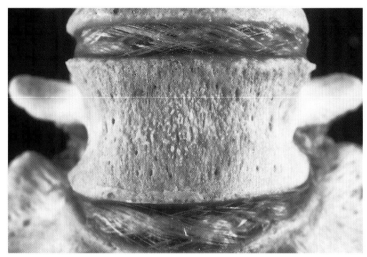

Figure 1.48 Photograph showing frontal view of L5 with the adjacent intervertebral disc. Note the oblique disposition of the collagen fibers of the annulus fibrosus in this macerated specimen, which allows for universal movement between the vertebral bodies.

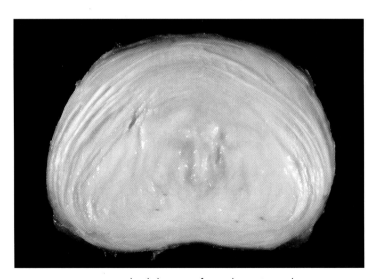

Figure 1.47 Intervertebral disc seen from above. Note the circumferential fibers in the annulus fibrosus. The nucleus pulposus (center) is rich in PG and water, and acts to resist compression. The circumferential fibers of the annulus prevent lateral displacement of the nucleus.

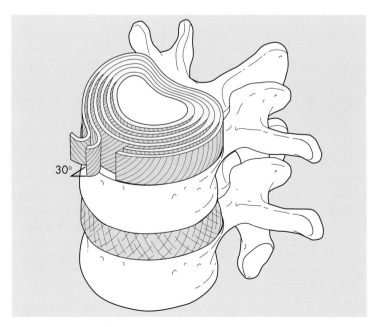

Figure 1.49 Schematic drawing of the intervertebral disc demonstrates the layered arrangement of collagen fibers in the annulus. The fibers of each layer run at an approximately 30° angle to the surface of the vertebral body and in a direction opposite to that of the adjacent layer.

cent vertebral bodies (Fig. 1.50). The antero-lateral component of the annulus, where the fibrous lamellae are stronger and more numerous, is almost twice the thickness of the posterior annulus. The nucleus pulposus typically occupies an eccentric position within the disc space, being closer to the posterior margin. The tissue of the nucleus is separated from that of the bone of the adjacent vertebrae by a clearly defined layer of hyaline cartilage which extends to the inner margins of the insertion of the annulus (Fig. 1.51).

On microscopic examination the nucleus pulposus shows chondrocytes as well as stellate and fusiform cells suspended in a loose myxoid fibrous matrix (Fig. 1.52).

Because no blood vessels are present in adult disc tissue, nutrients must reach the cells by diffusion from capillaries at the disc margins. The restricted flow of nutrients to the nucleus and inner annulus may contribute to or even underlie disc degeneration in the adult.

The third and final type of joint is the fibrous synarthrosis, such as the skull sutures, which are nonmovable joints filled with dense collagenized fibrous tissue (Fig. 1.53).

CARTILAGE

The articular ends of the bones are covered by hyaline cartilage, which is a nerveless, bloodless, firm and yet pliable tissue. Hyaline cartilage deforms under pressure but slowly recovers its original shape on removal of pressure (i.e. it has visco-elastic

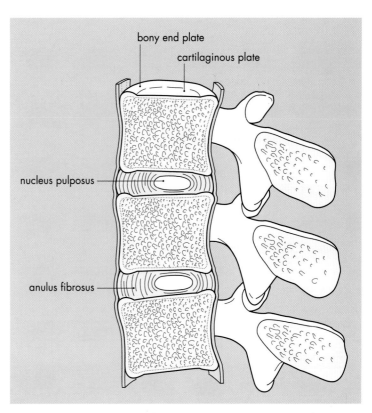

Figure 1.51 Intervertebral disc. Hyaline cartilage separates the tissue of the nucleus pulposus from that of the bone.

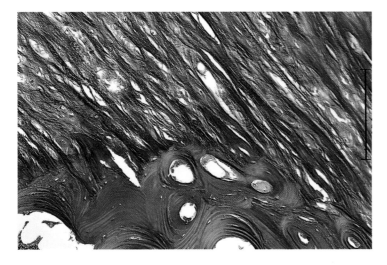

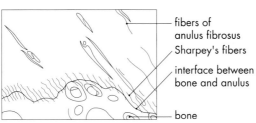

Figure 1.50 Photomicrograph showing the insertion of the fibers of the annulus fibrosus into the bone of the margins of the articular surface of the vertebral body. Where the collagen fibers of the annulus enter the bone (Sharpey's fibers) they are calcified (H&E stain, partially polarized light, × 4 obj.).

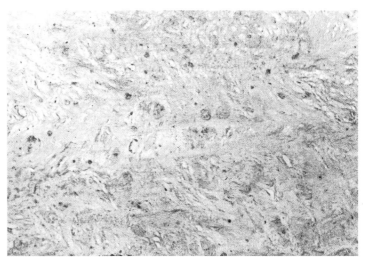

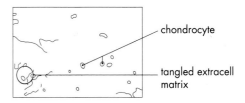

Figure 1.52 Photomicrograph of normal nucleus pulposus. The matrix is loose and fibrous, with scattered small stellate cells and occasional chondrocytes in clumps (H&E stain, × 4 obj.).

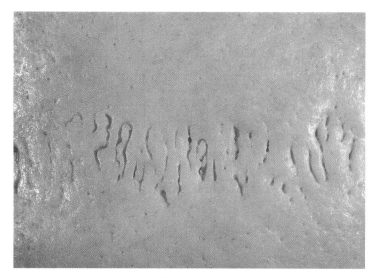

Figure 1.53 A photograph of the sagittal suture of the skull to demonstrate its interlocking pattern. (In the adult the sutures are generally partially obliterated by osseous fusion.)

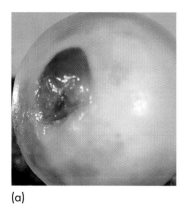
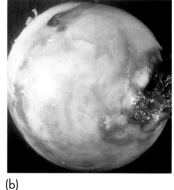

(a)   (b)

Figure 1.54 (a) Femoral head from an 18-year-old adolescent shows a translucent bluish-white cartilage and (b) from a 65-year-old patient shows an opaque, slightly yellowish cartilage.

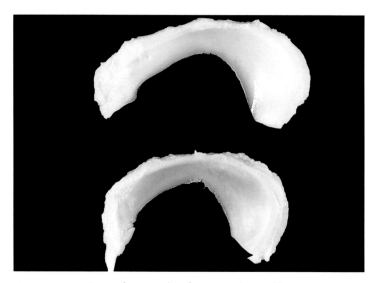

Figure 1.55 Gross photographs of menisci obtained from a young (upper) and an old (lower) patient. In contrast to the meniscus from the young patient, which has a bluish-white color and is supple, the meniscus from the old patient has a characteristically yellowish color and feels stiffer on palpation.

properties). In growing children cartilage is the precursor of the bony skeleton and also the means by which the bones increase in length.

In young people articular cartilage is translucent and bluish-white; in older individuals it is opaque and slightly yellowish (Fig. 1.54). This change with age in the appearance of articular cartilage is also seen in other connective tissues and is probably related to a number of factors, including dehydration of the tissues, increased numbers of cross-linkages in the collagen, and the accumulation of lipofuscin pigment in the tissues (Fig. 1.55).

On microscopic examination articular cartilage is characterized by its abundant glassy extracellular matrix with isolated, relatively sparse cells located in well-defined spaces (lacunae). It is often described as having four layers or zones: superficial (I), intermediate (II), deep (III), and calcified (IV). In the cell-rich superficial layer, zone I, the cells are relatively small and flat, oriented with their long axis parallel to the surface. In the intermediate zone II, the cells are larger and rounder, but also sparser and randomly distributed. In zone III or the deeper layer, the cells are even larger and have a tendency to form radial groups which apparently follow the pattern of collagen disposition. In the calcified zone IV, i.e. adjacent to the bone, the cells are mostly nonviable and the matrix heavily calcified (Figs 1.56 and 1.57).

That some fibrous system exists within normal articular cartilage can be demonstrated by pricking the surface with a pin, resulting in a split. If the pricking is repeated all over the surface, a constant pattern of split lines is revealed (Fig. 1.58). If the fissures reflect the internal fiber arrangement of the cartilage, then it can be inferred that on the surface the fibers run parallel to the surface and in the general direction of the split line.

If the superficial layer of the cartilage is pared away and the exposed surface pricked, instead of a split only a small, round hole appears (Fig. 1.59). If the cut edge of the cartilage is pricked, a vertical split line is produced and this occurs in all planes of the section (Fig. 1.60). These experiments indicate that in the deeper layers of the cartilage the fibers are predominantly vertical (Fig. 1.61).

Polarizing microscopy, transmission electron microscopy, and scanning electron microscopy all confirm that the principle orientation of collagen in articular cartilage is vertical through most of its thickness and horizontal at the surface (Fig. 1.62).

Electron microscopic studies show that in the surface layer the collagen fibers are closely packed, of fine diameter, and oriented parallel to the joint surface. The collagen content of cartilage progressively diminishes from the superficial to the deep layer and in deeper layers the collagen fibers are more widely separated, thicker in diameter, and vertically aligned in such a fashion as to form a web of arch-shaped structures. The fibers of zones II and III are continuous with those in the calcified layer of cartilage, but not with those of the underlying subchondral bone.

The very precise organization of collagen, as already described for the cartilage, bone, and annulus of the intervertebral disc, serves a mechanical function. The mechanical requirements of all connective tissues are similarly provided for by the microarchitectural arrangement of the collagen matrix. For example, the menisci of the knee are composed mainly of collagen, although some PG is also present. Microscopic examination of carefully oriented sections has shown that the principal orientation of the collagen fibers in the menisci is circumferential to withstand the circumferential tension developed during normal loading. The few small, radially disposed fibers probably act as ties to resist any

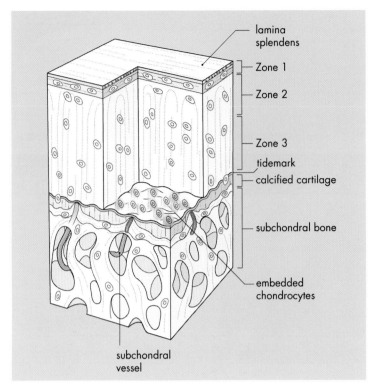

lamina
splendens

Zone 1

Zone 2

Zone 3

tidemark

calcified cartilage

subchondral bone

embedded
chondrocytes

subchondral
vessel

(a)

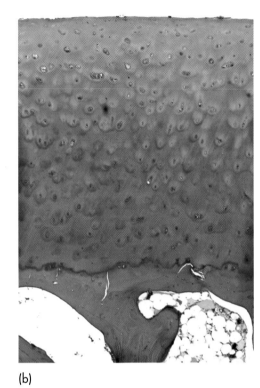

(b)

Figure 1.56
(a) The arrangement of adult articular cartilage.
(b) Photomicrograph of normal articular cartilage obtained from the femoral condyle of a middle-aged man (H&E, × 2.5 obj.).

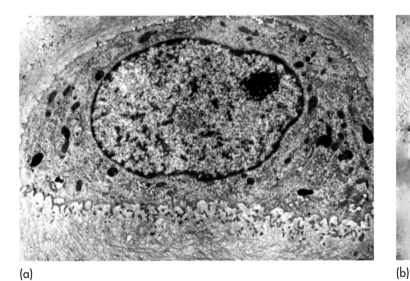

(a)

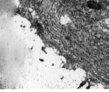

(b)

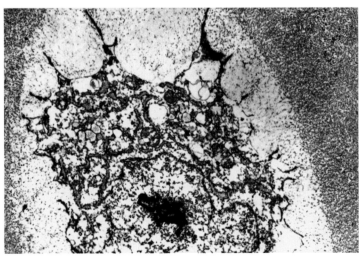

(c)

Figure 1.57 Electron photomicrographs to illustrate the typical appearance of chondrocytes at the surface, mid-zone and deep-zone of the articular cartilage. **(a)** At the surface the cell is typically flattened and shows more cell processes on the inferior surface (× 10,000). **(b)** In the mid-zone the cell is round and demonstrates a well-developed endoplasmic reticulum and Golgi apparatus (× 10,000). **(c)** The deep cells show vacuolization of the cytoplasm with shrinking and irregularity of the nucleus (× 10,000).

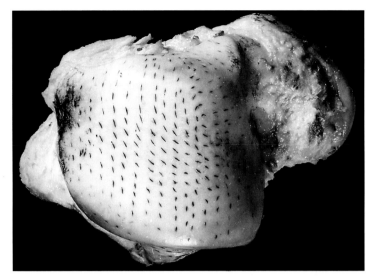

Figure 1.58   Photograph of the superior articular surface of the talus after the entire surface has been pricked with a pin dipped in Indian ink. Note the resulting pattern of split lines.

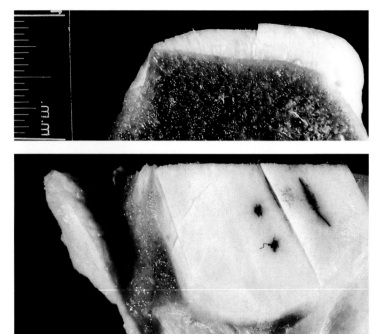

Figure 1.59   Photograph demonstrating that after the outer layer of cartilage is removed prior to pin insertion, only a round hole appears, rather than a split.

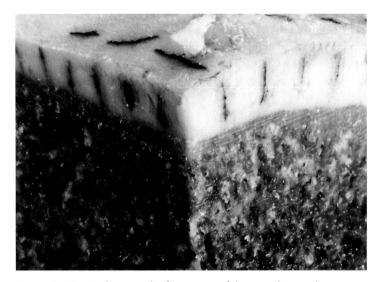

Figure 1.60   A photograph of a portion of the articular cartilage which has been sectioned vertically to show both the cut edge and the underlying bone. The direction of pin pricks made on the surface can be seen and additional pin pricks have been made on the cut edge, all of which result in vertical splits.

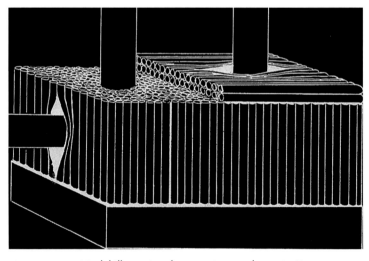

Figure 1.61   Model illustrating the experiments shown in Figures 1.58–1.60.

longitudinal splitting of the menisci that might result from undue compression (Fig. 1.63).

The amount of PG in the cartilage matrix relates to the mechanical requirements and varies from joint to joint, geographically within a single articular cartilage. The surface layers of the cartilage contain much less PG than the deeper layers. In the deeper layers there is a higher concentration of staining of the PGs with safranin O and methylene blue around the cells (the pericellular matrix) than between the cells (the intercellular matrix) (Fig. 1.64).

In histologic sections stained with hematoxylin–eosin, the junction between the calcified cartilage and the noncalcified cartilage is marked by a basophilic line known as the tidemark or calcification front and it will be described in more detail in

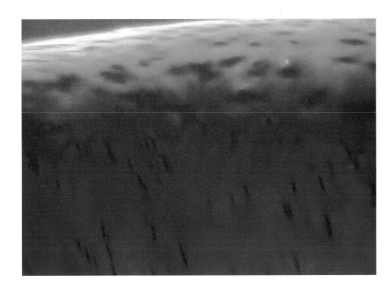

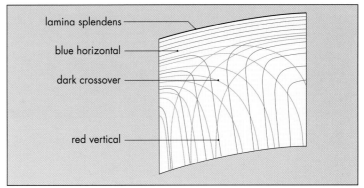

Figure 1.62 Photomicrograph of the articular cartilage using polarized light and a compensating filter. The fibers at the surface of the cartilage are seen in blue, the fibers in the lower part of the cartilage in red. Between the two layers there is less polarization, as can be seen. These observations can be interpreted as demonstrating that at the surface the fibers are horizontally disposed, in the deep part of the cartilage they are vertical, and in between there is a crossover of fibers (× 10 obj.). (See also Figures 12.55 and 12.56.)

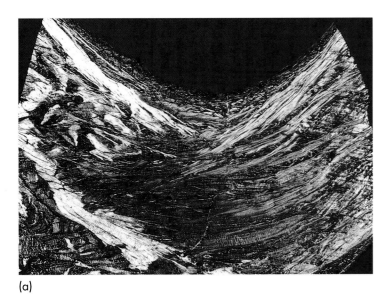

(a)

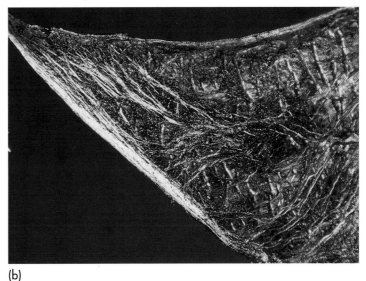

(b)

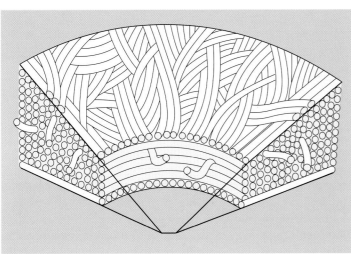

(c)

Figure 1.63 (a) Photomicrograph of a section cut along the length of the meniscus in its mid-zone demonstrates that the collagen fibers run circumferentially (polarized light, × 1 obj.). (b) Cross-section of the meniscus about halfway along its length demonstrates that most of the collagen fibers are cut crossways. However, especially on the tibial surface of the meniscus, the collagen fibers are cut lengthways, indicating their radial disposition (polarized light, × 1 obj.).
(c) Diagrammatic representation of the distribution of collagen fibers in the meniscus of a knee. Collagen is oriented throughout the connective tissues in such a way as maximally to resist the forces brought to bear on these tissues. The majority of the fibers are circumferentially arranged; a few radially arranged fibers, particularly on the tibial surface, resist lateral spread of the meniscus. In the meniscus, tension is generated between the anterior and posterior attachments.

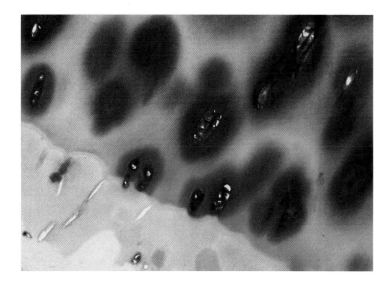

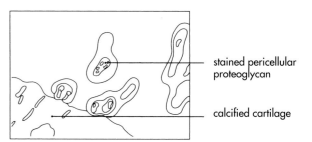

Figure 1.64   Portion of cartilage stained by methylene blue shows intense metachromasia around the chondrocytes in the deep part of the noncalcified cartilage. This represents staining of the PG. There is much less staining in the interterritorial matrix than around the cell. Even less staining is seen in the calcified cartilage (× 25 obj.).

stained pericellular proteoglycan

calcified cartilage

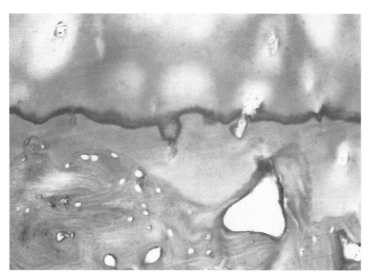

Figure 1.65   Photomicrograph of the junction of articular cartilage with bone shows the basophilic line (tidemark) that separates the noncalcified from the calcified cartilage. This line represents the mineralization front of the calcified cartilage. In normal adult cartilage it is clearly defined and relatively even, but in arthritic conditions the line may become widened and diffuse, and duplication of the line is a common finding (H&E, × 10 obj.).

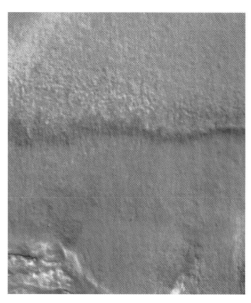

Figure 1.66 Photomicrograph demonstrates the tidemark at a somewhat higher power than in Figure 1.65. A granular appearance of the tidemark can be appreciated (H&E, × 25 obj., Nomarski optics).

Chapter 10, p. 241. This basophilic line clearly visible in the adult is not seen in the developing skeleton (Figs 1.65 and 1.66).

Mechanical failure in the cartilage rarely, if ever, gives rise to the separation of bone and cartilage. However, when failure occurs, it is seen as a horizontal cleft at the junction of the calcified and noncalcified cartilage (at the tidemark) (Figs 1.67 and 1.68). Presumably, shear failure occurs at the tidemark due to the considerable change in the rigidity of the cartilage at this junction.

The calcified cartilage layer is keyed into the irregular surface of the underlying bone (Fig. 1.69). The insertions of ligaments and tendons into the bone are effected by a similar keying, and at their insertions ligaments and tendons are also calcified (Fig. 1.70).

In addition to hyaline cartilage of which articular cartilage is composed, two other forms of cartilage have been described histologically. Fibrocartilage is a tissue in which the matrix contains a high proportion of collagen, but the cells are rounded with a halo of PG around them. It is found at the insertions of ligaments and tendons into the bone (Fig. 1.71), and on the inner side of tendons as they angle around pulleys, e.g. at the malleoli. Fibrocartilaginous metaplasia may be found in injured meniscus and other injured fibrous connective tissues, perhaps because the tissue is focally subjected to more compressive forces following

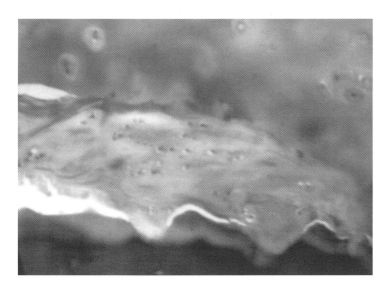

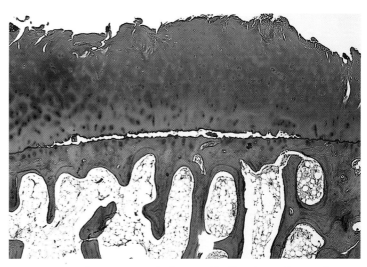

Figure 1.68 Photomicrograph showing fibrillated articular cartilage with underlying subchondral bone. Note the horizontal cleft, i.e. discontinuity, which has formed at the junction with the calcified cartilage just above the tidemark. (H&E, × 1.25 obj.).

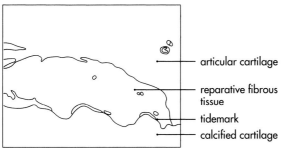

— articular cartilage

— reparative fibrous tissue

— tidemark

— calcified cartilage

Figure 1.67 Photomicrograph demonstrates a traumatic separation of the cartilage in the region of the tidemark. This defect has become filled by reparative fibrous tissue (H&E, × 10 obj.).

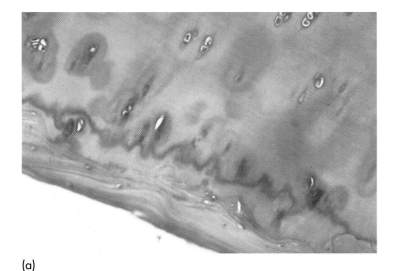

(a)

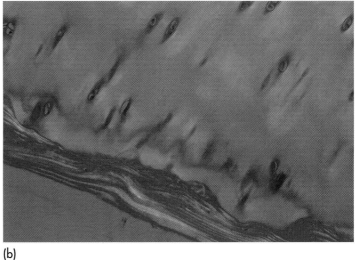

(b)

Figure 1.69 Photomicrographs of the bone–cartilage interface. (a) The tidemark, which indicates the upper edge of the calcified cartilage, can be seen as a wavy blue line, but the bone–cartilage interface is poorly visualized. (b) When the same histologic field is examined by polarized light, using a compensator filter, the bone, which is seen as red, and the cartilage, which is seen as blue, are easily differentiated and the tidemark can still be seen (H&E, × 10 obj.).

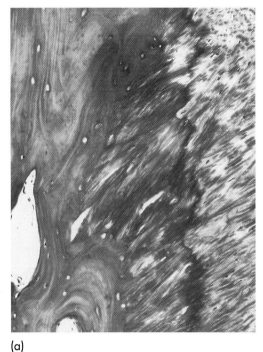

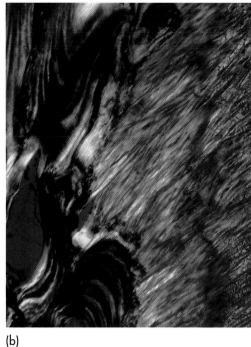

(a)

(b)

Figure 1.70 Photomicrographs of the insertion of the ligamentum flavum into bone. **(a)** The wavy blue line, which represents the edge of the calcified portion of the ligament, is clearly seen, although the interface of ligament and bone is not well visualized. **(b)** When the same histologic field is examined by polarized light, the interface of calcified ligament and bone is clearly demonstrated (H&E, × 10 obj.).

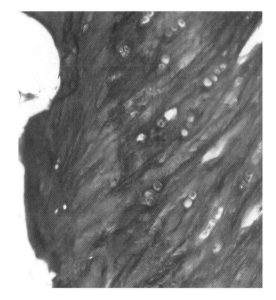

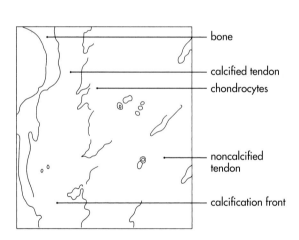

bone

calcified tendon

chondrocytes

noncalcified tendon

calcification front

Figure 1.71 Photomicrograph of a tendon insertion. Note that at the insertion, the cells of the tendon are rounded and lie in lacunae. This is described as fibrocartilaginous metaplasia. Elsewhere in a tendon the fibrocytes are flattened (H&E, × 10 obj.).

injury. The second type of nonhyaline cartilage, elastic cartilage, contains a high proportion of elastic tissue in the matrix. It is found in the ligamentum flavum, external ear, and epiglottis (Fig. 1.72), where some element of stretch is required in the tissue (normal collagen lengthens only very slightly, even under heavy loads).

Both fibrocartilage and elastic cartilage incorporate the term 'cartilage' because the cells are rounded and lie in lacunae, and staining will reveal some PG staining in the pericellular areas, which gives them a superficial resemblance to the cells of hyaline cartilage. However, the mechanical functions of these tissues are very different from those of hyaline cartilage. Both fibrocartilage

and elastic cartilage function principally as resistors of tension, with, however, some focal element of compression. On the other hand, hyaline cartilage is mainly subject to and resists compressive forces.

SYNOVIAL MEMBRANE

The synovial membrane lines the inner surface of the joint capsule and all other intra-articular structures, with the exception of articular cartilage and the meniscus; it consists of two components. The first is the synovial lining (or intimal layer) bounding the joint space; this is predominantly cellular. The second com-

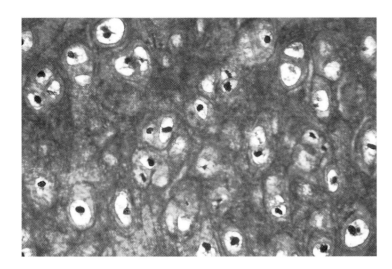

ponent is a supportive, or backing layer, formed of fibrous and adipose tissues in variable proportions.

The surface of the synovial lining is smooth, moist, and glistening, with a few small villi and fringe-like folds (Fig. 1.73). The cellular elements of the joint lining consist of a single row or sometimes multiple rows of closely packed intimal cells with large elliptical nuclei (synoviocytes) and deeper other connective-tissue cells, including fat cells, fibroblasts, histiocytes, and mast cells (which are omnipresent in connective tissue) (Figs 1.74 and 1.75).

Electron microscopic studies have revealed two principal types of synovial lining cells, which have been designated by Barland as types A and B. (Many cells have features of both types and have been called intermediate.) The less common cell (type A) has

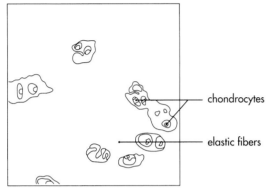

Figure 1.72   Photomicrograph of ear cartilage. Although the cells resemble those seen in hyaline cartilage, the matrix contains many elastic fibers. These fibers appear bright red in this section stained with phloxine and tartrazine (× 25 obj.).

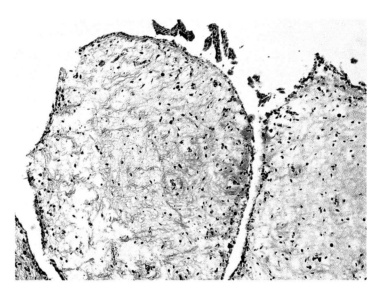

Figure 1.73   Photomicrograph of synovium showing the simple lining and the fibroadipose subsynovial tissue (H&E, × 4 obj.).

Figure 1.74   Photomicrograph of synovium showing a delicate synovial lining resting on a fibroadipose subintimal layer which is rich in capillaries, lymphatics, and nerve endings (H&E, × 25 obj.).

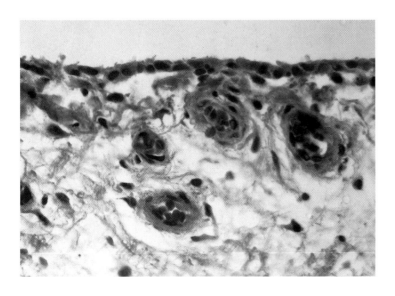

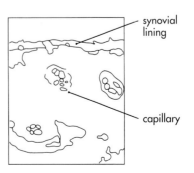

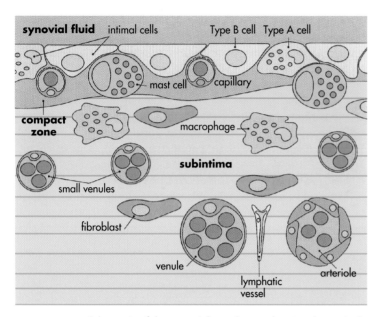

Figure 1.75   Schematic of the synovial membrane showing the typical arrangement of cells. The transudation of the synovial fluid requires specialized capillaries such as those seen in the renal glomeruli.

many of the features of a macrophage, and there is good evidence that it is structurally adapted for phagocytic functions (Fig. 1.76). The more common type B cells are richly endowed with rough endoplasmic reticulum, contain Golgi systems, and often show pinocytotic vesicles (Fig. 1.77). Normal synovial intima contains 25% of type A and 75% of type B cells.

The synovial membrane has three principal functions: secretion of synovial fluid hyaluronate (B cells); phagocytosis of waste material derived from the various components of the joint (A cells); and regulation of the movement of solutes, electrolytes, and proteins from the capillaries into the synovial fluid. Thus the synovium provides for the metabolic requirement of the joint chondrocytes and a regulatory mechanism for maintenance of the matrix.

In addition to lining the joints, synovial membrane lines the subcutaneous and subtendinous bursal sacs, which permit freedom of movement over a limited range, for the structures adjacent to the bursae. Synovial membrane also lines the sheaths that form around tendons wherever they pass under ligamentous bands or through osseofibrous tunnels.

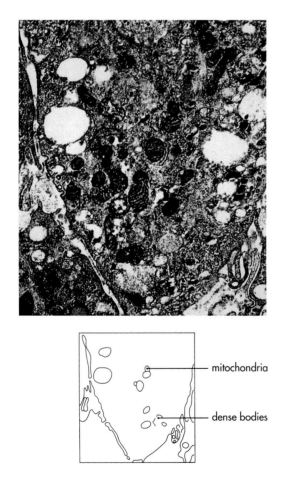

Figure 1.76   Electron micrograph of an A cell shows abundant mitochondria and dense inclusion bodies (× 10,000).

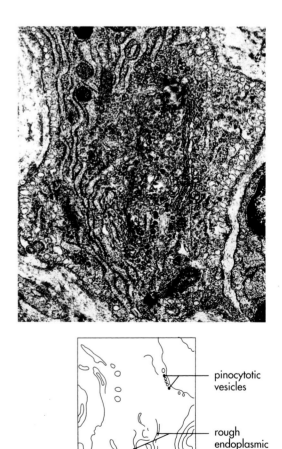

Figure 1.77   Electron micrograph of a B cell shows abundant rough endoplasmic reticulum and many pinocytotic vesicles (× 10,000).

BONE GROWTH AND DEVELOPMENT

Unlike most tissues, bone can grow only by apposition on the surface of an already existing substrate such as bone and/or calcified cartilage. As Hunter put it, 'Bones do not grow by fresh matter being put into all parts, so as to push the old matter to a greater distance but by new matter laid upon the external surface.'

In contrast to bone, cartilage grows by interstitial cellular proliferation and matrix formation. It is perhaps because of the capacity of cartilage for interstitial growth that most of the embryonic skeleton is first formed in the cartilage, and that cartilage proliferation plays such an important role in skeletal growth and modeling. (With the exception of the cranial vault, the skeleton first appears in the embryo as a cartilaginous structure.)

Before any bone formation occurs within the embryonic cartilage skeleton, it can be seen that the chondrocytes towards the middle of the individual skeletal parts are larger and more separated by interstitial matrix than those towards the ends, where the chondrocytes are fairly small and closely packed together (Fig. 1.78). As the cells in the center of the shaft continue to enlarge, the cartilage matrix lying between the cells becomes calcified, and the cells die (Fig. 1.79).

Although the mechanisms of calcification are not completely understood, it is clear that the regulation of cartilage calcification is essential to bone growth and modeling. The hypertrophic chondrocytes adjacent to the calcification front show electron microscopic alterations in their cytoplasmic structure and have been found to synthesize collagen type X, which appears to be an

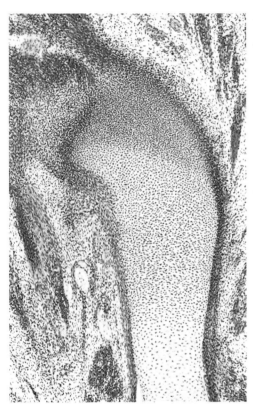

Figure 1.78
Photomicrograph of the upper end of the femur and hip joint in a 5-week fetus. The future bone is already modeled in cartilage and is covered by a condensation of mesenchymal cells, which will eventually become the periosteum. Note that the cells in the diaphysis of the cartilage model (at the lower end of the photograph) are larger and paler than those at the upper end (H&E, × 4 obj.).

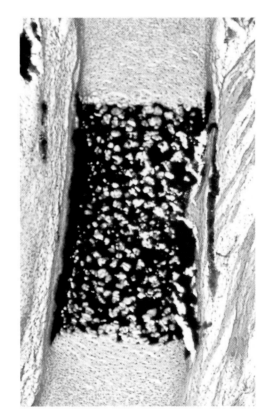

Figure 1.79
Photomicrograph of the shaft of a long bone in a 7-week fetus (undecalcified and stained with von Kossa stain). Note the calcification of the cartilage matrix (black) in the diaphysis (× 4 obj.).

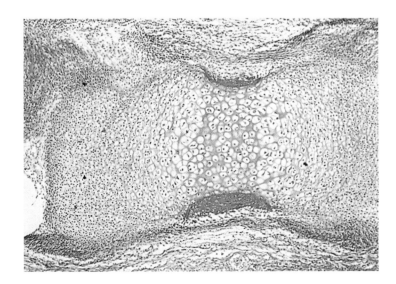

Figure 1.80 Photomicrograph of a section through a metacarpal from a 7-week fetus. In the diaphysis the cartilage matrix stains a deeper blue, indicating that it is calcified. Around the calcified cartilage matrix is a narrow cuff of immature bone (Trichrome stain, × 4 obj.).

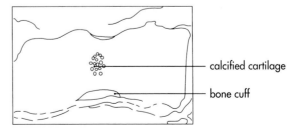

calcified cartilage

bone cuff

important mediator of vascular invasion. Still other factors involved may include extracellular matrix vesicles that provide sites for initial hydroxyapatite deposition, enzymes that increase local calcium and phosphate concentration, enzymes that degrade mineralization inhibitors or cause the formation of mineralization promotors. Other factors may inhibit or limit the extent of calcification, e.g. PGs and pyrophosphate.

Following calcification of the cartilage matrix, the periosteum surrounding this portion of the bone begins to produce from its cambium layer a primitive bone matrix, which is quickly formed into a cuff of bone (Fig. 1.80). Soon after these events, small capillaries penetrate the periosteum and the periosteal bone cuff into the calcified cartilage matrix, destroying the empty cartilage lacunae and establishing a vascular network throughout the calcified cartilage (Fig. 1.81). Cells, perhaps derived from the vessel walls, are seen to line up on the surface of the remaining calcified cartilage and deposit a bony matrix. This process of cartilage calcification, vascular invasion and deposition of bony matrix on the remaining calcified cartilage is known as endochondral ossification. It is the process through which cartilage is transformed into bone.

The bone first laid down, i.e. with a core of calcified cartilage and primitive bone on the surface, is commonly known as the primary spongiosa (Fig. 1.82; see also Fig. 1.95). As the primary

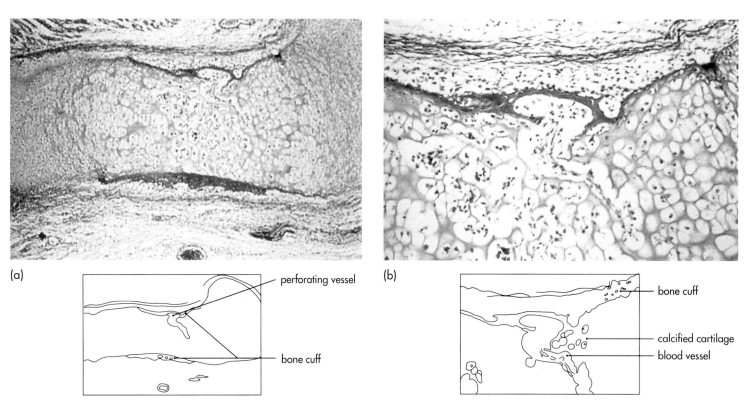

(a)

(b)

Figure 1.81   (a) Photomicrograph of a long bone removed from a 10-week fetus (Trichrome, × 4 obj.). (b) Close-up shows the calcified cartilage (below) and the diaphyseal bone cuff (above) covered by condensed mesenchymal tissue that forms the periosteum. Penetrating through the bone cuff into the calcified cartilage is a blood vessel. This blood vessel will eventually erode through the calcified cartilage entirely, bringing in osteoblasts to form the earliest primary spongiosa (Trichrome, × 16 obj.).

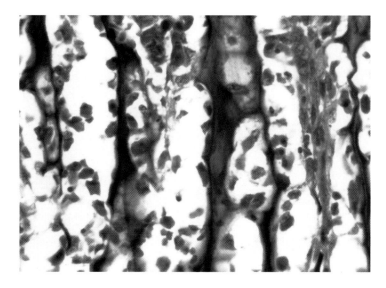

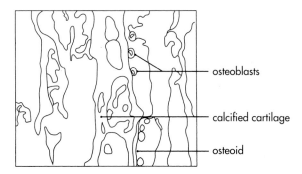

Figure 1.82   A portion of the primary spongiosa from the diaphysis of a long bone in a 10-week fetus. Notice the delicate cores of dark blue calcified cartilage covered by plump cells (osteoblasts), which are forming the seams of pink immature bone matrix (H&E, × 25 obj.).

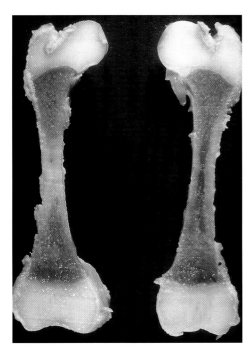

Figure 1.83 Gross photograph of a femur from a 6-month stillborn baby. At this stage the epiphyseal ends of the bone are still entirely cartilaginous.

spongiosa is remodeled and the calcified cartilage removed, the bone trabeculae come to be formed entirely of bone tissue; at this stage they are usually referred to as secondary spongiosa.

In the fetus, the process of endochondral ossification continues until a considerable portion of the shaft of a long bone has been converted into osseous tissue and only the ends of the bone are still formed of cartilage (Fig. 1.83). Throughout this process, the cartilage at the bone ends is continuously proliferating and enlarging by interstitial growth. As the cartilage cells in the epiphyseal bone ends approach the midshaft of the bone, they undergo enlargement and degeneration; subsequently the cartilage matrix calcifies, and eventually vascular invasion and the formation of more primary spongiosa occur. In this way the bone continuously grows in length (Figs 1.84 and 1.85).

During the early stages of skeletal development, the locations of joints are marked by a condensation of mesenchymal cells. Only after the fifth to eighth week of intrauterine life do these cells undergo flattening and apoptosis to form a joint cleft (Figs 1.86–1.88).

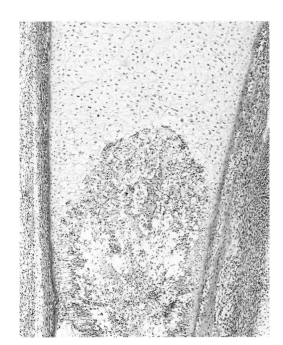

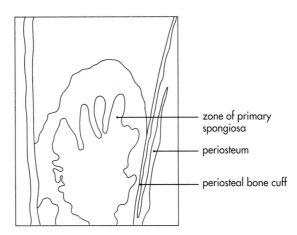

zone of primary spongiosa

periosteum

periosteal bone cuff

Figure 1.84 Photomicrograph of the upper end of the femur showing the junction between the newly formed bone and the epiphyseal cartilage. The bone grows in length by the process of endochondral ossification, in which the calcified cartilage is invaded by blood vessels and replaced by bone (H&E, × 10 obj.).

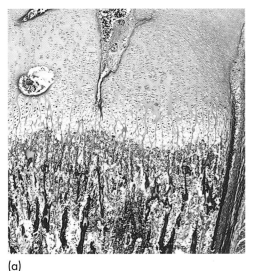

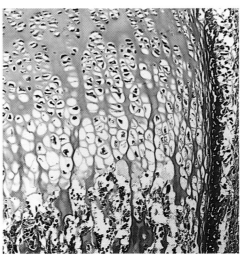

Figure 1.85 (a) Photomicrograph to show the zone where bony growth occurs. This is called the physis, and vascular invasion from the metaphysis results in the replacement of cartilage with bone during the growth process. Note that the periosteal bone extends beyond the growth plate, thereby mechanically stabilizing this zone. (This area shown in higher power in (b), is sometimes referred to as the groove of Ranvier; defects in this groove may explain the development of osteochondromas. See Chapter 17, p. 399)

(a)

(b)

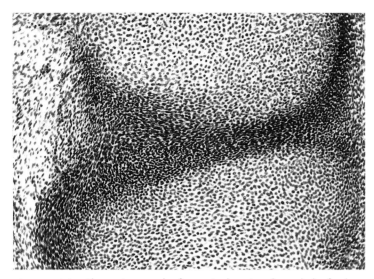

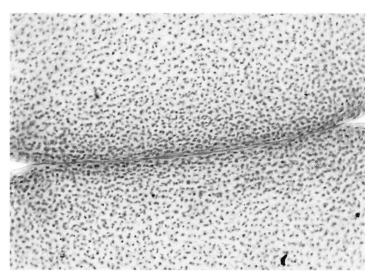

Figure 1.86   Photomicrograph of a sagittal section through the fetal knee joint at the sixth week of gestation, showing the condensation of the mesenchyme marking the future joint space (H&E, × 10 obj.).

Figure 1.87   Photomicrograph of a sagittal section through the knee joint at the ninth week of gestation, showing the development of the joint space from the periphery towards the center of the joint (H&E, × 10 obj.).

At some point during the growth period, usually during childhood, a secondary center of ossification is formed within the cartilaginous end of the bone (Figs 1.89–1.91). Calcification occurs initially at the middle of the secondary center. This area is then invaded by blood vessels carried through canals, that develop from invagination of the delicate surface perichondral covering of the epiphysis and the process of endochondral ossification ensues (Fig. 1.92). As the secondary center of ossification grows, the only remaining cartilage is that which covers the articular end of the bone (Fig. 1.93) and a thin layer or plate of cartilage lying between the secondary center of ossification and the main part of the bone shaft. This plate is the growth plate or physis (Figs 1.94–1.97).

The cartilage of the growth plates continues to proliferate and undergo endochondral ossification until apparent growth ceases during adolescence. At cessation of growth the epiphyseal plate is

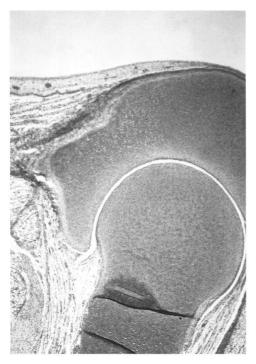

Figure 1.88 Photomicrograph of a section through the hip joint at the tenth week of gestation, showing a fully developed joint space (H&E, × 4 obj.).

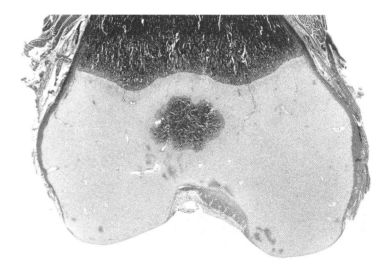

Figure 1.89   The secondary center of ossification is demonstrated in the lower end of the femur. This area increases in size by the process of maturation and calcification of the cartilage around the secondary center, with subsequent endochondral ossification (H&E, × 1 obj.).

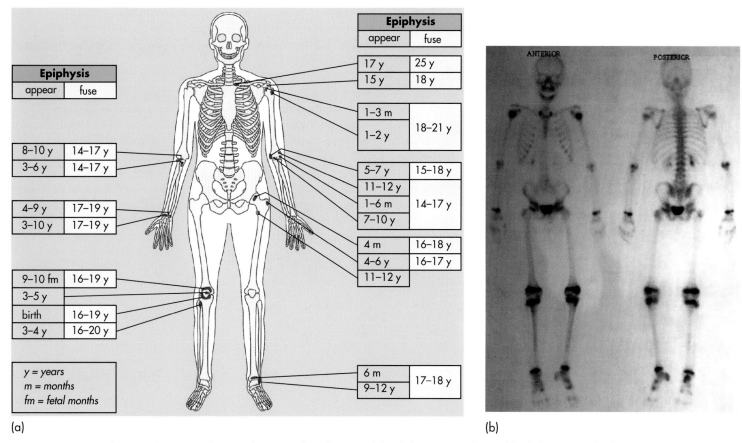

Epiphysis	
appear	fuse
17 y	25 y
15 y	18 y
1–3 m	18–21 y
1–2 y	
5–7 y	15–18 y
11–12 y	
1–6 m	14–17 y
7–10 y	
4 m	16–18 y
4–6 y	16–17 y
11–12 y	
6 m	17–18 y
9–12 y	

Epiphysis	
appear	fuse
8–10 y	14–17 y
3–6 y	14–17 y
4–9 y	17–19 y
3–10 y	17–19 y
9–10 fm	16–19 y
3–5 y	
birth	16–19 y
3–4 y	16–20 y

y = years
m = months
fm = fetal months

(a)

(b)

Figure 1.90   (a) Schematic diagram indicating the times of ossification of the skeleton. (b) In this total body bone scan the forming epiphyses are clearly identified by the intensity of isotope uptake.

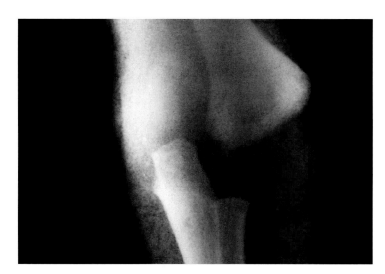

Figure 1.91   This radiograph of a 2-year-old child illustrates the importance of full awareness of the secondary centers of ossification. It might initially appear that there has been a dislocation of the elbow. However, since the ossification center of the capitulum is still in place, it can be inferred that the joint is intact and the displacement results from a fracture through the metaphyseal region of the humerus.

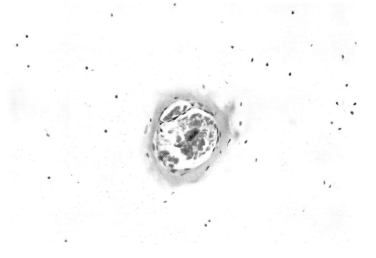

Figure 1.92   The vessels that feed the ossification center of the epiphysis are carried in canals through the epiphyseal cartilage; one of these canals is demonstrated here (H&E, × 25 obj.).

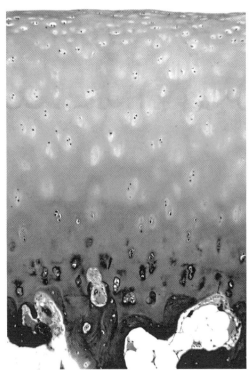

Figure 1.93
Photomicrograph of articular cartilage from an adolescent. Vascular ingrowth from the subchondral bone into the deep articular cartilage is associated with bone formation. Pericellular calcification is present around the deep chondrocytes, however, the tidemark is as yet only rudimentary (H&E, × 4 obj.).

perforated by blood vessels and becomes obliterated (Fig. 1.98). However, the growth plate scar continues in the form of a bone plate, seen on radiologic examination and in anatomic specimens throughout life (Fig. 1.99).

During the growth period acute illness may lead to a temporary cessation of growth, and the stigma of this cessation may remain for many years in the shaft of a bone as a linear density seen on radiographic images and known as a Harris line or growth arrest line, paralleling the epiphyseal scar (Fig. 1.100).

The bones of the skull, as well as some of the facial bones and most of the clavicle, form from undifferentiated connective-tissue cells (mesenchyme) in the same manner as the initial periosteal bone cuff, i.e. without a pre-existing cartilage model. These bones are termed membranous bones, and they grow only by the apposition of new bone on the surface. Membranous bones have no cartilaginous growth plates (Figs 1.101–1.103).

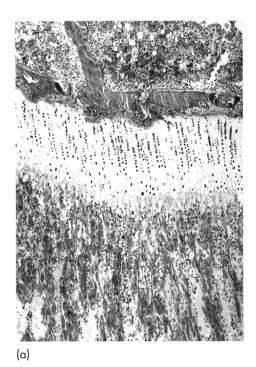

(a)

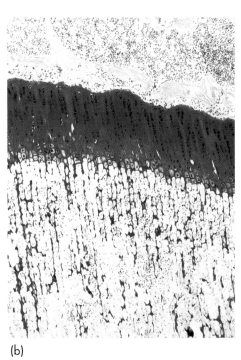

(b)

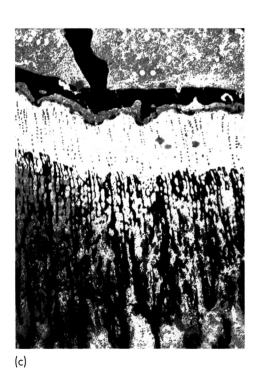

(c)

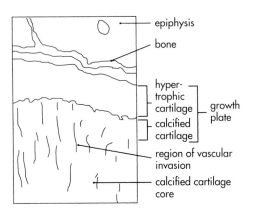

epiphysis

bone

hyper-
trophic
cartilage

calcified
cartilage

growth
plate

region of vascular
invasion

calcified cartilage
core

Figure 1.94   Photomicrograph demonstrating the appearance of the growth plate during active bone growth. At the top of the field is a portion of the epiphysis, and the cartilage cells in the growth plate which are closest to this region are proliferating cells. Further down the cells begin to palisade into vertical columns, and as they approach the metaphysis the cells hypertrophy and the matrix calcifies. The calcified matrix is invaded by blood vessels and bone forms on the residual calcified cores of cartilage. (**a**, H&E; **b**, Safranin O to show the distribution of PG; **c**, von Kossa to show the distribution of calcium; all × 4 obj.).

Figure 1.95 Diagram of the growth plate.

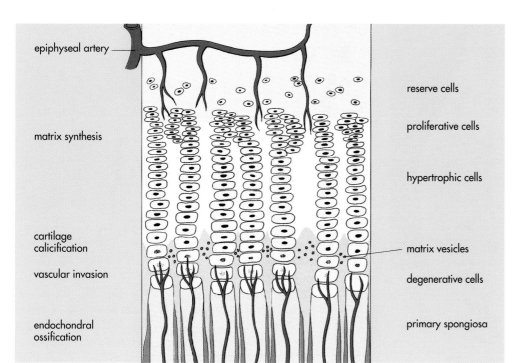

epiphyseal artery

matrix synthesis

cartilage calcification

vascular invasion

endochondral ossification

reserve cells

proliferative cells

hypertrophic cells

matrix vesicles

degenerative cells

primary spongiosa

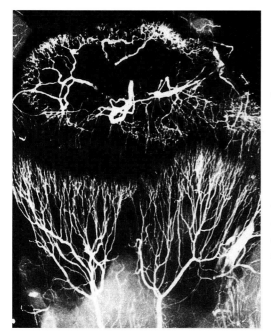

Figure 1.96 Specimen of the upper end of the tibia in an immature pig. The vessels have been injected with barium sulfate and the bone decalcified. The ramifying vessels in the metaphysis, which provide for endochondral ossification, are clearly seen.

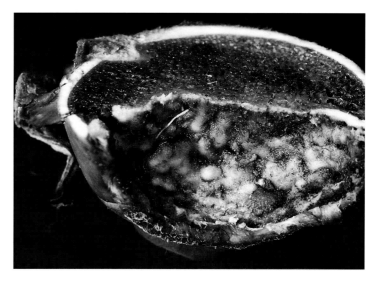

Figure 1.97 A bisected avulsed femoral head from an 8-year-old child. The photograph shows the cup-shaped metaphyseal surface of the growth plate and its knob-like protuberances, both of which help stabilize the epiphysis and prevent slippage during the growth period.

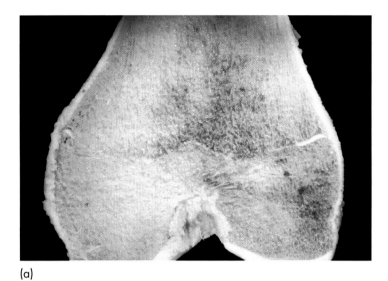

(a)

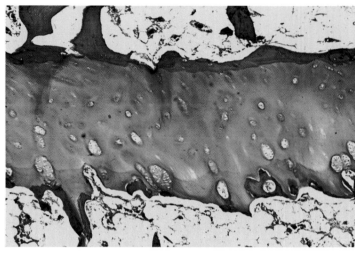

(b)

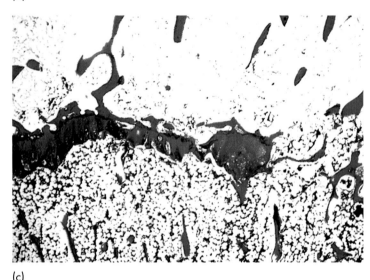

(c)

Figure 1.98   (a) A gross photograph of the distal femur of a 17-year-old male shows the residual growth plate, which is more intact towards the bone surface. (b) Photomicrograph of a portion of the more intact growth plate. Note the inactive metaphyseal surface (lower) (H&E, × 10 obj.). (c) In another area the growth plate is still open on the left side of the field, however, on the right side bony continuity has been established between the metaphysis and the epiphysis. At this point growth can be said to have ceased. In general, the plate first closes in its central portion, while the peripheral portion of the plate is the last part to close (H&E, × 4 obj.).

Figure 1.99   Radiograph of the ankle in an adult shows the epiphyseal scar in the lower end of the tibia.

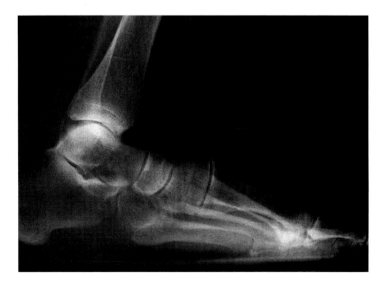

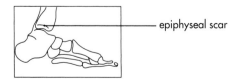

epiphyseal scar

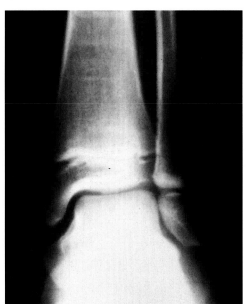

Figure 1.100
Radiograph of the tibia in a child with an open epiphyseal plate. In the shaft of the tibia a number of radiopaque lines (Harris lines) are clearly visible, representing episodes of growth arrest.

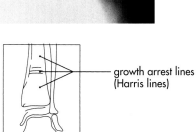

growth arrest lines
(Harris lines)

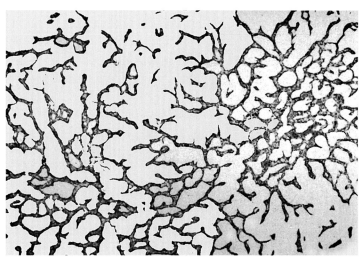

Figure 1.102   Drawing of a macerated specimen of the parietal bone obtained from an approximately 20-week fetus demonstrates how individual foci of secreted bone matrix fuse together initially to form a network of bone; later this network will develop into a plate.

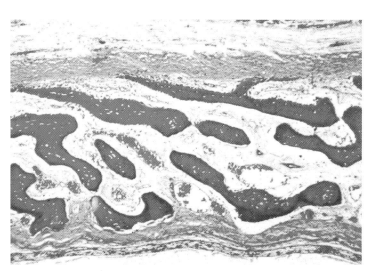

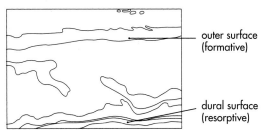

outer surface
(formative)

dural surface
(resorptive)

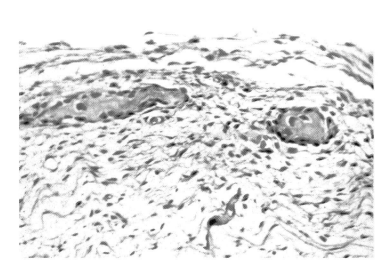

Figure 1.101   Photomicrograph of a section taken through the skull area of an 11-week fetus. The bone presents first as cell condensations which secrete an extracellular matrix of immature bone (H&E, × 16 obj.). Two islands of bone matrix are clearly seen in the upper third of the section.

Figure 1.103   Photomicrograph of a calvarial bone from a 19-week fetus shows a section through the bone plate. The dural surface is on the lower border of the field, and the epidermal surface is on the upper border. Note the resorptive activity along the dural surface and the blastic activity along the epidermal surface, which allows for expansion of the cranium (H&E, × 4 obj.).

METHODS OF EXAMINATION

The protocols used by the pathologist to examine diseased tissue are dealt with exhaustively in a number of texts and will not be discussed in detail here. However, for the general reader to better understand the limitations of tissue pathology some of the more important aspects of technique are dealt with in this chapter.

GROSS EXAMINATION

Bone specimens received by the surgical pathologist often consist only of fragments, and the anatomy is unrecognizable. When it is important to the diagnosis and subsequent management of the patient for the fragments to be differentiated, it is the surgeon's responsibility to ensure that the individual pieces are separately submitted and correctly labeled.

When a larger piece of bone is submitted for examination, anatomic landmarks should be carefully sought and if a photographic record is desirable, careful dissection of the soft tissue adherent to the bone surface is essential. Photographs without this step are likely to be less informative and visually disappointing (Fig. 2.1).

Cutting the specimen into thin slices (3–5 mm) allows both visualization of the interior of the bone and proper fixation of the tissue. Large specimens can be cut on a band saw, and smaller specimens on a small circular saw (Fig. 2.2). After using the saw, it is important to gently wash the cut surface of the bone tissue under running water. This ensures that any fragments of bone dust and other tissue debris generated by the sawing are washed out of the interstices of the marrow space. Unless this is done, microscopic artifacts may appear on the histological sections (see Fig. 2.25).

Visual examination of the cut surface is particularly helpful with tumors where it may be possible firstly to assess the viability of the tumor and, in some cases, to make a preliminary differential diagnosis based upon the consistency and type of matrix production (Fig. 2.3). We have found that a dissecting microscope mounted directly over the grossing area in the surgical pathology laboratory is useful for better visualization of the morbid anatomy and for correlating the gross appearance of a tissue

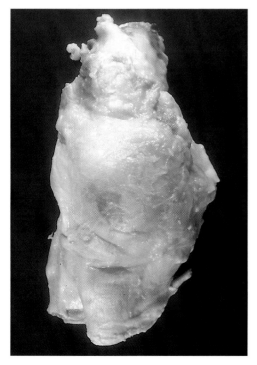
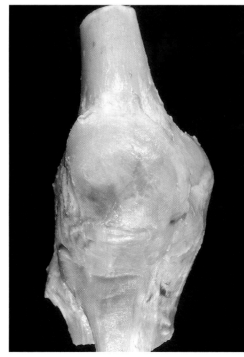

Figure 2.1 (a) Photograph of partially dissected knee joint. The residual soft tissues obscure the anatomy. (b) Once the remnants of muscle and fat are dissected away the gross anatomy is more obvious.

(a)   (b)

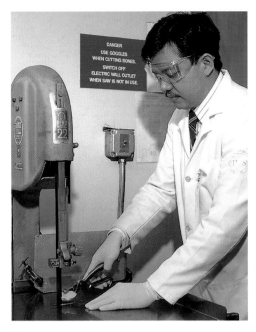

(a)

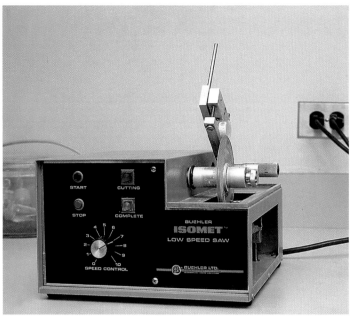

(b)

Figure 2.2   (a) A band saw is used to cut large specimens. Note that the soft tissue left attached to the bone is liable to catch in the saw blade and be torn. (b) Small pieces of bone can be cut on a circular saw, such as shown here, using a diamond blade and a micrometer screw to advance the specimen.

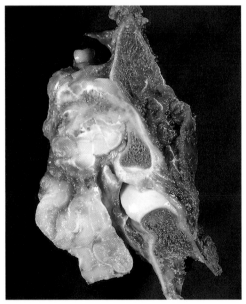

Figure 2.3   This patient had a large tumor projecting from the scapula surface. The glassy blue–white appearance is most consistent with a tumor of cartilaginous origin.

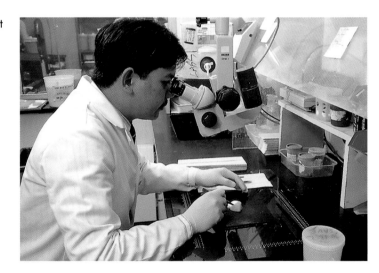

Figure 2.4   Photograph of the dissecting microscope used in the grossing area of the surgical pathology laboratory.

with the microscopic histology, for example, lymphoma, or in a metabolic disturbance, such as Gaucher's disease, in which the normal red or yellow marrow is replaced by a somewhat firmer pink, fleshy tissue. Bone necrosis is readily recognized, because of its opaque, yellow appearance in contrast to the translucent appearance of living bone tissue (Figs 2.4 and 2.5).

RADIOGRAPHIC EXAMINATION OF BONE SPECIMENS

The pathologist should also assess the texture and the porosity of the bone, whether increased or decreased from normal. Although this has often been done by a prosector who presses on the tissue with a thumb, porosity and texture are much better assessed radiographically and a valuable adjunct to the examination of bone specimens is the preparation of radiographs using low-voltage X-rays (Faxitron; Field Emission Corporation, McMinnville, OR) and industrial film (Kodalith Orthofilm type 3) (Fig. 2.6). The detail revealed by such films depends on the thickness of the specimen: the thinner the slice, the more detail will be revealed (Fig. 2.7). The radiograph is particularly useful for assessing alterations in bone texture and organization (Fig. 2.8). Fine-grain radiographs can also be helpful intraoperatively in lieu of a frozen section in finding the nidus of an osteoid osteoma (Fig. 2.9). In some cases the radiograph can be a useful guide in deciding which portions of the tissue to submit for microscopic examination (Fig. 2.10).

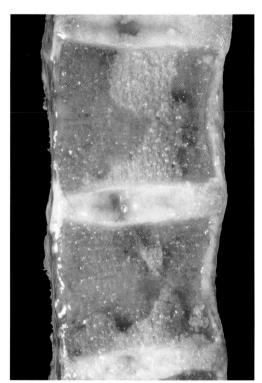

Figure 2.5
Segment of the spine from a child who died of leukemia. Within the vertebral bodies are geographic areas of necrosis that appear as yellow opacification of the bone and marrow. These are surrounded by a thin rim of hyperemic tissue. Note that the viable bone marrow has a fleshy tan color, reflecting the leukemic infiltrate.

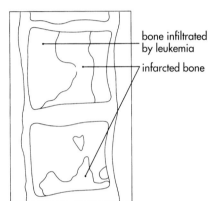

bone infiltrated by leukemia
infarcted bone

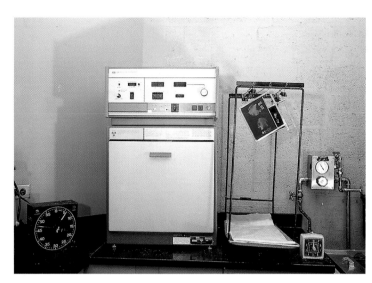

Figure 2.6 In a small darkroom adjacent to the surgical pathology laboratory is a low-voltage X-ray machine, shown here.

SPECIMEN PHOTOGRAPHY

Color images are useful both for research and teaching purposes. In either case, as mentioned earlier, before taking a photograph or obtaining a digital image the specimen must be adequately cleaned so that the bone and the area of the lesion are readily recognizable. It should be carefully washed and dried so that there are no abnormal highlights from reflections of the flood lamps, and also so that the lesion areas are clearly demarcated from normal tissue. The specimen should be aligned according to anatomic principles, and where indicated a scale should also be included in the image (Fig. 2.11).

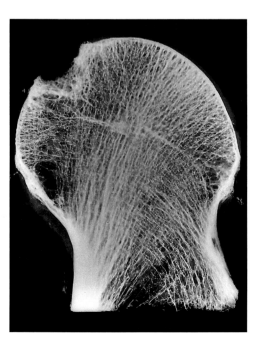

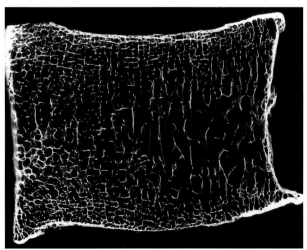

(b)

Figure 2.7 (a) Radiograph of a slice of the femoral head, 5 mm thick. (b) Radiograph of a slice of a vertebral body < 1 mm thick. Less overlay of structure results in improved discrimination.

(a)

osteopenic   normal   osteoblastic reaction

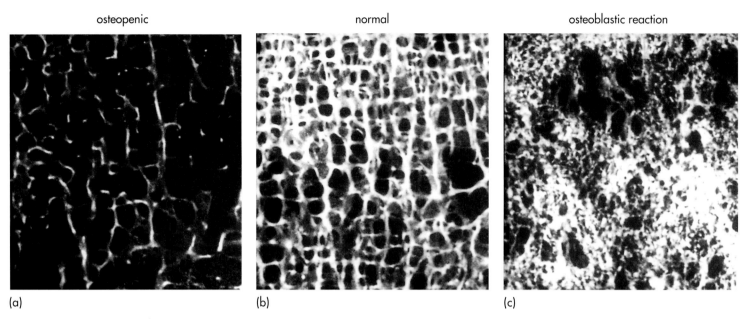

(a)   (b)   (c)

Figure 2.8   Radiographs of osteopenic (**a**), normal (**b**), and osteosclerotic (**c**) vertebrae demonstrate the relative radiolucency of osteoporosis (a) and density of metastatic cancer (c) The normal vertebra has readily identifiable vertical and horizontal bone trabeculae.

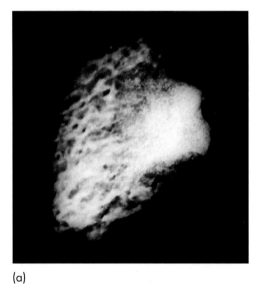

(a)

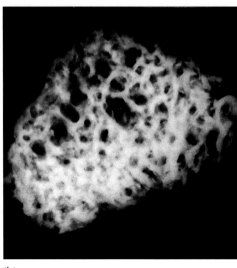

(b)

Figure 2.9   Thirteen fragments of bone were submitted from a patient with an osteoid osteoma. (**a**) Fragment 6, showing a portion of the nidus, recognizable by the dense, finely packed area of bone. (**b**) Comparatively, fragment 13 is entirely cancellous bone.

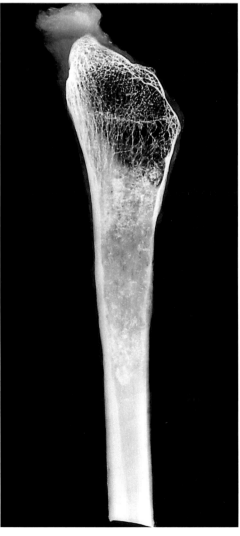

Figure 2.10   Radiograph of the upper end of a fibula resected because of an intraosseous tumor that proved to be a chondrosarcoma. The margins of the tumor are clearly seen on the radiograph, which therefore is an excellent guide to mapping of the section.

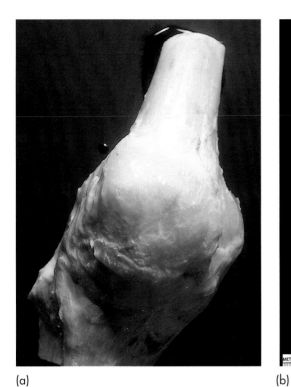

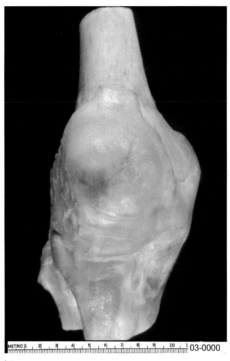

(a) (b)

Figure 2.11 (a) This photograph shows a number of photographic errors including a dirty background, slight lack of focus on the front of the patella, highlights caused by an improperly dried specimen, poor positioning, poor lighting, and no scale for identification. (b) A more correctly taken photograph of the same specimen for comparison.

For publication purposes, it is sometimes necessary to prepare black-and-white images, a generally difficult procedure owing to the uniformity of color normally present and especially because of the natural translucency of the tissue. White light, has a broad wavelength range, which results in variable penetration of light into a translucent object, thereby precluding a sharp focus. This problem can be largely overcome by the use of short-wave monochromatic light. We have found a black (ultraviolet – UV) light source to be inexpensive and to provide very satisfactory photographs (Figs 2.12 and 2.13).

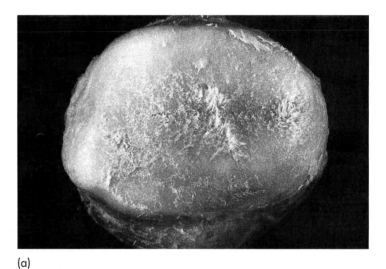

(a)

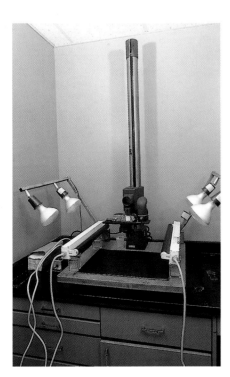

Figure 2.12 Illustration of the set-up used in our laboratory for UV photography. When in use, a developed X-ray film is used for the background to the specimen. Apart from the UV lights, the other lights in the room are switched off.

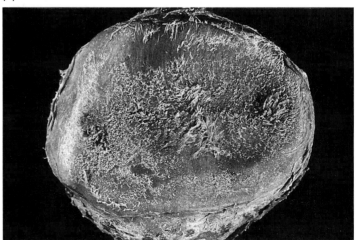

(b)

Figure 2.13 The articular surface of a patella with early degenerative joint disease. (a) Photograph taken with white light as illumination. (b) The same surface illuminated only with black (UV) light.

MICROSCOPIC EXAMINATION

PREPARATION OF TISSUE FOR MICROSCOPIC EXAMINATION

Preparation of tissue sections containing the maximum information depends on choice of the right piece of tissue and on proper processing of the tissue blocks.

To ensure adequate penetration of the processing fluids, the submitted tissues should not exceed 3–4 mm in thickness. It is important to use an adequate amount of fresh solution for fixation, because the fixative is being used up in the process. Far too frequently, specimens from the operating room are received barely covered by fixative, and irreversible tissue breakdown may have taken place as a result of inadequate fixation.

In general, the volume of fixative should be at least ten times the volume of the tissue. For most purposes, formalin provides adequate fixation. However, the formalin should be buffered to prevent the formation of formalin pigment, which can interfere with the proper interpretation of other pigments that may be present, such as iron or gold. Buffering the formalin also prevents the formation of formic acid, which might otherwise result in undesirable decalcification. It is worth noting that for immunoperoxidase stains, optimal fixation with formalin is probably achieved in less than 12 hours.

If decalcification is desired after adequate fixation of the tissue, 5% nitric acid will produce decalcification in a reasonable time with good preservation of the tissue. However, an adequate volume of acid should be used, approximately 10–20 times that of the tissue. Because the acid is neutralized as the calcium is removed from the bone, it should be changed frequently; in our laboratory we change the acid twice a day. To ensure access of the acid to the tissue, gentle agitation using a shaker is a helpful procedure (Fig. 2.14). [The adequacy of decalcification can be assessed by preparing radiographs of the specimens, which can be done with the tissues in their cassettes (Fig. 2.15).]

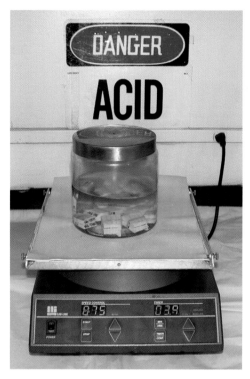

Figure 2.14
A shaker ensures adequate mixing of the acid and access of the acid to the surface of the bone.

After decalcification has been achieved, it is essential to wash the tissue adequately in running water for at least 12 hours, to ensure good differentiation of the hematoxylin–eosin (H&E) stain. If the bone tissue is overly decalcified, or if the acid is inadequately removed, poor staining will result.

For paraffin embedding of the tissue, the use of a vacuum, available in most modern processing machines, is strongly recommended to achieve better infiltration, thus making sectioning easier and ensuring better sections.

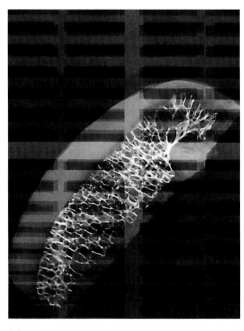

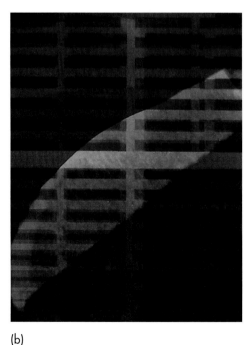

(a)   (b)

Figure 2.15   Radiograph of two bone specimens in their cassettes, showing the stages to complete decalcification.

The preparation of histologic sections of bones for routine microscopic examination has, in general, required the removal of the inorganic mineral component by acidic solutions, as just described. For this reason, the quantity and quality of mineralization have been impossible to assess. The technique of embedding bone in methylmethacrylate, although very time-consuming, not only allows thin histologic sections of bone to be cut without prior decalcification but also has the considerable advantage of achieving a better preservation of tissue relationships. [Because of the tough collagenous nature of the organic matrix, such preservation is often difficult to obtain when routine paraffin embedding is used (Fig. 2.16).]

Bone can be prepared for electron microscopy by fixing diced tissue in paraformaldehyde or in glutaraldehyde. The tissue can be decalcified using ethylenediamine tetra-acetic acid (EDTA), or the calcified tissue can be sectioned with a diamond knife.

STAINS

For most purposes a routine H&E-stained section is adequate. However, a variety of staining techniques may be used to demonstrate the different components of the matrix. Collagen can be demonstrated by a trichrome stain or by the van Gieson stain (Fig. 2.17). (Perhaps the most useful technique for examining collagen is polarized light microscopy.) The proteoglycans (PGs) can be demonstrated by the safranin O stain, alcian blue stain, and less specifically by toluidine blue and periodic acid–Schiff (PAS) (Fig. 2.18). Mineral components, can be demonstrated only in undemineralized tissue, and the mineral can be stained by two techniques: alizarin red, which stains the calcium components of the hydroxyapatite red, and the von Kossa method, which stains the phosphate component as well as other calcium salts (e.g. carbonate and oxalate), black (Fig. 2.19). [The distribution of

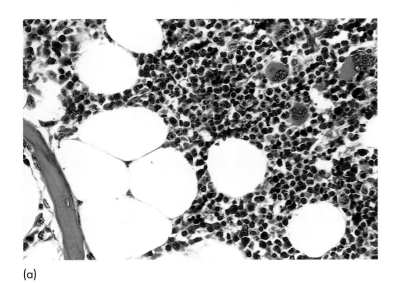
(a)

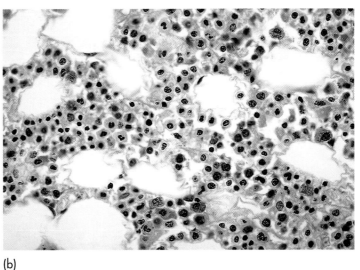
(b)

Figure 2.16   (a) Photomicrograph of a section of bone marrow decalcified and embedded in paraffin. (b) Photomicrograph of a section of bone marrow undecalcified and embedded in methylmethacrylate. Note that this is a thinner section than that demonstrated in (a) and therefore has more cytologic detail without obscuring overlay (both views, H&E, × 10 obj.).

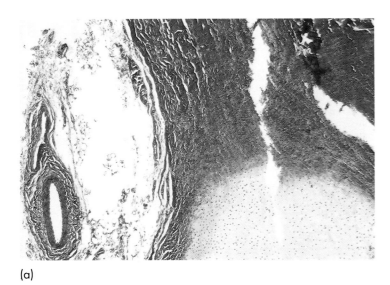
(a)

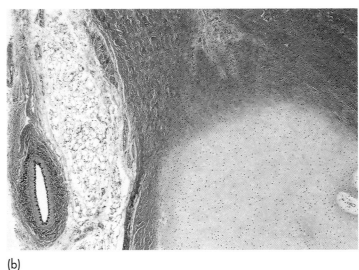
(b)

Figure 2.17   (a) Photomicrograph of a portion of developing cartilage, tendon and vascularized adipose tissue stained by Masson's trichrome stain. Muscle stains red, as seen in the media of the artery in the lower left, and collagen stains blue. (b) The same tissue stained with Verhoeff's elastic stain (van Gieson as counterstain), where the collagen stains red and the elastic tissue black. The muscle fibers stain yellow–green (× 4 obj.).

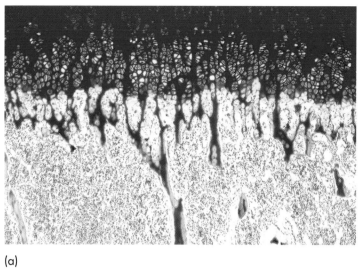

(a)

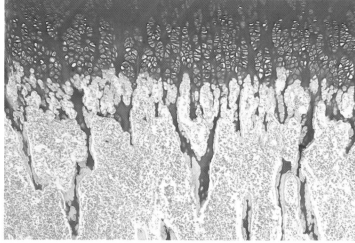

(b)

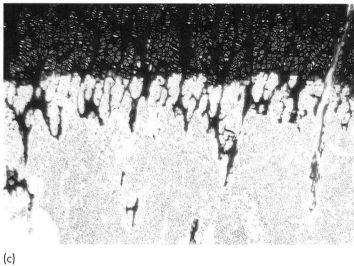

(c)

Figure 2.18   Photomicrograph of a portion of growth plate and underlying metaphysis. The PG in the matrix is stained red with safranin O (**a**), and blue with alcian blue (**b**). With toluidine blue (**c**), the cartilage is stained purple, i.e. the color of the dye is changed from blue to purple, which is described as metachromasia (× 4 obj.).

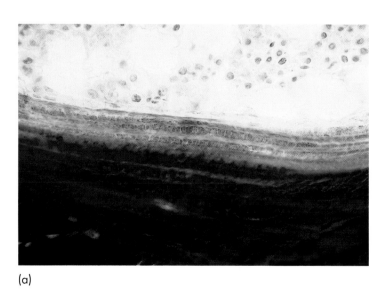

(a)

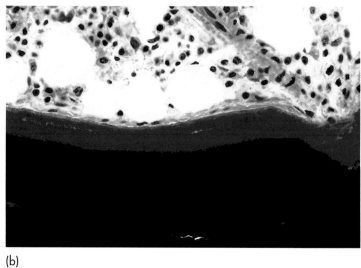

(b)

Figure 2.19   (**a**) Section of undecalcified bone stained with alizarin red, which stains the calcium salts red. The osteoid is counterstained with azure blue (alizarin red, × 10 obj.). (**b**) Section of undecalcified bone stained by von Kossa's method, in which the calcium salts are stained black. The osteoid is counterstained with acid fuchsin (von Kossa's, × 10 obj.).

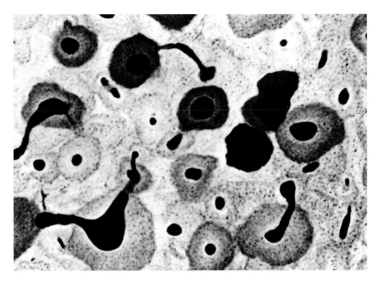

Figure 2.20 Microradiograph of a portion of cortical bone, to show the variation in the calcium content of various osteons and the generally increased calcium content of the interstitial osteons (× 10 obj.).

mineral in the tissue can also be studied by microradiography, using low-kilovoltage X-rays from an X-ray tube with a fine focal spot. These radiographs are prepared using thin slices of bone cut with a diamond saw at approximately 100 μm (Fig. 2.20). A fine-grained film (as is generally used with light photography) should be used to facilitate low-power microscopic examination. This will naturally require a correspondingly longer exposure time than is needed with a coarse-grained X-ray film.]

Osteoblasts and osteoclasts can be stained using alkaline phosphatase and tartrate-resistant acid phosphatase stains, respectively. These stains can be carried out on unfixed frozen sections or on glycol methacrylate sections prepared after brief fixation.

Immunohistochemistry

No procedure has revolutionized diagnostic histopathology as much as has the introduction of immunohistochemical staining. The technique is generally sensitive, specific and most importantly can be applied to routinely processed paraffin blocks (even after many years).

Like any technique there are pitfalls, including cross-reactivity, technical failures (including the failure to include proper positive

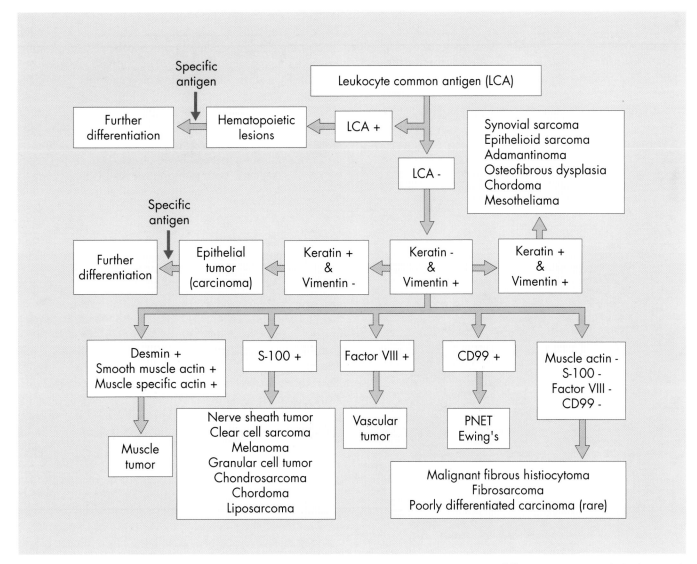

Figure 2.21 A flowchart illustrates how immunoperoxidase staining could be applied to a poorly differentiated tumor to help distinguish a lymphoid tumor from an epithelial tumor or a mesenchymal tumor.

and negative controls) and perhaps most importantly the failure to correlate the results with the H&E sections and clinical findings.

The objective in immunohistochemistry is a more precise characterization of the protein constituents of cells and matrix and the identification of the cell line of origin in undifferentiated or poorly differentiated tumors (Fig. 2.21).

The concentration of antigen in tumor cells may predict the aggressiveness of the tumor or, as in the case of estrogen receptors in breast cancer, the responsiveness to a particular type of therapy.

The most commonly used antibody markers are:

1. Those which distinguish the five major groups of intracytoplasmic intermediate filaments including vimentin (mesenchymal cells), cytokeratin (epithelial cells), desmin (muscle), glial fibrillary acidic protein (glial cells), and neurofilament protein (most neuronal cells)
2. Specific epithelial markers – epithelial membrane antigen
3. Muscle markers – in addition to desmin, actin, smooth-muscle actin
4. Vascular markers – factor VIII, CD34, ulex europaeus
5. Neural markers – includes S-100 protein, neuron-specific enolase, synaptophysin
6. Specific markers for lymphomas and small cell tumors.

Antibodies prepared against various collagen types and against constituents of PG aggregates have been used as investigative tools to study the distribution of the matrix constituents (Fig. 2.22).

A number of useful web sites are now available for information on both immunohistochemistry and cytogenetics.

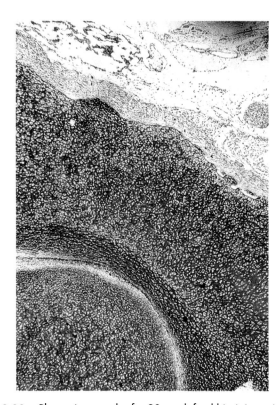

Figure 2.22 Photomicrograph of a 20-week fetal hip joint stained with a monoclonal antibody to type II collagen antibody (immunoperoxidase staining, × 4 obj.). (Courtesy of Dr German Steiner.)

Genetic markers

The majority of neoplastic tumors, both benign and malignant, are characterized by cytogenetic abnormalities. These abnormalities are believed to be the result of sequential genetic alterations in normal progenitor cells which in turn lead to a clonal expansion of phenotypically transformed cells.

Normal human cells contain twenty-two pairs of autosomal chromosomes and two sex chromosomes. Each chromosome has a long arm (q) and a short arm (p), and is characterized by alternating dark and light bands which can be stained using either Giemsa stain or a fluorescent stain (Quinacrine).

The transformed cells of a neoplastic tumor often contain multiple clonal genetic mutations, some of which, like deletions of large chromosomal segments, trisomy, or chromosome translocations, are visible in chromosome preparations. [In the description of translocation t(11;22)(q24:q12), t indicates a reciprocal exchange of material between two different chromosomal arms. The first set of parentheses contain the chromosomes involved and the second set the break points and arms of the chromosomes involved.] Other mutations such as substitution or deletions of individual DNA nucleotides cannot be detected optically in cytogenetic preparations.

Cytogenetics requires fresh viable tissue which must be transported, cultured, and maintained in a sterile state, all of which is difficult as a routine laboratory test. However, if a segment of DNA corresponding to a specific gene can be prepared and labeled, then it can become a probe for the gene in question. Most molecular cytogenetic methods in present use are based on in situ hybridization (ISH) using fluorescein as a label (FISH). Cocktails of probes that can target an entire chromosome are useful for demonstrating chromosomal translocations and deletions.

Genetic studies have proved to be particularly valuable in the differential diagnosis of lymphoma, small round-cell tumors such as Ewing's, and some spindle-cell tumors, e.g. more than 90% of synovial sarcomas, both monophasic and biphasic, are characterized by a reciprocal translocation of chromosomes x and 18 t(x;18)(p11;q11).

Fluorescence labeling

The autofluorescing antibiotics, known as the tetracyclines, have an affinity for mineral at actively mineralizing surfaces. They serve well as supravital in vivo markers of mineralization because they are clearly visualized when a section is examined using UV light. Two labels, usually of different tetracyclines, must be used to determine both the extent and the rate of mineralization. The protocol for tetracycline labeling used in our laboratory is as follows: 250 mg of oral oxytetracycline are given four times a day for 3 days. After an interval of 12 days, demeclocycline, 300 mg four times a day, is given for a further 3 days. The bone biopsy is then performed 4–7 days after the last dose of demeclocycline. The specimen is fixed in 70% alcohol, which helps to protect against leaching of both the label and mineral from the tissue. Unstained sections should be stored in the dark to prevent fading of the fluorescence before they are examined. At the time of examination they should be covered with optically inactive oil for optimal visualization of the label. In our experience, 5 μm-thick sections are adequate for the visualization of properly applied labels. In a normal biopsy, both single and double labels may be observed, and these labels are usually sharp and distinct (Fig. 2.23). In case of certain metabolic disturbances the labels have specific morphological features

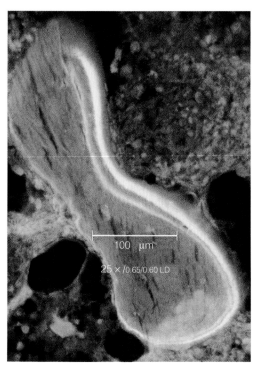

Figure 2.23 Photomicrograph showing two distinct tetracycline labels. The yellow label is demeclocycline, the green oxytetracycline. The scale is superimposed at the time of photography (UV, × 25 obj.).

that reflect the condition of the mineralizing bone–osteoid interface (see Chapter 8).

In addition to the commonly used transmitted light optical microscopy, a number of other techniques are particularly useful for examination of connective tissues. Differential interference contrast (DIC, or Nomarski optics) is especially valuable because it provides a pseudo-three-dimensional appearance to the tissue, which can be helpful in understanding the structure. In addition, this system gives some improvement of resolution, so that the resulting photographic images are clearer than those obtained with transmitted light microscopy (Fig. 2.24a and b).

Perhaps the most useful microscopic technique for the examination of connective tissues utilizes polarized light, not only because it clearly reveals the collagen fibers but also because it enables the determination of the orientation of the collagen and the study of the microarchitecture of the tissue (Fig. 2.24c). This information can be very helpful in the interpretation of disease states, e.g. in Paget's disease, or in delineating reparative scars.

An important diagnostic procedure in the clinical diagnosis of crystal synovitis is the examination of synovial fluid for crystals (see Chapter 12, p. 305 for a complete discussion of this procedure).

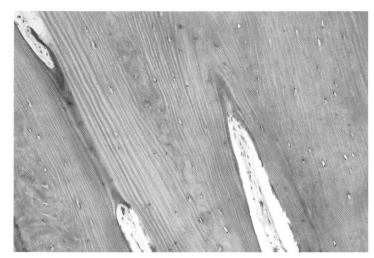

(a)

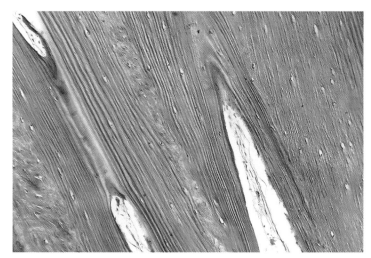

(b)

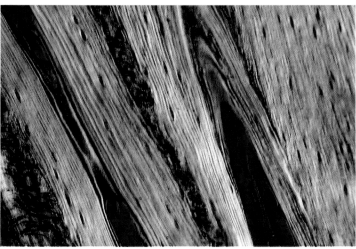

(c)

Figure 2.24 (a) Photomicrograph of a longitudinal section of cortical bone (H&E, × 10 obj.). (b) The same field as illustrated above, photographed using Nomarski optics (H&E, × 10 obj.), and (c) with polarized light (H&E, × 10 obj.).

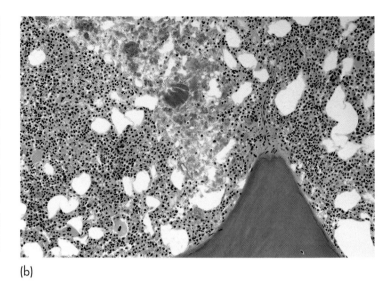

(a)   (b)

Figure 2.25   Two examples of bone dust artifact. This artifact is common and can be avoided by washing the tissue after it has been cut on the saw and by cutting deeply into the block (H&E, × 4 obj.).

The most common and one of the most troublesome artifacts encountered in sections of bone is the presence in the marrow space of irregular fragments of basophilic material that may be mistaken for tumor or some other morbid condition (Fig. 2.25). These fragments represent bone dust and other debris which is driven into the interstices of bone during the slicing process. This artifact can be avoided by washing the surface after sawing and by cutting into the paraffin block a little way before taking sections for microscopic examination. A decidedly rare artifact may occur from the acid decalcification of the bone. Under certain conditions a secondary calcium salt crystal may be deposited in the tissue in the form of calcium brushite (Fig. 2.26).

ROLE OF FROZEN SECTION IN ORTHOPAEDICS

Intraoperative frozen sections constitute an important tool in assisting a surgeon in his decision making. Whether for diagnosis or the evaluation of resection margins, the frozen section can help in determining the definitive surgical procedure for a particular case (Fig. 2.27).

With the increasing use of implant devices, it is important to differentiate between infection and a cellular reaction to implant debris, when treating failed prostheses. In the case of suspected neoplasia, frozen sections can usually differentiate between tumor, inflammation or necrotic tissue.

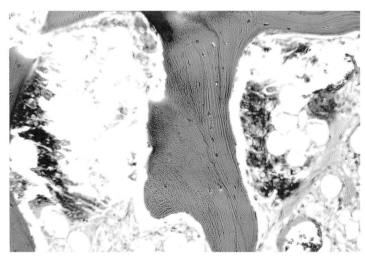

Figure 2.26   In this section taken from a totally necrotic femoral head, clusters of large needle-shaped crystals were present throughout the marrow spaces. These proved by X-ray defraction studies to be calcium brushite, an artifact occasionally seen in decalcified tissue (H&E, × 25 obj.).

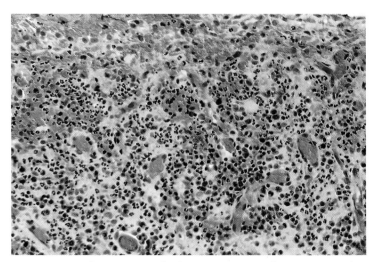

Figure 2.27   Photomicrograph of an intraoperative frozen section of synovium removed from a failed hip prosthesis shows a significant degree of acute inflammation consistent with infection (H&E, × 25 obj.).

The pitfalls of frozen section are inadequate tissue, tissue which is not representative of the entire lesion, tissues which are calcified and therefore difficult to adequately section without further processing and artifacts resulting from the surgical manipulation of the tissue or from poor freezing technique. (These artifacts tend to be particularly problematic in differentiating round-cell tumors from infection or spindle-cell tumors from exuberant granulation tissue.)

HISTOMORPHOMETRY

Histomorphometry is the quantification of tissue and cell features using thin sections. Because of its rigid nature, bone is more suitable for histomorphometry than most other tissues, as the tissue and cell relationships are not significantly altered during proper processing and thin sectioning.

There are essentially two reasons to perform histomorphome-

try on bone: first, to quantify cell activity in health and disease; and second, to study the structure of bone as a mechanical system under normal and abnormal conditions (see Chapter 8, p. 212).

Two methods have been used for the routine generation of histomorphometric values: manual and semiautomated methods. The manual method requires the use of integrating grids, usually set in the eyepiece of the microscope. In this method, the results of point and intercept counts provide the primary data from which the final figures are generated (Fig. 2.28). The semiautomated method employs a number of different computer-controlled procedures and devices for gathering and manipulating the primary data. In this method, an operator identifies the features of interest and the computer program automatically calculates the area and linear measurements and keeps track of the counts. Final results are then generated from these data (Fig. 2.29).

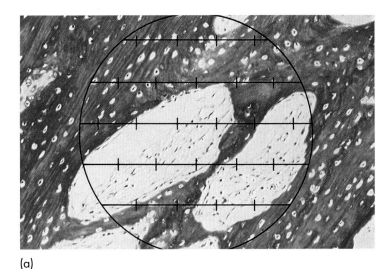

(a)

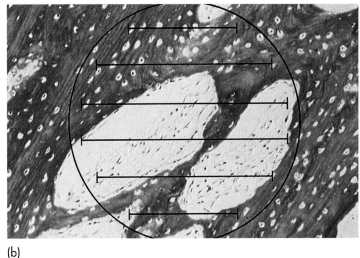

(b)

Figure 2.28 The types of integrating eyepieces employed to estimate various bone parameters. (**a**) The type I eyepiece is employed to estimate bone mass (volume). The eyepiece contains a series of lines on which are 25 points. Trabecular bone area is measured by recording the number of points that lie on bone. (**b**) The type II eyepiece contains a series of lines and is used to measure the extent of different bone surfaces. Total surface is recorded as the number of intersections of lines with bone surfaces, and each specific type of bone is estimated in a similar manner and expressed as a percentage of the total number of intersections.

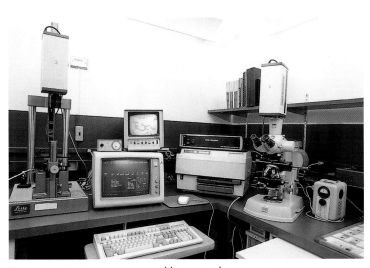

Figure 2.29 A semiautomated histomorphometry system.

Chapter 3

IMAGING TECHNIQUES, INTERPRETATION AND STRATEGIES

Imaging plays an important role in the identification, diagnosis and management of bone and soft-tissue diseases. Radiography is the longest established imaging modality and remains the cornerstone of musculoskeletal imaging. Definitive diagnoses of many bone and joint disorders, such as fractures, erosive arthritis and degenerative disease, can be made from radiographs alone, without recourse to more sophisticated techniques.

The range of imaging techniques has expanded greatly over the past 30–40 years, to include radionuclide (RN), computed tomography (CT), ultrasound (US) and magnetic resonance (MR) scanning. CT, MR and US have greatly improved the identification and characterization of soft-tissue lesions, often not visualized on radiographs. These techniques have their relative merits and limitations, and all require skill and experience in their execution and interpretation. For resources and imaging techniques to be used appropriately and effectively, there must be close collaboration between clinician, pathologist and radiologist, particularly when dealing with potentially malignant bone and soft-tissue tumors.

The role of musculoskeletal imaging includes:

- Confirmation of the presence of a skeletal lesion
- Definition of the characteristics of the lesion, to enable a pathological diagnosis to be made
- Performance of sequential investigation in a proper order, to refine the differential diagnosis of individual lesions
- Demonstration of the features, location and distribution of skeletal disorders
- Identification of 'don't touch' lesions, including lesions necessitating no further active investigation or treatment
- Distinction between benign and malignant lesions
- Staging of malignant tumors and identification of tumor recurrence
- Guidance for invasive procedures, such as targeted biopsy
- Monitoring progress of lesions
- Identification of complications of treatment
- Answering specific clinical queries
- Recognition of the limits of imaging.

Despite sophisticated developments in imaging, there continue to be radiological limitations in some tissue-specific diagnoses, particularly regarding tumor types and grades. Therefore correlation of a patient's radiological findings with the histopathologic and clinical assessment remains of paramount importance. Errors are less likely to be made if such teamwork, reliant on effective communication, is practised. For example, as the histopathologic grade of chondrosarcoma can vary within a single lesion, a sampling error can lead to an incorrect pathologic diagnosis of a benign lesion in patients with radiologic and clinical features of malignancy.

Effective communication is important in planning all stages of a patient's investigation and treatment. For example, the biopsy of suspicious lesions should be performed *after* imaging, as the presence of a cortical defect or hematoma following bone biopsy may erroneously raise the suspicion of malignancy on subsequent imaging. Similarly, biopsy of soft-tissue lesions should only be performed in consultation with surgeons experienced in the management of soft-tissue sarcomas, because biopsy through an inappropriate approach may adversely affect the subsequent resectability, and therefore prognosis, of the tumor.

IMAGING METHODS

TECHNIQUES THAT USE IONIZING RADIATION (X-RAYS)

Radiography

When radiography is performed, X-rays pass through the body. Some are absorbed, depending on the thickness and the atomic number of the tissues through which they pass. The remainder then exit the body, giving a differential pattern of X-rays, which falls onto the fluorescent screens of the radiographic cassette. The fluorescence emitted by these screens in response to the incident X-rays that pass through the patient results in the formation of silver crystals in the radiographic film held within the cassette. The film is then processed to give a radiographic image.

The use of fluorescent screens has been an important development. In the past, the formation of a radiographic image relied on the direct interaction between the X-rays and the radiographic film, without the use of screens. A much higher dose of radiation was therefore needed to form an image, and at greater risk to the patient.

A high proportion of X-rays are absorbed by material with a high atomic number, such as bone and calcium, giving a white, 'radiodense' appearance on the radiograph. In tissues where there is little absorption of X-rays, such as air and fat, more silver crystals are formed on the film, giving a black, 'radiolucent' appearance. Soft tissues such as muscle show intermediate X-ray transmission and appear grey on the processed film (Fig. 3.1). The intrinsic X-ray contrast of bone is particularly useful on radiographs, but other modalities, such as CT, US and MR, are often needed to assess the soft-tissue components of lesions.

Radiographs are two-dimensional (2D) images of three-dimensional (3D) anatomy, with superimposition of overlying structures in the path of the X-ray beam. In order to define clearly the anatomical site and extent of a bone lesion using radiography, at least two views [for example antero-posterior (AP) and lateral] are needed. Destruction of cortical bone is best seen where the X-ray beam is tangential, rather than perpendicular, to an area of cortical destruction (Figs 3.2a and b). Loss of trabecular bone is often more difficult to define. Up to 40% of the tra-

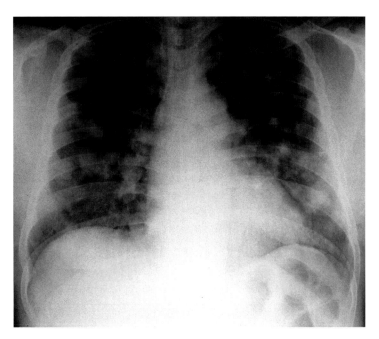

Figure 3.1   Postero-anterior (PA) chest radiograph. The bones appear radiodense (white); air in lungs appears radiolucent (black). Soft-tissue pulmonary metastases from bone sarcoma are radiodense within the lung.

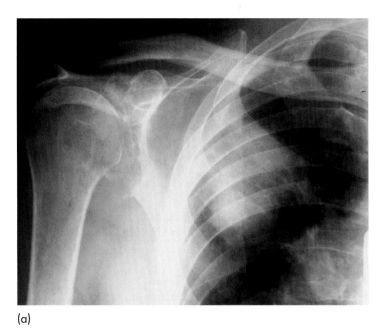

(a)

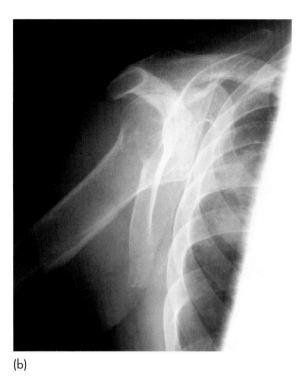

(b)

Figure 3.2   Metastasis in the proximal humerus. **(a)** Antero-posterior radiograph of the right shoulder showing an obvious destructive lesion of the glenoid. The cortical destruction is demonstrated because the X-ray beam is tangential to the cortex in this area. However **(b)** on the lateral projection the cortical bone destruction is not evident because the X-ray beam is vertical to the cortex. Note also in **(a)** a peripheral mass in the lung, which is the lung cancer, a primary malignancy from which the bone metastasis arose. There is also metastatic right hilar lymphadenopathy.

becular bone may be destroyed before its loss is evident on a radiograph. Radiography can therefore be insensitive to subtle bone destruction or abnormality (Figs 3.3a and b), and a normal radiograph does not reliably exclude the presence of a bone lesion. Detection of a lesion on radiographs may be particularly difficult in areas of complex anatomy, such as the wrist or foot, or where bone is obscured by overlying structures, such as the sacrum on an antero-posterior view of the pelvis (Figs 3.4a and b). In these cases, radionuclide bone scanning can be sensitive in identifying that a lesion is present, but may be limited in its specificity for defining the pathological etiology. Targeted cross-sectional imaging, using CT or MR, is then useful to subsequently define the pathology, the exact anatomical location and extent of the lesion.

When radiographic images are being examined, it is essential to optimize viewing conditions. Radiographs should be viewed on dedicated viewing boxes, with subdued background lighting. A bright light should be available to examine dark areas of the image and a magnifying glass may be useful, for example in the identification of early bone erosions.

Technological developments have led to the introduction of digital imaging, in which the image data are processed electronically, rather than in analog form. Digital images do not have the high spatial resolution of radiographic film–screen combinations, but have the advantages of greater exposure latitude, image enhancement, manipulation and storage. Digital images can be stored and transmitted electronically, providing the basis of filmless picture archiving and communication systems (PACS), or they can be printed on film if required.

Radiographic screening (fluoroscopy) allows imaging in real time, enabling dynamic studies that can examine motion or blood flow over time to be performed. Digital subtraction is used in fluoroscopy, particularly in angiography, but also in arthrography.

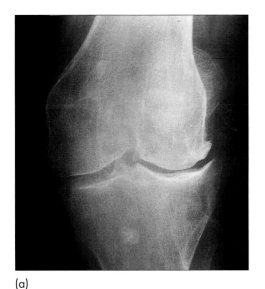

(a)

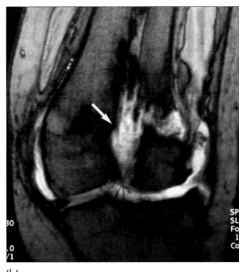

(b)

Figure 3.3 There was a history of trauma (patient fell down stairs) and the patient presented with pain in the knee. (a) Radiograph showed no fracture. (b) Coronal T_2-weighted MR image shows a high signal in a fracture (arrow) through the lateral femoral condyle, involving the joint surface, and associated with a joint effusion (high signal).

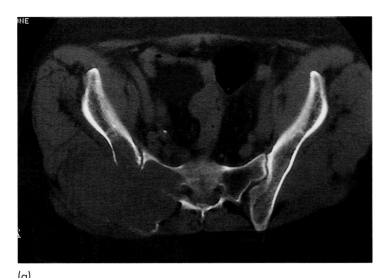

(a)

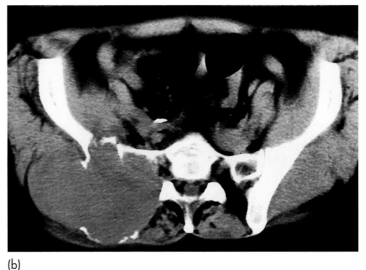

(b)

Figure 3.4 Bone sarcoma shown on pelvic CT scan. No abnormality could be identified on the pelvic radiograph, as the right sacral area was obscured by overlying abdominal gas. (a) Bone settings (level = 250 HU, window width = 1000 HU), demonstrating destruction of right sacral ala and postero-medial aspect of the ilium. (b) Soft-tissue settings (level = 50 HU, window width = 250 HU), showing large soft-tissue mass.

All techniques that use ionizing radiation must only be performed when there is clinical justification. Dose minimization techniques should be used with gonadal shielding where possible, particularly in children and young adults. Examinations should be tailored to the clinical indication, and unnecessary repetition should be avoided, as all examinations using ionizing radiation carry an element of risk.

Computed tomography

CT of the head transformed the practice of neuroradiology following its introduction in 1972 for brain imaging. The potential of CT for imaging the other parts of the body was soon realized. Body CT scanners were introduced in 1975, with one of their important clinical applications being in musculoskeletal disorders.

In CT, the X-ray beam is finely collimated, giving a fan-shaped beam with typical slice widths of 1–10 mm. The X-ray tube rotates around the patient and sensitive detectors record the X-rays that pass through the body. Powerful computers use the pattern of exiting X-rays to construct an image. This is viewed as a gray scale image, with the varying shades from black to white representing the range of X-ray attenuations of the tissues.

Tissues with high atomic numbers and X-ray attenuation values, such as bone, appear white; areas of low attenuation, such as air and fat, appear dark and other soft tissues, such as muscle, are depicted as shades of gray. The attenuation value of each picture and volume element (pixel and voxel, respectively) of the image can be described using Hounsfield units (HU). These form a numeric scale which uses the attenuation of X-rays by water as a reference point (0 HU), and which has both positive (e.g bone: 250–1000 HU) and negative (e.g. fat: −100 HU; air: −600 HU) values. A wide range of attenuation values can be measured on CT, whereas the human eye can appreciate only limited shades of gray. The attenuation level (the window level shows the mid-range of attenuations being viewed) and range (the window width shows the range of attenuations being viewed) must therefore be altered to optimize viewing of different tissue types, within the constraints of a visual image. The use of appropriate window settings and interrogation of the CT images on a workstation, rather than relying on hard-copy images (those recorded on film) for reporting, is essential to avoid missing lesions. To visualize soft tissues the window level would be set at 50 HU and the window width would be 500 HU; to visualize bone the window level might be set at 250 HU with a wide window width of 1000 HU, and when viewing the air-filled lungs the window level would be set in the region of −600 HU with a window width of 1000 HU (Figs 3.4a and b, and 3.5).

The use of contrast agents can aid diagnosis in CT. Orally administered dilute iodinated contrast media, given before scanning, are used to opacify the lumen of the bowel, to help distinguish bowel loops from soft-tissue masses. Intravenous contrast administration, given either as a pre-scan bolus or as a controlled pump infusion during the examination, can provide useful information regarding the vascularity of lesions and their relationship to adjacent vascular structures (Figs 3.5b, and 3.6a and b). Contrast media can also be administered via other routes, for example intrathecally, to give a CT myelogram, or into joints, to give CT arthrography.

The advantages of CT include the following:

- Ability to display cross-sectional anatomical data on CT transverse sections, which overcomes the problem of overlapping structures on 2D radiography
- Better than radiography for soft-tissue imaging [but not as good as magnetic resonance imaging (MRI)], as it gives higher soft-tissue contrast sensitivity
- CT imaging protocols can be optimized for specific clinical scenarios
- Quantitative data on composition (e.g. bone densitometry), dimensions or contrast enhancement can be provided
- Data can be manipulated to give multi-planar reconstructions (coronal, sagittal) or 3D images
- Good for assessing cortical bone.

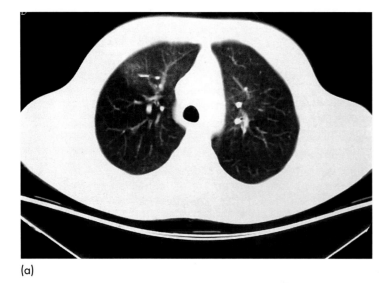

(a)

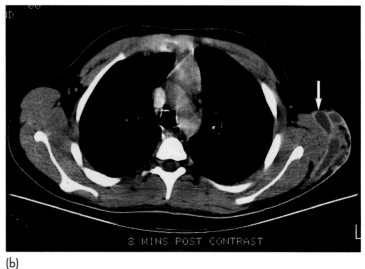

(b)

Figure 3.5   CT of the chest. (**a**) Lung window settings (level = −600 HU, window width = 1000 HU). (**b**) Soft-tissue settings (level = 50 HU, window width = 250 HU). Hemangioma of left chest wall (arrow) showing rim enhancement with contrast medium administered intravenously.

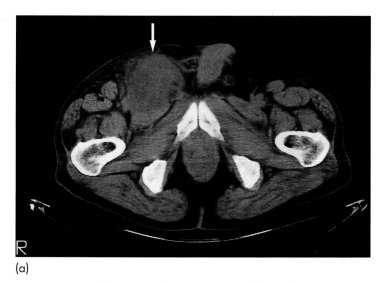
(a)

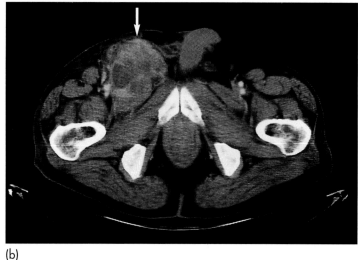
(b)

Figure 3.6   CT showing a soft-tissue sarcoma of the right groin (arrow). **(a)** Before contrast enhancement, a large soft-tissue mass is present that is heterogenous in attenuation. **(b)** After I.V. contrast administration, there is heterogeneous enhancement, indicating the tumor is fairly vascular; areas that fail to enhance indicate central necrosis or cystic components. The tumor margin abuts the neurovascular bundle laterally.

The disadvantages of CT include:

- Necessary use of significant doses of ionizing radiation; CT currently contributes a major proportion of medical radiation exposure
- Inferior soft-tissue contrast resolution to that of MRI.

Technological advancements (slip-ring technology) of continuous spiral and multi-slice imaging have led to reduced examination times (20 seconds to acquire 3D volume of the chest). These have also provided improved longitudinal spatial resolution, dynamic contrast-enhanced scanning and 3D volume acquisition (Figs 3.7a, b–f).

Radionuclide scanning

Radionuclide bone scanning was introduced in the early 1960s. Since that time, developments in radio-pharmaceutical agents and scanning techniques have led to significant improvements in the spatial resolution of radionuclide scan images.

In radionuclide bone scanning, Technetium-99m is used to label phosphate compounds, such as methylene diphosphonate (^{99m}Tc-MDP), which is then administered intravenously. ^{99m}Tc-MDP is chemi-absorbed onto hydroxyapatite crystals in bone. Its uptake is a reflection primarily of osteoblastic activity, but is also dependent on vascularity. Approximately 70% of the administered dose of radionuclide is excreted through the kidneys within 24 hours. Radiation exposure to the bladder can be minimized by ensuring that the patient is well hydrated and micturates frequently.

Photon emission from the whole skeleton or localized sites can be recorded using a scintillation camera. Initially, the radiopharmaceutical can be detected intravascularly, before pooling in soft tissues and then being taken up in bone over approximately 2 hours, where 50% of injected ^{99m}Tc-MDP localizes. This can be imaged as a 'triple-phase' examination with images obtained immediately (the flow images), after a few minutes (the blood pool images), and after approximately 4 hours (the static images) (Figs 3.8a–c). Depending on the indication for the scan, only the static images may be necessary.

Radionuclide scanning (RNS) is very sensitive to abnormalities in the skeleton. Any process that alters the balance between bone resorption and bone formation can cause abnormalities on the bone scan, with regions of increased osteoblastic activity ('hot spots') or decreased activity ('cold spots') (Figs 3.9a–c). RNS is very useful in the detection of pathologic changes at a symptomatic site, when radiography has shown no abnormality, as even small areas of increased activity are easy to detect. Photon-deficient lesions are difficult to detect and are often missed. This may be the case, for example, with myeloma, where a negative scan does not exclude the diagnosis, or with osteoclastic (lytic) metastases.

As a wide variety of conditions, both normal (epiphyses and metaphyses of the growth plate in children) and pathologic (primary and secondary bone tumors, osteomyelitis, fractures, metabolic bone disease and arthropathy), may all show increased activity, radionuclide scanning is non-specific. The distribution of abnormality may suggest particular processes: multiple 'hot spots' throughout the skeleton in the presence of normal radiography suggest metastases (Fig. 3.9c). Diffuse enlargement and increased activity of a single bone occurs in Paget's disease (Figs 3.9a and b) and focal abnormalities adjacent to joints may represent degenerative arthritis with hyperostosis (Figs 3.10a and b).

Single photon emission computed tomography (SPECT) applies tomographic technology to radionuclide scanning, enabling a cross-sectional image to be obtained. This enhances the conspicuity of lesions and is useful in their localization (Fig. 3.10b).

The advantages of RNS include:

- High sensitivity to increases in bone turnover
- Good survey technique for abnormality anywhere in the skeleton
- Role in the initial localization of bone lesions, enabling further imaging by other modalities to be targeted to the relevant anatomical site.

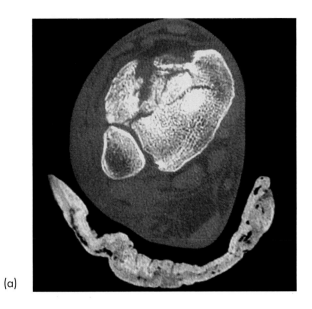

(a)

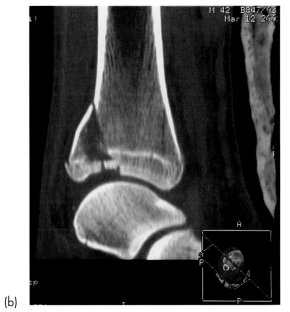

(b)

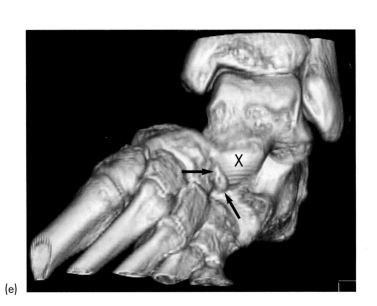

(c)

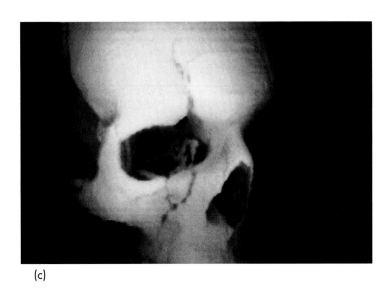

(d)

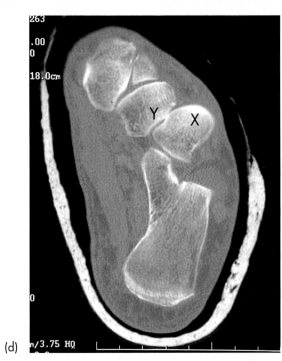

(e)

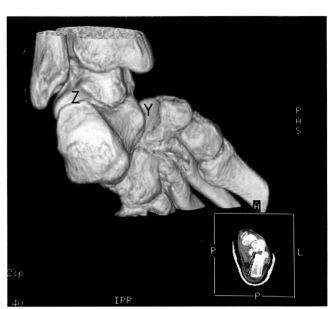

(f)

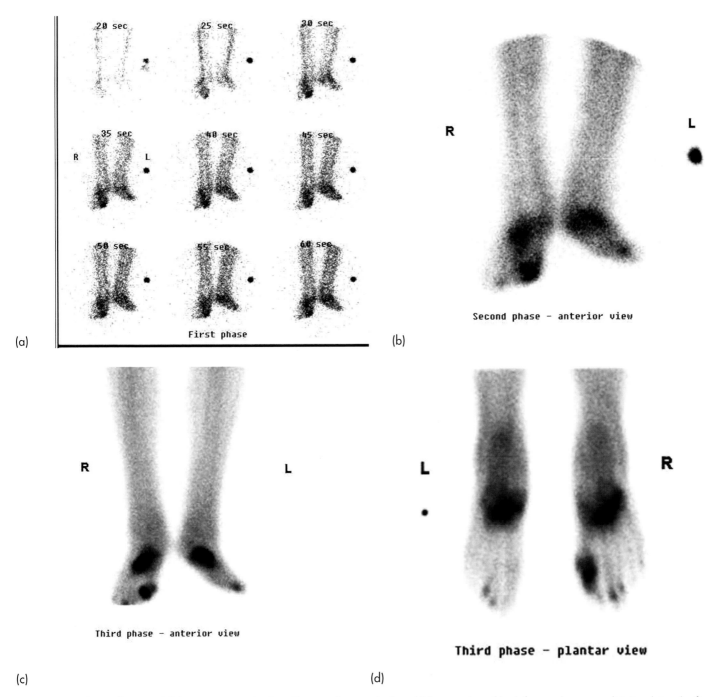

(a)

Second phase – anterior view

(b)

Third phase – anterior view

(c)

Third phase – plantar view

(d)

Figure 3.8   Three-phase RNS (**a**) in a patient who has Charcot changes in the mid foot portion of both feet and osteomyelitis involving the first metatarso-phalangeal joint of the right foot. Images have been obtained immediately (the flow images) (**a**), after a few minutes (the blood pool images) (**b**), and after approximately 4 hours (the static images) (**c** – anterior view; **d** – plantar view). There is increased blood flow and increased uptake of radionuclide in the bones of the mid-part of each foot (due to Charcot changes) and in the area of infection. Depending on the indication for the scan, only the static images may be necessary. (Courtesy of Dr Mary Prescott, Consultant Nuclear Medicine Physician, Manchester Royal Infirmary, UK.)

Figure 3.7   CT with multiplanar and 3D reconstructions: (**a**) Complex, comminuted fracture of the distal tibia in axial section and (**b**) in sagittal reconstruction which demonstrates more clearly the articular involvement. (**c**) 3D CT of the skull demonstrating a fracture extending through the right frontal region of the vault and maxilla, and involving the right orbit. Fracture dislocation of the hind foot. (**d–f**). (**d**) axial section through the hind foot showing talo-navicular dislocation, with lateral rotation of the head of the talus (X) from the concavity of the navicular (Y). (**e**) 3D reconstruction showing the exposed articular surface of the talar head (X), with a fracture of the lateral aspect of the navicular (arrows). (**f**) the posterior view shows associated subluxation of the posterior sub-talar joint as evidenced by exposure of the inferior articular surface (Z) of the talus, and dislocation of the talo-navicular joint, as evidenced by exposure of the concave joint surface of the navicular (Y).

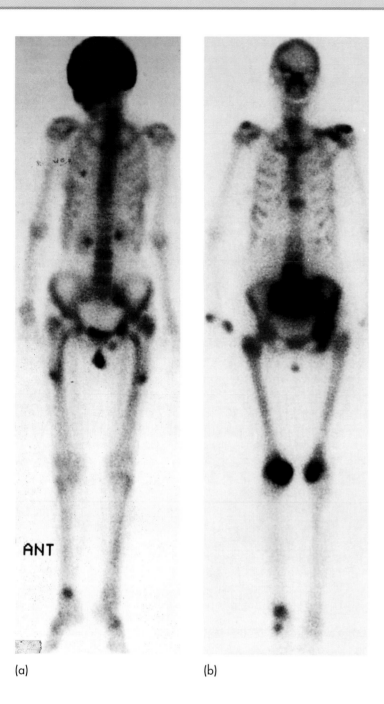

ANT

(a)

(b)

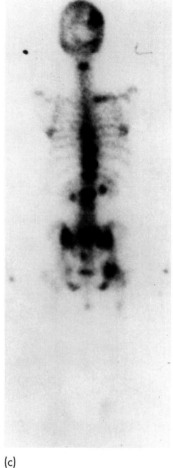

(c)

Figure 3.9 Radionuclide scans: 'hot-spots' due to areas of increased uptake of the radionuclide may be nonspecific, but there may be a characteristic distribution, as in Paget's disease of bone. (a) Generalized increased uptake in skull vault and bones of face (note also the bilateral hip replacements). (b) Increased uptake in the right skull base, left scapular, patellae, sacrum, and left hemi-pelvis. Such a distribution of having an entire bone involved is typical of Paget's disease. (c) There are areas of increased uptake in the skull, clavicle, spine and pelvis indicative of bone matastases.

The disadvantages of RNS include:

- Poor spatial resolution
- Non-specific appearance for areas of increased activity
- Can produce false-negative scans in myeloma and osteoclastic metastases
- Relatively high radiation dose, particularly to bone marrow, and in children.

TECHNIQUES THAT DO NOT USE IONIZING RADIATION

Ultrasonography

This technique has been in use since the late 1960s, initially in obstetric and antenatal practice. Its use has now disseminated to almost all radiological fields, with increasing musculoskeletal applications. US equipment has the advantages of being relatively inexpensive, small and mobile when compared with other imag-

ing hardware, but is highly dependent on the expertise of the operator for acquisition and interpretation of the US images.

During an US scan, sound waves are emitted from a transducer held against the skin surface. The use of lubricating gel couples the transducer to the patient, allowing the transmission of the sound waves into the body. The US waves are reflected at tissue interfaces within the patient and are detected back at the transducer. By timing the period elapsed from emission of the sound waves to the detection by the transducer, the depth to the echo-producing structure can be calculated. This information is displayed on a screen and can be recorded digitally or by using film, video or thermal paper images. The use of the Doppler principle enables qualitative and quantitative observation of vascularity and blood flow.

Not all of the sound waves are detected back at the transducer: some are lost due to scatter, absorption and reflection within the tissues. This attenuation depends partly on the frequency of the waves: high frequency waves show greater absorption than low

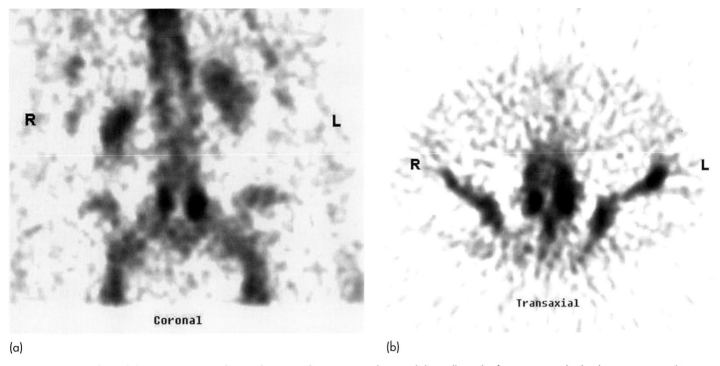

(a)   (b)

Figure 3.10 Radionuclide scan in osteoarthritis. There are degenerative changes bilaterally at the facet joints in the lumbar spine at L5/S1. (a) Coronal image showing increased uptake in both facet joints. (b) SPECT provides a cross-sectional transverse image for better anatomical localization. (Courtesy of Dr Mary Prescott, Consultant Nuclear Medicine Physician, Manchester Royal Infirmary, UK.)

frequency waves. High frequency US has the advantage of good spatial resolution, but because of high attenuation, it can only be used to visualize superficial structures. If deeper structures are to be visualized, lower frequency US has to be used, at the cost of poorer spatial resolution. Frequencies most commonly used for routine ultrasonography range between 3 and 14 MHz.

The examination of tendons is one of the commonest indications for musculoskeletal sonography, particularly around the shoulder, ankle and wrist. Normal tendons have an echogenic, fibrillar structure in the longitudinal plane and are ovoid in cross-section (Figs 3.11a–f). US has the considerable advantage over MR tendon imaging of allowing dynamic examination of these structures, with easy comparison with the contralateral limb.

US is also useful to confirm or refute the presence of a mass, whether perceived or occult. US can be helpful in confirming the presence of a mass, and possible defining its nature [cystic or solid (Figs 3.12a and b)]. Cystic lesions are clearly distinguishable from solid lesions by their hypo/anechoic appearances, their compressibility and the presence of posterior acoustic enhancement (Fig. 3.12g). Their location and relationships may suggest specific diagnoses, such as para-meniscal cysts or ganglia.

Many masses have nonspecific US appearances, whereas a few have more characteristic appearances. Neuromata, for example, are typically hypoechoic with a fusiform shape, and a neural 'tail' leading to and from the lesion. The presence of sinister clinical features, such as rapid growth or onset of pain, may necessitate examination with another modality, such as MRI, to examine for evidence of malignant pathology.

The sensitivity of US to the detection of fluid makes it particularly useful in the confirmation of joint effusions, particularly in deep joints such as the hip and the shoulder. US provides a useful technique for guided aspiration of effusions, and can also be used for real-time guidance of other procedures, such as therapeutic injections and soft-tissue biopsies.

The advantages of US are:

- Relatively low cost, compared to MRI and CT
- Multi-planar imaging
- Ability to perform dynamic scanning on active and passive movements (tendons, muscles, joints).
- Relatively portable and easily transportable equipment
- High level of patient acceptability
- No use of ionizing radiation
- Harmless at the intensities used in clinical practice.

The disadvantages of US include:

- Reliance on the skill and expertise of the operator in acquisition and interpretation of the images
- Long learning curve for developing skill in performing musculoskeletal US imaging and a relative lack of training opportunities in performing such scanning
- Relatively limited information gleaned of the pathologic composition of solid tumors
- Images are of limited value for objective interpretation by those who have not themselves performed the scans. This limits clinical acceptance of the technique and so slows changes in practice by referring clinicians who may not be familiar with US.

Magnetic resonance imaging

Magnetic resonance imaging (MRI) employs magnetic fields and radiowaves, rather than ionizing radiation. Materials placed in a magnetic field can absorb and re-emit radiowaves of a specific frequency. The application of magnetic fields and excitation radiofrequency pulses to a patient, with detection of the signal

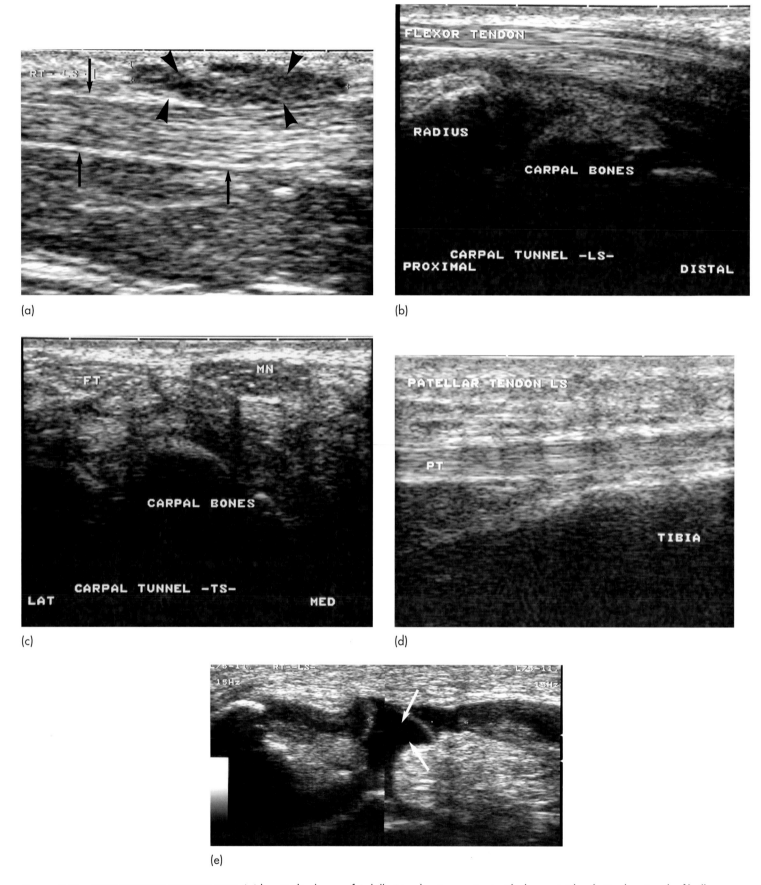

Figure 3.11   ULTRASOUND OF TENDONS: (a) longitudinal scan of Achilles' tendon in a patient with rheumatoid arthritis showing the fibrillar, echogenic structure of the tendon (arrow), above which is a less echogenic oval structure which is a rheumatoid nodule (arrowheads). (b) longitudinal and (c) transverse scans of the wrist showing the flexor tendon (FT) and the median nerve (MN); note that the tendon is more echogenic that the nerve. (d) Longitudinal scan of the intact patellar tendon (PT) – normal appearance. (e) longitudinal scan showing rupture of the patellar tendon (arrows). In the same patient there is an effusion in the knee joint (f) transverse scan showing anechoic fluid (effusion) in the suprapatellar pouch. (g) Longitudinal scan of the patellar tendon which contains calcification, seen as bright echoes (arrows), with posterior acoustic 'shadowing' (arrowheads).

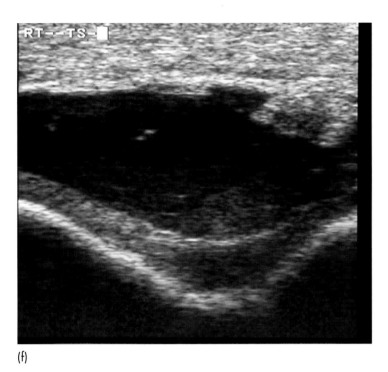

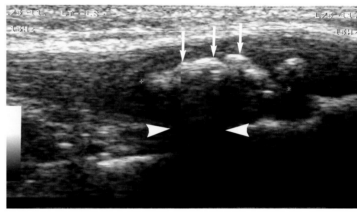

(f) (g)

Figure 3.11 (*contd*)   (**f**) Transverse scan showing anechoic fluid (effusion) in the suprapatellar pouch. (**g**) Longitudinal scan of the patellar tendon, which contains calcification seen as bright echoes (arrow), with posterior acoustic 'shadowing'.

emitted from the tissues of interest, can be used to build up an image.

Most MR sequences are tuned to detect hydrogen nuclei in water (protons). Images therefore reflect the relative concentrations of protons in tissues, by measuring the signals from individual volumes of tissue (voxels) in the patient and displaying these as a gray scale image.

Each proton spins like a top, around an axis. In the absence of a magnetic field, these axes are randomly orientated and produce no net magnetic effect. Inside the MR scanner, the static magnetic field causes the axes of rotation of the protons to align with the long axis of the magnet, with a slight excess orientated parallel to the field. As well as spinning, the protons also 'wobble,' or precess, around their long axes with a fixed frequency. The tilt in the spin axis of a proton splits its magnetization vector into both longitudinal and transverse components.

During MR imaging, radiofrequency pulses and magnetic field gradients are used to re-align the axes of rotation of the spinning protons and to pull their precession into step, or phase, with each other. When the excitation pulse is over, the protons spinning at an angle to the longitudinal axis of the scanner act like rotating magnets in a dynamo, inducing a tiny current in the surrounding coil, which can be detected and amplified to give a signal, and hence an image. The spinning protons then return to their original orientation.

Longitudinal relaxation occurs as their spin axes re-align to the long axis of the magnet. T_1 is defined as the time taken for the longitudinal magnetization vector to recover to 63% of its maximal value. This value varies, depending on how quickly protons give up energy to their surroundings. The greater the proportion of free water in a tissue, the longer the T_1 value for that tissue. As the precessing protons de-phase, the transverse component of the magnetization vector decreases exponentially, with a decrease in signal. T_2 is defined as the time taken for the MR signal to fall to 37% of its maximal value. The T_2 value is always shorter than the T_1 value of a tissue, and is also longest in tissues with a high proportion of free water, where there is less 'spin–spin' interaction.

The T_1 and T_2 values vary for different tissues and are therefore used for forming the image. The timing of excitation pulses and the collection of signal enable different sequence weighting. T_1-weighted images give maximum contrast between tissues dependent on proton density and T_1 values, with fat giving a high signal (bright, white signal) and fluid giving a low signal (dark, black signal). T_2-weighted images use longer times to detection of the signal and reflect T_2 contrast differences between tissues, as fluid appears brighter than fat. The relative signals of some different tissues on T_1- and T_2-weighted images are shown in Table 3.1, and those of hemorrhage are given in Table 3.2. The signal

Table 3.1   Signal intensities of tissues of the musculoskeletal system on T_1- and T_2-weighted magnetic resonance images (MRI). Structures of low signal intensity will appear black in the image; those of high signal intensity will appear white, and those of intermediate signal intensity will appear in ranges of gray between these two extremes.

Tissue	Signal – T_1-weighted image	Signal – T_2-weighted image
Fluid	Low	High
Fat	High	High
Muscle	Intermediate	Intermediate
Cartilage	Intermediate	High
Bone cortex	Low	Low

Table 3.2 The signal intensities of hemorrhage on MR images, on T_1-weighted (T_1-W) or T_2-weighted (T_2-W) sequences. Areas that give a high signal will appear white, those that give a low signal will appear black and those that give an intermediate signal will be shades of gray in between.

Age of hemorrhage	Approximate time	Blood product	T_1-W signal	T_2-W signal
Hyperacute	< 24 hours	Oxyhemoglobin	Intermediate	High
Acute	1–3 days	Deoxyhemoglobin	Low	Low
Subacute – early	> 3 days	Intracellular methemoglobin	High	Low
Subacute – late	> 7 days	Extracellular methemoglobin	High	High
Chronic	> 14 days	Hemosiderin/ferritin	Low	Low

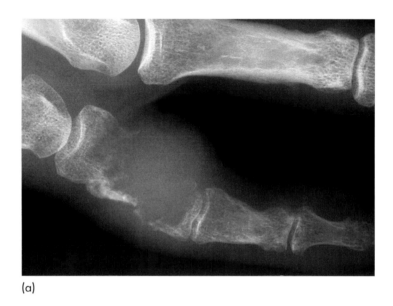

(a)

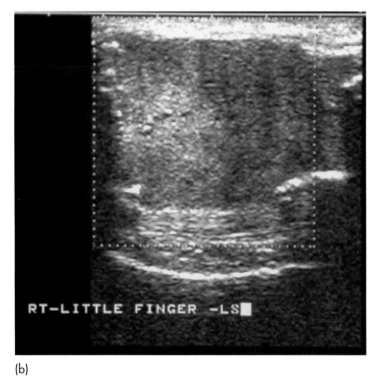

(b)

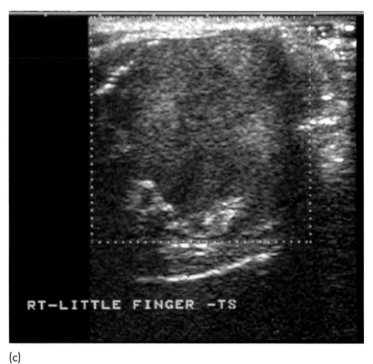

(c)

Figure 3.12 The patient presented with finger swelling. (a) The radiograph shows a destructive lesion of the proximal phalanx with associated soft-tissue swelling. There is a pathological fracture through the residual thin cortical rim. Ultrasound scan (b) longitudinal and (c) transverse scans show a round mass which has a fairly homogenous echo-texture and extends from the bone into the soft tissue, being only partially encased by the highly echogenic rim of cortical bone. This proved to be a solitary bone metastasis from a previously resected renal cell carcinoma.

characteristics of hemorrhage depend on the presence of differ-ent blood products according to the age of the bleed.

I.V. MR contrast media, containing chelated gadolinium (Gd DTPA), cause an increased signal on T_1-weighted images due to a paramagnetic effect. They are water soluble and are used to pro-duce increased ('positive') contrast between areas of high uptake and the surrounding tissues (Fig. 3.13). 'Negative' contrast media, such as iron oxide particles, are also used. These rely on ferromagnetic effects and give a reduced signal in areas of uptake.

(a)

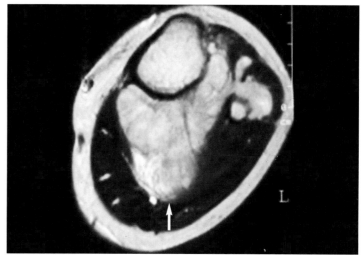

(b)

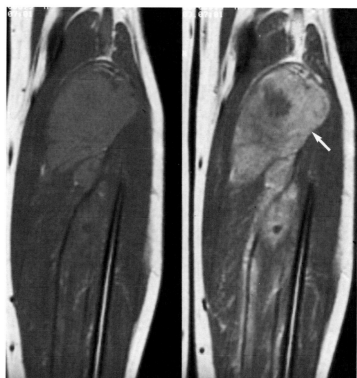

(d)

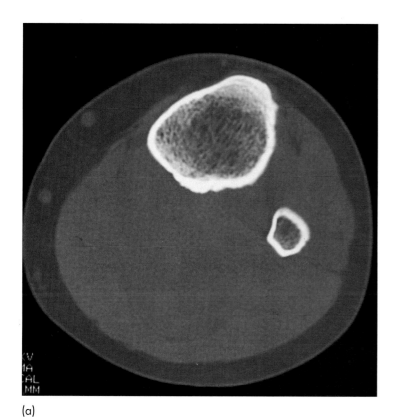

(c)

Figure 3.13   Soft-tissue sarcoma of the left calf; radiography showed no abnormality. (**a**) CT- a mass is present, but its margins are difficult to define because it has similar attenuation characteristics to adjacent normal muscle. MR (**b–d**) The tumor (arrow) is more clearly demonstrated by MR imaging: (**b**) transverse T_2-weighted image. (**c**) Coronal T_1-weighted image; (**d**) MR imaging – before (left) and after (right) contrast enhancement with Gd-labeled DTPA; these images demonstrate a large, vascular, soft-tissue tumor (arrow).

A great number of MR sequences have been developed to potentiate tissue contrast, and enhance the conspicuity of pathologic lesions. Short tau inversion recovery (STIR) sequences, for example, have a pulse designed to suppress the high signal from fat, making the high signals from fluid and edema more conspicuous, and pathologic lesions more obvious (Figs 3.3 and 3.14).

The high-contrast sensitivity of MR makes it the modality of choice for defining the soft-tissue margins of tumors and marrow changes within bones. It is therefore an important method of imaging the extent of tumors. MR images do give some indication of the pathologic nature of lesions, but may be nonspecific: edema for example gives a high signal, whatever the cause.

The advantages of MRI include:

- Capacity to image in any anatomical plane (multi-planar imaging)
- High soft-tissue contrast, with some indication of tissue composition
- No use of ionizing radiation
- Acquisition of 3D volume data using gradient echo sequences, with potential for multi-planar display
- Non-invasive imaging of blood vessels and other structures (e.g. bile and pancreatic ducts in MR cholangiopancreatography), without the use of contrast media or interventional methods.

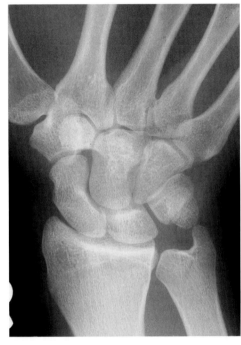

(a)

Figure 3.14 Occult fracture. Scaphoid fractures may not be evident on radiographs at presentation. (**a**) Radiograph in a patient suspected of having a scaphoid fracture; no fracture is identified. In such cases RNS or MRI are more sensitive imaging methods to identify such fractures. (**b**) T_1-weighted coronal image shows a thin oblique line (arrow) of reduced signal in the high signal of fatty marrow of the scaphoid, and patchy low signal in the lunate. (**c**) By using a coronal short tau inversion recovery (STIR) sequence, which suppresses the high signal from fat making the signal from fluid (edema) more obvious, the scaphoid fracture (arrow) becomes much more conspicuous, as does the bone 'bruise' (high signal) in the lunate.

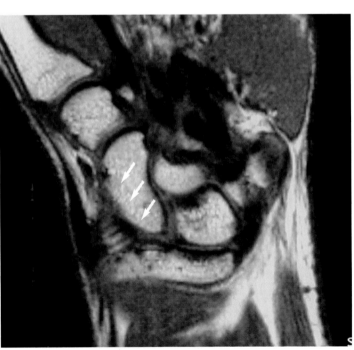

(b)

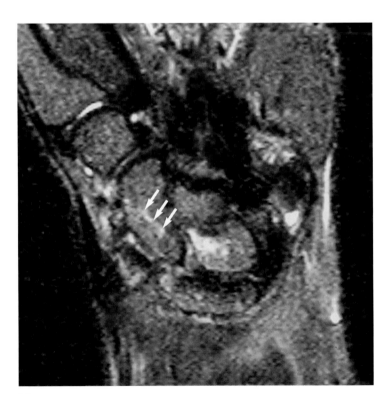

(c)

The disadvantages of MRI include:

- High cost of equipment
- Problems with image artifact from motion (e.g. of bowel, heart and respiration) and ferromagnetic objects
- Less good than CT for imaging cortical bone
- Contraindications to use (cardiac pacemakers, some cerebral aneurysmal clips, claustrophobia, first trimester of pregnancy, metallic foreign body in eye).

MORPHOLOGIC ABNORMALITIES OF BONE

The recognition of abnormal bone appearance is paramount in skeletal radiology, and requires familiarity and experience to enable distinction between a pathologic lesion and the wide range of radiographic normality. The distribution of an abnormality and the associated clinical and imaging features contribute to refine the differential diagnosis. Patient demographics and clinical/laboratory data are also vital in placing the imaging features into context.

The following section aims to illustrate this approach to morphological abnormalities of bone. Examples of characteristic distinguishing features are provided, rather than an exhaustive list of multiple etiologies, which are covered individually elsewhere in this textbook.

SCLEROSIS

Sclerosis is seen as an increase in bone density (white) on radiographs, in the context of appropriate radiographic exposure. This increased density may be due to defective osteoclast function (osteopetrosis), replacement of the marrow cavity by fibrosis (myelofibrosis) or increased osteoblastic activity (e.g. metastases). There is often cortical thickening, and the distinction between cortex and medulla may be lost.

Generalized sclerosis
Generalized osteosclerosis results from a range of conditions, but the identification of specific features helps to refute or confirm particular diagnoses. Osteopetrosis, for example, is a dysplastic condition associated with abnormal bone modeling, and a generalized increase in bone density (Figs 3.15a and b). A 'bone within a bone' appearance is characteristic of this condition. Myelofibrosis, in which progressive fibrosis of the bone marrow in middle-aged patients gives generalized bony sclerosis, is associated with splenomegaly and extramedullary hematopoiesis, whereas patients with fluorosis often have ossification of ligaments (enthesopathy).

Regional sclerosis
Paget's disease is a cause of regional osteosclerosis. The disease can affect any bone, single or multiple, but occurs most often in the pelvis, with characteristic thickening of the iliopectineal line. There is bone expansion, disordered trabecular pattern and sclerosis (Figs 3.15c and d). In the early phase of the disease there can be a lytic, or mixed lytic and sclerotic, appearance. Characteristically, Paget's disease extends from the end of a long bone, often with a 'flame-shaped' leading edge (cortical splitting), and may involve the whole bone. Bone softening results in bowing of weight-bearing bones, resulting from incremental fractures on the outer, convex margin. The skull is also often involved, and

may be thickened and sclerotic (leontiasis ossium in the maxilla) or lytic (osteoporosis circumscripta in the vault).

Patchy/focal sclerosis
The multiplicity and distribution of focal sclerotic lesions are useful in diagnosis. Osteoblastic metastases, most commonly from bronchial, prostatic and breast primary cancers, are usually multiple. Confusion may arise with other multiple lesions, such as those seen in osteopoikilosis, but the distribution of uniformly well-defined, small lesions in the ends of long bones is characteristic of osteopoikilosis. Melorheostosis is a rare osteosclerotic dysplasia in which there are irregular masses of sclerotic bone which 'flow' like 'dripping candle wax' from the bones of the limbs (Figs 15e and f).

OSTEOPENIA

Osteopenia is seen as a decrease in radiographic bone density, and reflects either a decreased quantity of bone (osteoporosis) or defective mineralization (reduced calcium per unit volume of osteoid) of bone (osteomalacia) and is used as a generic term to cover both of these entities.

Generalized osteopenia
Osteoporosis is a deficiency in the quantity of bone, resulting either from defective bone formation or an imbalance between bone accretion and resorption. It is seen most often in postmenopausal women.

Radiographically, there is thinning of the bony cortices, which may even show cortical tunneling, and resorption of secondary trabeculae, with prominence of remaining trabeculae, giving vertical striations, particularly in the vertebral bodies. As a consequence fractures occur with little or no trauma (insufficiency fractures), particularly in the spine, proximal femur and distal radius. In the spine, fractures result in wedge, end-plate or crush deformities of the vertebrae, causing thoracic kyphosis and loss of height (Fig. 3.16a). The diagnosis of osteoporosis from radiographs is unreliable in the absence of fractures, and quantitative measurements of bone density have therefore been developed such as dual-energy X-ray absorptiometry (DXA) and quantitative computed tomography (QCT). These can be applied to measure bone mineral density (BMD) in axial and peripheral skeletal sites.

Osteomalacia, or defective bone mineralization, is another cause of generalized osteopenia in adults and children. The pathognomonic features of rickets in childhood relate to defective enchondral ossification and are evident at the metaphyses (Figs 3.16b and c). In adults osteomalacia causes the diagnostic Looser's zone (Figs 3.16d and e). This linear lucent lesion is most often seen in the medial border of the femoral neck, but may also be seen in the pubic rami, lateral border of the scapulae, and ribs. Looser's zones occur perpendicular to the cortex, often have a sclerotic margin and can extend right across the affected bone, but heal with appropriate treatment. Causes of rickets in childhood, and osteomalacia in adults, include vitamin D deficiency, or more specifically deficiency of the active metabolite $1,25(OH)_2D$, hypophosphatemia, hypophosphatasia and severe systemic acidosis.

Regional osteopenia
Regional osteopenia often results from immobilization or disuse, such as after a fracture. This disuse osteoporosis occurs more

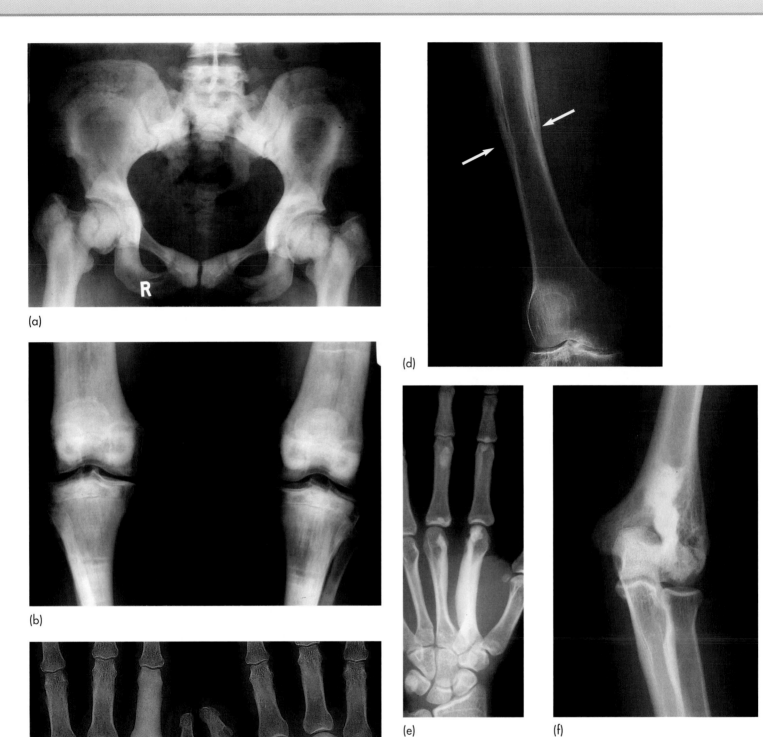

(a)

(b)

(c)

(d)

(e)

(f)

Figure 3.15 **Bone sclerosis: generalized**-osteopetrosis (**a–b**). (**a**) Pelvic radiograph and (**b**) AP radiograph of the knees show sclerotic bones and a 'bone within a bone' appearance. **Regional** (**c** and **d**) Paget's disease of bone. (**c**) Hands. Several metacarpals and phalanges are increased in density and size, with loss of cortico-medullary differentiation. (**d**) 'Flame edge' (arrows) due to splitting (lysis) of the cortex at the advancing edges of Paget's disease. Melorheostosis (**e–f**): Radiograph of (**e**) hand and (**f**) elbow, showing sclerotic masses of bone flowing like 'dripping candle wax' from the second metacarpal and distal humerus, respectively.

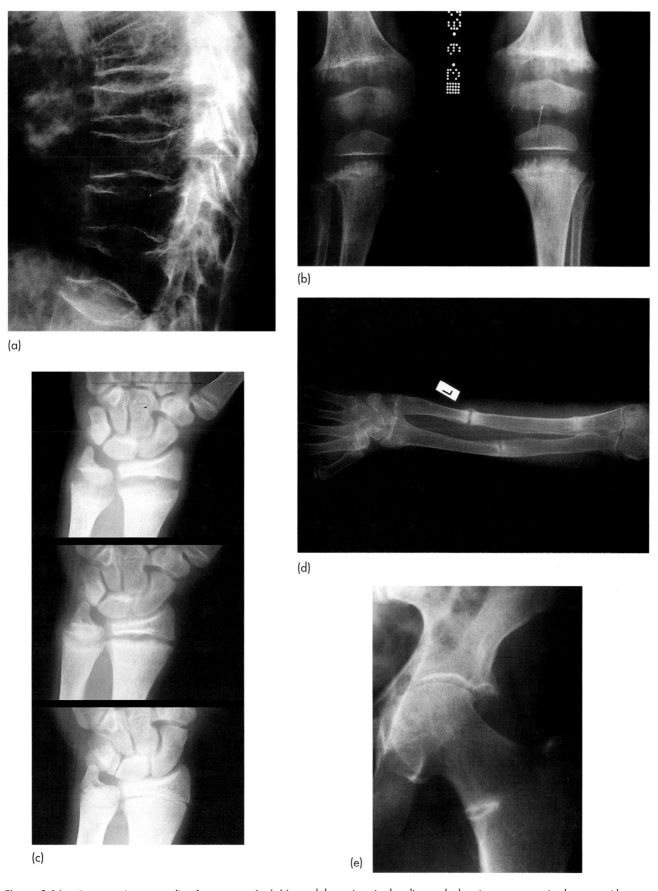

Figure 3.16 Osteopenia: generalized-osteoporosis. (**a**) Lateral thoracic spinal radiograph showing osteoporotic changes with reduced bone density, and multiple wedge or end-plate fractures. Note that the vertebral bodies are discernable only by the end-plates. (**b**) Rickets in a child showing bending of the bones (knock-knees), widening of the growth plate, and defective, irregular mineralization of the metaphyses, which are cupped and flared in shape. (**c**) Rickets in the metaphyses of the radius and ulna of the wrist, showing healing over a period of 4 months, following therapy. Osteomalacia. Loozer's zones in (**d**) Forearm and (**e**) femoral neck.

(Figure continues over page)

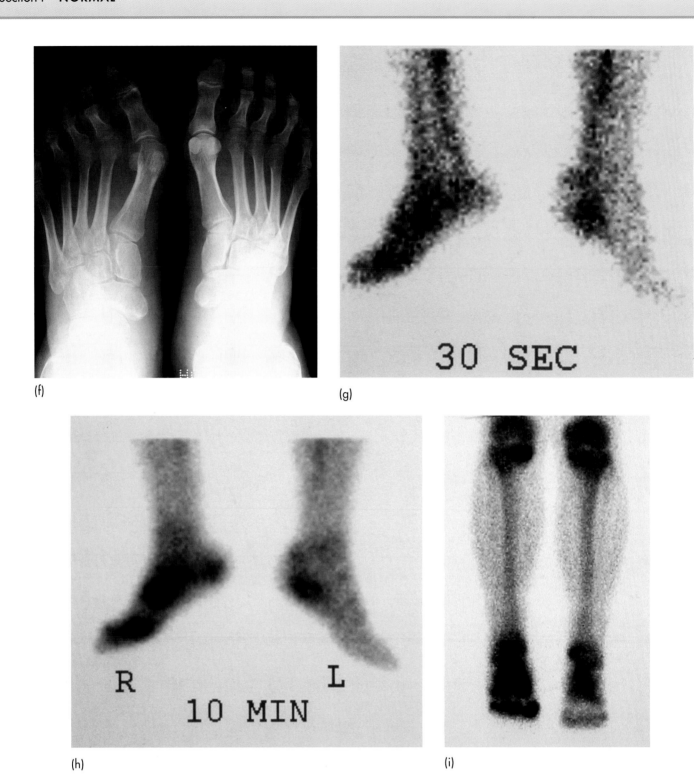

(f)

(g)

30 SEC

(h)

R   L

10 MIN

(i)

Figure 3.16 (*contd*)   Looser's zones are seen as translucent zones with sclerotic margins. Usual sites include the femoral necks, pubic rami, lateral borders of the scapulae, and ribs. Complete fractures can extend through Looser's zones, and these heal with appropriate treatment. **Regional:** (**f–i**) Sudeck's reflex sympathetic dystrophy in the right foot (**f**). Radiograph of the feet show that the bones of the right foot are reduced in density when compared to the left foot. Three phases of RNS radionuclide scans: (**g**) immediate – blood flow (**h**) blood pool and (**i**) static phases, respectively, show increased uptake in the right foot due to hyperemia and increased bone turnover.

rapidly than senile osteoporosis. The bone has a patchy, almost permeative, appearance, caused by osteoclastic bone resorption in the cortex and hyperemia. In reflex sympathetic dystrophy, (Sudeck's atrophy) a similar appearance can follow even relatively minor local or regional trauma and is accompanied by pain and soft-tissue swelling. There is increased uptake of radionuclide on the bone scan (Figs 3.16f–i). In erosive arthritides, such as rheumatoid arthritis (RA), hyperemia may result in peri-articular osteoporosis in affected joints.

Focal osteopenia

Transient osteoporosis of the hip is an example of a condition causing focal osteopenia. It is a rare disorder first described in women during the last trimester of pregnancy, but actually is seen most often in middle-aged men. The disease is characterized clinically by pain in the affected hip. Radiographically, there is osteopenia with no joint space narrowing, in the absence of other causes of synovitis or osteoporosis. Within a few months, the pain and the radiological abnormalities resolve spontaneously. MR and radionuclide bone scans are sensitive imaging techniques to identify this entity at an early stage.

ABNORMAL TRABECULAR PATTERN

An abnormal trabecular pattern is rarely seen in isolation; it usually occurs with abnormal bone density or shape.

GENERALIZED ABNORMAL TRABECULAR PATTERN

An abnormal trabecular pattern is found in osteoporosis, with decreased bone density, and in Paget's disease, typically with bone sclerosis and expansion (Figs 3.17a and b). Osteopathia striata, in which there may be widespread abnormalities as an incidental finding, characteristically shows longitudinally orientated striations in the appendicular skeleton and pelvis.

Conditions that cause marrow expansion, such as storage disorders and hemoglobinopathies, also cause abnormal trabecular appearances (Figs 3.17c–e). Identification of the typical radio-graphic and demographic features assist to define the specific diagnosis. In Gaucher's disease, most prevalent in Ashkenazi Jews, abnormal accumulation of lipid occurs in the reticulo-endothelial cells. In the bones, this results in endosteal cortical scalloping, resorption of spongy trabeculae and osteopenia. Erlenmeyer flask deformities of the distal femora are characteristic and fractures, osteonecrosis and infection may occur.

Patients with hemoglobinopathies share some features of Gaucher's disease. The bones may lose their normal tubulation (narrow shafts with wider ends) and show a net-like trabecular pattern caused by expansion of the marrow cavity (Figs 3.17c–e). In the skull, marrow expansion causes thickening of the vault, with a 'hair-on-end' appearance. Bone infarcts occur in sickle-cell disease and these can result in shortened and distorted bones if they involve the growth plate of the immature skeleton. There is also an increase in the occurrence of osteomyelitis, particularly due to *Salmonella*.

FOCAL ABNORMAL TRABECULAR PATTERN

Focal bone lesions can also be associated with trabecular abnormality. Hemangiomata, for example, show a striated pattern on radiography, especially when involving the vertebral body. These lesions show a spotty appearance on trans-axial CT, caused by sectioning across the thickened, vertical trabeculae, and give a characteristic fat signal on MRI (Figs 3.17f–h).

In the context of trauma, a focal abnormality of the trabecular pattern may be the only radiographic sign of fracture. This is particularly true in children, whose bones are relatively elastic,

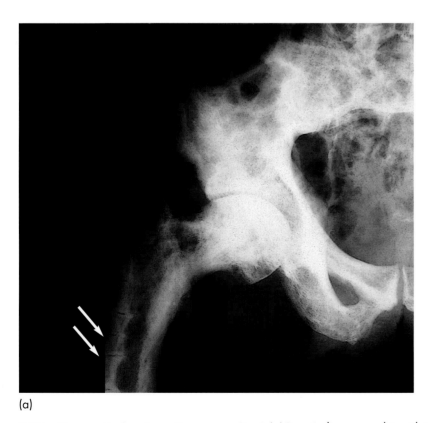

(a)

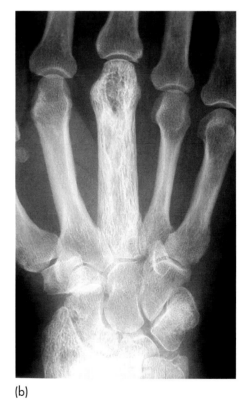

(b)

Figure 3.17   Abnormal trabecular pattern: generalized. (a) Paget's disease – pelvis with involvement of the right hemi-pelvis and right femur, which show a disordered trabecular pattern, mixed lysis and sclerosis and deformity (bending) of the bone affected due to bone softening. There are incremental fractures (arrows) along the outer cortex of the right femur. **(b)** Monostotic Paget's disease involving the third metacarpal, which is increased in size and has a disorganized and sclerotic trabecular pattern. Hematologic disorders.

(Figure continues over page)

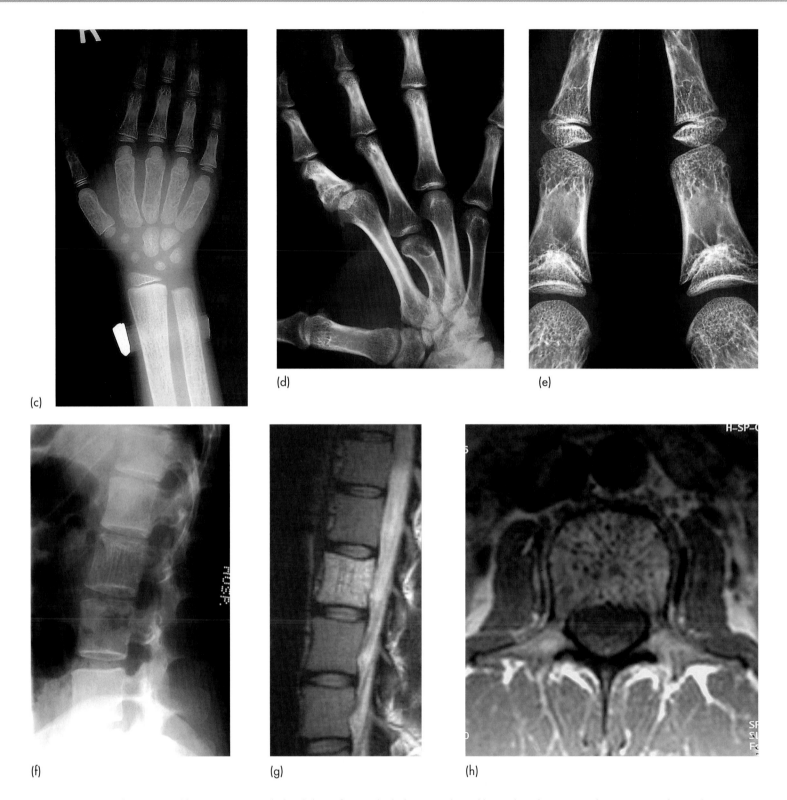

(c)

(d)

(e)

(f)

(g)

(h)

Figure 3.17 (*contd*)   **(c)** Hand bones are expanded with loss of normal tubulation and 'net-like' trabecular pattern due to marrow hyperplasia in thalassemia major. **(d)** Short third metacarpal in sickle-cell disease due to infarction at the growth plate and consequential defective growth in the affected bone. **(e)** 'Cone' epiphyses due to infarction of the mid-portion of the growth plates. **Focal (f–h)** hemangioma of bone: **(f)** Lateral spinal radiograph shows the second lumbar vertebral body is reduced in density and has prominent vertical trabecular striations. **(g)** Sagittal T_2-weighted MR shows increased signal from the body of L2 due to an increase in fat content. **(h)** Transverse T_1-weighted MR image shows a high signal from the fat, within which are prominent round trabeculae sectioned horizontally.

and can fracture with plastic deformation of the bone, without a visible cortical break. In adults, a band of relative sclerosis in a bone may reflect an impacted fracture, often less easily recognized than the more familiar lucent fracture line. Some fractures may be subtle, and not identified on radiographs; in such cases MRI, or alternatively RNS, are more sensitive techniques for confirming the presence of fracture, particularly in sites such as the femoral neck and scaphoid (Figs 3.3, 3.14a–c and 3.18).

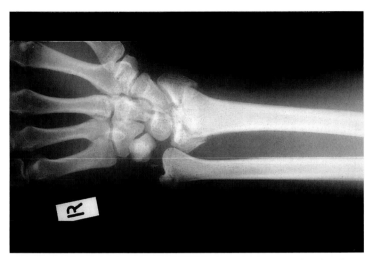

Figure 3.18   Traumatic, comminuted fracture through the distal radius, involving the joint surface; the latter will predispose to premature OA in later years. The bone is normal apart from the fracture. Some fractures may be subtle and not identified on radiographs; in such cases MRI (or alternatively RNS) may be a more sensitive imaging methods to confirm the presence of a fracture (see Figs 3.3 and 3.14).

BONE TUMORS AND TUMOR-LIKE BONE LESIONS

Patients with bone tumors can present to clinicians of various disciplines, most frequently to orthopaedic and accident and emergency departments. Timely interpretation of radiological examinations by appropriately trained personnel is important. Systematic review of the images is required to define the nature and extent of lesions and determine whether additional imaging is indicated.

Some bone tumors may be discovered incidentally when a radiograph is performed for another purpose. Alternatively, those with both benign and malignant lesions may present with acute pain or a pathologic fracture. Patients with certain tumors (e.g. osteoid osteoma) will present with chronic pain, whereas those with aggressive malignant lesions often present with an enlarging mass. In the context of localized symptoms and signs radiographs are performed of the relevant anatomical site.

The following features are of particular note in the differentiation of bone tumors:

- Patient age
- Anatomical site
- Margins of the lesion
- Cortical bone appearances

Table 3.3   Bone and soft-tissue tumors showing characteristic peaks in incidence at different ages

Decade of life	1st	2nd	3rd	4th	5th	6th	7th
Simple bone cyst	■						
Chondroblastoma		■					
Ewing's sarcoma	■	■	■				
Nonossifying fibroma	■	■					
Osteochondroma		■					
Osteoblastoma		■	■				
Osteosarcoma		■	■				■
Osteoid osteoma		■	■				
Aneurysmal bone cyst		■					
Chondromyxoid fibroma		■	■				
Giant-cell tumor			■	■			
Bone lymphoma			■	■	■		
Fibrosarcoma and malignant fibrous histiocytoma			■	■	■		
Osteoma				■	■		
Parosteal osteosarcoma			■	■			
Chondroma		■	■	■			
Chondrosarcoma				■	■	■	
Myeloma					■	■	■
Chordoma					■	■	
Hemangioma				■	■	■	

- Periosteal reaction
- Presence of a soft-tissue mass
- Presence of tumor matrix calcification or ossification
- Whether the lesion is single, or multiple
- Family history and predisposing conditions.

PATIENT AGE

Primary bone lesions occur within characteristic age distributions (Table 3.3). Certain tumors occur more frequently in the immature skeleton. For example, benign chondrogenic, osteogenic and fibrogenic tumors occur in the bones of children and young adults. Certain malignant tumors, such as osteosarcoma and Ewing's sarcoma, characteristically occur in the first 30 years of life. Other lesions, such as chondrosarcoma and myeloma, are much more common later in life.

SITE OF SKELETAL INVOLVEMENT

Bone tumors occur frequently in characteristic anatomical sites. For example, 50% of chondromas involve the small bones of the hands and feet (Fig. 3.19a), giant-cell tumors and primary osteosarcomas commonly occur around the knee, and chordomas occur exclusively in relation to the mid-line axial skeleton.

The position of the lesion in bone can also suggest the nature of its pathology: giant-cell tumors are typically juxta-articular and eccentric, chondroblastomas arise in the epiphyses, and chondromyxoid fibromas are typically located in the metaphyses of long bones (Figs 3.19b and c). Osteosarcomas arise either centrally or on the surface of the bone. Cartilage-capped exostoses tend to occur at the ends of long bones, as they are related to abnormalities of enchondral ossification, and are directed away from the adjacent growing end of the bone from which they arise.

MARGINS OF LESION

A narrow zone of transition between an area of bone destruction and normal bone, and a thin sclerotic or corticated rim are suggestive of benign etiology, such as an enchondroma (Figs 3.19a and 3.20a). The more aggressive or malignant a bone lesion, the wider and less distinct will be the transition zone between destruction and normal bone (Fig. 3.20c). Bone destruction may have a permeative or 'moth-eaten' pattern of destruction also indicative of an aggressive lesion (Fig. 3.20d).

Some locally aggressive lesions, such as giant-cell tumors and aneurysmal bone cysts, may have marginal features intermediate between these two extremes (Fig. 3.20b).

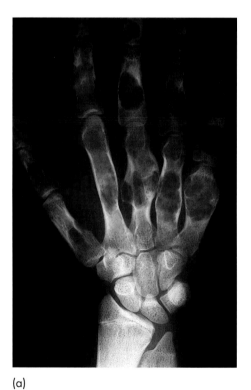

(a)

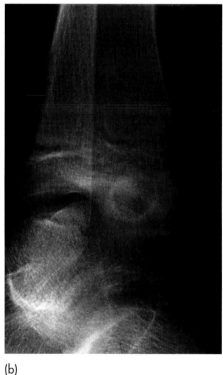

(b)

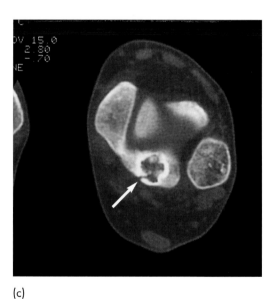

(c)

Figure 3.19   Bone tumors – site of involvement. (a) Chondromas – 50% of chondromas occur in the small bones of the hands and feet. Lesions are multiple (as illustrated) in Ollier's disease (dyschondromatosis). There can be associated disturbance of growth (there is shortening of the ulna). Multiple chondroma and angioma constitute Maffucci's syndrome. Chondroblastoma – these tumors are usually situated in the epiphysis. A 12-year-old girl complained of acute pain in the ankle. **(b)** Radiograph shows a round lytic lesion with sclerotic margins in the distal epiphysis of the tibia. **(c)** CT confirms the appearances and anatomical location more clearly. Note central matrix calcification characteristic of a tumor of cartilaginous origin. The reason for the acute pain is the presence of a pathologic fracture (arrow) through the cortex that is thinned by the tumor.

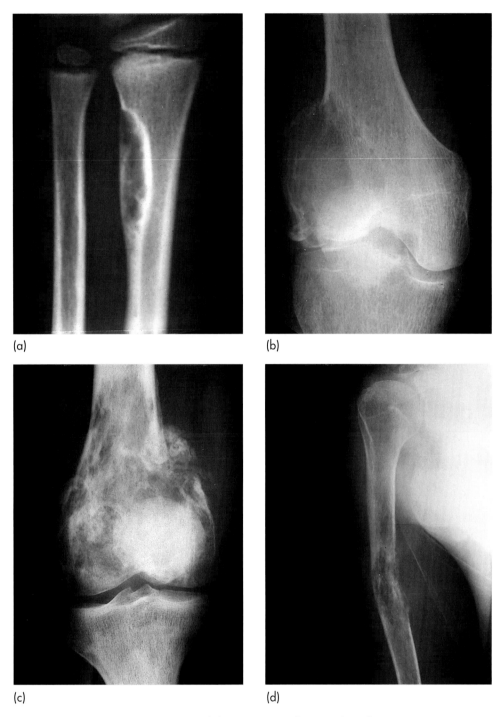

Figure 3.20   Margins of bone lesion. (a) Well-defined. Corticated – indicates non-aggressive, benign etiology (fibrous cortical defect in the distal radius). **(b) Intermediate.** Intermediate features of locally aggressive tumor with expansion and cortical destruction. Eccentric, subchondral destructive lesion in the lateral femoral condyle of the knee in a mature skeleton – giant-cell tumor with pathologic fracture. **(c)** and **(d) ill-defined, aggressive.** 'Moth-eaten' permeative pattern of bone destruction with wide zone of transition between normal and abnormal bone, indicative of an aggressive lesion – **(c)** malignant fibrous histiocytoma of the distal femur. **(d)** There is a permeative destructive lesion in the mid-humerus (metastasis from breast cancer) with an associated pathologic fracture.

CORTICAL BONE APPEARANCES

Benign lesions may cause some endosteal erosion of the bone cortex, but generally cause little expansion. If bone expansion does occur in benign lesions, a thin shell of cortex is usually retained. Disruption of the cortical rim can occur in benign lesions if a pathologic fracture has occurred, which may make differentiation between a benign or malignant pathology more difficult.

Aggressive and malignant lesions erode and destroy the bone cortex. When this occurs, a soft-tissue mass will be present and often there is an associated periosteal reaction.

PERIOSTEAL REACTIONS

Extension of an aggressive bone lesion beyond the confines of the bone is associated with cortical erosion and elevation of the periosteum at the margins of the lesion. This stimulates the periosteum to mineralize, and is seen radiographically as a 'Codman's triangle' (Figs 3.21a and b).

Periosteal reaction in benign tumors is unusual, unless a pathologic fracture has occurred.

SOFT-TISSUE MASS

An aggressive, rapidly growing tumor arising within a bone will extend into adjacent structures as a soft-tissue mass over a short period. The use of imaging is important to define this extension.

Such local staging is necessary to determine whether resection and limb salvage are feasible. MR is the modality of choice for such local staging (Fig. 3.22).

TUMOR MATRIX CALCIFICATION AND OSSIFICATION

Radiological features can give an indication of bone tumor tissue type. The matrix of osteogenic tumors may mineralize. In benign lesions (osteoma, osteochondroma), this matrix mineralization is ordered, forming trabeculae that can be traced from the tumor, through its margin, into the surrounding bone from which it arises (Figs 3.23a and b). The matrix of malignant osteosarcoma may also mineralize, but this occurs in a more haphazard fashion, forming clumps or 'sunray' spicules of calcification (Figs 3.21a and b).

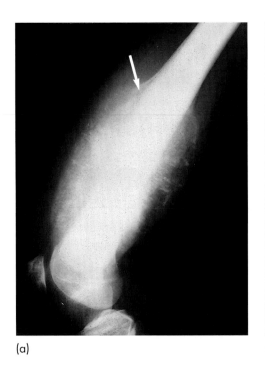

(a)

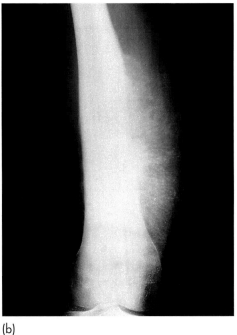

(b)

Figure 3.21 Periosteal reaction. (a and b) Malignant bone tumor, osteosarcoma of the distal femur with sclerosis, large soft-tissue mass and **(a)** elevated periosteal reaction at the proximal, anterior margin of tumor, giving a Codman's triangle (arrow), indicating an aggressive malignant lesion with a soft-tissue mass on the lateral view. **(b)** Frontal projection showing speculated 'sun ray' matrix ossification in a large soft-tissue mass.

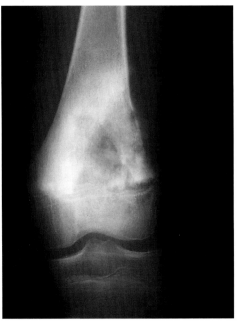

(a)

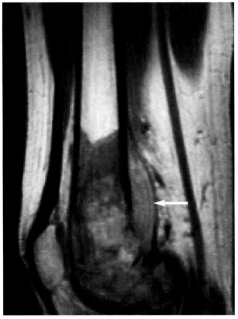

(b)

Figure 3.22 Soft-tissue mass – osteosarcoma: **(a)** Antero-posterior knee showing mixed sclerotic lesion of the distal femoral metaphysis; ill-defined margin between normal and abnormal bone; no obvious soft-tissue mass. **(b)** Coronal MR image (T$_1$-weighted) clearly defines the proximal tumor extent in the bone, as the tumor has a low signal compared to the high signal of normal marrow fat. There is also a breach in the posterior bone cortex and a soft-tissue mass (arrow).

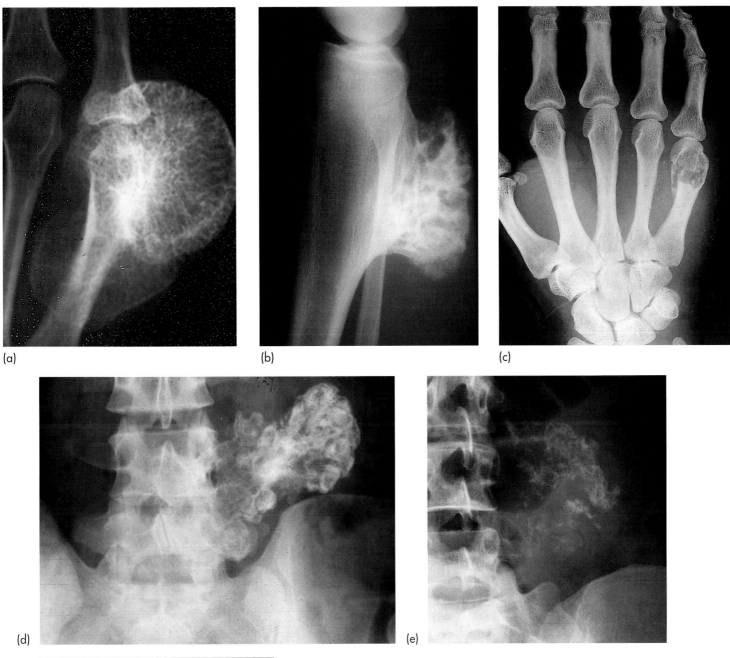

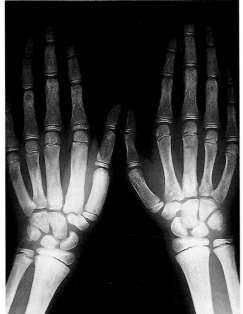

Figure 3.23   Matrix mineralization. (a) Ordered trabeculae in an osteoma of the fifth metacarpal. **(b)** Osteochondroma of the tibia with trabeculae and cortex in continuity from those of the bone of origin. Cartilaginous tumors. **(c)** Pathological fracture through a well-defined, benign (narrow zone of transition between normal and abnormal bone) lucent lesion with punctuate matrix calcification characteristic of a cartilaginous tumor (chondroma) of the fifth metacarpal. **(d)** Benign osteochondroma arising from the left lateral margin of the fifth lumbar vertebra. The margin of the mass is well defined, the matrix calcification is organized with evidence of trabeculae, and there is no evidence of bone destruction or soft-tissue mass. For comparison, **(e)** chondrosarcoma in the same anatomical site in a different patient. There is bone destruction (left transverse process of L4) and a large soft-tissue mass with ill-defined clumps of matrix calcification, features indicative of a malignant cartilage tumor. **(f)** Fibrous tumors do not contain calcification that is visible on radiographs, but in fibrous dysplasia the bone lesions may have a hazy 'ground glass' appearance as they are composed of abundant osseous trabeculae intermingled with fibrous tissue. The bone may appear sclerotic and increased in size with loss of the cortico-medullary differentiation, as illustrated in the radiograph of the hand of a child in which several metacarpals are affected.

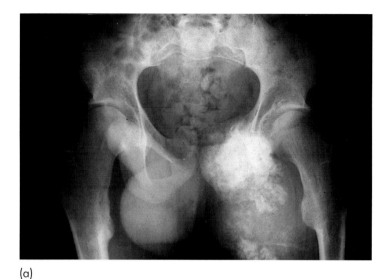

(a)

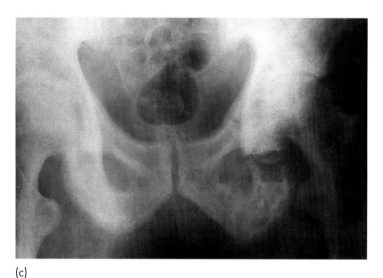

(c)

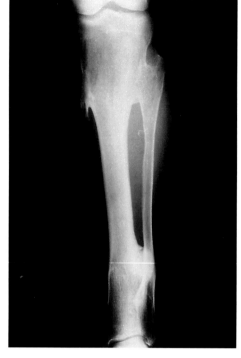

(b)

Figure 3.24   Lesions with a **family history** or in **pre-existing conditions:** Diaphyseal aclasis and chondrosarcoma. **(a)** Pelvic radiograph shows a large soft-tissue mass arising from the left superior pubic ramus; within this there are clumps of matrix calcification, features of a chondrosarcoma. There is some abnormal modeling of the right femoral neck and proximal and distal tibia, and there are multiple osteochondromas arising **(b)** from the tibia and fibula. Paget's disease and sarcoma. **(c)** There is sclerosis and a disordered trabecular pattern in the pelvis, indicating Paget's disease, with a pathologic fracture and bone destruction in the left ischium associated with the development of a sarcoma. MRI or CT would be the imaging techniques of choice to demonstrate the soft-tissue component of the tumor.

Cartilagenous tumors are generally radiolucent on radiographs, but can form well-defined conglomerate clumps of matrix calcification, seen as broken rings or snowflake shapes, often located centrally in the tumor (Figs 3.19c and 3.23c). Chondrosarcomas may also calcify, but this is more ill-defined in outline and is diffusely scattered throughout the tumor and its associated soft-tissue mass (Fig. 3.23e). Fibrous tumors do not contain calcification that is visible on radiographs. In fibrous dysplasia the bone lesions may have a hazy, 'ground glass' appearance because they contain an abundance of osseous trabeculae intermingled with fibrous tissue. These lesions can expand bone and cause sclerosis (Fig. 3.23f).

FAMILY HISTORY AND PRE-EXISTING CONDITIONS

In the small number of patients with multiple exostoses (diaphyseal aclasia), there is a strong family tendency and a higher incidence of chondrosarcoma (up to 27% in patients with multiple lesions who undergo surgery) (Figs 3.24a and b), compared with the incidence of malignant change in solitary lesions (2%). Previous radiotherapy and Paget's disease also predispose to the development of sarcoma in later life (Fig. 3.24c).

Specific clinical features may be associated with certain skeletal abnormalities. For example, in McCune–Albright's syndrome, polyostotic fibrous dysplasia is associated with precocious puberty and skin pigmentation; the association of nonossifying fibroma and café au lait spots is recognized as Jaffe–Campanacci syndrome.

IMAGING STRATEGIES IN BONE LESIONS, WITH PARTICULAR EMPHASIS ON BONE TUMORS

CLINICAL PRESENTATION

Asymptomatic presentation

Bone lesions are commonly identified as an incidental finding on a radiograph performed for other clinical reasons, such as trauma. From the radiographic appearances, it may be possible to deduce the pathologic entity. If appearances are indeterminate, comparison with any previous imaging may enable assessment of any interval change. A lesion showing no change over a period of years is likely to be benign, requiring no further action. It is important that normal variants, such as accessory ossification centers or asymmetric closure of synchondroses, are not mis-diagnosed as significant bone pathologies.

If the radiographic appearances of the lesion remain indeterminate, or if sinister pathology is suspected, further action is essential. A detailed clinical history and thorough physical examination of the patient should be made before embarking on further imaging, as these may reveal symptoms or signs relevant to the diagnosis: for example, a history of cancer or a palpable primary tumor suggests that a bone lesion is likely to be a metastasis.

In the absence of relevant history or abnormal physical signs, further imaging will be needed to determine the nature of the lesion. This may include MRI (or CT) to define additional features, helping to differentiate between benign and malignant pathologies. Alternatively a RN scan may be appropriate, to assess whether the lesion is single or multiple. The need for additional imaging, and its appropriate sequence, is best determined by discussion between the clinician and radiologist.

Ideally, the pathologist should also be involved: biopsy may be needed to confirm the definitive histologic diagnosis and familiarity with the case is helpful in pathologic diagnosis. There is a strong case for regular multidisciplinary meetings between clinicians, radiologists and pathologists to enhance the cooperative diagnosis and management of patients with bone tumors, and to extend the education and experience of those involved in their care.

Presentation with acute pain

Acute pain is most likely to be caused by a fracture, which may be pathologic and occur through an existing bone lesion (Fig. 3.20d). The symptomatic site should be radiographed with at least two views at right angles, with supplementary specialized projections as appropriate. The radiographic appearances may be diagnostic of a benign lesion, such as a simple bone cyst or enchondroma (Fig. 3.23c).

If the fracture has occurred through an aggressive lesion, the features (clinical and radiologic) require analysis to distinguish a bone tumor from other pathology. Further imaging may be relevant and biopsy is likely to be required, particularly if the lesion is solitary. The presence of a fracture may confuse both the imaging and histopathologic appearances. The pathologist should be informed of the presence of a fracture through a bone lesion and the site from which the biopsy was taken.

Presentation with chronic pain

Some bone lesions, such as osteoid osteoma, are characterized by pain that may have persisted for months or years. Juxta-articular bone tumors may stimulate a synovitis, causing pain and a joint effusion. Radiography of the symptomatic site forms the baseline imaging investigation. In the context of genuine symptoms and abnormal physical signs, such as tenderness or swelling, without demonstrable radiographic abnormality, further imaging is appropriate.

In this situation, RN scans have been used as a screening method to identify areas of increased bone activity. If a RN scan is normal, a significant bone lesion is highly unlikely and the patient may be reassured. The improved availability of MRI means that this is being used increasingly in the context of unexplained chronic pain as an investigation following initial radiography, in place of RN scanning, particularly when localized symptoms are present. MRI has the advantages over RN scanning

of superior anatomical detail and a lack of ionizing radiation, but cannot easily provide a screen for multiple skeletal lesions.

CT is particularly useful in showing fine bone detail. For this reason, CT is superior to MRI in the diagnosis of osteoid osteoma (Figs 3.25a–e). Neither radiographs nor RN scanning permit accurate localization of the nidus of the tumor in the context of extensive reactive sclerosis. In the absence of radiographic abnormality, RN scanning or MRI can be used to define the site and size of bone abnormality. Thin-section CT is then used to provide precise detail of the nidus, and can now be used to direct percutaneous treatment as an alternative to open surgery.

If the radiograph shows the characteristic features of a benign bone lesion, appropriate treatment can be planned. Cross-sectional imaging (using CT or MRI) may provide additional valuable information to the surgeon, particularly in malignant lesions. This information might include the exact site and extent of the lesion in three dimensions and the relationship of the lesion to adjacent articular surfaces and other anatomical structures, such as neurovascular bundles, all of which will influence the feasibility, approach and extent of surgery. Histologic confirmation of the lesion may be obtained before or during surgery.

Suspected bone metastases

If the radiographic features suggest a malignant lesion, distinction must be made between a primary bone tumor and metastases. RN scanning can confirm the presence of metastases by the presence of multiple 'hot spots' in a characteristic distribution throughout the skeleton (Fig. 3.9c), in which case no further imaging is required, particularly if the patient is known to have a primary malignant tumor.

If there is a solitary bone lesion that is suspicious, but not diagnostic, of a metastasis, biopsy should be performed for histologic confirmation and to determine subsequent clinical management. Biopsy may be performed using either image guidance, usually with CT (Fig. 3.28) or fluoroscopy, or an open, surgical technique.

PRIMARY MALIGNANT BONE TUMORS

The principle role of imaging, once features of a primary malignant bone tumor have been confirmed, is in tumor staging, both local and distant. Certain imaging features may suggest the tissue of origin, such as the matrix ossification of osteosarcoma or the ill-defined calcification within a soft-tissue mass of chondrosarcoma, but biopsy will be necessary to confirm the histological diagnosis.

Initial staging

Imaging plays an important role in the initial staging of bone tumors. It is useful in determining the potential resectability of the tumor, by defining its extent and showing any involvement of vital anatomical structures (such as neurovascular structures and major organs) that would exclude radical, but potentially curative, surgery. Limb-salvage procedures are being used increasingly in malignant tumors of the extremities. In these circumstances, the tumor is removed with a margin of surrounding normal tissue and the bone replaced by an endoprosthesis.

In order to plan the appropriate surgical excision and endoprosthesis, the surgeon managing such tumors requires accurate information of the intramedullary tumor component, the

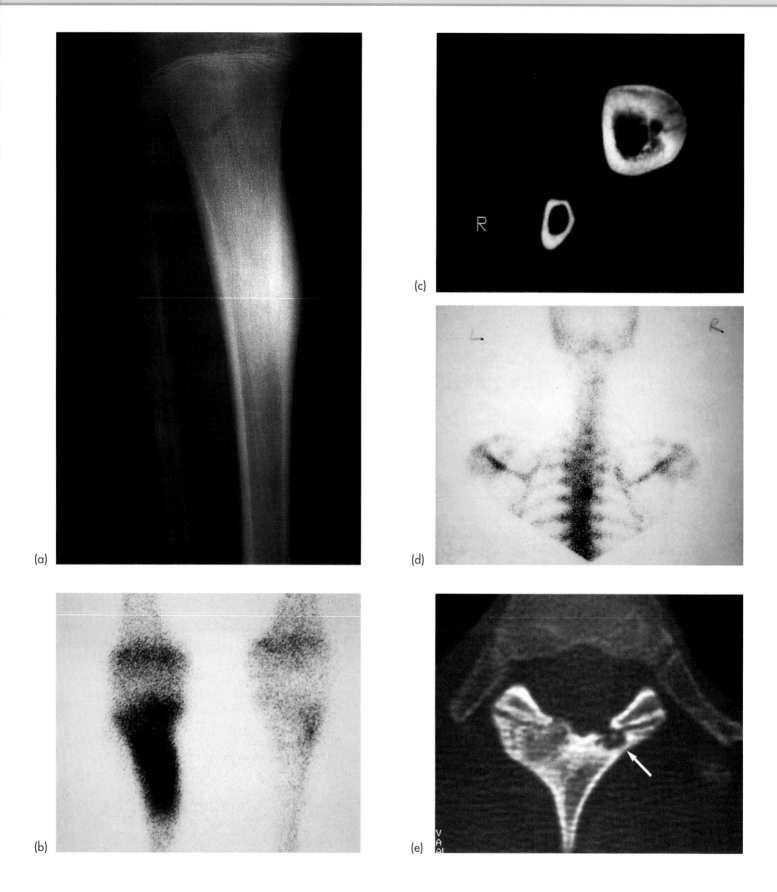

Figure 3.25 Osteoid osteoma of tibia. (a–c) A 17-year-old boy presented with a history of 18 months' pain in his right leg. (a) Radiograph showed diffuse sclerosis and periosteal reaction in the medial aspect of the tibial shaft. (b) Radionuclide scan shows extensive increased uptake in the proximal tibia. (c) CT is required (thin sections, 1–2 mm) to identify the site, characteristic features (low-attenuation nidus with central mineralization within the sclerotic bone, and extensive adjacent endosteal and periosteal sclerosis. This information is essential to the surgeon to ensure removal of the nidus, which is required for cure. (d and e) A patient of 18 years presented with backache. Radiographs showed no abnormality. (d) A radionuclide scan shows localized increased uptake in the thoracic spine and (e) CT confirms the characteristic appearance of an osteoid osteoma in the vertebral lamina on the left (arrow).

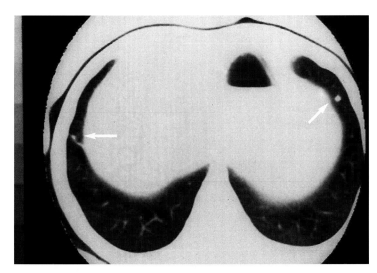

Figure 3.26 CT – lung metastases from Ewing's sarcoma. Malignant bone tumors metastasize to the lung. These may be evident on chest radiographs (see Fig. 3.1). However, metastases may be small and in areas of the lung not well seen on a chest radiograph (paravertebral and retrocardiac regions). Therefore, a normal chest radiograph does not exclude lung metastases and CT is a sensitive method of detecting such metastases. CT thorax showing two small soft-tissue nodules that are metastases (arrows) from Ewing's sarcoma. The chest radiograph was normal in this patient.

presence of any satellite lesions and the extent of soft-tissue tumor invasion in relation to the neurovascular structures and surrounding joints. MRI best provides this information (Figs 3.22a and b). CT can be substituted if MRI is unavailable, but the definition of the tumor/soft-tissue interface and marrow involvement demonstrated by CT is inferior to that of MRI (Figs 3.13a–d).

Malignant bone tumors most commonly metastasize to the lungs. High quality postero-anterior (PA) and lateral projections of the chest must be performed as part of the initial staging procedure. No other thoracic imaging is required if multiple pulmonary metastases are clearly identified on the chest radiograph (Fig. 3.1). However, the chest radiograph is not sensitive to the identification of small lung nodules, particularly those sited in the paravertebral and retrocardiac regions, or in the posterior costo-phrenic recesses. A normal chest radiograph therefore does not exclude the presence of lung metastases. Thoracic CT, the most sensitive method of detecting pulmonary metastases, should be performed if the chest radiograph is normal, or if a single pulmonary nodule of uncertain etiology is present (Fig. 3.26). MRI is not helpful in the identification of pulmonary metastases. Pulmonary osteosarcoma metastases that fail to regress with chemotherapy may be surgically resected, if single or few in number.

RN scanning is also carried out as part of osteosarcoma staging. Increased activity is present at the site of the primary tumor, with synchronous and metachronous tumors and bone metastases also evident as areas of increased skeletal uptake of radionuclide. Such increased uptake may also be evident in osteogenic metastases in the lymph nodes and lungs.

Assessment of treatment response

Adjuvant chemotherapy is used in the treatment of some malignant bone tumors, such as osteosarcoma, prior to surgical resection. Imaging, including MRI of the tumor and radiography or CT of the chest, is performed at initial staging and on completion of the course of chemotherapy. Assessment of the response to treatment is made in terms of reduction in size of the primary lesion and any regression of metastases. A reduction of 50% or more of the primary tumor volume and the development of heavy tumor matrix calcification after chemotherapy generally indicate a more favorable prognosis and may make the tumor easier to resect.

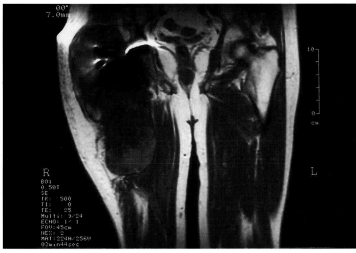

(a)

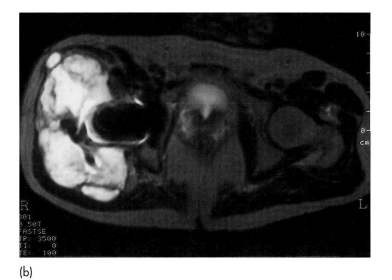

(b)

Figure 3.27 **Follow-up imaging:** MRI of a patient treated previously with an endoprosthesis for osteosarcoma of the proximal femur. Although there is artifact (signal void) from the ferromagnetic metal prosthesis in the proximal right femur, the quality of the image is still sufficient to identify extensive tumor recurrence in the right thigh. (a) Coronal T₁-weighted image – tumor recurrence in the thigh is low signal. (b) Transverse axial T₂-weighted image – the recurrent tumor mass is high signal.

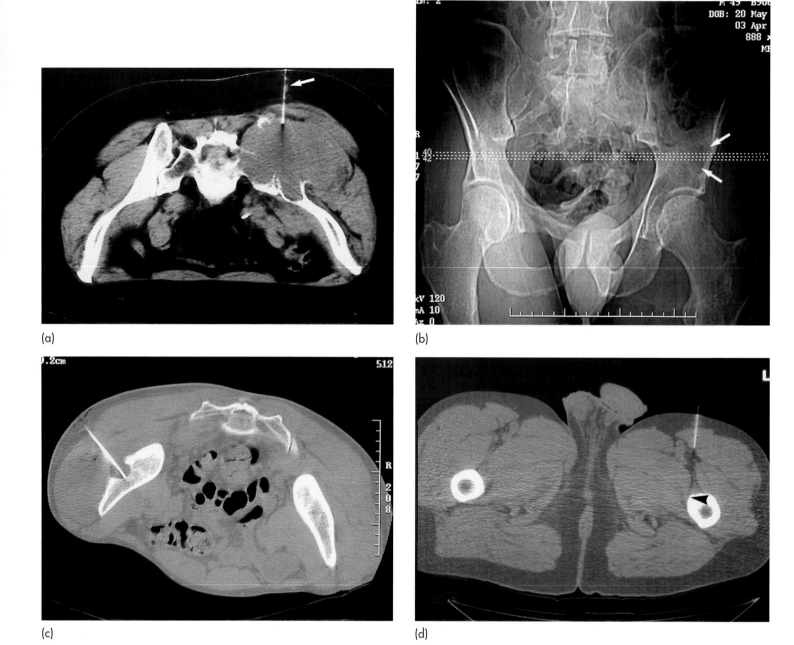

(a)

(b)

(c)

(d)

(e)

Figure 3.28   Image-guided procedures: (a) CT-guided biopsy (needle indicated by arrow) of a large lytic sarcoma involving the left sacrum and ilium. The patient is placed in a prone position on the CT scanner. CT guidance can be used for biopsy of smaller bone lesions. **(b)** CT scan projection radiograph with localizing line to identify the plane of the small lytic lesion (arrow) in the left ileum. **(c)** With the patient in the prone position the biopsy needle is directed to the lytic bone area. This proved to be a metastasis from lung cancer. Image-guided therapeutic procedures: **(d and e)** There is an osteoid osteoma in the antero-medial cortex of the left femur (arrow-head) and initially a needle **(d)** is used to define the ideal pathway to the lesion so as to avoid any important anatomical structures (vessels, nerves) and then in **(e)** the probe is advanced into the tumor for cryo-ablation.

Follow-up

Imaging is used in the surveillance that follows resection. Postoperative imaging is usually deferred for at least 3 months after surgery, because postoperative changes may be misinterpreted as tumor recurrence. Even after this time, it can be difficult to distinguish between tumor recurrence and postoperative changes, despite the use of dynamic contrast-enhanced MRI, and serial investigation or biopsy may be needed. The metal endoprostheses that are inserted at limb-salvage surgery cause considerable artifact both on MRI and CT, but useful information can nonetheless still be obtained with these imaging methods (Figs 3.27a and b).

Image-guided biopsy and therapy

Many bone tumors require biopsy for histological confirmation of the diagnosis. Biopsy can be performed at surgery ('open') or percutaneously ('closed'), either with image guidance or without ('blind'). Imaging can be used to identify the optimum site from which to obtain a tissue sample by avoiding predominantly necrotic or cystic components of lesions. Imaging techniques, most often fluoroscopy and CT (Figs 3.28a–c), but also US and more recently open MRI systems, can be used to guide closed biopsy procedures, ensuring accurate needle placement.

Biopsy should only be performed following consultation with the specialized tumor surgeon, to avoid inadvertent up-grading of the tumor due to an inappropriate approach. Close co-operation with the pathologist is also required: success depends not only on obtaining an adequate tissue sample, but also on the histopathologic interpretation of a relatively small volume of tissue obtained at biopsy.

Therapeutic procedures are being increasingly performed using image guidance. Osteoid osteoma, for example, is now commonly treated by CT-guided biopsy and removal of the nidus by radiofrequency ablation or cryotherapy (Figs 3.28d and e). These procedures obviate the need for open surgical resection, which often results in slower clinical recovery.

Angiography is no longer used routinely in the diagnosis and staging of bone tumors, but embolization can be used to reduce the vascularity of a tumor prior to surgery, or to treat arterial tumor hemorrhage. Chemotherapeutic agents can also be infused through intra-arterial catheters placed selectively in the vessels that supply the tumor. Such interventional vascular procedures are rarely required in the management of primary bone tumors.

Differential diagnosis

Other pathologies may resemble bone tumors, both clinically and radiologically. Infection, in particular, may have radiologically aggressive appearances, with bone destruction or sclerosis, periosteal reaction and a soft-tissue component (Figs 3.29a and b). Clinical features, such as pyrexia, raised inflammatory markers and leucocytosis may favor the diagnosis of osteomyelitis, but biopsy may be needed to confirm the correct diagnosis. It is good practice to include a microbiologic sample whenever a bone biopsy of a suspected tumor is performed, to exclude an unexpected diagnosis of infection and avoid unnecessary repeat procedures, should the histopathology prove to be negative. Some metabolic bone disorders (for example hyperparathyroidism) are associated with bone cysts or subperiosteal erosions, which can be mistaken for primary bone tumors.

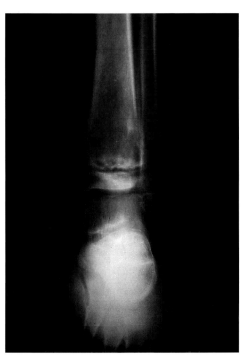
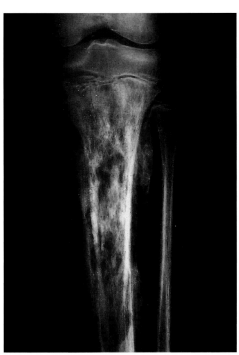

Figure 3.29 Infection: Osteomyelitis may have features resembling those of bone tumors and biopsy may be required for a definitive diagnosis. **Acute.** (a) Osteomyelitis of the distal tibia – there is bone destruction in the metaphyseal region and periosteal reaction seen as faint calcification in the soft tissue adjacent to the bone cortex. **Chronic.** (b) Osteomyelitis of the proximal tibia – there is extensive lysis and sclerosis extending along the tibial shaft, with consolidated periosteal reaction, giving a 'bone within a bone' appearance.

(a)   (b)

IMAGING STRATEGIES IN SOFT-TISSUE TUMORS

Soft-tissue tumors commonly present with a mass. In benign tumors, the mass is usually painless and may have been present for months or even years, with little change in size. Benign soft-tissue masses are more common than sarcomas, with at least a 50–100-fold higher incidence than malignant lesions. Soft-tissue sarcomas are rare, accounting for only 0.8–1% of malignancies. They may present with pain and a swelling, the latter increasing in size with time. Soft-tissue lesions caused by trauma (myositis ossificans) (Figs 3.30a–c) and infection must be differentiated from tumors.

The role of imaging in soft-tissue masses is to:

- Confirm the presence of a mass
- Define the tissue composition and nature of a mass – relevant to management, either conservative or surgical
- Identify the anatomical location and extent of the mass – relevant to biopsy site and resectability
- Differentiate between benign and malignant etiology.

In soft-tissue sarcoma, imaging also contributes to:

- Local staging
- Identification of metastases
- Assessment of tumor and metastatic response to treatment
- Identification of tumor recurrence.

Radiographs are usually not helpful in the imaging of soft-tissue tumors and may be entirely normal, unless the mass is large, contains fat or calcification, or causes abnormality of adjacent bone. US is a good screening method in the initial assessment of soft-tissue masses, particularly those that are small and relatively superficial, providing a simple method of confirming whether a soft-tissue abnormality is present. US can indicate whether a mass is cystic, solid or vascular. US allows assessment of the mass during muscle contraction, and changes in position can be used to define the relationship of a mass to surrounding structures. Confident characterization is possible for certain masses (e.g. neuromas and ganglia).

CT can be used to identify soft-tissue tumors and define their composition, but the limited contrast resolution of the technique means that interfaces between tumor and normal soft-tissue structures can be difficult to delineate. MRI is the modality of choice for characterizing soft-tissue tumors: The high contrast sensitivity of MRI makes even small lesions conspicuous (Fig. 3.31).

Some benign soft-tissue tumors have characteristic appearances on MRI and do not require biopsy or treatment (e.g. lipomas, hemangiomas, cysts and ganglia) (Figs 3.32a–e). Developmental anomalies or hypertrophied structures can be confirmed as the cause of a palpable mass.

Benign tumors typically have a well-defined margin. Many such tumors have homogenous signal intensity and show little enhancement with Gd-labeled DTPA. The signal intensities on T_1- and T_2-weighted MRI sequences give an indication of tissue composition. Myxomas, cysts and ganglia give a low or intermediate signal on T_1-weighted images and a higher signal on T_2-weighted sequences, whereas lipomas and subacute hematomas give a high signal on both T_1- and T_2-weighted sequences.

Malignant soft-tissue tumors are often large, with irregular, indistinct margins and heterogeneous signal intensity (Figs 3.32a–e). They usually show prominent patchy enhancement with gadolinium-labeled DTPA, sometimes with cystic or necrotic, non-enhancing central components. Most soft-tissue tumors are iso-intense to muscle on T_1-weighted MRI sequences. Tumors give a high signal on T_1-weighted images if they contain areas of fat, melanin, proteinaceous material or subacute hemorrhage.

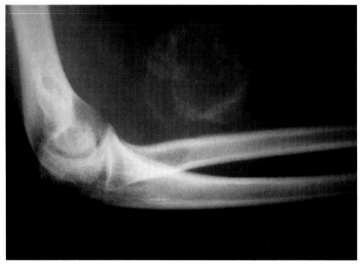

(a)

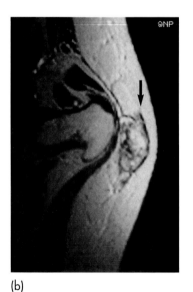

(b)

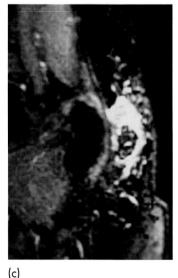

(c)

Figure 3.30 This must be differentiated from soft-tissue sarcoma. (**a**) Lateral radiograph of the forearm of a girl who suffered from epilepsy and had a convulsion. Over the next 2–4 weeks a hard mass developed in her arm. There is circumferential calcification in the periphery of a soft-tissue mass, lying anterior to the radius and ulna; this is characteristic of traumatic myositis ossificans, and can be differentiated from tumor calcification, as the latter usually lies centrally in the soft-tissue mass. In a different patient (**b** and **c**), who developed a swelling over the left greater trochanter following trauma, faint calcification was evident on the radiograph of the area. (**b**) T_1-weighted coronal MR image shows a mass (arrow) within the fat adjacent to the trochanter (**c**). Inversion recovery fat-suppressed T_2-weighted MRI confirms that there is extensive edema (high signal) around the lesion, confirming the traumatic etiology.

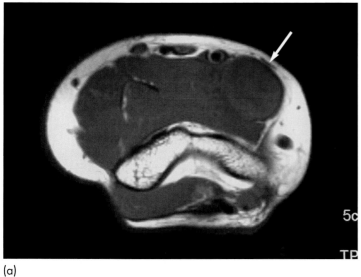

(a)

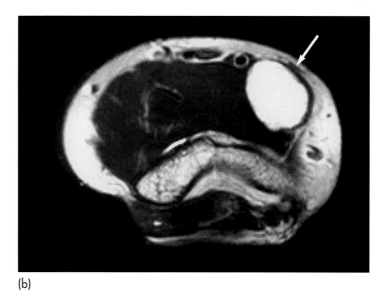

(b)

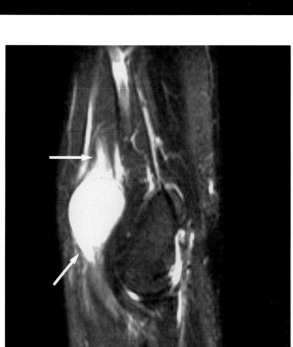

(c)

Figure 3.31 Neuroma. MRI images (a) pre- and (b) post-Gd DTPA. Transverse T$_1$-weighted images showing a well-defined soft-tissue mass (arrow), which is a low to intermediate signal, and showing enhancement following contrast medium (b). (c) Sagittal STIR sequence (fat suppression) shows the tumor to be high in signal, with characteristic 'tails' at the proximal and distal ends of the tumor.

Calcified or predominantly fibrous tumors give a low signal on all MRI sequences. Most sarcomas give a high signal on T$_2$-weighted images, due to their increased free water content, as a result of high vascular permeability and edema.

Many soft-tissue masses have indeterminate features on MR images. All such lesions should be presumed to be malignant until proven otherwise by pathologic evaluation. Closed biopsies, with small-tumor samples, can give misleading results, due to sampling error: soft-tissue tumors often show regional variation in grade. As with bone tumors, inappropriately sited biopsies and inadequate resected margins can compromise subsequent effective limb-salvage surgery and adversely affect prognosis. Therefore biopsy, whether open or closed, must be performed only after consultation with the experienced surgeon who will perform

the definitive surgery, and collaboration between clinician, radiologist and pathologist is essential.

The staging, prognosis and management of a patient are dependent on the size and location of the tumor, and the presence of lymph node or distant metastases. Surgical excision is by a local procedure (either by intralesional, marginal or radical resection) or amputation. Limb-salvage procedures are performed where feasible.

MR imaging is the modality of choice for the definition of local tumor extent. Potential resectability depends on the tumor's location, its relationship to adjacent structures and whether or not the tumor is limited to a single anatomical compartment. Regional lymph node metastases causing lymphadenopathy may be evident on MRI. The relevant sites of regional lymph node

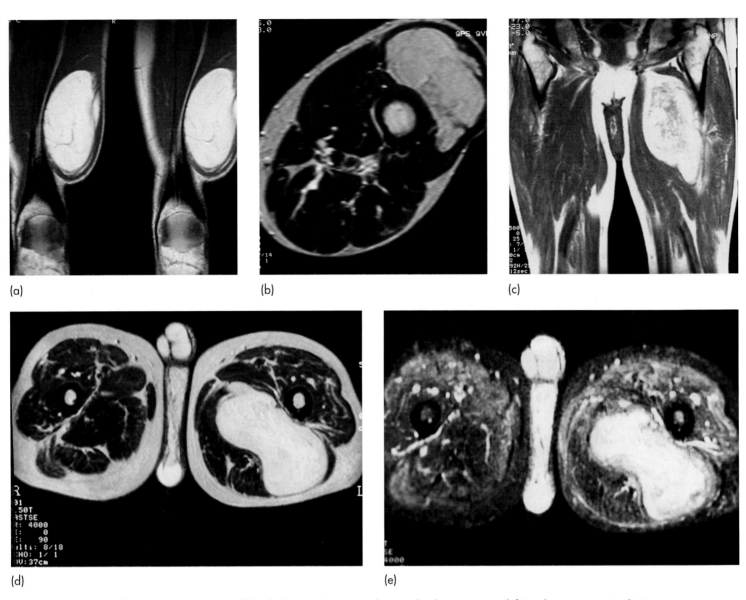

(a)

(b)

(c)

(d)

(e)

Figure 3.32 Fatty soft-tissue tumors. Lipoma of the thigh. MRI. **(a)** Coronal T$_1$-weighted pre-contrast (left) and postcontrast (right) images. **(b)** Transverse T$_2$-weighted image. The tumor is of uniform signal intensity, which is similar to that of the normal subcutaneous fat, and showed no enhancement with contrast medium (Gd-labeled DTPA). These are the features of a lipoma. Liposarcoma of the left thigh **(c–e)** MR: **(c)** Coronal T$_1$-weighted image and **(d)** transverse T$_2$-weighted image confirm a large soft-tissue mass with signal characteristics similar to those of subcutaneous fat. However, there are areas of low signal intensity within the tumor, suggesting soft-tissue components other than fat and this is confirmed by **(e)** an inversion recovery sequence in which the fat signal is suppressed, but a considerable proportion of the tumor tissue components do not suppress, confirming that they are not simply fat. These features indicate a liposarcoma.

drainage should be included on imaging and scrutinized accordingly, but nodal size is a poor predictor of metastatic involvement.

The commonest site of distant metastases from sarcoma is to the lung. High-quality chest radiographs are performed, which may be diagnostic of metastases. If chest radiographs are normal, or equivocal, thoracic CT is required for confirmation or exclusion of lung metastases.

MRI is also used in the identification of tumor recurrence. Follow-up MRI should be deferred for at least 3 months after surgery to allow postoperative changes to resolve. Differentiation between tumor recurrence and postoperative fibrosis may be dif-

ficult. Paramagnetic contrast agents may help in differentiation, but serial examination to assess change in size, and biopsy may be needed in difficult cases.

A great number of MRI sequences have been developed to potentiate tissue contrast and enhance the conspicuity of pathologic lesions. The high-contrast sensitivity of MRI makes it the modality of choice for defining the soft-tissue margins of tumors and marrow changes within bones. MRI is therefore an important method of imaging to define the extent of tumors. MR images do give some indication of the pathologic nature of lesions, but may be non-specific: edema, for example, gives a high signal on MRI, whatever the cause.

JOINT DISORDERS

Abnormalities of joints can occur as a consequence of degenerative, erosive, or inflammatory (e.g. infective) arthritis, or be associated with metabolic disorders (e.g. hemochromatosis or gout) (Figs 33a and b). In RA, an erosive arthropathy, narrowing of the joint space caused by destruction of articular cartilage is an early feature. As the affected joints are inflamed and hyperemic, there is peri-articular soft-tissue swelling, particularly at the proximal interphalangeal joints, and osteopenia. Synovial hypertrophy

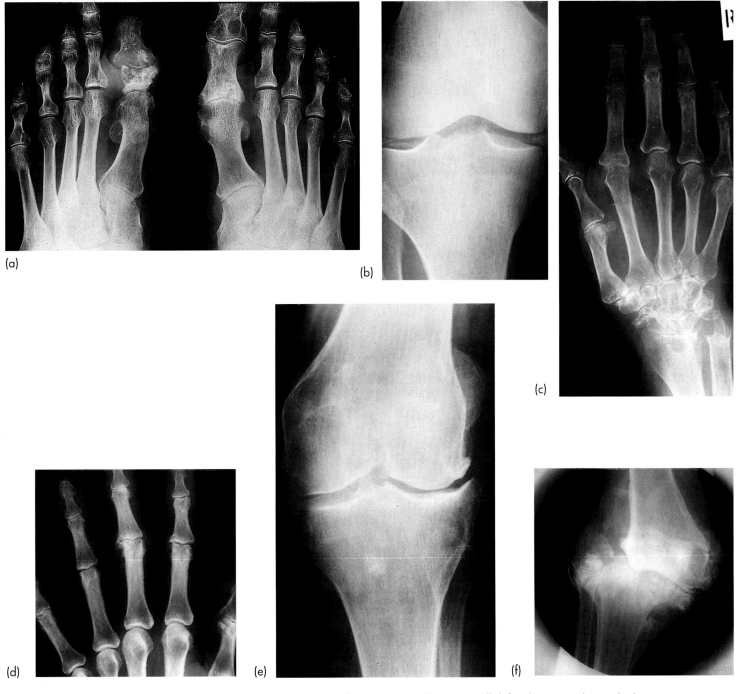

Figure 3.33   Joint disorders: (a) Gout – particularly involves joints of the great toes. There are well-defined, corticated ('punched out') areas present in the distal phalanx of the left great toe. Occasionally, bone destruction may occur due to tophaceous deposits, as is evident in the proximal phalanx of the right first toe. (b) Crystal deposition disease – chondrocalcinosis ('pseudogout'). There is calcification in the articular cartilage and menisci of the knee. (c) Erosive arthritis (rheumatoid arthritis) with peri-articular osteopenia, narrowing of joint spaces due to destruction of articular cartilage and juxta-articular erosions, particularly in the carpus, metacarpophalangeal and proximal interphalangeal joints. (d) Degenerative arthritis (OA) – hand radiograph with some narrowing of the interphalangeal joints and osteophytes, particularly in the middle finger; but no peri-articular porosis, as is characteristic of an erosive arthritis. In the knee: (e) Antero-posterior knee – weight-bearing – to identify narrowing of the joint space which may not be evident on supine films. There are also lateral marginal osteophytes. (f) Neuropathic: Charcot joint. There is complete derangement of the knee, which is subluxed with juxta-articular bone destruction, sclerosis and bone debris in the soft tissues.

causes juxta-articular bone destruction (erosions) (Fig. 3.33c). Such erosions can involve any joint, but most commonly involve the metacarpophalangeal and proximal interphalangeal joints, and may be evident initially in the feet and the styloid process of the ulna. MRI is a more sensitive imaging method than radiography to identify pannus and erosions. Ligamentous damage and laxity cause joint subluxation and even dislocation. In RA there is little reactive new bone formation, unlike in degenerative joint disease, where osteophytes and subchondral sclerosis are common features. However, in juvenile chronic arthritis, bony ankylosis of some affected joints can occur.

Other erosive arthropathies, where rheumatoid factor is not present in the serum (seronegative arthropathies), have radiographic features that can closely resemble those of RA, but tend not to cause peri-articular osteopenia. Such conditions include Reiter's disease, ankylosing spondylitis, and psoriatic arthropathy. These diseases have features that distinguish them from RA; there is usually bilateral (but often asymmetric) sacroiliitis and there may be associated paraspinal ossification. Reiter's disease (uveitis, urethritis, arthritis) more commonly involves the lower limbs and is often associated with periosteal reaction (periostitis), and psoriatic arthritis frequently involves the distal interphalangeal joints.

Destruction of articular cartilage and consequent narrowing of the joint space is a late feature in degenerative joint disease (osteoarthritis). There is reactive new bone formation, causing osteosclerosis and osteophytes, but no peri-articular osteopenia (Figs 3.33d and e). Juxta-articular cysts also occur and generally have a corticated margin, not a feature of the erosions of RA.

Septic arthropathy is characterized by pain and limited joint movement. An effusion is generally present; ultrasonography is a useful technique to confirm this and can be used to guide joint aspiration, which is usually required to reach a definitive diagnosis. On imaging there can be peri-articular osteopenia, loss of joint space, synovial thickening, and bone destruction. Rapid reduction in joint space over a short period (2–4 weeks) on serial radiographs should always suggest infection as the cause. Similarly, rapid reduction in disc space in the spine suggests an infective etiology. Timely diagnosis and correct therapy are essential in septic arthritis to avoid extensive bone and joint destruction with the clinical consequences that result (pain, deformity, ankylosis, and secondary osteoarthritis). MRI is a sensitive imaging technique for the diagnosis of inflammatory arthritis and the associated soft-tissue and bone changes.

When the deep pain sensation is disturbed or absent (e.g. in asymbolia, neurosyphilis, diabetes), very florid joint destruction can occur (Charcot joints) (Fig. 3.33e). There is complete derangement of the joint, which may be subluxed or dislocated, with extensive sclerosis, hyperostosis, bone destruction, and fragmentation. In the feet of patients with diabetic neuropathy these features may be indistinguishable from osteomyelitis, and may also coexist with infection.

RESPONSE TO INJURY

INJURY AND REPAIR

The publication in 1858 of Virchow's, *Die Cellularpathologie in ihrer Begründung auf physiologische und pathologische Gewebelehre* (The Cellular Basis of Disease and Its Foundations in Physiology and Tissue Pathology), brought a completely new understanding of the fundamental nature of disease. For the first time, the cell was seen as the basic unit of the living organism, and alterations in cellular function as being responsible for disease states. The study of disease was no longer limited to gross anatomical description. The new pathology depended on the correlation of clinical findings and cellular biology.

One of the most fundamental questions in medicine is: what happens to a cell, and to the tissue of which the cell is a unit after injury and how much injury can the cell sustain and how does the body deal with the injured cells and effect repair?

EFFECTS OF INJURY

A commonly used term in pathology reports is 'degeneration' or 'degenerative change'. This terminology is more emotive than substantive. The clinician would be better informed if a pathology report detailed the etiology of and the response to the injury. For example, instead of 'fragment of degenerated intervertebral disc,' a more descriptive diagnosis might be 'fragment of lacerated anulus fibrosus with granulation tissue and early scarring'.

Degeneration is defined in the Oxford Dictionary as 'A morbid change in the structure of parts consisting in a disintegration of tissue or in a substitution of a lower for a higher form of structure.' Although degeneration resulting from injury is a major topic of this chapter, it is important to bear in mind that injury is not the only cause of degeneration; degeneration is also the end result of disuse and of getting older.

Injury may be physical (mechanical trauma, extremes in temperature, or ionizing radiation), chemical (e.g. the quinolone antibiotics have been associated with rupture of the Achilles and other tendons), or biologic, either intrinsic (metabolic, immunologic) or extrinsic (bacteria, viruses, fungi, or other organisms). Regardless of the etiology, two effects can be expected: a local effect at the site of injury and a general effect on the body as a whole (e.g. shock following severe hemorrhage in association with an open fracture).

The cell is a complex structure in which the basic processes of energy conversion, protein synthesis, and other vital activities are constantly taking place (Fig. 4.1). Each cell exists in an ever-changing environment, and its ability to adapt to new conditions determines its continued functional activity. Injury to the cell occurs when conditions in the local environment are such that the cell is unable to maintain its physiologic equilibrium.

The results of injury are altered synthesis (anabolism) and/or altered breakdown (catabolism). The nature of the injurious agent and the duration of its application determine which process predominates. If only transient alterations occur in the intracellular or extracellular regulatory mechanisms, the cell may revert to its normal basal state when the adverse conditions cease. A more severe yet sublethal injury may result in adaptive changes, recognizable microscopically as hypertrophy, atrophy, or hyperplasia. When the insult is lethal, the necrosis (death) of the cell can be recognized microscopically by loss of staining, disintegration of the nucleus, and breakdown of the cell membranes.

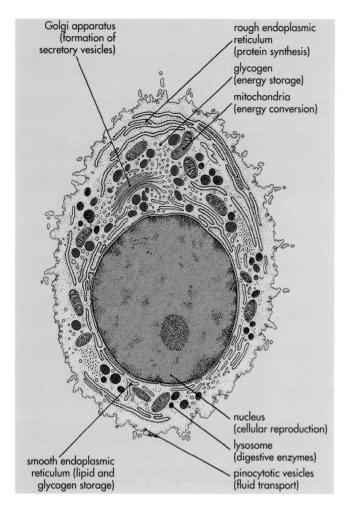

Figure 4.1   Diagram of a cell showing the basic cytoplasmic organelles and their function.

Because of the variability in injurious agents and the widely differing susceptibility of various tissues, it is difficult to generalize about the morphologic effects. However, mechanical injury usually causes cell disruption; freezing depresses cell metabolism and ultimately leads to the formation of destructive intracytoplasmic ice crystals; heat increases rates of metabolism, enzyme inactivation, protein coagulation, and even tissue charring. The effects of ionizing radiation are focused mostly on the nucleus, where it causes chromosome breakage and gene mutation. Chemicals act both locally and systemically by interfering with metabolic processes in the cell, especially by inactivation of enzymes and denaturation of intracellular protein. Finally, many microorganisms manufacture toxins that disturb cell metabolism.

Other considerations also influence the effects of injury: the intensity of application and the site of injury (for example, anoxia rapidly produces irreversible damage to brain cells and cardiac muscle, whereas connective tissue can usually withstand anoxia for considerable periods of time). Lastly, the effects of injury are influenced by the individual's general health, including nutritional state, presence or absence of drugs in the body, and so on.

HISTOLOGIC OBSERVATIONS

The most commonly observed microscopic change associated with altered cell homeostasis is a change in cell volume. This results from the cell's loss of ability to regulate electrolyte and fluid metabolism, owing to altered function of the mitochondria and the cell membrane.

Hypoxia, which affects lipoprotein as well as protein synthesis and secretion, may lead to accumulation of lipid droplets and of amorphous eosinophilic material in both the cell and extracellular space (Fig. 4.2).

A fundamental characteristic of living cells is their ability to sense and to adapt to changes in the environment. This ability to

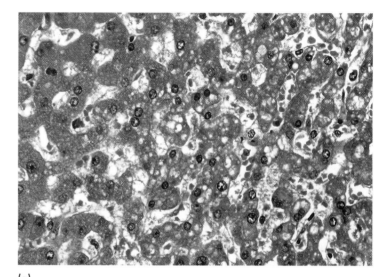

(a)

(b)

Figure 4.2   Cell changes due to hypoxia are well demonstrated in these photomicrographs of the centrilobular part of the liver. **(a)** In the upper left, normal liver tissue can be seen, while in the middle and lower right some vacuolization is apparent within the cytoplasm and there is swelling of the cell outline. **(b)** In tissue adjacent to the central veins, congestion of the liver sinuses is readily apparent, with marked vacuolization and some shrinkage and darkening of nuclei also in evidence. This appearance is characteristic and indicative of chronic anoxic conditions (H&E, × 25 obj.).

adjust enables cells to survive under conditions that might otherwise prove lethal. Such adaptations, which include atrophy, hypertrophy, and hyperplasia, are commonly observed in the course of many disease processes (Fig. 4.3).

Atrophy

Atrophy refers to a decrease in the size and activity of a cell, which occurs as an adaptation to diminished use, or as a result of a reduction in blood supply, poor nutrition, or a decrease in normal hormonal stimulation. Cell atrophy is usually accompanied by shrinkage of the affected organ. In parenchymal organs, atrophy may result solely from a decrease in cell size. However, in the later stages of disease the decrease in cell size may also be accompanied by actual loss of cells (Fig. 4.4).

Atrophy in connective tissue is made obvious by changes in the quantity and quality of the extracellular matrix. For example loss of bone tissue (osteopenia) or loss of cartilage turgor (chondromalacia).

Hypertrophy

Hypertrophy refers to an increase in cell size caused by augmentation of the intracellular organelles, especially the endoplasmic reticulum; as a result, protein synthesis is generally enhanced (Fig. 4.4). Hypertrophy is frequently a compensatory reaction, as in the heart muscles of patients with increased cardiac workload who develop an increased number of myofibrils. In an athlete, not only is there hypertrophy of the skeletal muscle, but also a related increase in bone density (Fig. 4.5).

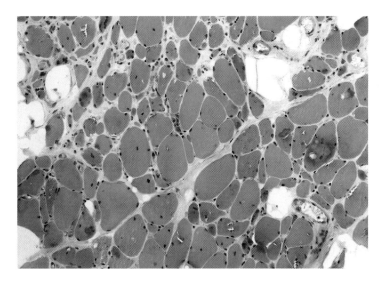

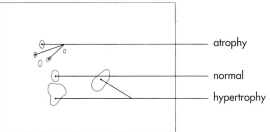

Figure 4.4 In this photomicrograph of abnormal skeletal muscle, small, atrophied fibers as well as some with increased diameter are present (H&E, × 4 obj.).

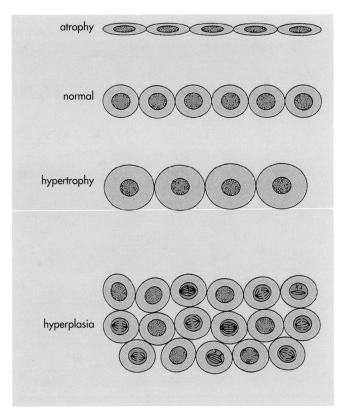

Figure 4.3 Diagrammatic representation of atrophy, hypertrophy, and hyperplasia.

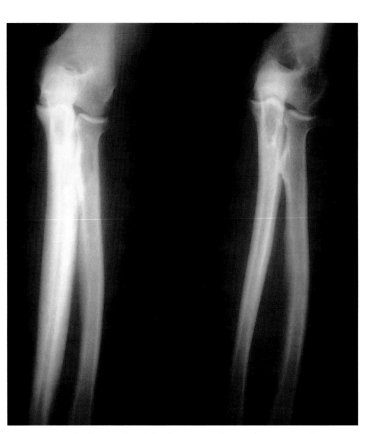

Figure 4.5 Radiographs of the forearms of a competition rodeo cowboy who specialized in bareback bronco and bull riding, show a marked hypertrophy of the right ulna typical of such athletes. (Courtesy of Dr Guerdon Greenway, Dallas, TX.)

Hyperplasia

An example of hyperplasia, an increase in the number of cells, is commonly seen in the synovium of patients with arthritis. The accelerated breakdown of the joint constituents (cartilage and bone) that occurs in all forms of arthritis leads to enhanced phagocytosis by the synovium. This increased activity is associ-

ated with augmentation of the synovial lining cells, thus increasing not only the thickness of the synovial lining but also the absolute area of the synovium, which is frequently thrown up into papillary projections that extend into the joint cavity (Fig. 4.6).

Necrosis

Necrosis is a passive process resulting in a breakdown of ordered structure and function following irreversible traumatic damage. Cell necrosis (death) is usually recognized microscopically by changes in the nucleus. These changes include swelling of the nucleus, which is followed by condensation of the nuclear chromatin (pyknosis) and finally by dissolution of the nucleus (karyolysis) (Fig. 4.7).

The gross and microscopic appearance of necrotic cells depends on the organ involved and the type and extent of injury. In tissue necrosis associated with sudden and complete cessation of the blood supply (an infarct), the affected tissue usually has a loss of translucency, i.e. an opaque appearance on gross examination and a firm consistency, like a hard-boiled egg. Microscopic examination of infarcted tissue usually reveals maintenance of structural anatomy, with preservation of the ghost-like outlines of the cells (Fig. 4.8). On the other hand, in most bacterial

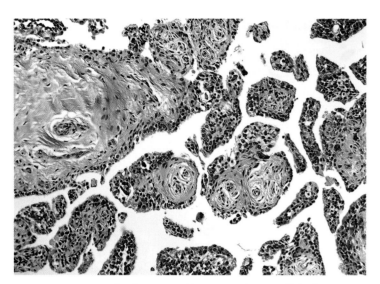

Figure 4.6 Normally, the synovial lining is only one cell thick; however, in this photomicrograph of the synovial lining from a patient with chronic osteoarthritis, one can readily see a marked proliferation of synoviocytes, characteristic of a hyperplastic condition (H&E, × 4 obj.).

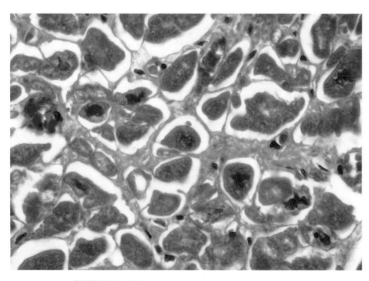

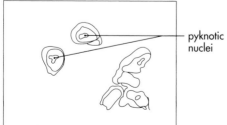

pyknotic nuclei

Figure 4.7 High-power photomicrograph of necrotizing myocardium shows a number of dense, shrunken and fragmented (pyknotic) nuclei, characteristic of cell necrosis (H&E, × 40 obj.).

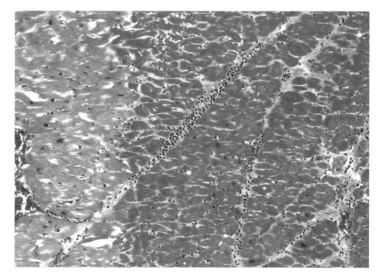

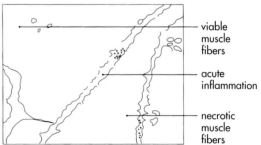

viable muscle fibers

acute inflammation

necrotic muscle fibers

Figure 4.8 The right side of this photomicrograph of myocardial tissue exhibits fibers with granular, eosinophilic cytoplasm devoid of nuclei. In addition, acute inflammatory infiltration between the muscle fibers and along the course of the myocardial capillaries can be seen. All of these features are characteristic of necrotic tissue. By contrast, note the pale cytoplasm and intact nuclei in the normal, viable tissue on the left (H&E, × 4 obj.).

injuries the cells are totally broken down, resulting in soft necrotic tissue in which no structural elements of the cell are recognizable (Fig. 4.9).

In the connective tissue because the nonviable extracellular matrix, which gives form to the tissue, is often unchanged cell necrosis may be easily overlooked. In a bone, the most obvious evidence of cellular necrosis is seen in the marrow, either as fat necrosis and dystrophic calcification or as ghosting of the hematopoietic tissue (Fig. 4.10). On the other hand, changes in the osteocytes may be difficult to recognize (Fig. 4.11) and in general it can be said that evaluation of the viability of the osteocytes is a poor way to diagnose bone necrosis. In cartilage, ghosting and sometimes calcification of the chondrocytes is a frequent finding in arthritis (Fig. 4.12). Inflammatory arthritis is often characterized by gross enlargement of the chondrocyte lacunae referred to as Weichselbaum's lacunae, which contain either pyknotic nuclei or no obvious cellular elements (Fig. 4.13).

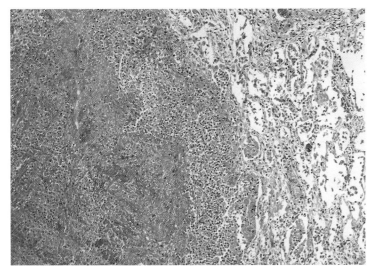

Figure 4.9   Photomicrograph showing cell degradation within an abscess. Note that at the periphery of the abscess (at right) there is an infiltration of acute inflammatory cells as well as fibrin. However, towards the center of the abscess there is complete loss of tissue architecture, with an accumulation of cell debris and acute inflammatory cells (H&E, × 4 obj.).

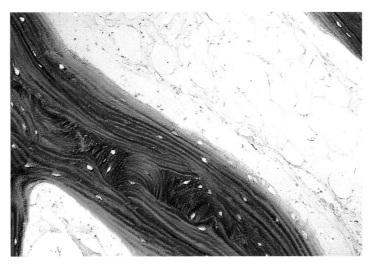

Figure 4.11   Necrotic cancellous bone. There is no hematoxylin staining of the fat cells in the marrow or of the osteocytes in the bone, although the ghosts of the cells remain. Recognition may be difficult in such cases without areas of viable bone for comparison (H&E, × 10 obj.).

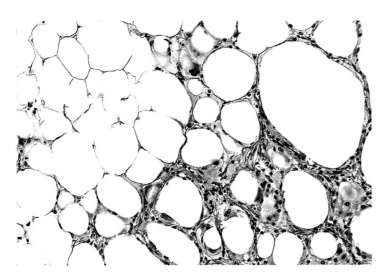

Figure 4.10   Photomicrograph showing stages of necrosis in the fatty marrow. In the upper left there is complete necrosis; on the right, ischemia has resulted in breakdown of the fat cells, with reactive chronic inflammation and foamy histiocytes (H&E, × 10 obj.).

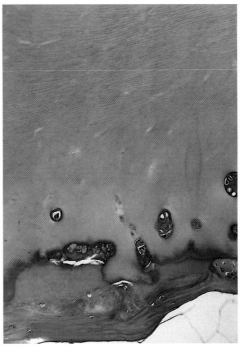

Figure 4.12 Photomicrograph revealing necrosis of virtually all chondrocytes in the articular cartilage. Isolated clones of chondrocytes are still staining with hematoxylin–eosin adjacent to the tidemark (H&E, × 4 obj.).

Figure 4.13
Photomicrograph illustrating the dissolution of the matrix that occurs around dying chondrocytes in cases of inflammatory arthritis (typically rheumatoid arthritis). Chondrocyte lacunae with this alteration in appearance are known as Weichselbaum's lacunae (H&E, × 10 obj.).

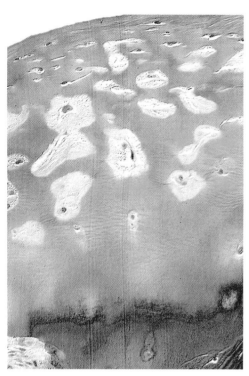

Apoptosis

In addition ·to the passive cell death following traumatic injury there is another and fundamentally different form of cell death that is genetically determined. This process balances new cell formation, through the process of mitoses, with programed cell death or apoptosis. Apoptosis is actively involved in development, and in the continuing lifelong replacement of tissues. Apoptosis also plays a role in some pathologic states including tissue injury in diseases of cellular immunity.

Unlike necrosis, which is generally associated with an obvious inflammatory response, apoptosis is difficult to observe by ordinary microscopic technique, even in very active cellular epithelial linings.

Apoptotic bodies can be recognized in paraffin-embedded sections as small round or oval cytoplasmic masses which are usually eosinophilic and may contain nuclear fragments. However, the small size of apoptotic bodies together with their short half-life renders them inconspicuous in histologic sections, even if the rate of cell deletion is high (Fig. 4.14). Immunohistologic techniques have been developed, which assist in the recognition of apoptotic cells. However, these techniques might be unreliable and it is recommended that a molecular or fluorescence-based assay is used to specify the type of cell death occurring (Fig. 4.15).

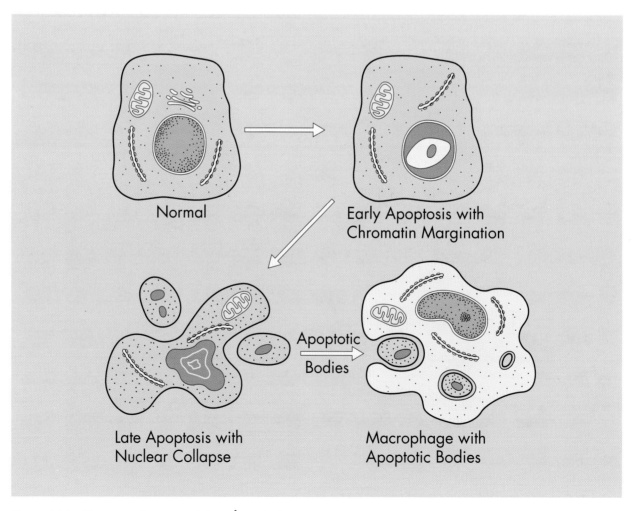

Normal

Early Apoptosis with Chromatin Margination

Apoptotic Bodies

Late Apoptosis with Nuclear Collapse

Macrophage with Apoptotic Bodies

Figure 4.14 Diagrammatic representation of apoptosis.

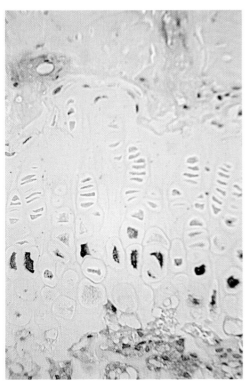

Figure 4.15
Photomicrograph of femoral epiphyseal growth plate of a young rat stained by the TdT-mediated biotinylated-dUTP nick end labeling (TUNEL) technique to demonstrate apoptotic cells in the hypertrophic zone. Note that no counterstain has been used (×25 obj.). (Courtesy of Dr Stephen Doty).

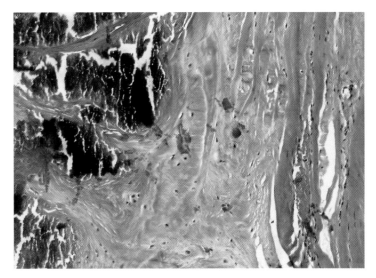

Figure 4.16 Photomicrograph shows extensive calcification in the capsule of the shoulder joint. Such dystrophic calcification is a common complication of tissue necrosis following injury (H&E, ×10 obj.).

Apoptosis has been associated with various orthopaedic pathologies. In rheumatoid arthritis, the hyperplastic synovial lining increases both through enhanced proliferation, inflammatory cell migration, as well as decreased apoptosis.

The chondrocytic production of nitric oxide (NO) and other inflammatory mediators, such as eicosanoids and cytokines is increased in osteoarthritis. The excessive production of NO inhibits matrix synthesis and promotes the mechanism of cytokine-induced apoptosis of the chondrocytes.

In the postnatal and adult skeleton, apoptosis is integral to physiological bone turnover, repair, and regeneration. The balance of osteoblast proliferation, differentiation, and apoptosis determines the size of the osteoblast population at any given time. The osteocytes appear to use some molecular signaling pathways such as the generation of NO and prostaglandins as well as directing cell–cell communication via gap junctions. They may also regulate the removal of damaged or redundant bone through mechanisms linked to their own apoptosis or via the secretion of specialized cellular attachment proteins such as osteopontin.

Certain features of growth cartilage development and mineralization are shared with aging and degenerative cartilage. These include chondrocyte proliferation, hypertrophy and increased apoptosis. Parathyroid hormone-related protein (PTHrP), one of the central mediators of endochondral development, is also abundant in osteoarthritic cartilage.

Calcification

Dead tissue that does not undergo rapid absorption frequently becomes calcified. This type of calcification, which is not related to a generalized disturbance in calcium homeostasis, as occurs with hyperparathyroidism (discussed in Chapter 8, p. 216), is called dystrophic calcification. It is common in areas of infarction, fat necrosis, and also the caseous necrosis of tuberculosis. Of particular interest to orthopaedic surgeons is the calcification commonly found in areas of injured tendons or ligaments (Fig. 4.16).

The association of crystal deposition with senile osteoarthritis is well recognized and there have been recent advances in understanding the mechanisms whereby calcium crystals contribute to cartilage damage. These may be related to the induction of proto-oncogenes, which in turn lead to crystal-induced modulation of normal gene expression in the chondrocytes.

Injury to the extracellular matrix

The extracellular matrix, which is composed of collagen, proteoglycan (PG), various noncollagenous proteins, and inorganic constituents, is a nonviable material. Nevertheless, it shows the effects of both mechanical and chemical injury. Fibrillation of the cartilage is an example of mechanical injury with disruption of the collagen framework (Fig. 4.17). The so-called 'hyalinization' of collagen is caused by chemical (usually enzymatic) breakdown of the fibrillar structure, especially of the intermolecular and possibly the intramolecular cross-linkage of the collagen molecules (Fig. 4.18).

Such injured matrices invariably have altered mechanical properties. The fibrillated cartilage does not function as well as normal cartilage, either in the transmission of load or in providing a low-friction articulating surface. The 'hyalinized' collagen, with its weakened cross-links, has lost much of its tensile strength. On the other hand unless structural changes of the bone matrix have occurred, a piece of 'dead bone' (i.e. one in which both marrow cells and bone cells are dead), is perhaps as strong as a similar piece of viable bone.

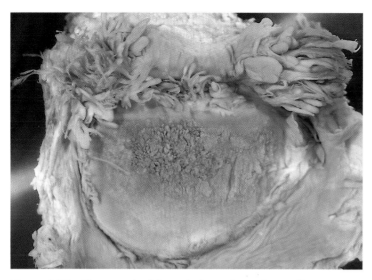

Figure 4.17 Photograph of the articular surface of a patella, illustrating loss of integrity due to collagen disruption or fibrillation. Around the edge of the patella there is a striking synovial hyperplasia. The brownish discoloration of the synovium and cartilage is secondary to old hemorrhage.

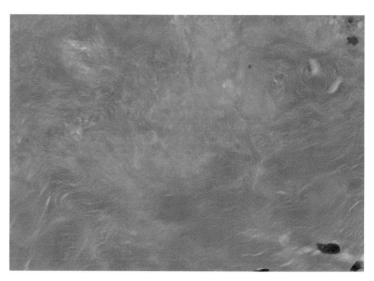

Figure 4.18 Photomicrograph of fibrous tissue to show loss of nuclei and smudging, or hyalinization, of the collagen matrix (H&E, × 50 obj.).

RESPONSE TO INJURY

The inflammatory reaction comprises the collective responses of the body, to both local and systemic injury. These responses include: removal and/or sequestration of the necrotic tissue and injurious agents; defense against further injury; and replacement of injured cells with possible restoration of tissue architecture by reparative tissue. Thus the inflammatory reaction is not confined to the acute, local cellular response, which is a popular misconception; it involves the entire body's defense mechanism and is not completed until a homeostatic state has been restored.

The sequence of events after a limited local injury is firstly vascular dilatation and increased blood flow. The blood vessel wall becomes more permeable. White blood cells attach themselves to the vascular endothelium and pass through the wall of the vessel into the extravascular space. These observations, first made in the nineteenth century by Julius Cohnheim, explain Celsus' four cardinal signs of inflammation:

1. Redness, caused by vasodilatation
2. Heat, the result of increased blood flow
3. Swelling, caused by exudation of fluids and cells into the extravascular spaces
4. Pain, the result of irritation of the nerve endings.

Swelling, caused by the accumulation of protein-rich fluid (or exudate) in the injured tissue, is always present to a greater or lesser degree during the acute stage of inflammation and occurs because the vessels of the inflamed tissue are directly injured or because they become more permeable.

Increased permeability of the vessels is brought about by substances released from and/or produced by the damaged tissue. These substances, which are referred to as inflammatory mediators, have two sources: the cells and plasma.

In cells, the mediators are either preformed or are newly synthesized in response to the injurious agent. Preformed mediators include histamine, serotonin (mast cells and basophils) and lysosomal enzymes (leukocytes and monocytes). Newly synthesized mediators are produced principally by leukocytes, monocytes and endothelial cells and include NO, platelet-activating factor, leukotrienes, prostaglandins and cytokines. In the plasma the two primary mediators are the various components of complement and factor XII (Hageman factor).

The complex interactions of these various substances which affect most aspects of normal physiology as well as pathophysiology are beyond the scope of this book and are the subject of many monographs.

The accumulation and activation of leukocytes are central events in virtually all forms of inflammation and deficiencies in these processes generally lead to a compromised host reaction. The migration (diapedesis) of leukocytes through the wall of the capillary and venule is an active rather than a passive phenomenon. Even after fluid exudation has passed its peak, leukocyte migration continues, presumably as a result of a persistent chemotactic effect of the injurious agent and the injured tissue (Fig. 4.19).

Although Cohnheim described the migration of white blood cells through the vessel walls, it was Elie Metchnikoff who, a few years later, determined the function of these cells. He observed that they were capable of engulfing foreign matter, including bacteria, and he called this process phagocytosis. Because both large and small cells are involved in phagocytic activity, he called the large cells macrophages and the small cells microphages [now referred to as polymorphonuclear leukocytes (PMNs) or neutrophils] (Fig. 4.20).

The type of cell seen microscopically in the cell infiltrate depends firstly on the nature of the injury (e.g. bacterial injury results in a marked neutrophilic infiltrate, whereas a mechanical injury does not) and secondly on the elapsed time since injury. Within the first few hours, and up to a day or so, the predominant cells in the tissue exudate are PMNs. However, after a period

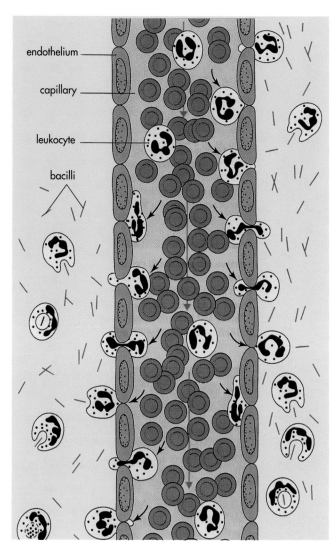

Figure 4.19 Schematic diagram illustrates the migration of leukocytes across the vascular endothelium into the adjacent tissue. Once in the tissue, the leukocytes may encounter and engulf any existing microbes by means of phagocytosis.

labels on figure: endothelium, capillary, leukocyte, bacilli

A chronic inflammatory response also results from certain bacterial infections, including tuberculosis and syphilis, as well as with fungal infection. Persistent inflammatory stimuli lead to chronic inflammation, which is characteristic of autoimmune diseases (e.g. rheumatoid arthritis and systemic lupus erythematosus) and the introduction of foreign bodies.

Most forms of acute and chronic inflammation depend on the recruitment of humoral and cellular components of the immune system. Immunologically mediated elimination of foreign material requires a number of steps. First, the material to be eliminated (i.e. antigen) is recognized as being 'foreign'. Specific recognition is mediated by immunoglobulins (i.e. antibodies) or by receptors on T-lymphocytes that bind to specific determinants (epitopes). Nonspecific recognition (i.e. of denatured proteins or endotoxins) can be mediated by the alternative complement pathway or by phagocytes. The binding of a recognition component of the immune system to an antigen generally initiates production of proinflammatory substances which alter blood flow, increase vascular permeability, augment adherence of circulating leukocytes to vascular endothelium and promote migration of leukocytes into tissues. The actual destruction of antigens is mediated by phagocytic cells. Such cells may migrate freely, e.g. leukocytes, or may exist at fixed tissue sites as components of the mononuclear phagocyte system (e.g. Kupffer's cells in the liver and type-A synovial lining cells).

For the most part the processes of the immune system lead to the elimination of antigens without producing clinically detectable inflammation. The development of clinical inflammation indicates either an unusually large amount of antigen, a virulent antigen, or a depressed immune response.

The initial phase of the inflammatory reaction serves as a defense and a means for removal or sequestration of necrotic tissue; the final component of the inflammatory reaction is repair. Amongst the most important mediators of the inflammatory response are the cytokines, which are mostly the product of sensitized lymphocytes and are involved in every stage of wound healing (Fig. 4.24). Some of the factors which affect bone and cartilage growth and repair include transforming growth factor beta (TGF-β), insulin-like growth factor (IGF), platelet-derived growth factor (PDGF), β2-microglobulin, bone morphogenetic protein (BMP), interleukin-1 (IL-1) and tumor necrosis factor (TNF).

Eventual restoration of the damaged area may involve cell regeneration of tissue similar to the original, or replacement by fibrous connective tissue (scar tissue); but usually a combination of these two processes occurs. In general, the epithelium of the skin, the gastrointestinal tract, and the respiratory tract, as well as the connective tissues all regenerate well. However the more specialized and differentiated tissues are, the more limited their regenerative capacity. It is important to recognize that regeneration of tissue does not imply restoration of anatomy and in the case of the connective tissues especially, failure to restore anatomy may lead to failure of function.

Perhaps the most characteristic early histologic finding in the reparative stage of the inflammatory response is the proliferation of capillaries and fibroblasts that comprise granulation tissue (Fig. 4.25). In granulation tissue, the fibroblasts produce the structural extracellular matrix, composed of collagen, PG, and other noncollagenous proteins which give body and strength to the new scar tissue.

The clinician should take every opportunity to promote regu-

of 24–48 hours, more of the cells in the exudate are seen to be mononuclear – lymphocytes and macrophages. This biphasic response may be the result of a sequential action by specific chemical mediators.

Polymorphonuclear and mononuclear phagocytes migrate into the damaged tissues, where they engulf and digest bacteria and necrotic cells (Fig. 4.21). Phagocytes are equipped for this task by their possession of large numbers of cytoplasmic granules, including large dense granules (lysosomes), which contain various enzymes such as acid phosphatase, an antibacterial substance called lysozyme, and peroxidase.

The acute inflammatory reaction may either subside, as is usually the case, or, in the presence of continuing cell injury, it may persist and become chronic. On microscopic examination, chronic inflammation is distinguished from acute inflammation by a marked increase in the number of mononuclear cells in the inflamed area. These mononuclear cells include macrophages, lymphocytes, and plasma cells (Figs 4.22 and 4.23).

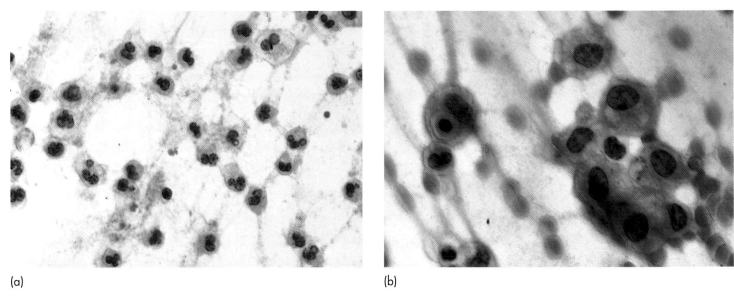

(a)

(b)

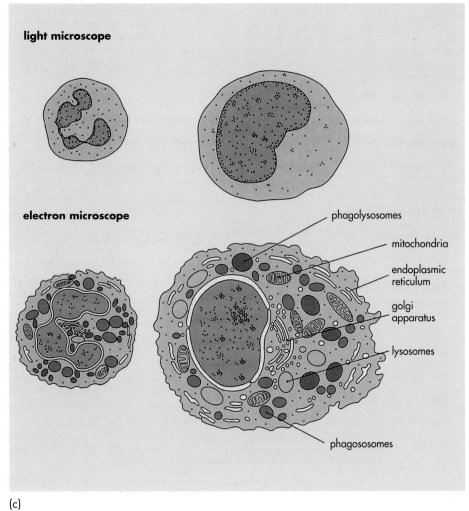

light microscope

electron microscope

phagolysosomes

mitochondria

endoplasmic
reticulum

golgi
apparatus

lysosomes

phagososomes

(c)

Figure 4.20 Photomicrographs of PMN leukocytes
(a) and histiocytes (b) (H&E, × 100 obj.).
(c) Diagrammatic representations of the light
microscopic and electron microscopic characteristics
of a PMN leukocyte (left) and a histiocyte (right).

lated healing; the prevention both of delayed healing and excessive scarring are equally important. Therapeutic measures include wound debridement, adequate administration of antibiotics, use of nonreactive suture material, and good surgical technique. The avoidance or at least the limitation of drugs that suppress the inflammatory reaction [e.g. cortisone and non-steroidal anti-inflammatory drugs (NSAIDs)] is important, and adequate intake of substances necessary for wound healing (protein and vitamin C) is essential. (However, there are cases in which the use of corticosteroids may be necessary to suppress excessive scar formation.)

During most of the inflammatory response, the exudative and reparative events take place simultaneously, although the exudative features predominate in the early stages of the process, and

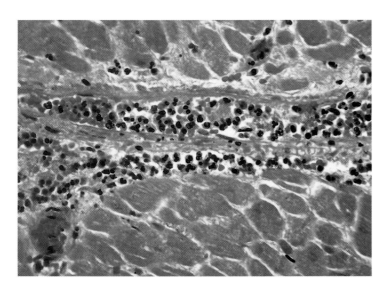

Figure 4.21 This photomicrograph illustrates the events during an acute inflammatory reaction brought on by tissue necrosis (in this case, specifically, by myocardial infarction). A small capillary is congested with blood and with many more PMNs than would normally be expected. These PMNs have infiltrated the vessel wall by diapedesis and are now seen in the perivascular tissue (H&E, × 32 obj.).

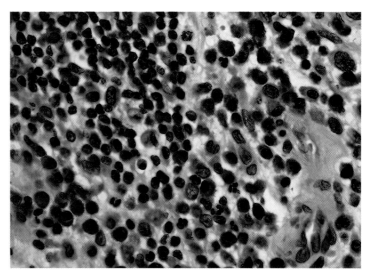

Figure 4.23 This high-power photomicrograph reveals perivascular chronic inflammatory infiltrate of lymphocytes and plasma cells (H&E, × 100 obj.).

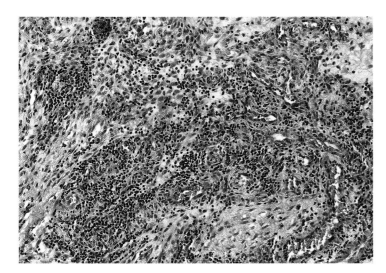

Figure 4.22 In this photomicrograph, a chronic inflammatory reaction is characterized by an extensive infiltration of mononuclear cells (H&E, × 10 obj.).

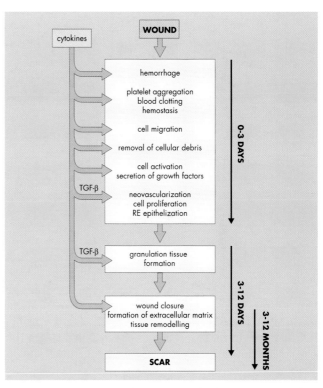

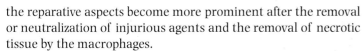

Figure 4.24 Numerous cytokines are involved in every stage of wound healing, however, it appears that TGF-β is a major factor in matrix protein synthesis and the formation of granulation tissue.

the reparative aspects become more prominent after the removal or neutralization of injurious agents and the removal of necrotic tissue by the macrophages.

Following is a series of discussion on repair of connective tissues after trauma.

SURGICAL WOUND HEALING

In the case of a surgical wound, all tissue in the path of the knife blade (including the epithelium, fibrous connective tissues, blood vessels, nerves and fat) is injured either reversibly or irreversibly. When the wound edges have been apposed and the sutures applied, a thin clot fills the space between the apposed wound edges and, in the absence of bacterial contamination, the acute inflammatory response is limited. The macrophages rapidly mobilize to remove red blood cells, fibrin, and damaged tissue. Meanwhile, the fibroblasts on either side of the wound hypertrophy and migrate, together with capillary sprouts, and within a few days circulation is re-established across the margins of the wound.

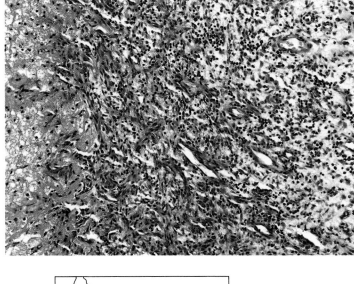

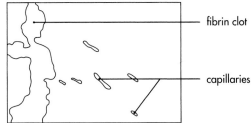

fibrin clot

capillaries

Figure 4.25 Photomicrograph of granulation tissue in an early stage of repair. Note the fibrin clot on the left, and the proliferating fibroblasts and capillaries interspersed with chronic inflammatory cells towards the right (H&E, × 4 obj.).

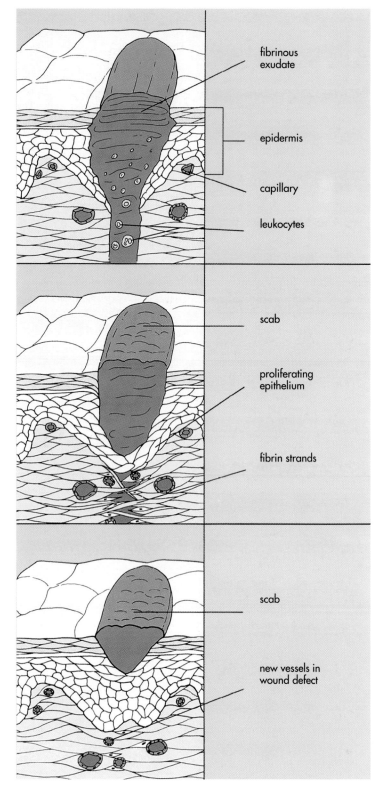

fibrinous exudate

epidermis

capillary

leukocytes

scab

proliferating epithelium

fibrin strands

scab

new vessels in wound defect

Figure 4.26 Schematic diagram illustrates the healing process in epithelial tissue after ulceration. The wound is first filled with a fibrinous exudate composed of acute inflammatory cells. This is gradually replaced by granulation tissue, with proliferating epithelium extending from the margins of the wound, over the granulation tissue, and beneath the residual fibrin of the surface. As the epithelium completely re-covers the wound, the dried-up layer of fibrin forms a scab, which eventually falls off.

As the fibroblasts lay down collagen, the cellular inflammatory infiltrate diminishes. The epithelial cells at the surface begin to undergo mitosis and to migrate over the vascularized granulation tissue. In the case of a nonlinear wound, as the epithelial cells migrate over the granulation tissue they extend beneath the fibrin clot (scab) that closes off the surface of the wound. When the epithelium is firmly re-established underneath the scab, the scab sloughs off (Fig. 4.26).

The suture material used to appose the wound edges frequently causes a foreign body giant-cell reaction. In our experience this has been most severe with some types of absorbable sutures where the suture material breaks up into myriads of fragments (Fig. 4.27). The suture may also act as a track along which bacteria may travel. If infection is thus induced, healing is delayed until the infection has been overcome. Healing may also be delayed if there is poor circulation in the area, or if the patient is severely debilitated.

MUSCLES

Contrary to widespread belief, muscle tissue regenerates well, but the restoration of normal structure and function is very dependent on the type of injury sustained. In severe infections the muscle fibers may be extensively destroyed. However, the sarcolemmal sheaths usually remain intact and rapid regeneration of muscle cells within the sheaths occurs, so that the function of the muscle may be completely restored (Fig. 4.28).

After the transection of a muscle, muscle fibers may regenerate either by growth from undamaged stumps or by growth of new, independent fibers. The nuclei for both of these processes are derived from the satellite or reserve cells found in the endomy-

sium. However as the muscle fibers regenerate and grow, there is also an ingrowth into the damaged muscle of capillaries and fibroblasts, with accompanying production of collagen; this scarring usually overrides and prevents muscle fiber regeneration (Fig. 4.29). In muscle regeneration and healing, much depends on the correct alignment of the supportive structures by meticulous surgical restoration.

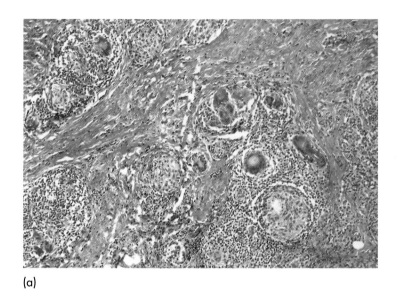

(a)

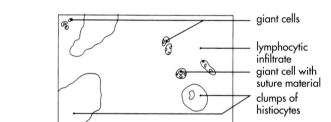

giant cells

lymphocytic infiltrate

giant cell with suture material

clumps of histiocytes

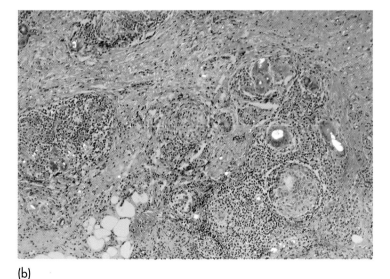

(b)

Figure 4.27 The introduction of foreign matter into tissue frequently leads to a chronic inflammatory reaction, with proliferating macrophages digesting the foreign material. Photomicrograph (a) shows giant cells and chronic inflammatory cells, giving the appearance of a granulomatous inflammation. However, under polarized light (b), one can clearly see the fragments of suture material that gave rise to this reaction (H&E, × 4 obj.).

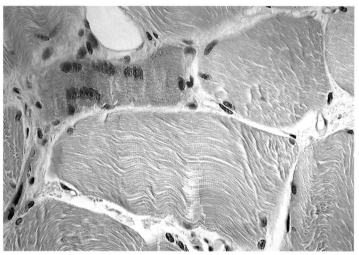

Figure 4.28 Photomicrograph shows a regenerating muscle fiber (upper left). Note the basophilic cytoplasm and the centrally located nuclei (H&E, × 40 obj.).

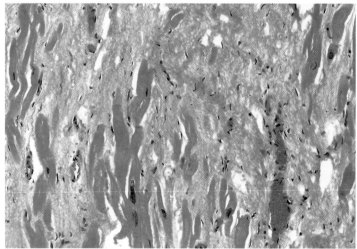

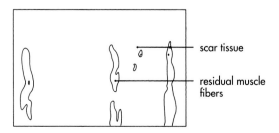

scar tissue

residual muscle fibers

Figure 4.29 Photomicrograph of damaged myocardial tissue shows extensive fibrous scarring, with only a few muscle fibers enmeshed in the dense scar tissue. This scarring blocks any potential for regeneration and restoration of the muscle tissue (H&E, × 25 obj.).

Compartment syndrome (Volkmann's ischemic contracture)

Compartment syndrome, that is, swelling and ultimate loss of viability of a muscle group, is caused by compromised circulation within a confined anatomic space. The condition most commonly involves the anterior tibial compartment of the leg, the volar compartment of the forearm, or the interosseous compartments of the hand (Fig. 4.30).

In general, compartment syndrome results from trauma to an extremity (usually a fracture or crush injury; recently, the disorder has also been seen in patients suffering from i.v. drug overdose). Vascular occlusion from either direct injury or increased pressure within the anatomic compartment leads to diminished tissue viability and function. Pain and swelling are prominent symptoms. Muscle necrosis ensues, and eventually the original tissue is replaced by dense, fibrous connective tissue, with subsequent deformity and loss of function. Microscopic findings depend on the stage at which the tissue is obtained. Muscle necrosis, granulation, scar tissue, and calcification may all be present (Fig. 4.31).

Treatment of the acute condition is aimed at relieving the pressure by fasciotomy, the removal of tight bandages, or whatever is appropriate to the circumstances.

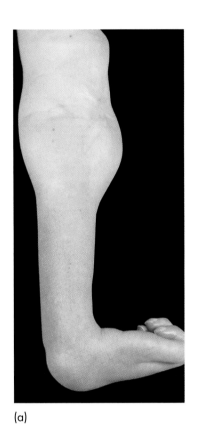

(a)

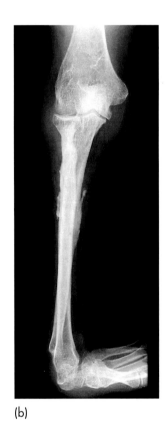

(b)

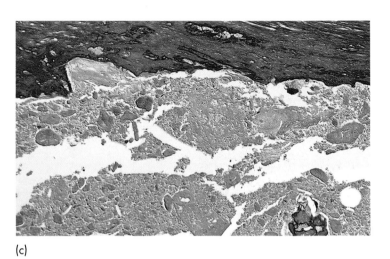

(c)

Figure 4.30 (a) Clinical photograph of the arm in an untreated patient who developed compartment syndrome after multiple injuries to the elbow and forearm some months earlier. Note the severe flexion contractures. (b) Radiograph of the arm shown in (a). In addition to evidence of traumatic arthritis, there is also some shortening of the ulna and mature bone formation around the ulna and radius in the upper third of the forearm. (c) Photomicrograph shows that the involved tissue is entirely necrotic. The purple-stained areas have calcified (H&E, × 4 obj.).

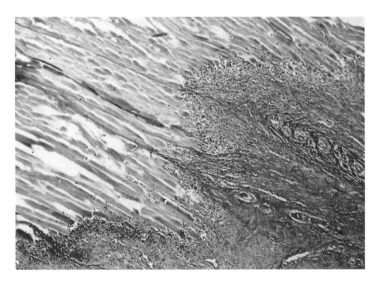

Figure 4.31 Histologic section through a part of the muscle mass of the anterior tibial compartment involved in compartment syndrome reveals extensive muscle necrosis, with, on the right, an inflammatory reaction and fibrous replacement at the margin of the infarcted tissue (H&E, × 4 obj.).

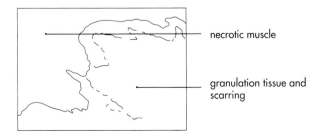

necrotic muscle

granulation tissue and scarring

TENDONS AND LIGAMENTS

Rupture of a tendon or ligament in a healthy individual is extremely rare, occurring only in association with a severe injury or with chronic repetitive injury. The slow application of excessive load usually results in an avulsion of the tendinous or ligamentous insertion and includes the bone. The rapid application of excessive load in a tendon usually results in a separation at the musculo-tendinous junction. Risk factors for spontaneous (i.e. low threshold) rupture include fluoroquinolone or steroid therapy; hypercholesterolemia; rheumatoid arthritis; Marfan's syndrome, Ehlers–Danlos syndrome, and other connective tissue diseases.

Tendons may heal either as a result of proliferation of the tenoblasts from the cut ends of the tendon, or more likely, as a result of vascular ingrowth and proliferation of fibroblasts derived from the surrounding tissues that were injured at the same time as the tendon. Because the surrounding tissues contribute so much to the healing of a tendon, adhesions are very common. To avoid this complication, the repair of lacerated tendons in the hand requires meticulous atraumatic technique. With rupture of the Achilles tendon or of the cruciate ligament, functional restoration usually requires apposition and suturing of the cut ends (Figs 4.32 and 4.33).

PERIPHERAL NERVES

When a nerve fiber is divided, the peripheral portion rapidly undergoes myelin degeneration and axonal fragmentation. The lipid debris is removed by macrophages mobilized from the surrounding tissues (Wallerian degeneration). In the central stump, the nerve fibers retract and the axons adjacent to the cut degenerate. However, within 24 hours of section, new axonal sprouts from the central stump can usually be demonstrated, together with proliferation of Schwann cells from both the central and peripheral stumps (Fig. 4.34). With careful microsurgical approximation of the nerve, reinnervation may be achieved. The most important requirement of successful nerve regeneration following repair is the maintenance of the neurotubules along which the new axonal sprouts can pass.

Carpal tunnel syndrome

Carpal tunnel syndrome is an entrapment neuropathy caused by pressure on the median nerve as it passes under the transverse carpal ligament and over the hollow of the carpal bones (Fig. 4.35). Patients usually complain of night pain, often accompanied by paresthesia in the distribution of the median nerve. In advanced cases, wasting of the thenar muscles may occur. The cause of the increased pressure varies, but most often it results from post-traumatic fibrosis or synovitis. Occasionally carpal tunnel syndrome may herald rheumatoid arthritis or other synovial disease and, on rare occasions, it has been found to result from amyloid deposits (a discussion on the difficulties of diagnosing amyloid in connective tissue will be found in Chapter 9. p. 224).

Microscopic examination of the transverse carpal ligament usually reveals nonspecific fibrosis and occasional fibrocartilaginous metaplasia. This syndrome is treated by surgical division of the transverse carpal ligament. At operation, the nerve is often seen to be congested above the ligament, and constricted and pale where it lies under the ligament (Fig. 4.36).

Two conditions that may be related to carpal tunnel syndrome

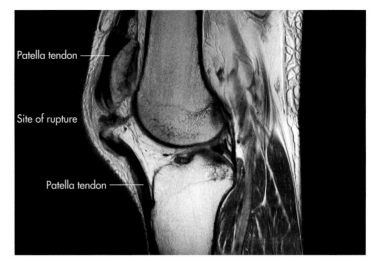

(a)

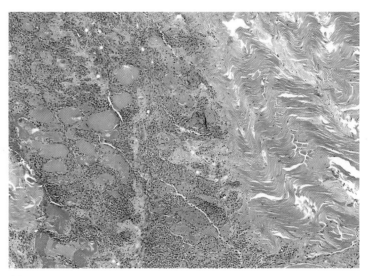

(b)

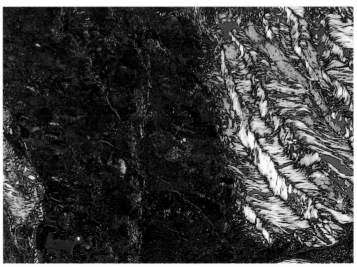

(c)

Figure 4.32 (a) Magnetic resonance image of a knee which demonstrates a rupture of the patella tendon. (b) Photomicrograph of acutely ruptured tendon to show the interruption of the collagen bundles and an acute inflammatory response (H&E, × 10 obj.). (c) Same field photographed with polarized light to highlight the discontinuity of the tendon collagen.

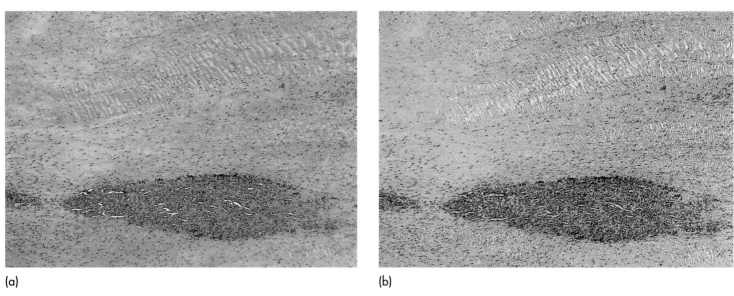

(a)   (b)

Figure 4.33   (**a**) Photomicrograph of a segment of ruptured tendon in the healing phase. Cellular collagenous tissue has largely filled in the traumatic defect. One focus of vascular granulation tissue is still present. Part of the original tendon is seen towards the top of the picture. (**b**) Same field photographed with polarized light to highlight the tendon collagen (H&E, × 10 obj.).

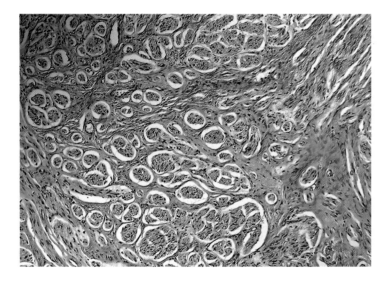

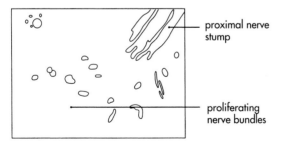

Figure 4.34   After nerve damage, the proximal stump of the damaged nerve demonstrates proliferation of Schwann cells and eventually of axons. Unless the nerve fascicles are meticulously approximated, adequate restoration of the nerve fibers will not occur. This photomicrograph shows the proximal stump at right, and a tangled mass of proliferating (regenerative) Schwann cells and axons at left (H&E, × 4 obj.).

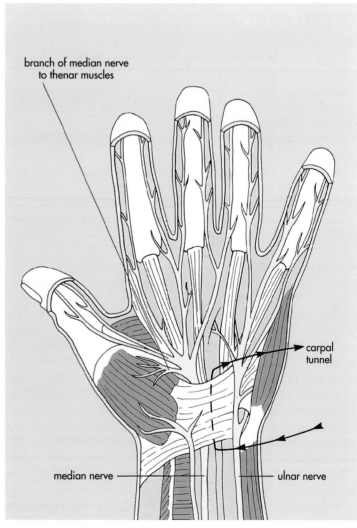

Figure 4.35   This diagram of a dissected hand shows the median nerve passing through the carpal tunnel and under the transverse carpal ligament.

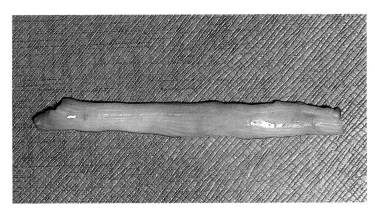

Figure 4.36   Gross photograph of a segment of the median nerve, resected at autopsy from the part of the nerve that had entered the carpal tunnel. Note the slight constriction and pale appearance in the area of the nerve that had coursed under the transverse carpal ligament (on the left) as compared with the pink appearance of the slightly swollen nerve proximal to the ligament (on the right).

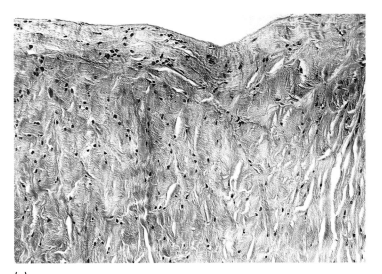

(a)

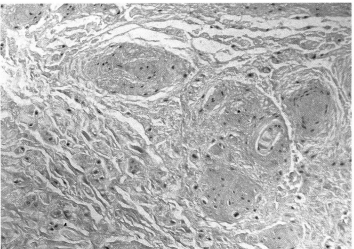

(b)

Figure 4.37   (a) Photomicrograph of a portion of tissue excised from the thickened tendon sheath in a case of trigger finger. Note the fibrocartilaginous metaplasia of the subsynovial tissue (H&E with Nomarski, × 10 obj.). (b) In another field of the thickened tendon sheath, there is a more disorganized fibrocartilaginous matrix (H&E, × 10 obj.).

are trigger finger and de Quervain's disease (stenosing tenovaginitis of the common tendon sheath of the abductor pollicis longus and the extensor pollicis brevis). In both of these conditions the free movement of the tendon is blocked by a focal thickening of the tendon sheath, which results from fibrocartilaginous metaplasia (Fig. 4.37). The treatment is excision.

BONE

Bone injury (fracture)

Fracture of the bone results from a combination of mechanical injury, failure of neuromuscular coordination and the strength of the bone itself. Many fractures seen in hospital practice are in elderly people; in these patients, fractures of the vertebral bodies, femoral neck, and wrist are common, usually as the result of osteoporosis together with an increased liability to falls resulting from a deterioration in neuromuscular coordination.

A recently recognized fracture mostly seen in elderly individuals is a subchondral insufficiency fracture usually occurring in the femoral head or medial femoral condyle of the knee. These lesions are discussed in more detail in Chapter 11, p. 273.

Children with meningomyelocele may present with severe periarticular fractures resulting in a Charcot joint which may on occasion simulate a malignant tumor (Fig. 4.38).

Pathological fractures result from weakening of the bone caused by local disease such as tumor or infection. In such a case the underlying disease process may be masked by the fracture callus and therefore not readily be apparent to the attending physician.

Child abuse and even abuse of the elderly often lead to nonaccidental injury fractures. These fractures may be present without there necessarily being any external evidence of trauma. In children such fractures need to be distinguished from pathologic fracture secondary to an underlying metabolic disturbance such as osteogenesis imperfecta.

The minor injuries of everyday life may result in individual trabecular fractures in cancellous bone, microfractures (Figs 4.39 and 4.40). Repetitive stress to the bone, as occurs in hikers, long-distance runners, and very commonly in dancers, may result in cumulative microfractures and the development of stress (or fatigue) fractures usually in the feet or in the tibia (shin splints) (Figs 4.41 and 4.42). Such lesions occur without a history of significant mechanical trauma, and therefore may be misinterpreted by the clinician, radiologist, or pathologist as a neoplasm. Repeated trauma at ligamentous and tendinous insertions that results in an avulsion fracture may also exhibit a pseudosarcomatous appearance, both radiographically and histologically. In young adolescents, such injuries are most likely to occur in and around the pelvis, particularly at the origins of the adductor muscles along the inferior pubic ramus adjacent to the symphysis pubis; the lower head of the rectus femoris just above the acetabulum; and the origins of the hamstring muscles at the ischial tuberosity, as well as the insertions of the gluteus at the greater trochanter and the psoas at the lesser trochanter (Fig. 4.43).

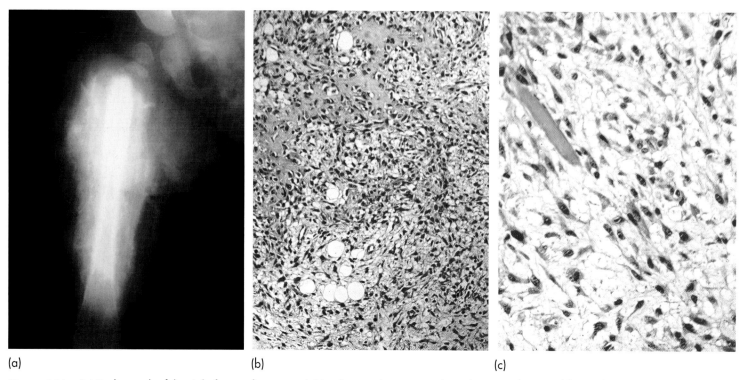

(a)   (b)   (c)

Figure 4.38 (a) Radiograph of the right femur of a young child with a myelomeningocele and a recent history of fever of unknown origin. Because of the swelling and redness of the leg, the radiograph was interpreted as either osteomyelitis or a primary malignant tumor; it is however the result of a fracture. (b) Low-power photomicrograph shows islands of immature fracture callus with proliferating fibroblastic tissue (H&E, × 10 obj.). (c) The higher power photomicrograph confirms the absence of inflammatory cells or a malignant tumor (H&E, × 25 obj.). (Courtesy of Dr Julius Smith).

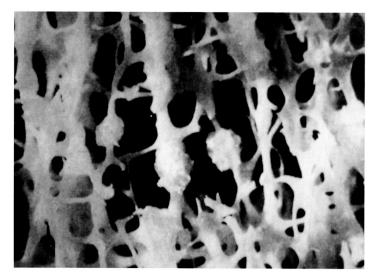

Figure 4.39 Enlarged photograph of an area of subarticular cancellous bone, showing three microfractures, which are recognized by the presence of cocoon-like microcallus attached to the trabeculae.

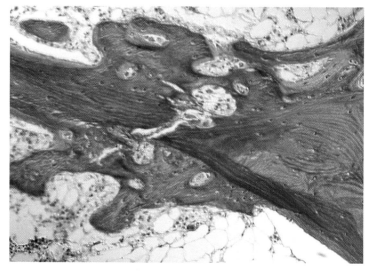

Figure 4.40 Photomicrograph of a microfracture through a single trabecula. Note the fracture line, the resorption at the fracture line, and the surrounding reactive immature bone of the microcallus (H&E, Nomarski optics, × 4 obj.).

Repeated trauma at the insertion of the adductor muscles of the thigh may lead to the formation of a bony spur on the lower medial aspect of the femur, often referred to as a rider's spur because it is commonly seen in those who ride horseback.

In children around the ages of 10 and 11 years, avulsion fractures are also seen at the tibial tubercle, where the effects of the injury and eventual repair result in the lesion known as Osgood–Schlatter disease (Fig. 4.44).

Because bone is a composite material and is also anisotropic (see Chapter 1, pp. 6 and 14), the gross appearance of a fracture depends on the microstructure of the bone tissue. Bone's most important structural features, in terms of fracture propagation

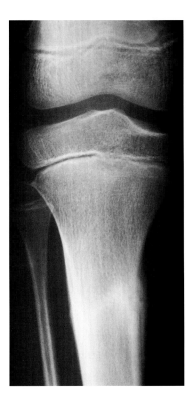

Figure 4.41 In this young individual (open growth plate), an area of sclerosis is apparent on the medial side of the tibia. Overlying the sclerotic area is a periosteal reaction extending down the shaft of the tibia. A horizontal lucent line in the sclerotic zone marks the fracture line.

are its many weak interfaces, which include both the cement lines as well as the osteocyte lacunae and canaliculi dispersed throughout the matrix. The osteocyte lacunae can act as sites of crack initiation, and the cement lines provide the major planes of fracture propagation (Fig. 4.45). The alignment of the cement lines in the cortical bone is predominantly longitudinal and is partially responsible for the obliquity of most fractures in the shafts of long bones. In diseases in which the microstructure of bone is markedly disturbed (e.g. in osteopetrosis or Paget's disease, the transverse pattern of fractures in a long bone reflect the disturbance in microarchitecture).

The direction in which a load is applied also determines the direction of the fracture. In general, tensile loads cause flat fractures, whereas compressive loads result in oblique fractures, usually with greater damage to the bone. Bending forces cause fractures which combine the features of tensile and compressive fractures, and torsional loads usually lead to helical fractures (Fig. 4.46).

Bone fracture repair

Fortunately, the healing of bone is one of the great successes of nature. Under favorable conditions and provided the fractured ends are properly aligned, bone can regenerate and remodel to function optimally.

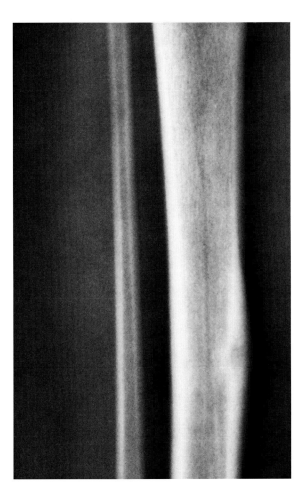

Figure 4.42 Clinical radiograph of a stress fracture of the leg. A patient with this type of fracture usually does not have a history of trauma, and presents clinically with pain and swelling in the affected parts after strenuous physical activity. The periosteal elevation, combined with a lack of displacement or obvious fracture line through the bone, may lead to this fracture being misdiagnosed radiographically as a tumor. Even if a biopsy is obtained, the hypercellular appearance of the callus may lead the pathologist to believe that this is a cellular bone-forming neoplasm or, as in this case, an osteoid osteoma.

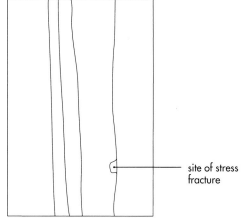

site of stress fracture

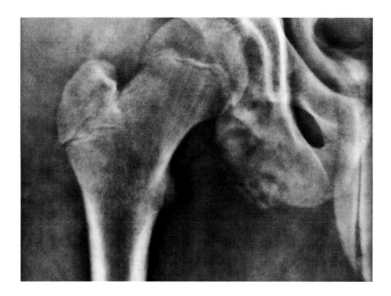

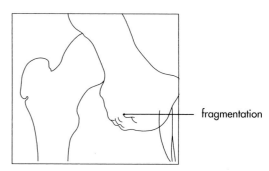

Figure 4.43   Clinical radiograph shows an avulsion fracture in the pelvis. Note the fragmentation due to avulsion injury of the ischial tuberosity. This fracture, like the stress fracture in Figure 4.42 may easily be misdiagnosed as a tumor, either radiographically or microscopically.

fragmentation

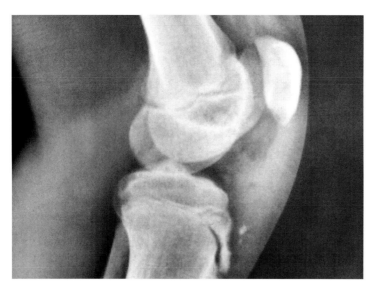

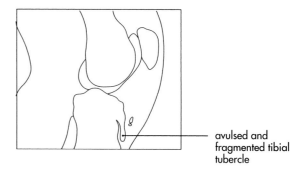

Figure 4.44   Clinical radiograph of the knee in a 12-year-old child shows fragmentation and avulsion of the tibial tubercle. This condition, known as Osgood–Schlatter disease, is almost certainly post-traumatic.

avulsed and fragmented tibial tubercle

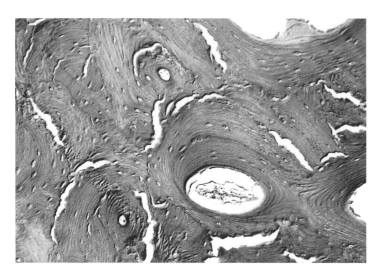

Figure 4.45   As bone fracture develops, the propagation of cracks is likely to follow the cement lines. In this photomicrograph, the cement lines are indicated by cracks which have developed during tissue sectioning (H&E, × 10 obj.).

The single most important factor in the primary healing of a fracture is complete immobilization of the fractured bone ends. In nature, this immobilization is achieved through the production of immature bone and cartilage matrix by the cambial layer of cells in the periosteum, and from undifferentiated mesenchymal cells in the soft tissues around the broken ends of the bone. This immature reparative tissue is referred to as the fracture callus (Fig. 4.47).

The amount of callus produced depends on a number of factors, including the degree of instability and the vascularity of the injured bone. The amount of callus is usually increased in unstable fractures, where the callus often contains much cartilage tissue (Figs 4.48 and 4.49). In poorly vascularized areas of the skeleton (e.g. the midshaft of the tibia), callus formation may be scant; consequently, healing may be delayed, sometimes indefinitely. This delay often gives rise to chronic nonunion of the fracture site (Fig. 4.50).

When a fracture occurs, the amount of injury sustained by the bone itself and by the surrounding soft tissues depends on the direction and magnitude of the force applied. The bone fragments

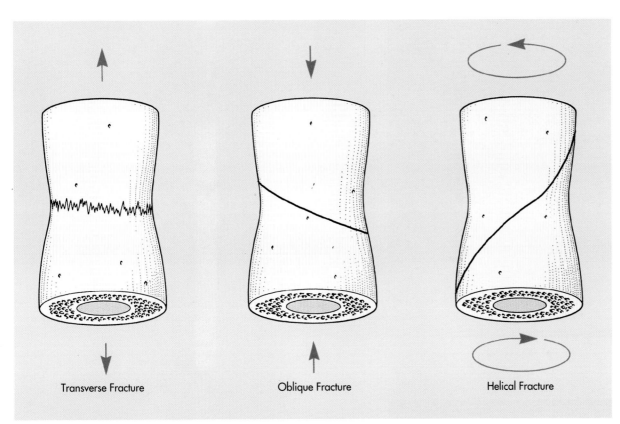

Transverse Fracture   Oblique Fracture   Helical Fracture

Figure 4.46   These diagrams illustrate three different kinds of fractures, and how they are caused. (Left) Transverse fracture, caused by traction (pulling force). (Center) Oblique fracture caused by compression. (Right) Helical fracture, caused by torsion. These differences in the pattern of fracture will apply not only to a whole bone but to an individual trabeculum.

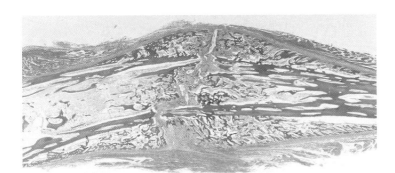

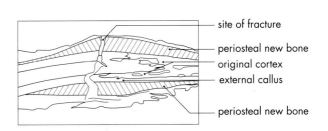

site of fracture
periosteal new bone
original cortex
external callus
periosteal new bone

Figure 4.47   Low-power photomicrograph shows reparative new bone that has formed in the soft tissue and periosteum surrounding a fractured rib. Restoration of bone cortex and medulla depends on complete immobilization of the fracture site, which is accomplished naturally through the formation of external callus. However, when a fracture is treated by rigid internal fixation, external callus may not be evident because it is not necessary (H&E, × 1.5 obj.).

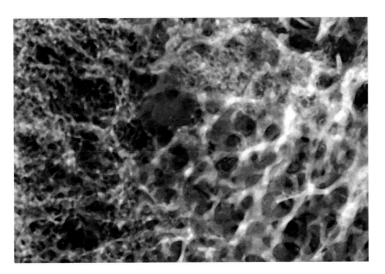

Figure 4.48   Fine grain radiograph to show the fine trabecular pattern of callus (left) as compared to normal cancellous bone at the right (magnification × 4).

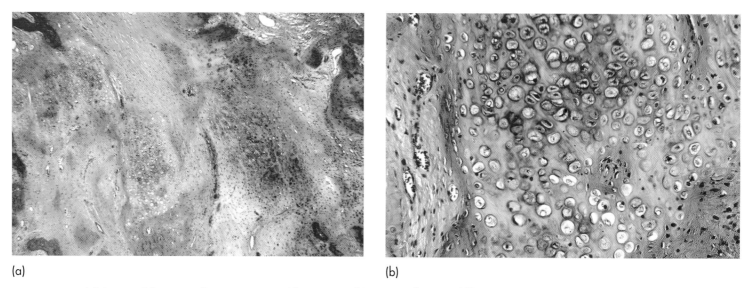

(a)   (b)

Figure 4.49   (a) A normal fracture callus contains variable amounts of bone, cartilage, and fibrous tissue depending on the stability, vascularity and extent of injury (H&E, × 4 obj.). (b) When a fracture is unstable or when the fracture site is poorly vascularized, an abundance of cartilage will be found, as seen in this photomicrograph (H&E, × 25 obj.).

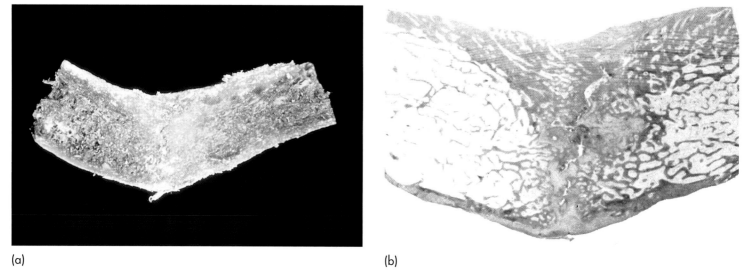

(a)   (b)

Figure 4.50   Healing may be delayed in a poorly vascularized or extremely unstable fracture, and sometimes may not even occur at all. In such a case, a false joint or pseudoarthrosis is formed. (a) Gross specimen of a long-term nonunion bone. (b) Microscopic examination will reveal dense fibrous connective tissue and lack of bony union (H&E, × 1.5 obj.).

may be displaced. The fracture line may be single (a simple fracture) or the bone may be broken into many fragments (a comminuted fracture). If the skin over the fractured bone is also broken, the injury is considered a compound fracture, and infection is a common complication. In some cases, soft tissue may become interposed between the fractured ends of the bone, causing healing to be significantly delayed. For all these reasons, the histologic appearance of the reparative tissue surrounding a fracture is variable.

Tissue obtained within a few days of injury usually shows areas of hemorrhage and acute tissue damage (Fig. 4.51). The bone and bone marrow on either side of the fracture undergo necrosis, the extent of which depends on the local anatomy (Fig.

4.52). Fractures of the femoral neck, of some of the carpal and tarsal bones, and of the patella frequently demonstrate widespread bone necrosis because the local vascular supply is severely compromised (Fig. 4.53). In a comminuted fracture the separate bone fragments are also likely to undergo necrosis. If bone and/or soft-tissue necrosis is extensive, healing will be delayed.

Microscopic examination of tissue from a 2-week-old fracture callus generally shows markedly cellular tissue, usually hypervascular, which produces irregular islands and trabeculae of immature bone (Figs 4.54 and 4.55). The hypercellularity and the disordered organization may produce a pseudosarcomatous appearance (Figs 4.56 and 4.57) and because a biopsy is not likely to be performed unless the clinician has failed to recognize

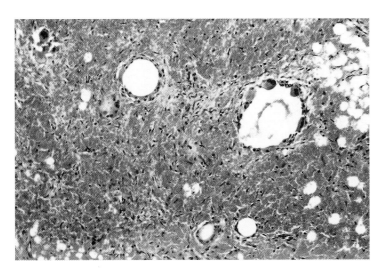

Figure 4.51   Photomicrograph of tissue obtained from the area around a fracture site shows extensive hemorrhage and a large fat cyst surrounded by giant cells, characteristic of fat necrosis (H&E, × 10 obj.).

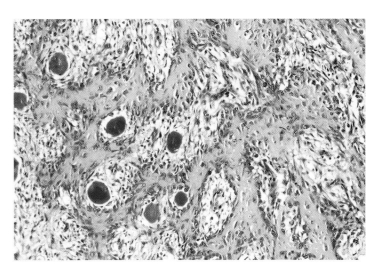

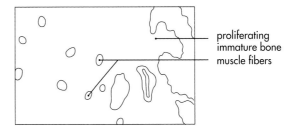

proliferating immature bone
muscle fibers

Figure 4.54   Photomicrograph of a fracture callus obtained from the soft tissue around a 2-week-old fracture demonstrates proliferating trabeculae of immature cellular bone growing around and between muscle fibers, staining red in this preparation. This histologic finding could be misdiagnosed as an infiltrating bone-forming tumor (phloxine and tartrazine, × 10 obj.).

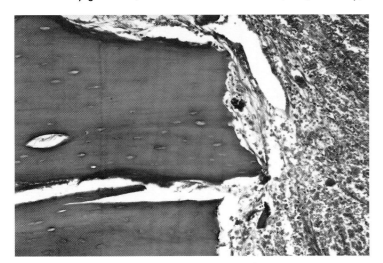

Figure 4.52   Photomicrograph of the broken end of a bone taken one week after the fracture demonstrates both hemorrhage and bone necrosis. Note that the osteocyte lacunae in the bone are completely empty. Some tissue necrosis will always be present following significant injury (H&E, × 1 obj.).

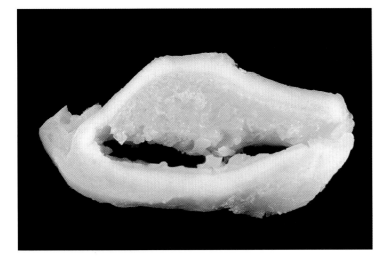

Figure 4.53   After injury, the blood supply may be so compromised as to cause complete necrosis of the affected tissue. In this gross specimen, complete osteonecrosis of the carpal lunate bone has occurred. The necrotic bone is recognized by its opaque yellow appearance.

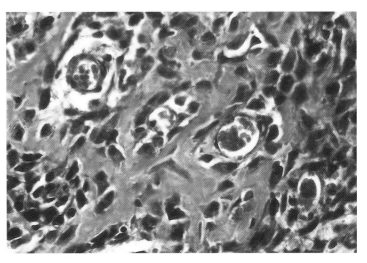

Figure 4.55   Higher-power photomicrograph demonstrates the cellularity and immature appearance of early fracture callus (H&E, × 32 obj.).

the traumatic origin of the patient's complaints, the pseudosarcomatous appearance of the callus can easily lead to errors in interpretation by the pathologist. It cannot be too strongly emphasized that because stress fractures without an obvious history of injury are common in young people (the same age group as osteosarcomas), recognition of the true nature of the problem is important and, on occasion, is among the most difficult problems in differential diagnosis (Fig. 4.58).

Once the callus is sufficient to immobilize the fracture site, repair occurs between the fractured cortical and medullary bones. When union has been achieved, the callus is remodeled and eventually disappears.

Very little callus is produced when a fracture is treated with rigid internal or external surgical fixation, where primary healing of the bone proceeds without the abundant external callus seen in association with unstable fractures.

Many factors influence the repair of a fracture. These include the particular bone involved (the tibia being especially difficult), the portion of the bone involved (the diaphysis is worse than the metaphysis), the type of fracture (comminuted vs simple), the

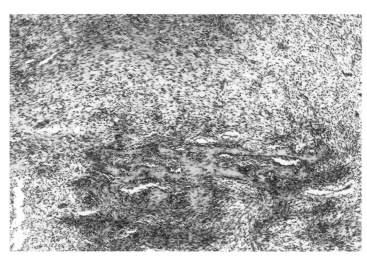

Figure 4.56   Lower-power photomicrograph demonstrates the hypercellular, proliferative appearance of callus, which in this case shows only minimal bone matrix formation. The pseudosarcomatous appearance of this tissue may lead to misdiagnosis (H&E, × 10 obj.).

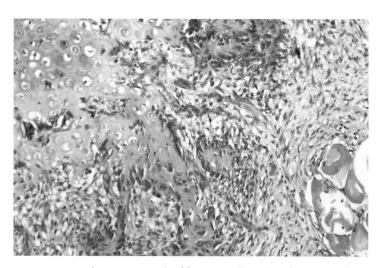

Figure 4.57   Photomicrograph of fracture callus taken from around a 10-day-old fracture. Note the proliferating cartilage and immature bone to the left, and the degenerate muscle fibers to the right (H&E, × 10 obj.).

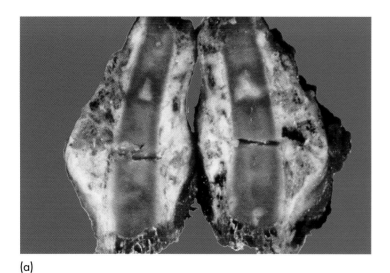

(a)

Figure 4.58   A segment of the costochondral junction was resected from an elderly patient who presented with a swelling in the chest wall (**a**). Radiographic examination revealed a localized dense mass, which was interpreted by both the clinician and the radiologist as a neoplasm. However, the histologic preparation of the resected specimen (**b**) shows a fracture through the calcified costal cartilage, surrounded by a mass of reactive bone and scar tissue (H&E, × 1.5 obj.).

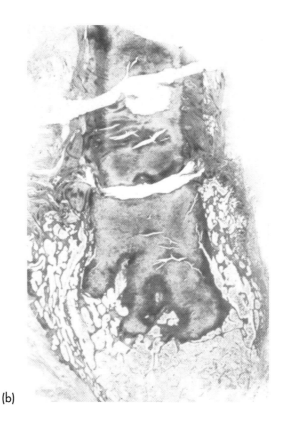

(b)

degree of soft-tissue injury, interposition of soft tissue between the fractured bone ends, and the stability of the site after fixation. Evaluation of fracture repair in any clinical study must consider the effects of these factors. When there is nonunion of a previous fracture or when large bone defects are present, grafting with autografts (from another anatomic site in the same patient), allografts (from other human subjects), or xenografts (from animals) is an accepted practice (Fig. 4.59).

Histologic evidence from experimental studies of fracture repair and ectopic ossification indicates the necessity of a rigid calcified framework for lamellar bone to be deposited. The composition of this framework may be calcified cartilage, calcified woven bone, or even foci of dystrophic calcification. When such a framework exists and lamellar bone is produced, it is said to be osteoconductive, playing the role of a filler to assist in the bridging of a gap (usually a fracture line). Most bone grafts act in this way (Fig. 4.60), however, it has been shown that certain proteins (BMPs) derived from bone and bone marrow are osteoinductive, i.e. they stimulate the formation of bone matrix by the cell. A mixture of xenograft material (osteoconductive) and admixed bone marrow (osteoinductive) will work better as a graft than a xenograft alone.

Fractures can also lead to systemic complications, including shock syndrome and myoglobinuria, the latter occurring when there is significant muscle injury. Associated with all fractures is a disruption of the bone marrow, with the potential for embolization of the fatty marrow through the locally damaged venous system. Fat embolization becomes a clinical problem in severe multiple fractures and extensive orthopedic surgery, e.g. bilateral joint replacements and may result in petechial hemorrhages, cerebral ischemia, and/or pulmonary insufficiency (Fig. 4.61).

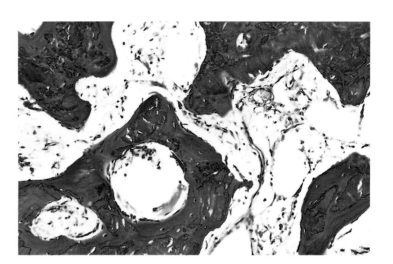

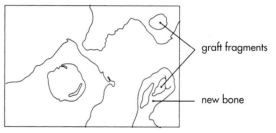

Figure 4.60 Photomicrograph of tissue obtained from an area previously grafted with bone tissue broken into very small pieces. New bone has formed and surrounds the fragments of grafted bone (H&E, × 4 obj.).

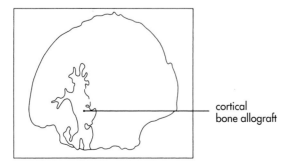

Figure 4.59 This patient with a history of segmental avascular necrosis of the femoral head had been treated with a cortical bone allograft 18 months before the resection of the femoral head. This cut section through the femoral head clearly shows the graft has been incorporated.

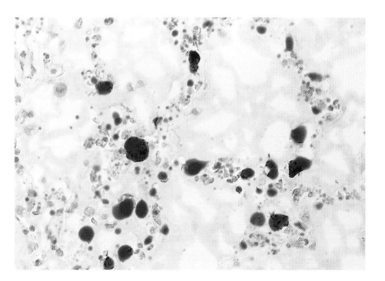

Figure 4.61 Photomicrograph of lung tissue showing globules of fat in the alveolar walls (frozen section; oil red O stain, × 4 obj.).

The effects of fat emboli on the tissues are, first, mechanical obstruction of the capillary bed and, second, an inflammatory response resulting from breakdown of the fat into free fatty acids.

Congenital pseudoarthroses

A pseudoarthrosis (false joint) usually occurs in adult life as a complication of a fracture. However, it may also manifest at birth or during infancy, commonly in the shaft of the tibia (or rarely the ulna). The lesion is usually observed at the level of the junction of the middle and lower third of the bone shaft. This type of pseudoarthrosis is considered congenital and constitutes a distinct orthopedic entity.

Radiographic evaluation of an infant with congenital pseudoarthrosis reveals discontinuity in the diaphysis of the affected bone, associated with a characteristic tapering of the bone ends at the site of the pseudoarthrosis (Fig. 4.62). Histologic examination reveals dense, fibrous connective tissue filling the defect (Fig. 4.63).

Neurofibromatosis is present in a high percentage of children with this condition, and as many as 10% of patients with neurofibromatosis have the disorder. Nevertheless, neurofibromas are not usually recognized on microscopic examination of histologic specimens from the involved site. These lesions usually prove to be very refractory to treatment.

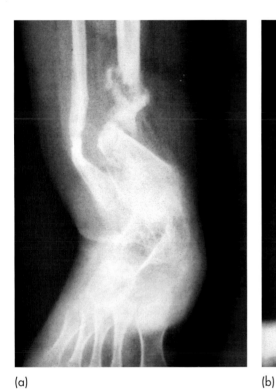
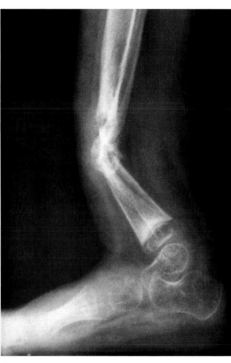

(a) (b)

Figure 4.62 (a) Antero-posterior radiograph of a young boy with congenital pseudoarthrosis of the tibia and fibula. The appearance of the lesion at the junction of the middle and lower third of the bones and the tapering of the bone ends are characteristically found in patients with congenital pseudoarthrosis. (b) Lateral radiograph of the case shown in (a).

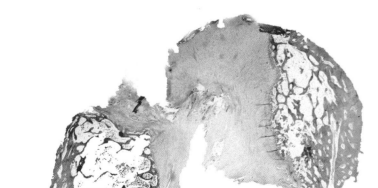

Figure 4.63 Histologic section of a congenital pseudoarthrosis of the clavicle shows that the gap in the bone is filled with dense, fibrous connective tissue, with no significant new bone formation (H&E, × 1 obj.).

CARTILAGE

Healing of cartilage is adversely affected by two factors: its avascularity, its low cell-to-matrix ratio and, in contrast to the appositional growth of bone, its interstitial pattern of growth. Nevertheless, it is essential to recognize that cartilage cells can indeed proliferate, and that in arthritis, in which the cartilage is damaged, cartilage regeneration with both cartilage cell proliferation (Figs 4.64 and 4.65) and cartilage matrix production is a regular feature. Similar processes also occur at the borders of a traumatic cartilaginous defect (Figs 4.66 to 4.68).

The ability of cartilage cells to produce an adequate matrix and to restore functional tissue probably depends on their mechanical environment. After an injury to the articular surface, as might occur in an athletic injury, continued irritation will probably result in worsening of the condition. (Cartilage repair will be discussed at greater length in Chapter 10, p. 247.)

MENISCI OF THE KNEE

The menisci are composed mainly of collagen, although some PG is also present. The amount of PG is increased dramatically in the injured degenerate meniscus and is associated histologically with cartilaginous metaplasia in the injured tissue. Examination of carefully oriented sections has revealed that the principal orientation of the collagen fibers in the menisci is circumferential (see Fig. 1.66). The few small, radially disposed fibers that do occur exist primarily on the tibial surface. The circumferential orientation of most of the collagen fibers is designed to withstand the circumferential tension within the meniscus during normal loading. The radially disposed fibers probably act as ties to resist longitudinal splitting of the menisci that might result from undue compression.

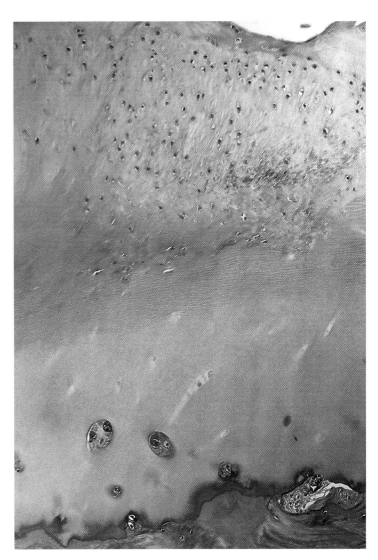

Figure 4.65   Photomicrograph of cartilage obtained from the knee joint of a patient with osteoarthritis shows cellular reparative cartilage at the surface overlying pre-existing cartilage, which is largely necrotic with few remaining viable cells (H&E, × 10 obj.).

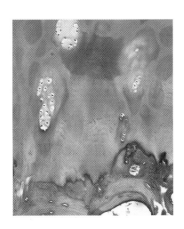

Figure 4.64   After injury to cartilage tissue resulting in cell death, proliferation of clones of reparative chondrocytes may appear, as seen in this photomicrograph (H&E, × 25 obj.).

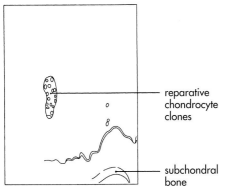

reparative chondrocyte clones

subchondral bone

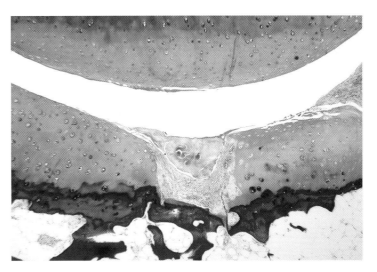

Figure 4.66   A traumatic injury to the convex surface of an interphalangeal joint has resulted in displacement of the subchondral bone plate. At the site of injury there is necrotic cartilage and viable dense fibrous connective tissue (H&E, × 2.5 obj.).

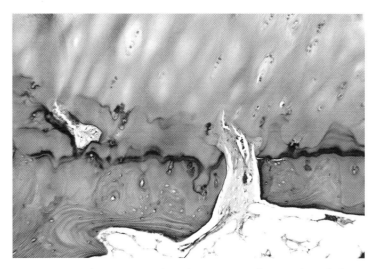

Figure 4.67 Photomicrograph to demonstrate a fracture through the subchondral bone plate with some reactive fibrous tissue filling the gap (H&E, × 10 obj.).

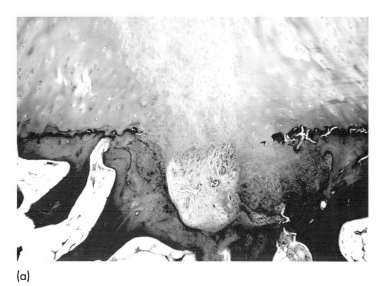

(a)

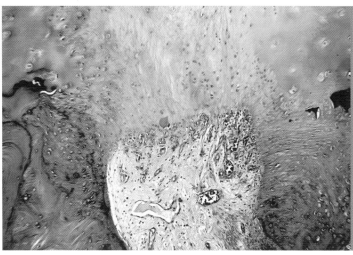

(b)

Figure 4.68 (a) A traumatic cartilage defect being filled with reparative fibrocartilage and granulation tissue from the subchondral marrow space (H&E, × 2.5 obj.). (b) Higher power of the fibrocartilage and granulation tissue (H&E, × 10 obj.).

The menisci of young individuals are usually white, have a translucent quality, and are supple on palpation. The menisci in older individuals lose their translucency, become more opaque and yellow in color, and feel less supple (see Fig. 1.55).

Lacerations of the meniscus cause symptoms that require surgical treatment in two groups of patients: young active patients in whom injury is frequently related to athletic activity, and older individuals in whom degeneration leads to laceration. In older individuals a good deal of fraying of the inner edge of the menisci is a frequent occurrence.

Most significant lacerations take place in the posterior horn of the meniscus and, more commonly, in the medial meniscus. They usually occur as clefts that run along the circumferentially directed collagen fibers (Fig. 4.69). Extension of the tear may lead to the bucket-handle deformity (Fig. 4.70). Over time, such a

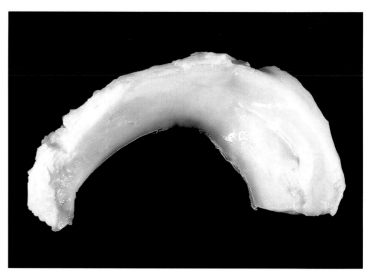

Figure 4.69 Gross photograph of a medial meniscus with an early tear in the posterior horn. These tears characteristically occur as clefts in the substance of the meniscus and run in the direction of the collagen fibers.

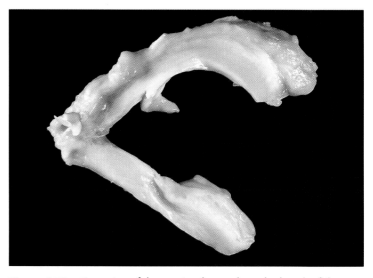

Figure 4.70 Extension of the meniscal tear along the length of the meniscus may result in a bucket-handle tear, as demonstrated here.

cleft may extend to the medial margin of the meniscus and create a tag, which eventually may become quite smooth (Fig. 4.71). Sometimes, the meniscus shows peripheral detachment, again usually posteriorly. A horizontal cleavage in the posterior horn of the meniscus is found at autopsy in over 50% of older individuals (Fig. 4.72).

The advent of initially arthrography, later magnetic resonance imaging (MRI) and arthroscopy has greatly improved the clinical diagnosis of tears in the menisci. These techniques help to localize tears and, when the scope of the injury is limited, can facilitate partial meniscectomy.

In histologic sections of torn menisci, evidence of both injury and repair may be seen, with the findings likely to be time depen-

dent (Fig. 4.73). In sections of a torn meniscus it is not unusual to see cartilaginous metaplasia probably resulting from the altered loading pattern (Fig. 4.74). It is difficult to determine

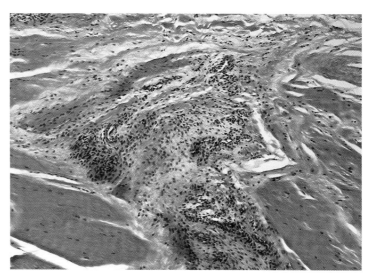

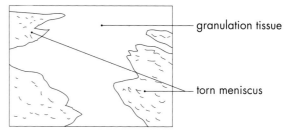

Figure 4.73   Photomicrograph of an area of laceration in a meniscus. On both the right and left side, intact collagen fibers can be seen, while in the center a defect filled with granulation tissue is evident. Repair is much more likely to be seen in the peripheral third of the substance of the meniscus, where the tissue is vascularized (H&E, x 10 obj.).

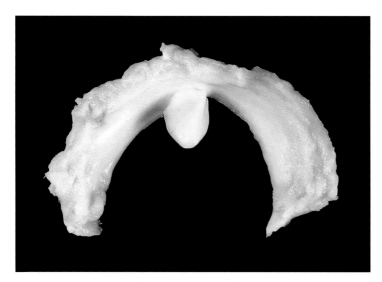

Figure 4.71   Occasionally, a tear such as that shown in Figure 4.69 will extend onto the medial margin and form a tag that extends into the joint space. Such a tag may become smoothed off at its margins, as seen in this specimen.

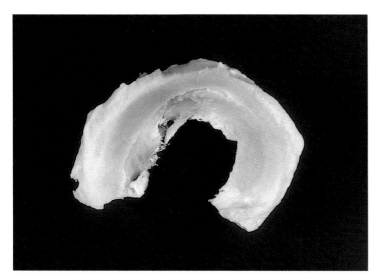

Figure 4.72   The lateral meniscus removed from an older individual. Notice the yellow discoloration; fraying of the inner margin is present together with some small clefts.

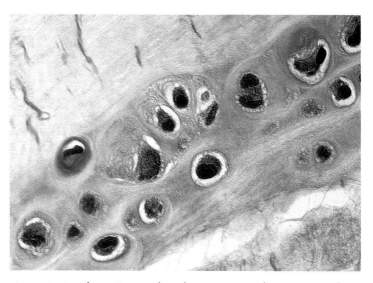

Figure 4.74   Photomicrograph to demonstrate cartilaginous metaplasia within injured meniscal tissue. This alteration is probably the result of local alterations in loading from predominantly tensile to predominantly compressive (H&E, × 40 obj.).

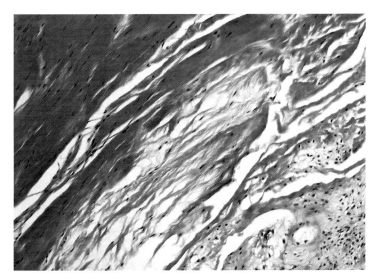

Figure 4.75   Photomicrograph of meniscal tissue shows foci of normal-appearing collagen at the upper left; collagen fibers, which are frayed, in the middle; and myxomatous tissue, possibly the result of degenerative changes, at lower right (H&E, × 25 obj.).

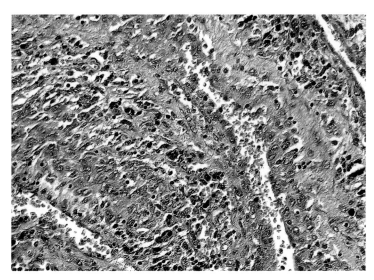

Figure 4.76   Photomicrograph of synovial tissue obtained from a knee joint about 1–2 months after injury to the joint. The synovial lining is both hypertrophied and hyperplastic. There is extensive hemosiderin deposition in the subsynovial tissue (H&E, Nomarski optics, × 10 obj.).

whether histologic degenerative changes observed at meniscectomy result from or contribute to the tear (Fig. 4.75).

SYNOVIUM

Injury to any of the joint structures necessarily affects the synovium. Traumatic synovitis is usually characterized microscopically by evidence of hemorrhage (hemosiderin staining), hypertrophy and hyperplasia of the synovial lining cells, mild chronic inflammation, and occasionally by included fragments of detached bone and cartilage (Fig. 4.76). Sometimes the severity of the synovial response may obscure the underlying traumatic etiology.

SUMMARY

Mechanical trauma is a major cause of skeletal malfunction. Trauma also plays a contributory role in a number of other morbid conditions, including but not limited to osteoarthritis, slipped capital femoral epiphysis, myositis ossificans, and interdigital (Morton's) neuroma of the foot, all of which will be discussed in greater detail later.

The response to injury (the inflammatory response) is effected mainly through the vascular system; its purpose is to restore the body to its status quo. In the case of minor injuries that frequently befall all of us, the status quo is indeed restored. In the case of more severe injury, however, a new status quo with resulting disability is more likely to occur. Effective management of such disabilities is dependent on a thorough understanding of pathogenesis.

BONE AND JOINT INFECTION

Clinically significant inflammation is most frequently the result of infection. However it is important to remember that inflammation also occurs in response to other pathologic processes, including trauma, some metabolic diseases (e.g. gout), and even neoplasia. Because it is so common, the physician understandably thinks first of infection when signs of inflammation are present; however, it is important to rule out other possible etiologies.

It was only in the late 19th century that the clinical picture of bone marrow infection (osteomyelitis) became recognized for what it is. Before the era of antibiotics, bone and joint infections were both common and serious clinical problems resulting in high rates of morbidity and mortality. In the present day, the incidence of osteomyelitis, and its associated mortality, has decreased dramatically; however, even with antibiotic use, the morbidity rate remains high.

The proper diagnosis and management of osteomyelitis depends on a careful correlation of clinical, radiologic, and histopathologic findings. Occasionally, there are problems with differential diagnosis, especially when differentiating osteomyelitis from round-cell tumors and eosinophilic granuloma. Diagnostic problems are encountered not only radiologically and clinically (a Ewing tumor may present with fever and increased sedimentation rate), but also microscopically, especially with small crushed specimens, where tumor cells and inflammatory cells may be difficult to distinguish (Figs 5.1 and 5.2). In such cases, the diagnosis of osteomyelitis may depend on intra-operative cultures in combination with the patient's subsequent postoperative course. The importance of taking an adequate amount of culture material and its prompt inoculation into the transport medium cannot be overemphasized.

The majority of bone and joint infections are either pyogenic (characterized by neutrophilic infiltration and pus formation) or granulomatous (characterized by multiple nodules or granules in tissue). In general, pyogenic disease is more common in bone, whereas granulomatous infections are more often found in joints.

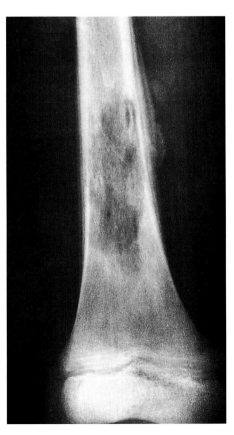

Figure 5.1 A 7-year-old boy had pain in his right leg for 3 weeks. Antero-posterior radiograph demonstrates a lesion in the medullary portion of the distal femoral diaphysis with a moth-eaten type of bone destruction, associated with a lamellated periosteal reaction. These radiographic features may suggest a diagnosis of Ewing's sarcoma; however, the lack of a definite soft tissue mass and the short symptomatic period points to the diagnosis of osteomyelitis, which was confirmed by biopsy and culture.

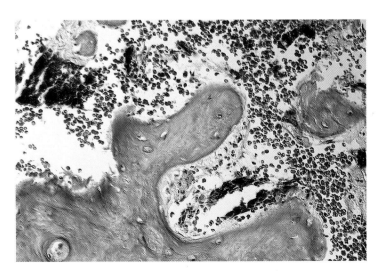

Figure 5.2 Photomicrograph of tissue shows nests of dark hyperchromatic cells crushed at the time of biopsy, rendering accurate microscopic diagnosis impossible in this histologic field (H&E, × 10 obj.).

PYOGENIC AND OTHER NONGRANULOMATOUS INFECTIONS

CLINICAL CONSIDERATIONS

Infection of skeletal tissue results from microbes that are either blood borne (hematogenous infection) or implanted directly into the bone. The latter most often occurs as a complication of a compound fracture or of surgery.

Hematogenous osteomyelitis

Children comprise the majority of patients with acute hematogenous osteomyelitis. As in adults, only one type of bacteria are usually recovered. In children over the age of 1 year, *Staphylococcus aureus*, *Streptococcus pyogenes* and *Haemophilus influenzae* are the most commonly isolated microbes. After 4 years of age, the incidence of osteomyelitis caused by *H. influenzae* decreases in incidence.

The most frequent sites of pediatric osteomyelitis are areas of rapid growth and increased risk of trauma: the distal femur, proximal tibia, proximal femur, proximal humerus, and distal radius (Fig. 5.3). There is some evidence that the large caliber of the metaphyseal veins in children results in a marked slowing of blood flow, predisposing traumatized tissue to thrombosis and subsequent colonization of the area by blood-borne bacteria (Fig. 5.4).

Hematogenous osteomyelitis is uncommon in healthy adults. However, with increasing numbers of debilitated individuals (i.e. those with chronic immune deficiency disease or drug addiction), adults with osteomyelitis are being seen with greater frequency. *S. aureus* is the most commonly isolated pathogen in these individuals, although infections with *S. epidermidis*, Gram-negative rods and yeasts such as *Candida* are also seen.

Studies of osteomyelitis in i.v. drug users (IDUs) reveal that almost 90% are bacterial in origin with a predominance of pyogenic infections. *S. aureus* and streptococci are the most frequently encountered pathogens. Gram-negative bacilli, particularly *P. aeruginosa* are well known, although less common, infecting organisms. Polymicrobial infections may occur. Infecting bacteria are carried into the blood from the skin as well as injected from unclean hypodermic needles. Additionally, the injected drugs are often 'cut' and thereby contaminated with other particulate matter. The resulting microvascular occlusion provides a ready site for bacterial colonization. Clinical symptoms and signs are often subtle with fever and chills conspicuously absent in most IDU patients. Local pain may be the sole clinical finding and thus the diagnosis of osteomyelitis may be delayed. The focus of osteomyelitis is usually the spine (Fig. 5.5) or the pelvis, although the disease may occur anywhere in the skeletal system (sometimes in unusual sites such as the clavicle). When long bones are involved, radiographic changes include lyses of affected bone as well as sclerosis and periosteal reaction (sometimes in an onion-skin pattern), which result in a misleading diagnostic picture of malignancy.

In elderly individuals, especially those with genitourinary infections, opportunistic bacteria selected out by repeated antibiotic use, usually *P. aeruginosa*, gain access to the spine possibly via Batson's venous plexus (Fig. 5.6). Another group of elderly patients in whom osteomyelitis may be a problem are those with peripheral vascular insufficiency, which in many cases is associated with diabetes. In these patients the infection usually involves the small bones of the feet. The etiology is frequently polymicrobial; likely suspects include *S. aureus, S. agalactiae* (Group B streptococci), *Enterococcus* (Group D streptococci), Gram-negative bacteria as well as anaerobic Gram-positive cocci.

Adults with bone infections often present only with pain; thus, a diagnosis of osteomyelitis may not be obvious. As already mentioned, the accompanying radiographic bone changes are easily misinterpreted by the radiologist as a malignant tumor (Fig. 5.7). The clinical diagnosis may be further confused by negative cultures resulting from inappropriate empirical use of antibiotics.

Neonatal osteomyelitis

Neonatal osteomyelitis, which also commonly involves the joint adjacent to the involved bone, is usually the result of hematogenous infection by one of three organisms: *S. aureus, S. agalactiae*, or *Escherichia coli*. *S. agalactiæ* is commonly found in the vagina, and the unborn child presumably becomes infected during delivery. *E. coli*, a common contaminant at the time of delivery, can become pathogenic in neonates because of the infant's immature immune system.

In the case of *S. aureus* and *E. coli* infection, about 40% of the neonatal patients show polyostotic involvement (Fig. 5.8) (Polyostotic involvement with osteomyelitis is extremely rare except in the neonate). When *Streptococcus* is the causative organism, usually only a single bone is involved. In some cases of neonatal osteomyelitis, the absence of systemic symptoms (because of immunologic incompetence) can delay the clinical diagnosis.

Osteomyelitis resulting from direct inoculation of bacteria

Now that acute hematogenous osteomyelitis of childhood, which used to be regularly seen in orthopaedic practice is much less frequent, post-traumatic osteomyelitis has become the more com-

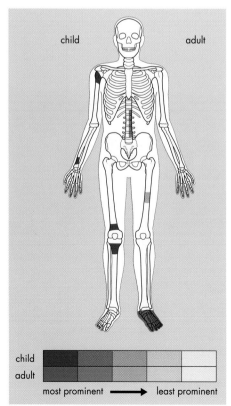

Figure 5.3 Distribution of osteomyelitis in children and adults.

child   adult

child
adult

most prominent ➡ least prominent

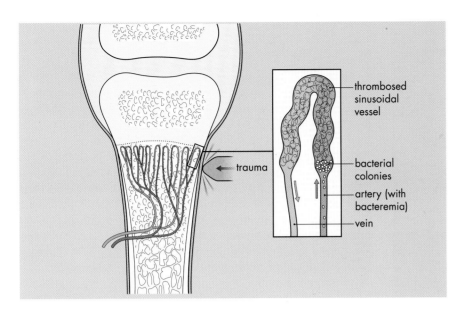

Figure 5.4   After mechanical trauma to the bone in children, the large venous channels in the metaphysis are liable to thrombose (see vein on right). In the presence of bacteria from infection elsewhere in the body, such a site of thrombosis can act as a nidus for bacterial growth and subsequent development of osteomyelitis.

thrombosed sinusoidal vessel

bacterial colonies

artery (with bacteremia)

vein

trauma

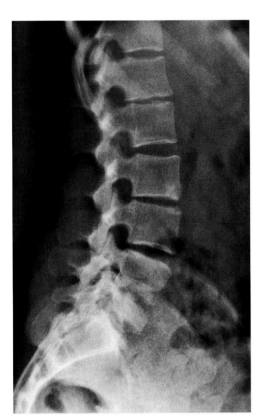

Figure 5.5   Radiograph of a lateral portion of the spine in a young drug addict shows bone destruction anteriorly on both sides of the disc between L2 and L3 and extensive destruction at L4-L5 and L5-S1, with collapse of L5. Bacteriologic culture showed that the offending organism in this case was *Staphylococcus aureus*.

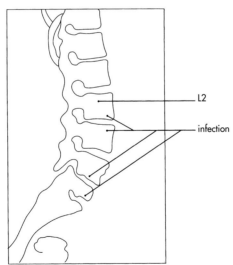

L2

infection

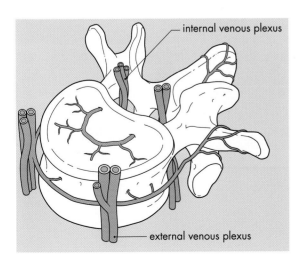

internal venous plexus

external venous plexus

Figure 5.6   The veins of the vertebral column form intricate plexuses around the column, along the spinal canal, and through the bone substance. These venous plexuses, also known as Batson's plexus, communicate freely with the segmental systemic veins and portal system. Because of these anastomoses and also the lack of valves in these veins, retrograde flow frequently occurs and may result in metastatic infection, as well as metastatic tumors, affecting the vertebral bodies, spinal cord, brain, and skull.

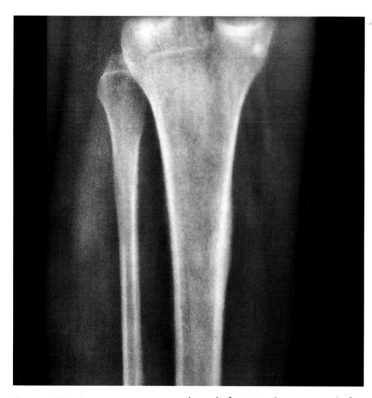

Figure 5.7 A young woman complained of pain in the upper end of the tibia. A radiograph shows periosteal reaction at the junction of the upper and middle third of the tibia. Clinical examination of the area revealed tenderness and swelling; the patient's general health appeared to be good. The differential diagnosis was between a round-cell tumor or infection. Biopsy and culture proved the lesion to be infective in nature.

mon clinical problem. Post-traumatic osteomyelitis usually results from puncture wounds, traffic accidents, and surgery (Figs 5.9 and 5.10).

Most traffic accidents involve high-impact collisions causing compound and comminuted fractures. A significant amount of foreign material, including metallic debris, pieces of clothing, soil, etc., is usually found in these wounds. It is important to recognize the polymicrobial nature of the infection in accident cases. *Staphylococcus* and *Streptococcus* infection can be expected; in addition, Gram-negative organisms (including *Pseudomonas*) are often present. The most important first step when treating these patients is removal of all foreign and dead matter. If this step is omitted, elimination of the infection becomes difficult, if not impossible. Potent, preferably targeted, antibiotic treatment should be administered for as short a period as possible. Antibiotic selection should reflect local susceptibility patterns.

When osteomyelitis is a complication of a fracture, it is important to completely immobilize the fracture fragments. Without immobilization, it is virtually impossible to re-establish the vascular supply necessary to adequately deal with the infected and inflamed tissues (Fig. 5.11).

Iatrogenic infections may be a direct result of surgical intervention, associated with the internal fixation of a simple or compound fracture, or, with prosthetic joint replacement. (More than 500,000 prosthetic joint replacements are performed each year in the USA alone.) After a total joint replacement procedure, infection may occur as an acute complication of the operation or may present insidiously many months (or even years) later (Fig. 5.12). The causative organisms commonly identified in such cases are *Staphylococcus* (both coagulase negative and coagulase positive), Gram-negative organisms such as *Pseudomonas* species

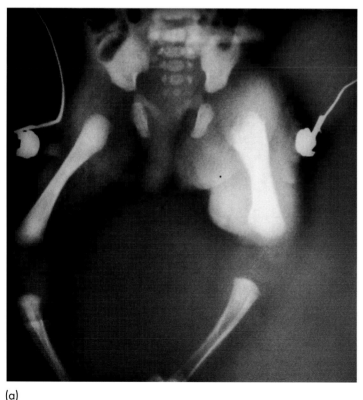

(a)

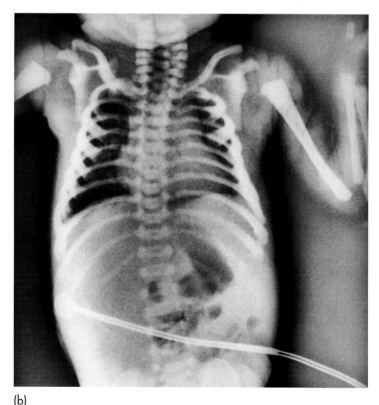

(b)

Figure 5.8 Polyostotic involvement in neonatal osteomyelitis. Radiograph of the lower limbs of a newborn child (a) shows marked periosteal reaction all along the left femur. Radiograph of the chest (b) shows involvement of some ribs as well as the right clavicle.

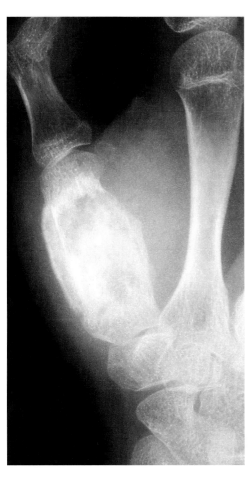

Figure 5.9
Radiograph of the left thumb of a 15-year-old boy with recent swelling of the first metacarpal following a penetrating injury. The radiograph shows patchy sclerosis and mature periosteal bone formation secondary to infection. (Courtesy of Dr Alex Norman.)

or *E. coli*, and a variety of anaerobic organisms may also be found. Improved surgical technique, the use of hood, suit and laminar flow have dramatically reduced the incidence of infection to less than 0.5% for both hips and knees in our institution. (A further discussion of infection associated with total joint replacement will be found in Chapter 14, p. 333.)

In rare cases actinomycosis (*Actinomyces israeli*) may gain access to the bone through a puncture wound and such a case is illustrated in Figures 5.13 and 5.14.

Chronic osteomyelitis

With the mortality rate reduced to almost zero, few people die from hematogenous osteomyelitis; however, between 15% and 30% of patients go on to develop chronic disease. Chronic osteomyelitis is frequently the result of either inadequate antibiotic treatment or incomplete surgical debridement of necrotic bone. Necrotic bone within the affected area (the sequestrum) protects bacteria from even high levels of appropriate antibiotics. Furthermore, recent data implicate bacterial bio films – formation of sessile microbial communities with inherent resistance to antimicrobial agents – in the genesis of chronic osteomyelitis. Occasionally bio films developing on dead tissue such as the sequestra of dead bone, give rise to non-sessile colonies that multiply rapidly and disperse. The bio film acts as a 'nidus' of infection and acute disease results when host defenses cannot eliminate the released bacteria. Bio films associated with osteomyelitis are usually comprised of a mixture of various bacterial and fungal species and the disease is not resolved until the

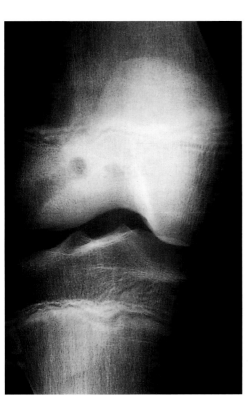

Figure 5.10
Radiograph of the right knee of a 13-year-old boy with a recent history of pain and stiffness in the knee following a fall in which the skin was punctured. The lytic area within the otherwise dense femoral epiphysis proved at biopsy to be an abscess. (Courtesy of Dr Alex Norman.)

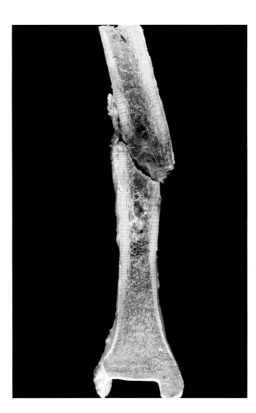

Figure 5.11
Photograph of tibia amputated for an infected nonunion of a compound fracture of the mid-diaphysis.

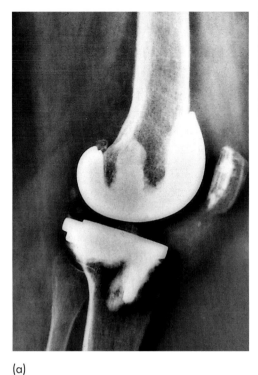
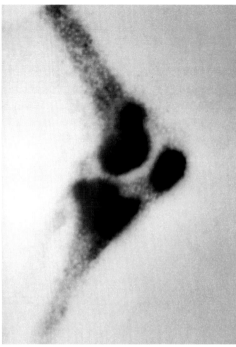

(a)   (b)

Figure 5.12   Radiograph of a patient with a total knee prosthesis inserted 18 months previously (**a**). The patient had recently experienced increasing pain in the knee; evidence of osteolysis can be seen around the prosthesis, particularly in the tibial component. Such osteolysis can result from either infection or mechanical loosening. An isotope scan (**b**) shows intense uptake around all the components of the knee joint, typical of infection. Increased isotope uptake would also occur with prosthetic loosening, however, one would expect it to be limited to the component that had been loosened (usually, in the case of the knee, the tibial component) and to be focal at the sites of maximal movement of the prosthesis.

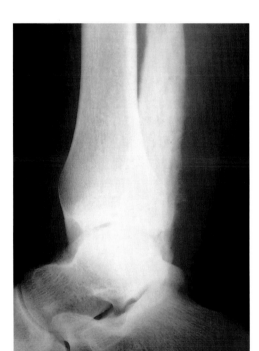

Figure 5.13 Radiograph of the ankle of a middle-aged shepherd with a sclerotic lesion of the lower fibula which on biopsy proved to be due to actinomycosis. (Courtesy of Dr Juan Roig.)

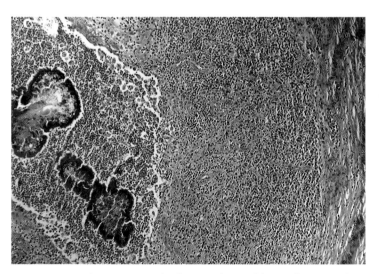

Figure 5.14   Photomicrograph of tissue obtained from a lesion similar to that shown in Figure 5.13 demonstrates an acute and chronic inflammatory reaction surrounding the typical eosinophilic 'sulfur' granule seen in association with actinomycosis (H&E, × 10 obj.). (Courtesy of Dr Miguel Calvo.)

sessile population is surgically removed. Indeed, *Staphylococcus* species of the same phage type as the original infecting bacteria have been isolated from patients with relapsing osteomyelitis years after the initial infection.

Squamous-cell carcinoma in association with a chronic fistula (Marjolin's ulcer) has been reported to be a late sequela of chronic osteomyelitis in about 1% of patients, occurring up to 30–40 years after the original infection (Fig. 5.15). Systemic amyloidosis may also be a complication of chronic osteomyelitis.

Hypertrophic pulmonary osteoarthropathy (Marie–Bamberger syndrome)

Hypertrophic pulmonary osteoarthropathy involves the formation of symmetrical periosteal new bone along the diaphyses of

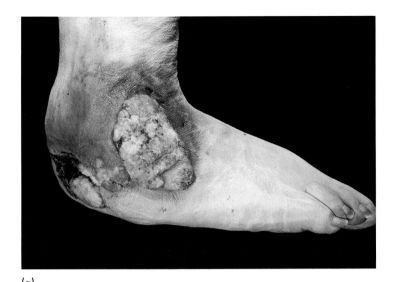

(a)

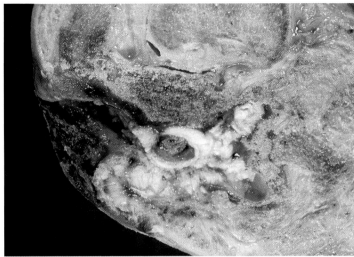

(b)

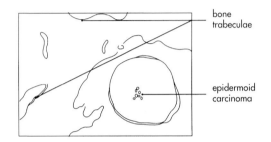

(c)

Figure 5.15 (a) Gross photograph of the foot and ankle in a patient with longstanding osteomyelitis. Overgrowth of partially ulcerated hyperkeratotic skin is seen in the area of the ankle joint. (b) Sagittal section shows a draining sinus from the infected bone opening onto the ulcerated skin. There is invasion of firm white tissue from the skin surface into the underlying soft tissue and bone. (c) Photomicrograph of the bone shows that the bone is being invaded by a well-differentiated epidermoid carcinoma (H&E, × 10 obj.).

the bones of the appendicular skeleton. This condition is seen in association with both chronic inflammation and neoplastic diseases of the lung and, less commonly, of other organs. The classic presentation is an adult with complaints of arthralgia and/or aching bone pain, with or without clubbing of the fingers and toes.

The striking radiographic feature of hypertrophic pulmonary osteoarthropathy is symmetrical 'onion-skin periostitis' of the shafts of long bones, which is confined to the diaphyses but progresses proximally. Densities in the sites of insertions of ligaments and tendons have also been noted. The patient's level of serum alkaline phosphatase may be elevated. Although the joints do not show significant radiographic change, patients may have painful effusions that are characteristically noninflammatory. The arthralgia is usually relieved by aspirin.

On microscopic examination of the affected bone, there is marked periosteal new bone formation. The outer layer of the periosteum may show a mononuclear cell infiltrate. No endosteal bone deposition is seen. Sections of the clubbed finger shows no bone formation but increased and hypervascular soft tissue (Fig. 5.16).

The etiology of pulmonary osteoarthropathy remains obscure. Treatment should be directed at the underlying disease.

Chronic recurrent multifocal osteomyelitis

Chronic recurrent multifocal osteomyelitis (CRMO), a variant of osteomyelitis affecting children and young adults, is characterized by the insidious onset of low-grade fever, local swelling, and pain in affected bones. Radiologic findings suggest osteomyelitis and bone-seeking isotopes may reveal multiple asymptomatic sites of involvement. The lesions occur mainly in the metaphyses of tubular bones, as well as the clavicles, and are sometimes symmetrically distributed. Cultures are consistently negative. Consequently the suspicion of a round-cell malignancy, especially because of periosteal new bone formation in the region of the clavicle, is frequently entertained (Fig. 5.17).

The clinical course of this obscure disease is characterized by periods of intermittent exacerbations and improvements over a period of several years. Some patients have associated recurrent skin lesions (pustulosis palmoplantaris) that closely parallel the exacerbations of the bone lesions. Acute inflammation, with polymorphonuclear leukocyte predominance, occurs in the early phases of the disease, and fibrosis of the marrow with chronic inflammation occurs in later phases. Microscopically, the most common finding is subacute or chronic osteomyelitis with a predominance of plasma cells. Fragments of necrotic bone with associated multinucleated giant cells, are a common finding (Fig. 5.18).

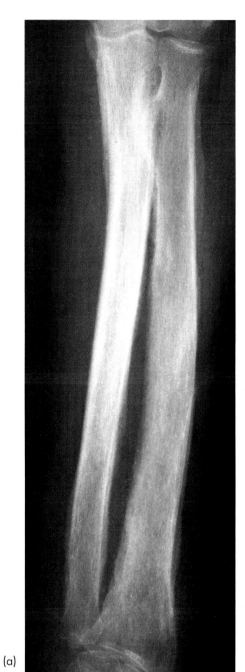

(a)

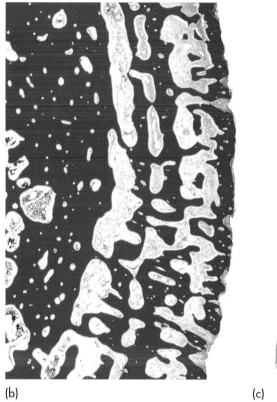

(b)

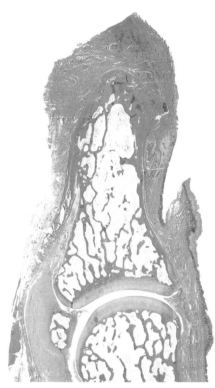

(c)

Figure 5.16   (**a**) Radiograph of the forearm in a patient with carcinoma of the lung shows periosteal bone formation on both the radius and the ulna. In this patient all the long bones demonstrated dramatic periosteal new bone. (**b**) Photomicrograph of a biopsy of cortical bone from a patient with pulmonary osteoarthropathy. Note the three layers of new periosteal bone (H&E, × 4 obj.). (**c**) Photomicrograph of a section through an affected terminal phalanx shows marked increased hypervascularity of the soft tissue beneath the nail bed (H&E, × 1 obj.).

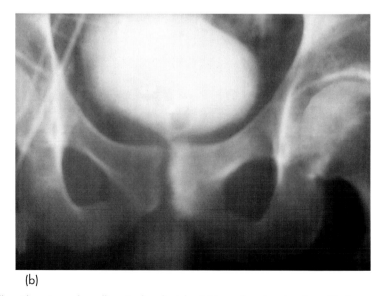

(a)

(b)

Figure 5.17   (**a**) Radiograph of a 23-year-old male who presented initially with pain and swelling in the clavicle. (**b**) Later he also developed lesions in the first and third ribs as well as in the pubis.

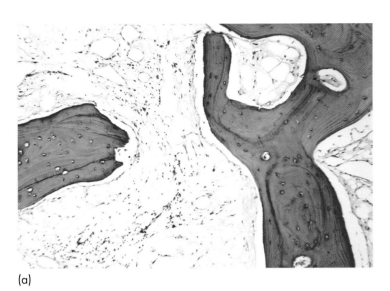

(a)

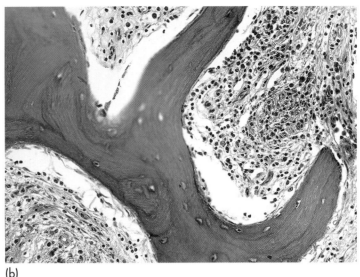

(b)

Figure 5.18 (a) Photomicrograph of a bone biopsy obtained from the clavicle of the case illustrated in Figure 5.17 (H&E, × 4 obj.). (b) At a higher power it can be seen that there is marrow fibrosis as well as an infiltration of chronic inflammatory cells. As is typical in such cases, no organisms could be isolated (H&E, × 10 obj.). (Case published with permission of Dr Howard Dorfman.)

Infantile cortical hyperostosis (Caffey's disease)

Infantile cortical hyperostosis (ICH) is a disease of infants who present with a classic triad of hyperirritability, soft-tissue swelling, and palpable hard masses over multiple and often symmetric bones. Patients may be feverish and acutely ill; the disease often follows a recent upper respiratory tract infection. Radiography reveals diffuse, usually symmetric cortical thicken-

ing. Many bones are affected, but especially the mandible, clavicle, and ribs. Involvement of the long bones occurs less often, and the vertebral column and tubular bones of the hands and feet are usually spared. Histologic examination of tissue from affected areas reveals a thickened periosteum, often with marked periosteal new bone formation and mild infiltration by chronic inflammatory cells (Fig. 5.19).

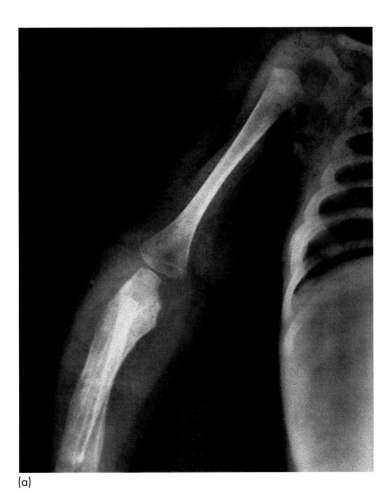

(a)

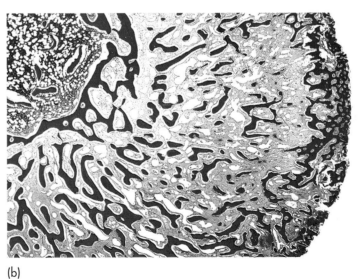

(b)

Figure 5.19 (a) Radiograph of an infant admitted to the hospital with fever and enlargement of the forearm shows extensive periosteal new bone formation causing enlargement of the ulna. In addition, there was thickening and widening of the seventh rib, as well as bilateral thickening of the mandible (not shown here). (b) Histologic section of tissue affected by infantile cortical hyperostosis reveals extensive periosteal new bone formation, with vascularized fibrous tissue lying between the bone spicules. Although not seen here, a scattering of chronic inflammatory cells is commonly found (H&E, × 1.25 obj.).

Laboratory findings in patients with ICH may include an increased erythrocyte sedimentation rate, anemia, and leukocytosis with a shift to the left. These findings are highly suggestive of an infection; however, in the vast majority of cases no organism has been isolated.

Infantile cortical hyperostosis usually follows a protracted course with several exacerbations and remissions, but spontaneous recovery usually occurs in a few months.

Septic arthritis

Joint infection may be caused by hematogenous infection of the synovium, by decompression of contiguous osteomyelitis (Figs 5.20–5.22), or may be a consequence of direct inoculation of organisms into a joint following trauma. Septic arthritis is common in neonates and infants, affecting most commonly the hip, and less commonly the knee, or ankle. The reason the hip is more commonly involved is because of the low attachment of the hip capsule onto the neck of the femur, so that the metaphysis is intracapsular, thus facilitating the spread of infection into the joint. In these patients, severe residual growth disturbance often results from damage to the growth cartilage. For this reason, the importance of early diagnosis and treatment cannot be overemphasized (Fig. 5.23). Another group of patients particularly susceptible to developing septic arthritis are debilitated older adults with rheumatoid arthritis or other chronic inflammatory joint diseases.

The diagnosis is established by joint aspiration, preferably assisted by radiologic image intensification and performed under strict antiseptic conditions. The aspirate should be sent immediately to the laboratory for direct smear, aerobic and anaerobic cultures, and antibiotic sensitivity analysis. To increase the likelihood of bacterial growth, the aspirate should be inoculated into the medium as soon as possible. (The phenomenon of an apparently sterile infection may well result from difficulties in recovering and growing the bacteria.) The hip joint, situated deep in the body, is difficult to examine as well as to aspirate, and therefore the diagnosis of septic arthritis in this joint tends to be delayed, particularly in newborns and infants.

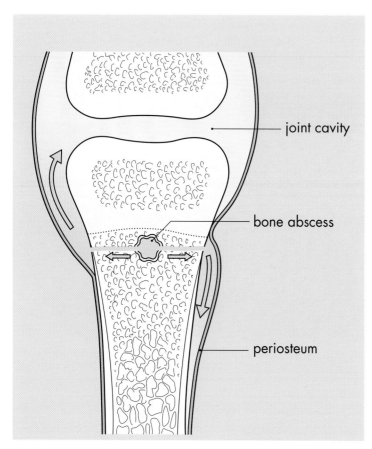

Figure 5.20 In patients with osteomyelitis, infected fluid material tracks through the bone to the bone surface, initially elevating the periosteum, and finally breaking through the periosteum into the soft tissues to drain onto the skin surface. In instances where the capsule of the joint is attached below the growth plate (as in the hip), the infection may extend directly into the joint cavity, giving rise to secondary septic arthritis.

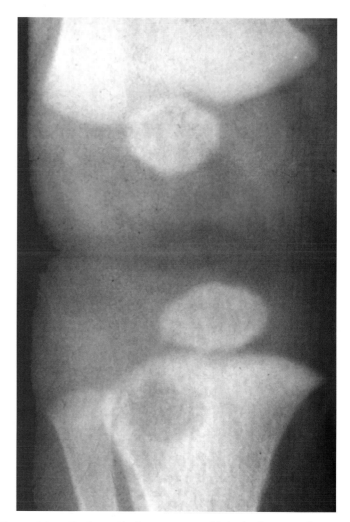

Figure 5.21 Radiograph showing an established infection in the upper tibial metaphysis of a 5-month-old boy with a history of a painful swelling and fever. Note the eccentric metaphyseal lytic defect and the periosteal reaction. Note also that there is no involvement of the joint, which would be expected with a similar lesion in the hip. (In the absence of fever, a differential diagnosis of eosinophilic granuloma would have to be considered.) (Courtesy of Dr Alex Norman.)

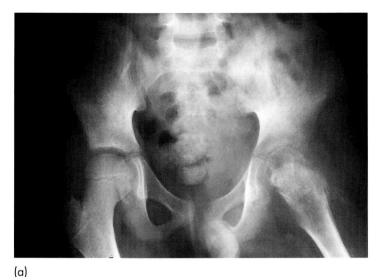

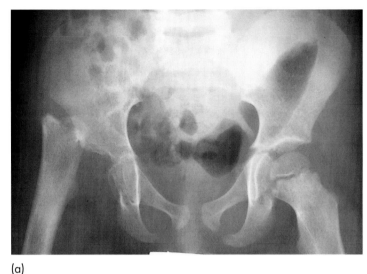

(a)

(a)

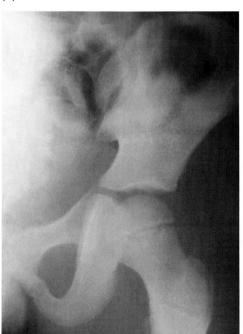

Figure 5.22 (a) In this 11-year-old boy, there is marked joint space narrowing in the left hip as well as patchy osteoporosis, typical of infection in the upper femoral metaphysis. A radiograph obtained 3 weeks before (b) at the time of the onset of symptoms shows no obvious changes. (Courtesy of Dr Alex Norman.)

(b)

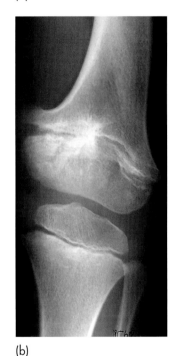

Figure 5.23 (a) Radiograph of a 3-year-old boy with multiple sites of osteomyelitis. In the upper femur, the capital femoral epiphysis and growth plate have been destroyed, leading to dislocation of the upper end of the femur and dysplasia of the acetabulum. (b) Radiograph of the deformed knee of the same boy at age 6, which shows a disturbance of the growth plate of the lower femur with focal fusion, which led eventually to marked limb shortening. (Courtesy of Dr Alex Norman.)

(b)

Cartilage is particularly susceptible to the action of enzymes released by bacteria and disintegrating inflammatory cells, and consequently is rapidly destroyed in patients with septic arthritis (Fig. 5.24). For this reason, treatment of the disease consists of immediate surgical incision and drainage, followed by immobilization of the affected joint. Antibiotic therapy alone is usually insufficient.

Joint infection following sexually transmitted disease

Suppurative arthritis, which was once a frequent complication of gonorrhea, is now decidedly rare, presumably as a result of early and efficient chemotherapy. However, it is an important diagnostic alternative to bear in mind, because the true nature of the disease is likely to be missed unless a careful history is taken. As with other forms of bacterial arthritis, the knee joints are usually the first to be affected, but multiple joint involvement is much more common in patients with gonorrhea than in those with other types of infection. Unlike other *Neisseria*, *N. gonorrhoeae* do not grow well on simple nutrient agar or at reduced temperatures. Furthermore, they do not tolerate drying; thus, care should be taken to inoculate patient samples immediately onto the appropriate agar medium. In recent years, DNA-based tests have become common. The advantages of DNA-based tests over culture include more rapid results, equal or better sensitivity and ease of sample taking.

Transient inflammatory arthritis may be a complication of the acute stage of gonorrhea. However, in these cases the arthritis is not caused by bacterial infection of the joint but rather is an immunologic response, often associated with a genetic predisposition. A similar type of arthritis may also complicate cases of nonspecific urethritis and acquired immune deficiency syndrome (AIDS).

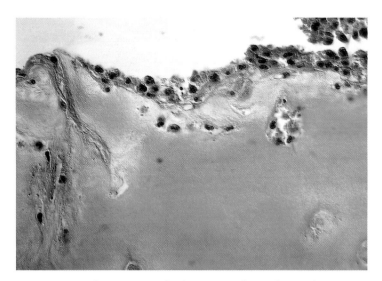

Figure 5.24 Photomicrograph of a portion of articular cartilage obtained from an acutely inflamed joint to show polymorphonuclear leukocytes on the cartilage surface and underlying erosion of the matrix (H&E, × 25 obj.).

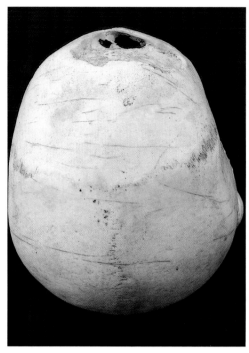

Figure 5.25 Photograph of the cranium showing thinning and fenestration of the frontal bone, in this case secondary to a syphilitic gumma.

Patients with syphilis may also develop arthritis, either as a result of the extension of gummatous osteitis into a joint or as a complication of congenital syphilis. (Charcot's joint, a rapidly destructive noninfectious arthritis which frequently complicates tabes dorsalis, is discussed in Chapter 11, p. 259)

In the tertiary stage of syphilis, chronic necrotizing and destructive osteomyelitis characterized by heavy infiltration of plasma cells used to be a common occurrence. These lesions, referred to as gumma were usually seen in the skull and the long tubular bones (Fig. 5.25). Non-gummatous syphilitic periosteitis, a frequent complication of acquired syphilis, may be accompanied only by mild inflammation, comprising mainly fibrosis and perivascular chronic inflammation. Therefore, its infectious nature can easily be overlooked (Fig. 5.26).

Pyogenic spondylitis

Pyogenic osteomyelitis of the vertebral column is rare in comparison with infections of the appendicular skeleton, and constitutes less than 1% of all cases of osteomyelitis. The disease can be seen at any age but is most common after the sixth decade. It should always be considered in the differential diagnosis of back pain in the elderly. As already mentioned, the predisposing factors include systemic urinary tract infection, diabetes, and i.v. drug abuse. The lumbar spine is involved twice as frequently as the thoracic spine; the cervical spine is only rarely affected. This variation is probably associated with the source of the primary infection, as well as the route of infection via Batson's plexus.

Depending on the virulence of the infectious agent, pyogenic spondylitis may manifest as back pain, radiculopathy, or systemic signs of acute infection. Usually, however, the patient presents only with vague localizing symptoms and general malaise. Untreated infection may ultimately result in significant deformity of the spine and severe neurologic deficit.

An abscess in the vertebral body can spread posteriorly to involve the posterior arch and the neural canal, resulting in

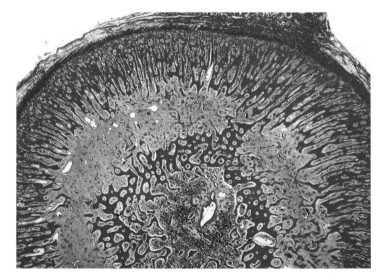

Figure 5.26 Photomicrograph showing severe periostitis with fibrosis and chronic inflammation secondary to syphilitic infection (H&E, × 1 obj.).

meningitis or may violate the anterior cortex and ligamentous structures to form paravertebral soft-tissue abscesses. Retropharyngeal abscesses may arise from cervical infections, and an abscess in the paraspinal muscle may follow thoracic infections. In the lumbar region, an abscess in the psoas sheath may spread to the groin or even to the popliteal fossa. The adjacent vertebra is often infected by spread along the vertebral ligaments; in these circumstances the intervertebral disc becomes sequestrated, and may eventually be destroyed (Figs 5.27 and 5.28).

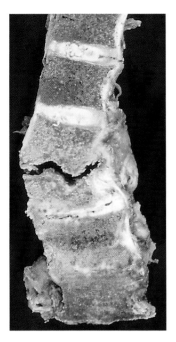
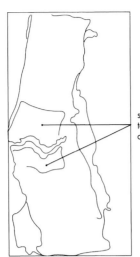

segmental collapse due
to complete destruction
of the disc

Figure 5.27   Photograph of sagittal section through the thoracolumbar spine of a patient with pyogenic spondylitis, showing involvement of few vertebral segments. Mild kyphotic deformity is apparent. Note the complete destruction of the disc by the disease process. (Courtesy Dr Krishnan K. Unni.)

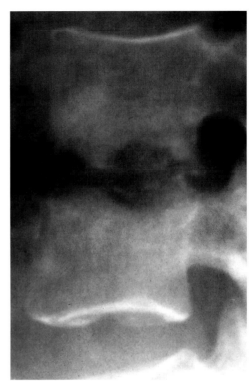

(a)

RADIOGRAPHIC DIAGNOSIS

Morphologic changes in individuals with infectious disease cannot be demonstrated on radiographs until the disease is well established, i.e. significant bone destruction has occurred, and there is reactive new bone formation. Such difficulties in radiologic diagnosis have been partly solved by other imaging modalities, permitting earlier detection of osteomyelitic foci. For example in the early stages of osteomyelitis and septic arthritis, changes can usually be observed with MRI (Fig. 5.29).

In clinical studies, radionuclide uptake has been shown to occur in a sizable percentage of cases 10–14 days before changes are evident on radiographs. [Of the many radioactive substances used, technetium polyphosphates appear to produce the best results (Fig. 5.30).] Despite its usefulness, radionuclide imaging has important limitations. First, in some patients multiple 'hot spots' are detected in the bones at an early stage of *S. aureus* septicemia, but these 'spots' do not necessarily progress to clinical osteomyelitis. (It is not known whether these areas represent false-positive results or aborted bone infection.) Second, experimental and clinical studies have documented rare cases of osteomyelitis that have been confirmed by bacteriologic and histologic studies, even though bone scans were initially negative. (This phenomenon may be explained by impaired blood supply to or infarction of the infected area.) Third, technetium polyphosphate bone scanning performed after fracture or bone surgery does not differentiate bone repair from bone infection.

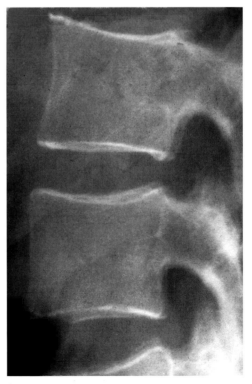

(b)

Figure 5.28   (a) Radiograph of the lumbar spine of a 55-year-old female to demonstrate the typical appearance of established late-stage septic spondylitis, which in this case was due to *E. coli* secondary to genitourinary infection. There is destruction of the adjacent vertebral end-plates of L3 and L4 with some bone sclerosis. A radiograph taken 2 months previously (b) shows no obvious evidence of disease. (Courtesy of Dr Alex Norman.)

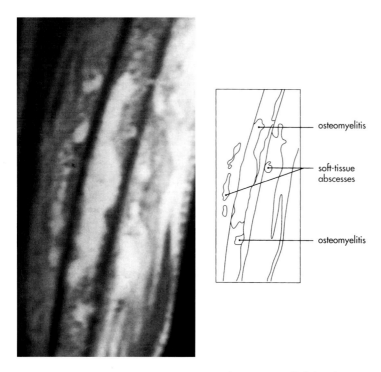

Figure 5.29   Magnetic resonance image showing a well-defined area of increased signal intensity in the medullary space of the midshaft of the femur, representing osteomyelitis in this i.v. drug abuser. There are soft-tissue inflammatory changes with multiple small abscesses adjacent to the femur.

BACTERIOLOGIC DIAGNOSIS

The conclusive diagnosis of septic arthritis or osteomyelitis depends on the isolation of the pathogen from the lesion or from blood cultures (Fig. 5.31). However, the blood culture may be positive only in about 50% of patients with acute, untreated hematogenous osteomyelitis. In patients for whom osteomyelitis is a likely diagnosis on the basis of clinical data, direct bone aspiration or surgical biopsy should be carried out when blood culture has been negative. The importance of immediate inoculation into the medium of the material suspected of being infected cannot be overemphasized. Delay in getting the material from the operating room to the microbiology laboratory, and consequently in plating out and inoculating medium from swabs and tissue obtained from the diseased area, may lead to a reduced number of viable organisms, and therefore to a false-negative culture.

MORBID ANATOMY OF OSTEOMYELITIS

The presence of bacteria in a bone does not necessarily lead to osteomyelitis and it is generally believed that trauma is an important associated prerequisite, perhaps because it produces venostasis or thrombosis and thus provides a nidus for bacterial growth.

As with most infections, the clinical course of bone infection depends on the interaction between the injurious agent and the host tissue. In other words, the severity of the disease in a patient with osteomyelitis depends on the virulence of the infecting organism, the site of infection, and the patient's age and general health.

The initial local response to infection with pyogenic bacteria is acute inflammation, resulting in production of a fluid exudate containing polymorphonuclear leukocytes (neutrophils) and fibrin (Figs 5.32 and 5.33). Continuing exudation raises the tissue pressure and, because the bone is unable to expand, this pressure cannot be relieved by swelling, as is possible in most tissues. Instead, the only potential space – the vascular space – is compromised, leading to widespread bone death (Fig. 5.34). Indeed,

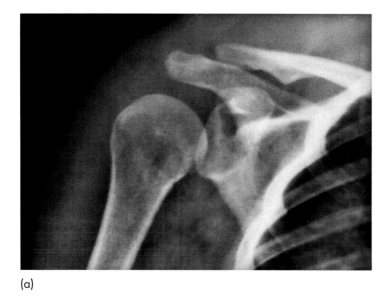

(a)

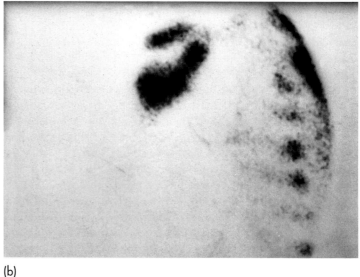

(b)

Figure 5.30   Radiograph of the shoulder in a patient with fever, and pain and tenderness at the upper end of the humerus (**a**). Although some osteolysis may be present, it is difficult to define a lesion. No obvious periosteal reaction has occurred. However, in the isotope scan intense uptake of radioactive isotope is evident at the upper end of the humerus (**b**). (A scan frequently demonstrates the presence of osteomyelitis before any changes are evident on radiographs.)

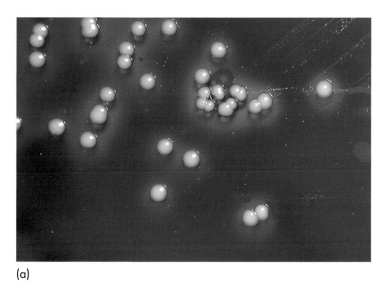

(a)

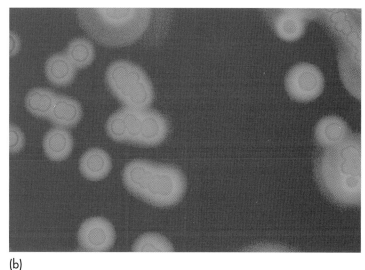

(b)

Figure 5.31 (**a**) Colonies of *S. aureus* illuminated to show their color and growth characteristics on blood agar. (**b**) Transilluminated to show hemolysis of the blood agar plate around each colony.

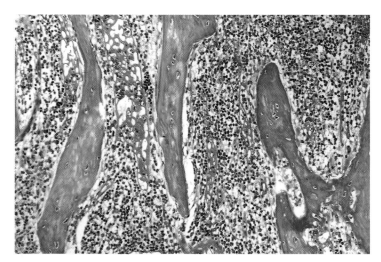

Figure 5.32 Photomicrograph to illustrate the acute phase of osteomyelitis. The marrow space is filled with acute inflammatory cells but no obvious bone destruction or necrosis is yet evident (H&E, × 10 obj.).

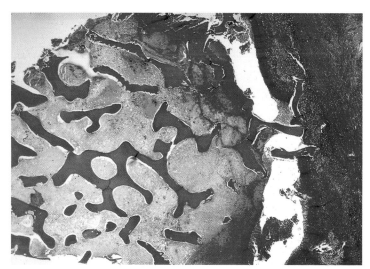

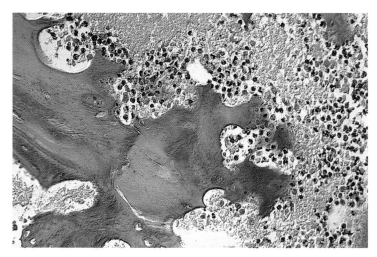

Figure 5.33 Photomicrograph of biopsy tissue from a case of osteomyelitis at a slightly later stage than in Figure 5.32 demonstrates a polymorphonuclear leukocyte infiltrate with focal areas of fibrinous exudate. The bone is necrotic and shows focal surface erosion secondary to enzymatic digestion (H&E, × 25 obj.).

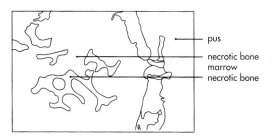

pus

necrotic bone
marrow
necrotic bone

Figure 5.34 Photomicrograph demonstrates an area of necrotic bone surrounded by an acute inflammatory exudate (pus). A focus of necrotic bone such as this allows the sequestration of bacteria, and, unless it is surgically removed, antibiotic therapy may not prevent the development of chronic relapsing osteomyelitis (H&E, × 4 obj.).

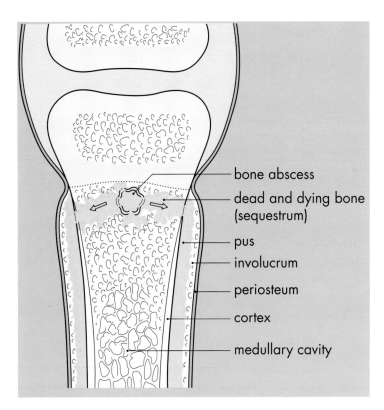

- bone abscess
- dead and dying bone (sequestrum)
- pus
- involucrum
- periosteum
- cortex
- medullary cavity

Figure 5.35 As illustrated in this diagram, increased pressure in the medullary cavity eventually results in extension of the inflammatory exudate through the haversian systems of the cortex and beneath the periosteum. The elevated periosteum will lay down a sleeve of new bone (the involucrum) around the infected bone (the sequestrum) segment. In children, this reaction is likely to be prominent, in adults, much less so.

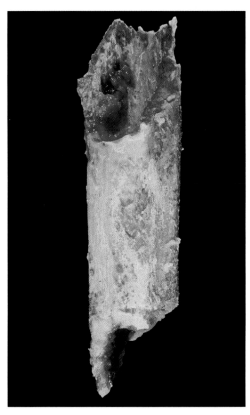

Figure 5.37 Gross photograph of a sequestrum removed from a patient with chronic osteomyelitis of the femur. It is important to remove such a focus of dead bone from an individual with osteomyelitis if persistent chronic infection is to be avoided.

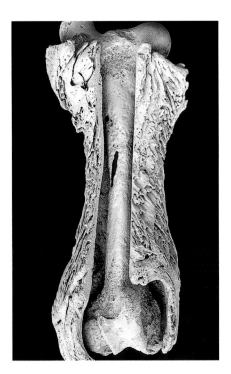

Figure 5.36 Gross photograph of a femur from a young cow with osteomyelitis of the femur. The periosteal reaction has resulted in an extensive sleeve of new bone (the involucrum) which surrounds the necrotic, partially destroyed diaphysis of the femur (the sequestrum).

the major clinical problem in treating patients with osteomyelitis is the extent of the osteonecrosis, which interferes with the access of antibiotics.

In the natural course of events, the exudate is forced through the medullary canal and the haversian systems of the cortical bone to the bone surface. In children, the cortex is thin and the periosteum only loosely attached, so it is easily elevated (Fig. 5.35). New bone from the cambium layer of the periosteum produces a sleeve of reactive bone (the involucrum) around the affected bone segment. In very young children, the involucrum may be quite massive (Fig. 5.36). In adults (because the periosteum is firmly attached to the cortical bone), the periosteal elevation and new bone formation may be minimal. In children, the necrotic medullary bone becomes isolated within a large cavity and is referred to as the sequestrum (Fig. 5.37). The sequestrum may consist of a mere wafer of cortex, the devascularized cancellous bone having been absorbed, or it may be a large piece of bone or many small pieces. In adults, a large involucrum and the associated sequestrum formation are much less common. In untreated cases, the pus frequently extends beyond the confines of the periosteum into the soft tissue and ultimately through the skin, forming a draining sinus (Fig. 5.38).

The extent of the bone affected varies from case to case. When the entire diaphysis is surrounded by pus, it becomes completely necrotic. If only a small area is devascularized, the affected area may be gradually resorbed and an abscess (Brodie's abscess) will form (Fig. 5.39). The radiographic differential diagnosis of Brodie's abscess might include osteoid osteoma, eosinophilic granuloma, and malignant small-cell tumors (Fig. 5.40).

Bone infection does not result in localized abscesses in most patients because necrotic bone undergoes resorption only when

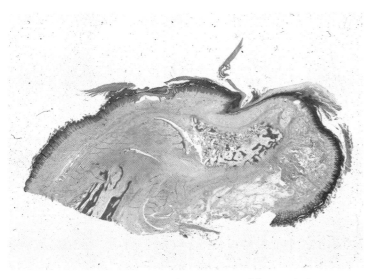

Figure 5.38 Photomicrograph of a toe removed from a diabetic patient who had developed osteomyelitis. The inflammatory response has led to destruction of the bone, the distal interphalangeal joint, and a sinus tract opening onto the skin dorsally (H&E, × 1 obj.).

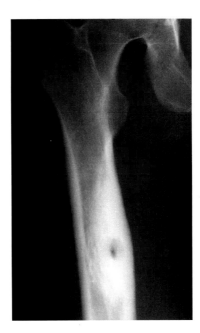

Figure 5.40 Radiograph to show a bone abscess in the upper femoral shaft of a 33-year-old male demonstrating massive bone sclerosis and mature periosteal bone formation. The lack of central calcification in the lytic area together with the age of the patient make a diagnosis of osteoid osteoma less likely. (Courtesy of Dr Alex Norman.)

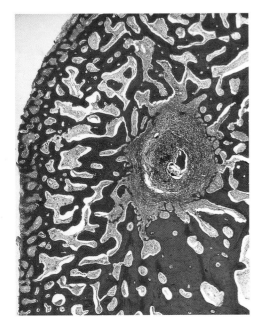

Figure 5.39 Photomicrograph of a cortical abscess, excised from the femoral neck of a 12-year-old boy, which was mistaken clinically and radiographically for an osteoid osteoma (H&E, × 1 obj.).

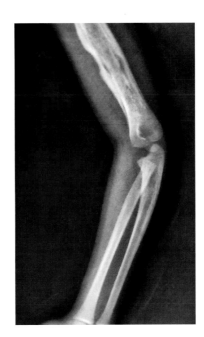

Figure 5.41 Radiograph of the arm in a patient with sickle-cell disease shows permeative bone destruction of the humerus, with involucrum formation and extensive sequestration. At surgery, these complications were shown to be due to infection.

there are viable marrow cells to secrete the necessary enzymes and provide active osteoclast phagocytosis.

Osteomyelitis often accompanies disease that results in vascular insufficiency as in, for example, sickle-cell anemia, in which patients often experience repeated bone infections (Fig. 5.41). In almost all cases, the infecting organisms are Gram-negative rods, most commonly *Salmonella* (approximately 80%). However, Gram-positive bacteria, particularly *S. aureus* are also routinely found in these patients. Because the presenting symptoms in individuals with sickle-cell disease are often insidious and mimic those of marrow crisis, early culture of blood and stool is recom-

mended. Presumptive antibiotic therapy should include agents active against *Salmonella* species. [It should be noted that not all instances of *Salmonella* osteomyelitis are encountered in patients with sickle-cell disease (Fig. 5.42).]

Two other bone diseases that may be complicated by ischemia and infection are Gaucher's disease and osteopetrosis. In patients with Gaucher's disease, osteomyelitis sometimes follows a biopsy procedure. Therefore, if a biopsy is performed on such patients the strictest asepsis is necessary (and even antibiotic coverage should be considered). In patients with osteopetrosis, the jaw is often affected, probably via tooth infections.

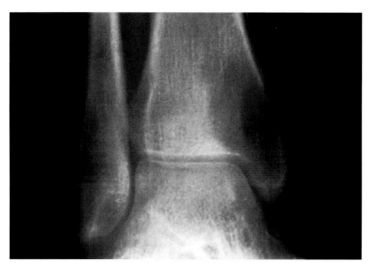

Figure 5.42   Radiograph of a middle-aged woman who was in good general health except for pain in the right ankle. The X-ray was interpreted as being most consistent with a giant-cell tumor. Biopsy proved the lesion to be inflammatory, and *Salmonella typhosa* was isolated by culture.

GRANULOMATOUS INFLAMMATION OF BONES AND JOINTS

MYCOBACTERIAL INFECTION (TUBERCULOSIS)

Clinical considerations

In 1779, Percival Pott described the clinical presentation of paraplegia associated with the characteristic gibbus formation that bears his name. We now know that Pott's disease is most commonly associated with granulomatous inflammation due to mycobacterial infection.

Approximately 1% of patients with granulomatous inflammation develop musculoskeletal complications and the most common site of skeletal involvement is the spine, because the most common primary foci are in the lungs and bowel. Before the advent of modern chemotherapy for mycobacterium tuberculosis, and before the elimination of bovine tuberculosis in most of the western world, bone and joint tuberculosis was one of the most common indications for admission to an orthopaedic service. In less developed countries this is still the case. In developed countries, however, tuberculosis has become unusual enough that there is a real risk that it may remain clinically undetected. In many instances, the true nature of the disease becomes apparent only after the pathologist has examined the tissue. There is increased risk for mycobacterial infection in individuals with chronic debilitating conditions including narcotic addicts, therapeutically immunosuppressed patients and those with AIDS. In

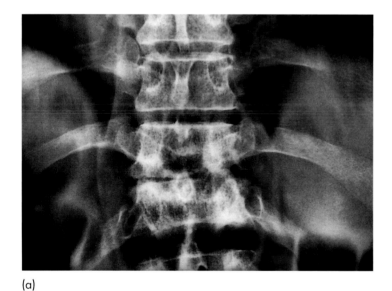

(a)

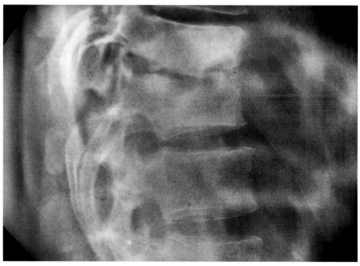

(b)

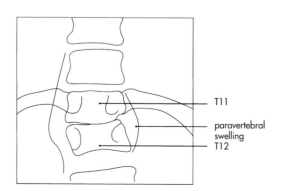

T11

paravertebral swelling

T12

Figure 5.43   Antero-posterior radiograph of the spine (**a**) shows narrowing and destruction of the intervertebral disc at the level of T11–T12. Note also the paravertebral soft-tissue swelling. In the lateral radiograph (**b**), destructive bone disease is seen anteriorly in the 11th and 12th thoracic vertebrae. This lesion was proved to be due to tuberculosis.

the latter group miliary mycobacterial disease may present as an acute febrile illness. However, in most patients the onset of symptoms is likely to be insidious and includes local pain as well as systemic signs of chronic debilitating illness.

Osseous disease is caused by metastatic spread of the mycobacterium from elsewhere in the body, usually from the lungs. In most patients, bony foci of infection coexist with arthritis, and multiple skeletal lesions are not uncommon. Skeletal manifestation of infection most often occurs in the spine (Figs 5.43 and 5.44); the next most commonly affected area is the hip (Figs 5.45 and 5.46), followed by the knee (Fig. 5.47). However, any joint may be involved, including those of the hand.

In general, osseous disease is most common in patients under the age of 25 years and both sexes are equally affected. The spine and hip are more commonly affected in children, and the knee is more common in adults.

The lower thoracic spine is the most frequent site of tuberculous spondylitis, and involvement of several vertebral bodies occurs in 50% of cases. The disease often begins in one vertebral body and spreads underneath the spinal ligaments to affect other vertebrae. In untreated patients, this course of events eventually leads to vertebral collapse and angulation of the vertebral column (Fig. 5.48).

At the time of presentation, the patient with tuberculous spondylitis may have radiculopathy caused by compression of the spinal cord or nerve roots. The disease may also spread to the meninges, with subsequent tuberculous meningitis.

Paraplegia was the most serious complication before the advent of antibiotic therapy. Paraplegia is caused by extension of the disease process into the peridural space with resultant pressure on the cord. This may be accentuated by the mechanical

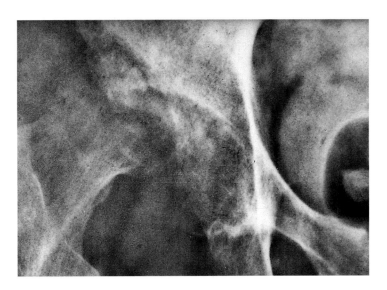

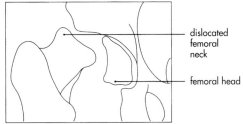

dislocated femoral neck

femoral head

Figure 5.45 Radiograph of a patient with longstanding pain and limitation of motion in the right hip. Destructive joint disease with involvement of the bone is evident in both the femoral head and the acetabulum. In addition, a dislocation of the femoral neck has occurred. These are common manifestations of tuberculosis.

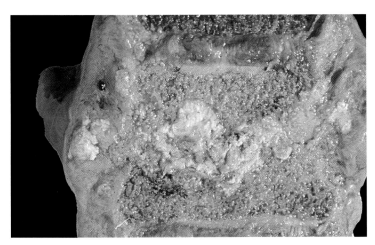

Figure 5.44 Gross photograph of a portion of the spine removed at necropsy from a patient with tuberculosis reveals destruction of the intervertebral disc space and contiguous bone, and the presence of a cheesy necrotic tissue (caseation necrosis). The caseating tissue extends into the soft tissue on either side of the spinal column.

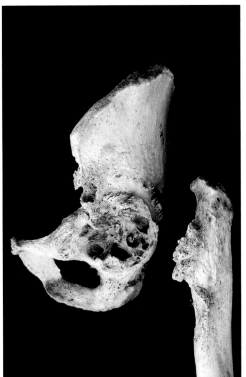

Figure 5.46 Macerated bone specimen obtained at necropsy demonstrates destructive disease of the hip joint in a patient with tuberculosis. Total destruction of the femoral head has occurred, with only a stump of the femoral neck remaining attached to the shaft of the femur.

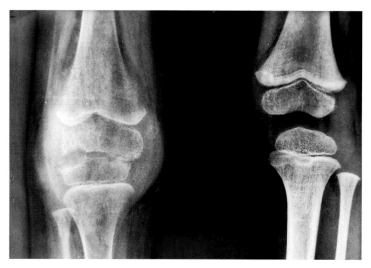

Figure 5.47   Radiograph of the knees in a child complaining of pain, swelling, and limitation of motion in the right knee. Note the narrowing of the joint, resulting from the destruction of cartilage and bone, that is evident in the right knee (the destruction is particularly obvious at the margins of the joint). In addition to the destructive changes, the radiograph also shows marked soft-tissue swelling. These changes were caused by tuberculosis.

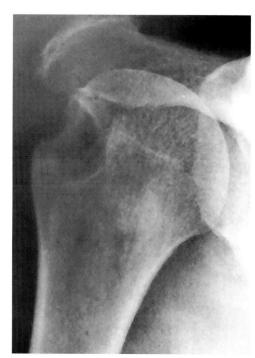

Figure 5.49
Radiograph showing a well-defined lytic lesion in the outer aspect of the humeral head, which encroaches upon both the epiphysis and metaphysis. This lesion proved on biopsy to be due to tuberculosis.

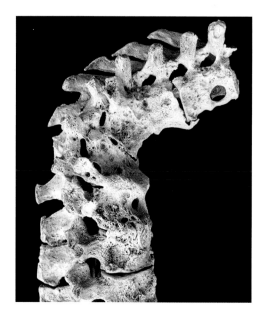

Figure 5.48
Macerated specimen of spine removed at autopsy from a patient with chronic tuberculosis. In addition to extensive bone destruction, severe kyphosis and fusion of several vertebral bodies are seen.

pressure associated with bone deformity. Dislocation of affected segments may lead to sudden paraplegia.

Because the initial lesion is most often seen in the lower thoracic spine, the psoas muscle sheath is frequently involved in the process. Patients may present with a fluctuant swelling, or cold abscess, in the groin or elsewhere as the result of tracking of the infected material from the paraspinal area.

Radiographic findings

Radiographic examination of an involved joint shows osteopenia and soft-tissue swelling early in the disease. These changes are followed by marginal erosion of the bone and destruction of the subchondral bone, with narrowing of the joint space.

In non-weight-bearing joints such as the shoulder, but also occasionally in the knee joint, subchondral lysis may occur without obvious joint destruction and narrowing. In such cases, which are sometimes referred to as 'caries sicca', the lesion may mimic a tumor radiographically, and so in children may be mistaken for a chondroblastoma (Fig. 5.49).

In the spine, radiographic examination may show focal bony destruction with disc involvement and vertebral collapse. Unlike pyogenic osteomyelitis, reactive new bone and hypertrophied osteophyte around the infected focus are not common.

The primary granulomatous abscess may be located in the vertebral body either anteriorly, paradiscally, or centrally, giving rise to three characteristic radiographic presentations (Fig. 5.50).

The anterior lesion, which accounts for approximately 20% of cases, usually leads to cortical bone destruction under the anterior longitudinal ligament. As the ligament lifts off the vertebral margin, infection spreads to the adjacent vertebral segment.

The paradiscal lesion, which accounts for over half of the cases, begins in the vertebral metaphysis and erodes through the cartilaginous end-plate, extending around and sequestrating the disc to extend into the adjacent vertebra. Disc space narrowing, bone destruction with subsequent kyphotic deformity, and eventual intervertebral body fusion occur, usually after 1–2 years.

The central lesion, which accounts for the remaining cases, begins in the mid-portion of the vertebral body. It then spreads to involve the entire vertebral body, leading to vertebral collapse and usually to pronounced gibbus deformity (Fig. 5.51).

Pathologic findings

Gross examination of the areas affected by tuberculosis is likely to show thickened edematous tissue, frequently studded with grayish small nodules, sometimes with white opaque centers (granulomas). These granulomas often become confluent and produce larger areas of white necrotic material, so-called caseation (or

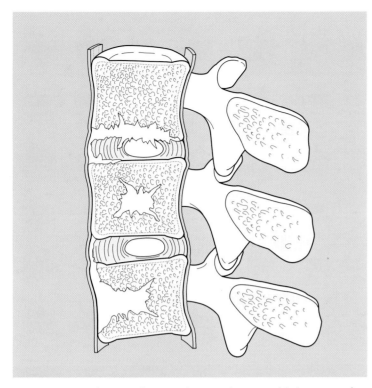

Figure 5.50 Schematic drawing showing three possible locations of the primary focus of tuberculosis infection in the vertebral body. Each results in a characteristic radiographic presentation.

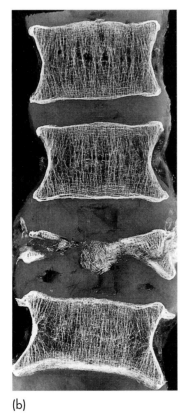

(a)   (b)

Figure 5.51 (a) Frontal section through the thoracolumbar spine of a 67-year-old male. There is complete collapse of L3 secondary to tuberculosis, which initially involved the mid-portion of the vertebral body. (b) Specimen radiograph of illustration (a).

cheesy) necrosis. In the joint separation of the articular cartilage, dissected from the underlying bone by granulomatous tissue, is a characteristic feature. In the later stages of untreated disease, ankylosis is a frequent complication.

On microscopic examination, the typical granuloma (Figs 5.52 and 5.53) consists of a central necrotic area surrounded by pale histiocytes, sometimes referred to as epithelioid cells. Among the epithelioid cells are some scattered giant cells, the nuclei of which are typically arranged at the margin of the cell (Langerhans' giant cells). At the periphery of the tubercle is a rim of mixed chronic inflammatory cells. Often the granulomas are confluent, resulting in extensive central caseation necrosis. The acid-fast

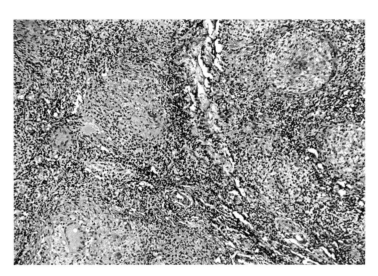

Figure 5.52 Photomicrograph of granulomatous tissue obtained from the synovium of a knee joint in a patient with tuberculosis. Many focal giant cells, nodular collections of histiocytes, and an infiltration of chronic inflammatory cells are present. In this section, caseation necrosis is not present (H&E, × 4 obj.).

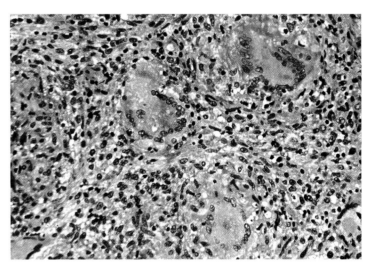

Figure 5.53 Photomicrograph showing the typical appearance of the giant cells in tuberculosis, with peripherally arranged nuclei – the so-called Langerhans' giant cells (H&E, × 10 obj.).

bacilli (AFB) can be demonstrated with the Ziehl–Neelsen stain, and are characteristically seen in the giant cells and at the margin of the caseous area.

ATYPICAL MYCOBACTERIAL DISEASE

Patients who are severely immunocompromised, in particular those with advanced human immunodeficiency virus (HIV) infection, are at risk for disseminated mycobacterial disease usually, but not always, *Mycobacterium avium* complex. Bone infection in these patients, as in others with severe immunodeficiency diseases, can be difficult to detect because local redness and swelling may be absent and the patient afebrile. Typical granulomas may not form and microscopically, only large numbers of histiocytes with admixed chronic inflammatory cells may be present. However, acid-fast staining reveals large numbers of intracellular mycobacteria – many more than are seen in a patient with the more typical presentation of tuberculosis (Fig. 5.54). In general though, diagnosis invariably depends on imaging techniques in conjunction with a well-educated guess.

In addition to *M. avium-intracellulare*, nontuberculous mycobacteria causing osteoarticular infections include *M. fortuitum* group, *M. marinum*, *M. kansasii*, *M. abscessus*, and *M. chelonae*. All nontuberculous mycobacteria are ubiquitous in the environment (soil, water, animals, and birds) and, while generally less pathogenic than *M. tuberculosis*, they do cause a variety of infections. Notably though, as with most infecting microbes, the intrinsic virulence of mycobacterial species is not the sole factor determining clinical outcome. The genetic background as well as the immune status of the infected individual play an important role in the expression of mycobacterial disease.

Nontuberculosis mycobacteria can cause a variety of chronic granulomatous infections affecting tendon sheaths, bursae, bones and joints after direct inoculation through accidental trauma, surgical incision, puncture wounds, or injections. Not surprisingly then, there have been a number of recent reports of acupuncture mycobacteriosis due to *M. chelonae* – an organism commonly colonizing instruments or growing in contaminated water and difficult to kill with regular cleaning and disinfection methods. An association may not be made between the inoculating procedure (i.e. acupuncture) and the clinical illness because the infection has such a long incubation period.

Osteomyelitis can also follow infection with *Mycobacterium marinum*, a common aquatic organism. The bacteria are inoculated into traumatized skin exposed to contaminated water (or fish) and clinical disease typically begins with small papules which become suppurative. Infection, which can take up to 4 weeks to develop, is usually localized to distal portions of the upper extremities and resolves spontaneously. However, dissemination to bursa, joints and bone has been reported in both immunocompetent and immunocompromised people and *M. marinum* infection can easily be misdiagnosed as gout, rheumatoid arthritis, tendinitis, or sterile abscesses. Antibiotic therapy can prove difficult because the organism is resistant to many conventional antimicrobial agents.

Management of nontuberculosis mycobacterial bone and joint infections always require surgical debridement. Drug therapy for specific pathogens is also essential. Identification of the organisms increasingly focuses on rapid diagnostic systems [including high-performance liquid chromatography (HPLC), polymerase chain reaction (PCR) and genetic probes].

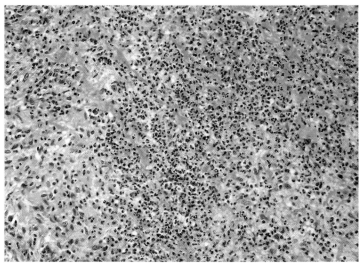

(a)

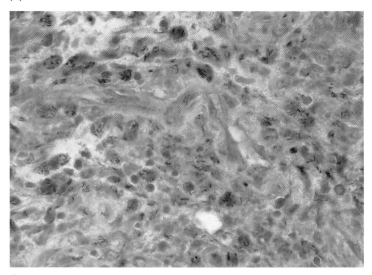

(b)

Figure 5.54   (a) Photomicrograph of tissue obtained from a periarticular abscess in a middle-aged male who had renal transplantation and immunosuppressive therapy. Microscopically there is a heavy infiltration of acute inflammatory cells with many admixed large histiocytic cells. No granulomas are recognized (H&E, × 10 obj.). (b) An acid-fast bacilli (AFB) stain shows an abundance of organisms, mostly intracellular. This is a typical microscopic presentation for atypical mycobacterial infection (Ziehl–Neelsen, × 50 obj.).

SARCOIDOSIS

About 10% of patients with sarcoidosis have an episode of joint involvement. In most cases this is a migratory acute polyarticular disease, often symmetrical and of only a few weeks' duration. Hilar lymphadenopathy and erythema nodosum are frequently associated. In a small number of patients, a chronic granulomatous arthritis is present. This may involve a large joint and is generally monoarticular. The lesion is most likely to be mistaken for tuberculosis (Fig. 5.55). However, certain histologic features help to distinguish sarcoidosis from tuberculosis: the formation of well-delineated tight granulomas, the lack of

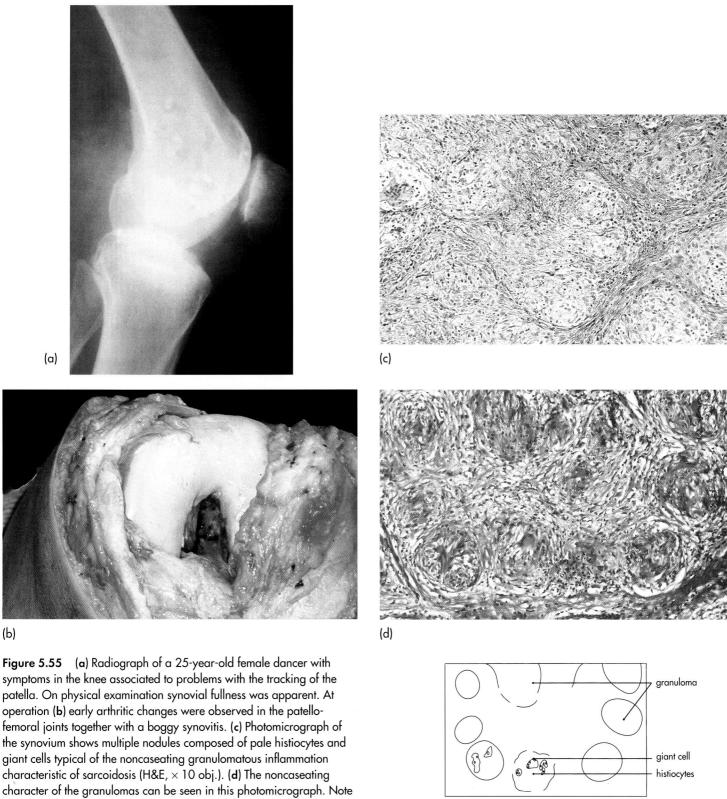

(a)

(b)

(c)

(d)

Figure 5.55 (a) Radiograph of a 25-year-old female dancer with symptoms in the knee associated to problems with the tracking of the patella. On physical examination synovial fullness was apparent. At operation (b) early arthritic changes were observed in the patello-femoral joints together with a boggy synovitis. (c) Photomicrograph of the synovium shows multiple nodules composed of pale histiocytes and giant cells typical of the noncaseating granulomatous inflammation characteristic of sarcoidosis (H&E, × 10 obj.). (d) The noncaseating character of the granulomas can be seen in this photomicrograph. Note also the lack of lymphocytic cuffing of the granulomas. The rarity of sarcoidosis in large joints is likely to result in misinterpretation of the lesion as some other form of granulomatous inflammation, as was the case in this patient, who was treated with antitubercular drugs for 18 months without improvement, until the correct diagnosis of sarcoidosis was made (H&E, × 25 obj.).

granuloma

giant cell
histiocytes

caseation necrosis, the increased prominence of large, pale epithelioid cells with fewer chronic inflammatory cells, and the absence of AFB. (With regard to the last point, it should be noted that it is frequently difficult to demonstrate AFB in patients with bone and joint tuberculosis. In any individual suspected of having granulomatous tissue, smears should be taken for direct examination, and cultures for tuberculosis, brucellosis, fungus, and atypical mycobacteria should be prepared. In general, a firm diagnosis can be made only when positive cultures have been obtained.)

About 5% of patients with early acute or subacute sarcoidosis will be found to have asymptomatic bone changes on routine radiography of the hands, feet and occasionally in other bones (Figs 5.56 and 5.57). The most common clinical findings in sarcoid dactylitis are soft-tissue swelling over the affected digits, with tenderness and stiffness of the adjacent joints; the overlying skin may be erythematous. When the terminal phalanges are involved, the nails may show thickening and ridging. In severe cases, the affected bones may be completely resorbed, leading to virtual disappearance of the phalanges, sometimes complicated by pathologic fractures and marked deformity.

MYCOTIC INFECTIONS

As with tuberculosis infections, fungal infections are likely to be seen more frequently in debilitated patients, especially young immunocompromised individuals. The spine, as well as other bones and joints, can be affected by mycotic infections, with the lung being the usual portal of entry. The radiographic and pathologic features are similar to those of tuberculosis. For this reason, when granulomatous infection is found or suspected, it is important to make direct smears and to prepare cultures not only for acid-fast organisms but also for fungi. Common fungal conditions that have been found to be responsible for granulomatous infections include blastomycosis, coccidioidomycosis, cryptococcosis, candidiasis and sporotrichosis.

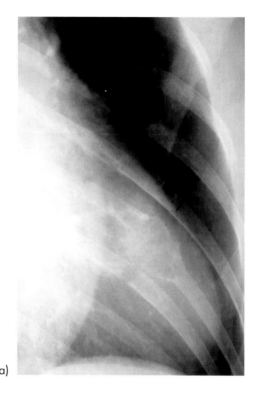

(a)

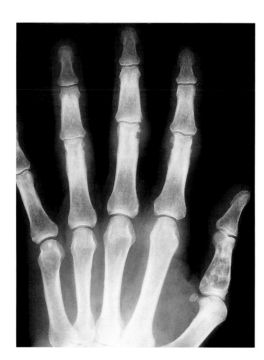

Figure 5.56 Radiograph of the hand in a patient with sarcoidosis demonstrates the two types of lesions that can be seen in this condition. Punched-out cortical erosions, some with obvious overlying soft-tissue lesions, are evident at the distal end of the proximal phalanx in the index, middle, and ring fingers. In the thumb is a central lytic lesion of the proximal phalanx, similar in appearance to the lesions of dactylitis tuberculosa seen in young adults.

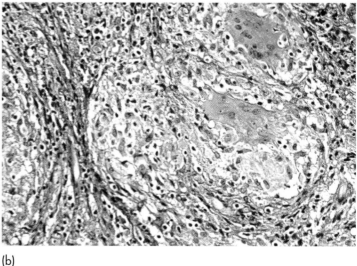

(b)

Figure 5.57 A 52-year-old woman with pleuritic pain showed on x-ray examination (a) lytic lesion in the 5th and 7th rib. Biopsy (b) revealed granulomatous inflammation consistent with sarcoidosis (H&E, × 10 obj.).

Blastomycosis

Blastomycosis is endemic in the south-eastern and south central states of the USA as well as Canadian provinces that border the Great Lakes. *Blastomyces dermatitidis* is the asexual stage of *Ajellomyces dermatitidis*. *Blastomyces dermatitidis* is dimorphic – growing as mycelial form at room temperature and transforming into a yeast form at 37°C. Initial infection is through the lungs and generally subclinical. The organism may be carried throughout the body via blood, culminating in disease with protean manifestations. The most common skeletal sites are the vertebrae, ribs, tibia, and the tarsal and carpal bones. Vertebral disease is easily confused with tuberculosis, with anterior involvement of the vertebral body, interspace destruction and development of large paraspinous abscesses. Therefore, if the vertebrae are involved, radiographic differentiation from tuberculous spondylitis can be difficult (Fig. 5.58). Microscopic examination of a stained smear of sputum, pleural fluid, or pus from the affected part will reveal the characteristic thick-walled, budding yeast cells.

Coccidioidomycosis

Coccidioidomycosis, also known as San Joaquin Valley fever, is caused by the fungus *Coccidioides immitis*. There is a high incidence of this disease in the arid south-western USA. The bone lesions are usually lytic, with indiscriminate involvement and destruction of vertebral bodies, neural arches, and even contiguous ribs. Late changes of vertebral collapse may render differentiation from tuberculous spondylitis difficult (Figs 5.59 and 5.60).

Cryptococcosis

Skeletal cryptococcosis often occurs secondary to cases of chronic meningoencephalitis caused by *C. neoformans*. The pelvis, femur, spine, and tibia are among the most common sites of involvement. Patients usually present with pain, swelling, and tenderness over the affected part. Radiographically, these lesions present as radiolucencies with or without local subperiosteal new bone formation. Histologically, the lesions reveal granulation tissue containing multinuclear giant cells, lymphocytes, and histiocytes. The presence of the yeast-like cryptococci may also be demonstrated.

Other fungal infections

Sporotrichosis infection may result from the direct contamination of a joint by a puncture wound from the thorn of a contaminated plant (often a rose).

Patients with long-term indwelling i.v. catheters (e.g. for parenteral nutrition) occasionally develop bone and joint infections due to *Candida* or *Aspergillus*.

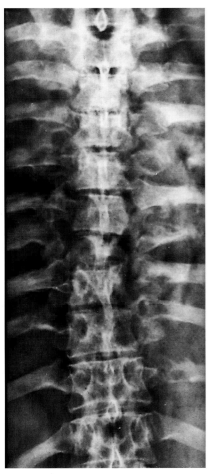

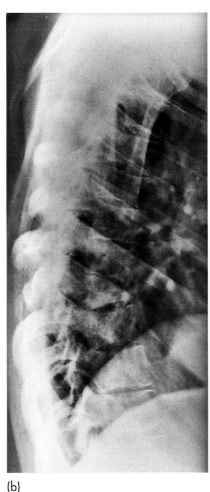

(a)   (b)

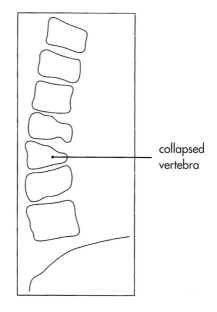

Figure 5.58 Anteroposterior (**a**) and lateral (**b**) radiographs of the thoracic spine demonstrate multiple destructive lesions involving several vertebral bodies, some of which are partially collapsed. Biopsy proved this to be due to blastomycosis.

collapsed vertebra

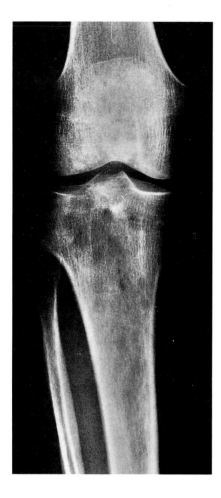

Figure 5.59 Radiograph of the knee of a 60-year-old man complaining of mild pain for a few months. The film shows a poorly defined lytic lesion extending from the articular surface of the tibia into the diaphysis. The cortex appears to be intact. Biopsy proved this to be the result of infection with coccidioidomycosis. (Courtesy of Dr A. Roessner.)

Because blood cultures are likely to be negative, biopsy may be necessary for diagnosis of fungal infections.

PARASITIC INFECTIONS

Echinococcal cysts

Echinococcal cysts (hydatid cysts) are commonly seen in the bones of patients from sheep-raising countries in which the disease is endemic (Spain, Greece, and the Middle East). The cyst is often seen initially at the epiphyseal end of the bone, usually affecting the spongiosa because localization is dependent on hematogenous dissemination. It should be noted that hydatid echinococcosis developing intraosseously does not resemble the classic unilocular hydatid of soft tissue. Rather, it is usually a multiloculated lesion, with an irregular outline that can be easily confused with a tumor on radiographs (Fig. 5.61). This is because the resistance offered by the osseous tissue causes the larva to develop by exogenous budding, resulting in the presence of many small cysts growing outside the original focus of implantation (Fig. 5.62). Scolices rarely develop in these cysts, and therefore, they are usually sterile (Fig. 5.63). Only when the cyst erupts to the surrounding soft tissue does the lesion assume the more conventional large unilocular appearance.

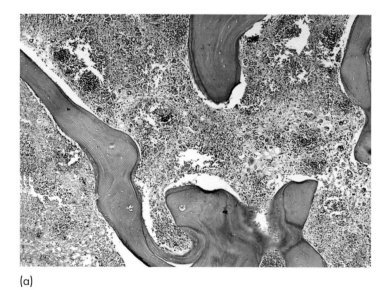

(a)

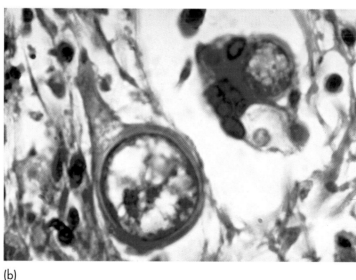

(b)

Figure 5.60   (a) Low-power photomicrograph of tissue obtained from a patient with chronic spinal disease resulting from infection with *Coccidioides immitis*. The marrow space is infiltrated by chronic inflammatory tissue (H&E, × 4 obj.). (b) High-power view of the same tissue reveals two rounded, thick-walled fungal organisms containing endospores (H&E, × 100 obj.).

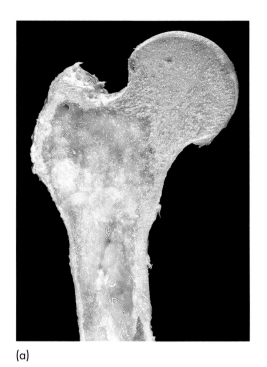

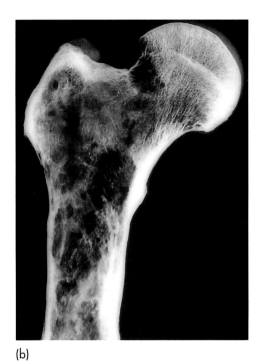

(a)

(b)

Figure 5.61   (a) Gross photograph of the upper end of a femur removed at necropsy from a patient with hydatid disease. The medullary cavity is filled with glistening white nodular tissue, which on closer examination is found to be made up of fibrous walled cysts. (b) Radiograph of the same specimen shows a multiloculated lytic appearance and irregular thinning of the cortices. In those parts of the world where the occurrence of hydatid disease is rare, such radiographic findings will probably be interpreted by the radiologist as a tumor.

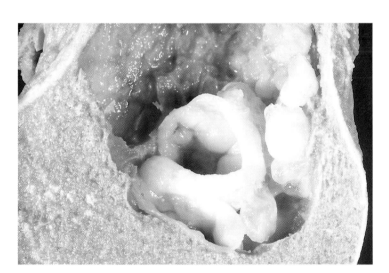

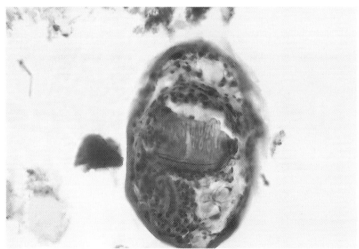

Figure 5.62   Gross photograph of the many small cysts that are characteristic of echinococcal infestation of the bone.

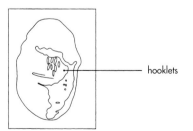

hooklets

Figure 5.63   Photomicrograph of material removed from a hydatid cyst reveals a scolex with hooklets (H&E, × 100 obj.).

METABOLIC DISTURBANCES

DISEASES RESULTING FROM ABNORMAL SYNTHESIS OF MATRIX COMPONENTS

The final adult size of an individual (height, weight, build) is the result of many complex factors, both intrinsic (genetic), and extrinsic (such as diet and activity level). Perhaps the most important determinants of size are the total number of connective tissue cells involved in production of the extracellular matrix, and the quantity of extracellular matrix produced by each of the connective tissue cells. Especially important to skeletal size, is the optimal functioning of the epiphyseal growth plate during the period of development.

As previously discussed in Chapter 1, p. 6, the mechanical properties of the connective tissues depend on the synthesis by osteoblasts, chondroblasts and fibroblasts of organic matrix constituents including collagen, proteoglycan (PG), and other non-collagenous proteins, both of the right type and in the right amount.

Disturbances in collagen synthesis may be congenital, as in osteogenesis imperfecta (OI), or acquired, as in scurvy. The disturbance may be intracellular, as in both OI and scurvy, or extracellular, as in some cases of Ehlers–Danlos syndrome (Fig. 6.1). However, whether congenital or acquired, pretranslational or post-translational, all of these conditions give rise to abnormalities in the connective tissue matrices that affect the mechanical properties of the skeleton.

The mechanical properties of the bony skeleton also depend on the calcification of the organic matrix. This, in turn, depends not only on adequate amounts of calcium and inorganic phosphates in the tissue fluid but also on the exercise of cellular control by means of the positive and negative influences of many substances, including alkaline phosphatase.

In this chapter, the most important of the diseases resulting from disturbances in both organic and inorganic matrix synthesis will be discussed.

DISTURBANCES IN COLLAGEN SYNTHESIS

OSTEOGENESIS IMPERFECTA

Clinical evaluation
OI is the most commonly recognized congenital disease affecting the production of collagen. It involves the bone matrix as well as other connective tissues. The disease comprises a number of distinct syndromes having in common propensity to fracture and

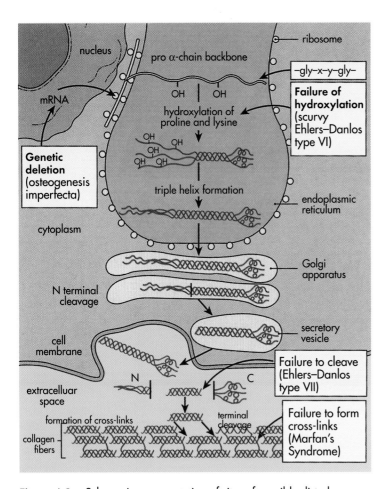

Figure 6.1   Schematic representation of sites of possible disturbances in collagen synthesis leading to various disorders.

clinical evidence of osteopenia. Some of these syndromes are inherited as an autosomal dominant trait, others as a recessive trait, and still others occur as spontaneous mutations. Many patients have poorly formed dentin, hearing loss and Ehlers–Danlos-like features; however, it is the susceptibility to fracture that gives rise to most of their clinical problems. On the basis of clinical as well as genetic features, six distinct groups have been described.

- Type I, the largest group, has an autosomal dominant inheritance with moderate osteoporosis and gray-blue sclera. The disease is mild and often the patient is at the low end of normal height.
- Type II is lethal before or soon after birth, and has an autosomal recessive mode of inheritance. There is severe osteoporosis and the long bones are said to be characteristically broad and crumpled.
- Type III, a severe clinical form of the disease in children surviving the perinatal period, results in multiple fractures and progressive deformities. In these patients, the scleral color is almost normal, and both autosomal dominant and recessive inheritance patterns have been observed.
- Type IV has an autosomal dominant pattern of inheritance of osteoporosis which is of varying severity and associated with normal scleral color.
- Type V is a form of autosomal dominant OI which does not appear to be associated with collagen type I mutations and has

been reported to be associated with hyperplastic callus formation.

- Type VI OI is a moderate to severe form of disease with accumulation of osteoid due to a mineralization defect in the absence of a disturbance of mineral metabolism. No mutations have been found in type VI OI and type I collagen protein analyses are reported to be normal. Qualitative histology of iliac crest bone biopsy specimens has shown an absence of the birefringent pattern of normal lamellar bone under polarized light, often with a 'fish-scale' pattern thought to be similar in appearance to fibrogenesis imperfecta.

These various syndromes have certain clinical features in common. The majority of patients are short in stature, and the most severely affected cases are dwarfed. There is an increased propensity to fracture due to osteopenia. However, the incidence of fracture varies considerably depending on the severity of the disease and age; fractures are more common in children than in adults (Fig. 6.2). The standard treatment of fractures by immobilization results in disuse osteoporosis, which in patients with OI, further increases the tendency to fracture, thereby setting up a vicious cycle (Fig. 6.3). Thus, once a fracture has occurred, these unfortunate individuals have a tendency towards repeated fractures in the same area.

The presence in many patients of blue sclerae (Fig. 6.4), poorly formed dentin (Fig. 6.5), and ligamentous laxity confirm that the disease is not confined to the skeleton but is rather a generalized disorder of the connective tissues. Collagen synthesis by the osteoblasts and other connective tissue cells is deficient quantitatively (Fig. 6.6) and has been shown to differ qualitatively, at least in some patients. Based on linkage analysis it has been concluded that 90% of typical familial cases of OI are linked to abnormalities in collagen type I genes. Mutations in OI affect the type I collagen loci COL1A1 and COL1A2. The commonest are nucleotide

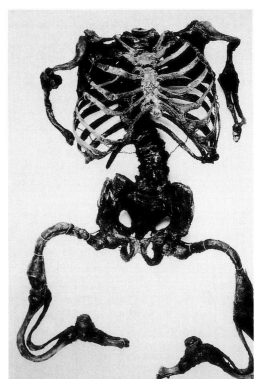

Figure 6.2
Skeleton of an older child with OI congenita, who died after massive hemorrhage from a blow to the head. There are postfracture deformities in all four limbs, together with scoliosis, chest and pelvic deformities.

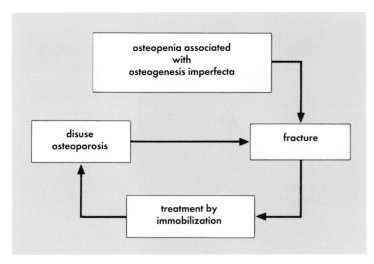

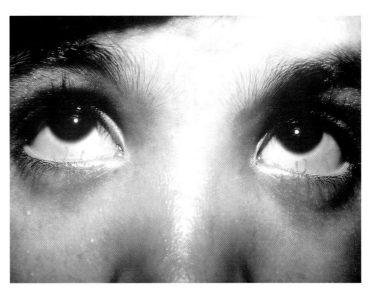

Figure 6.3   The standard treatment of fractures by immobilization results in disuse osteoporosis, which especially in these patients with already weakened bone, increases the tendency to further fracture.

Figure 6.4   OI: clinical photograph showing blue sclerae. The color results in part from the thinness of the sclerae.

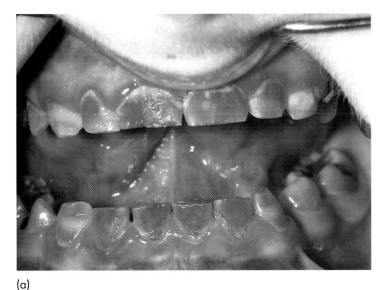

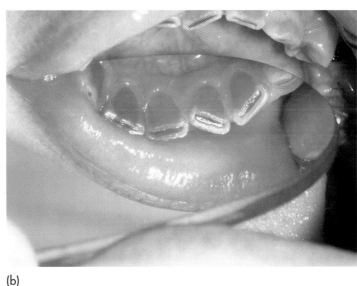

(a)   (b)

Figure 6.5   Two examples of the appearance of teeth in patients with OI. **(a)** Brown, short teeth result from failure in the formation of dentin (dentinogenesis imperfecta). **(b)** When seen from above the enamel appears to be normal.

substitutions or less commonly splicings or small deletions. However, familial cases are a minority of severe cases and the prevalence of collagen mutations in most severely affected OI patients is currently unknown.

Two clinical presentations of OI are readily recognizable. The more severe type, manifest at birth, is associated with generalized osteoporosis, multiple fractures with deformities, micromelia, and caput membranacea (Fig. 6.7). Patients afflicted by the less severe (tarda) type have far fewer fractures, usually two or fewer per year during the growing period, although the other stigmata of the disease (e.g. ligamentous laxity, blue sclerae, deafness, dentinogenesis imperfecta) are usually present. The less severely affected cases, which may or may not be manifest at birth, can be

clinically separated into two groups according to the degree of functional disability (Fig. 6.8). Patients in the first group have deformities, usually confined to the lower limbs, which limit ambulation. Those in the second group, although short, are without significant limb deformity and are therefore functionally much less disabled.

Radiographic features

The radiologic appearance in a case of OI depends on the severity of the clinical disease, but the hallmark of the disease is osteopenia, which is associated in most cases with evidence of multiple fractures and, in severe disease, deformities (Fig. 6.9). The entire skeleton is affected.

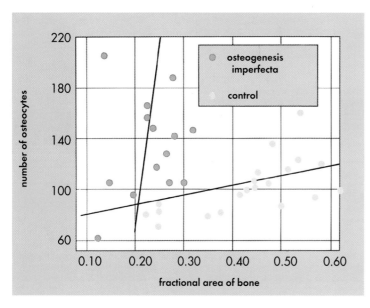

Figure 6.6 Graph showing that the number of osteocytes per unit area of bone is always greater in OI patients than in age-matched controls. Stated another way, the volume of territorial matrix around each osteocyte is smaller in OI than in age-matched controls.

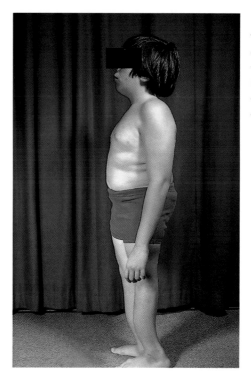

Figure 6.8 Patient with OI tarda shows anterior bowing of the tibia and short lower limbs. In comparison, the upper limbs appear to be relatively normal.

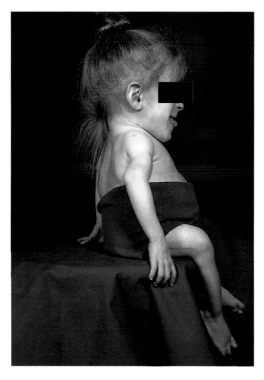

Figure 6.7 Patient with severe OI shows deformity of all four limbs and increased antero-posterior diameter of the chest. Also note the spinal deformity.

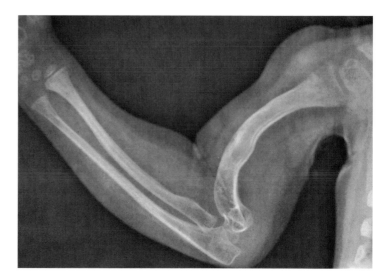

Figure 6.9 Radiograph of upper extremity in a patient with severe OI shows osteoporosis, slender bones, and multiple healed fractures.

In the spine, platyspondyly and biconcavity are evidence of compression fractures in the vertebral bodies, and in many cases these multiple fractures give rise to kyphoscoliosis (Fig. 6.10). Odontoid fractures are a rare complication, occurring mostly in children. In the severely affected patient, the pelvis is often markedly deformed and sometimes referred to as being triradiate in appearance.

The skull films reveal a large vault with temporal bulging and typically a small triangular face beneath. Multiple centers of ossification may be observed in the skull, particularly in the occipital portion (wormian bones) (Fig. 6.11). Occasionally, there is a 'hair-on-end' appearance. Basilar impression with deformity and encroachment upon the foramen magnum may lead to compression of the medulla oblongata.

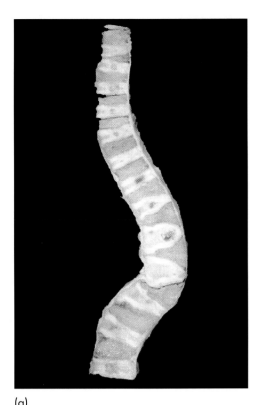

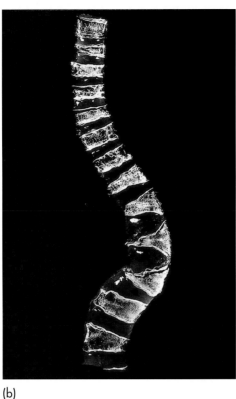

(a)   (b)

Figure 6.10   (a) Dissected specimen of spine shows scoliosis subsequent to multiple compression fractures. (b) Specimen radiograph of spine demonstrates the underlying osteoporosis.

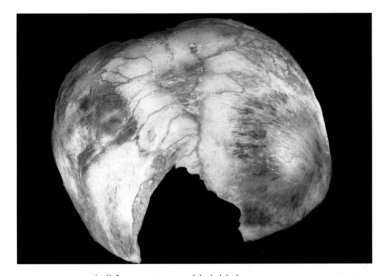

Figure 6.11   Skull from a 9-year-old child shows an open posterior fontanelle and multiple wormian bones.

In the lethal type II OI, the long bones are wide in diameter with thin shell-like cortices and multiple fractures, with telescoping of the bones. In most cases of severe clinical OI however, the long bones are very slender (Fig. 6.12). The ribs may be so attenuated that one sees a ribbon-like configuration suggestive of neurofibromatosis.

Fractures vary in number, depending on the severity of the disease, but they are commonest in the lower limbs. Usually they heal at the normal rate. The number of fractures sustained each year is maximal in the growing period and decreases after adolescence. Fractures again become a problem with aging and the onset of senile osteoporosis. Hyperplastic callus develops in a few cases (type V) resulting in excessive swelling, heat, throbbing pain, and tenderness. It is important to distinguish hyperplastic callus from acute osteomyelitis and osteosarcoma (Fig. 6.13).

Many patients, particularly those with the severe form of the disease will be treated with intramedullary rods, which both correct deformity and help to prevent further fracture. Complications associated with this procedure include breakage of the rod, cutting out of the bone at one end of the rod associated with the continuing growth of the bone, and migration of the rod. Infection around the rods is very rare.

The radiographic differential diagnosis of OI in the newborn might include congenital hypophosphatasia, although in that condition the alkaline phosphatase level is abnormally low. In a young child, the differential diagnosis might include 'battered baby syndrome' or the early stages of leukemia. In the preadolescent, the self-limiting condition of juvenile osteoporosis might have to be considered.

Approximately 50% of the growing (epiphyseal) ends of the bones in children with moderate to severe OI whose roentgenograms the author has reviewed have a collection of rounded, scalloped radiolucencies with sclerotic margins. In some cases this is accompanied by a balloned-out epiphysis and metaphysis, giving a 'popcorn bag' appearance similar to that described by Fairbank as cystic (Fig. 6.14). These lesions are seen only in the long bones, most commonly in those of the leg with equal incidence on the right and left sides of the body. In all instances where such lesions occur, the cartilaginous growth plate is irregular and either partially, or completely absent. In the cases with 'popcorn' epiphyses, films obtained during the

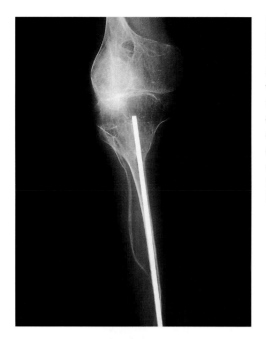

Figure 6.12 Radiograph of the leg of a patient with severe clinical OI, which has been treated by rodding of the tibia. The extreme attenuation and ribbon-like quality of the bones is obvious in the fibula.

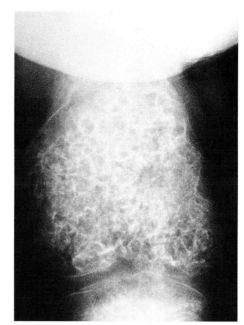

Figure 6.14 Radiograph of knee joint in an 8-year-old child with severe OI. The epiphysis and metaphysis of the femur contain nodular 'popcorn' lesions with radiolucent centers and radiodense margins. No growth plate is seen in the femur. In the tibia, the growth plate is visualized but the central portion is disrupted. The buttock image obscures the femoral diaphysis.

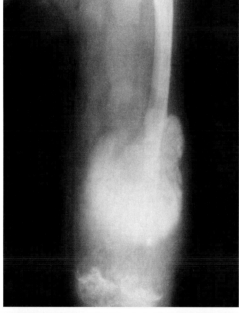

(a)

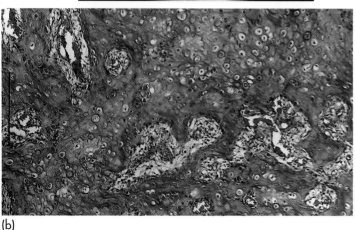

(b)

Figure 6.13 (a) Radiograph of the femur of an adolescent patient with OI, who developed a rapidly growing, hyperemic tumor following injury. Radiographically, the tumor might suggest a neoplasm. (b) Photomicrograph of a biopsy obtained from the mass demonstrates a cellular mass of immature bone and cartilage consistent with fracture callus (H&E, × 10 obj.).

neonatal period show normal epiphyses and growth plates, indicating that the lesions are not congenital (Fig. 6.15). Films taken after the adult state has been achieved were available for review in 40% of the patients, and in all of these cases the epiphyseal changes had resolved. A summary of the radiographic findings is shown in Table 6.1.

Pathologic features

Gross examination of the bones reveals a generalized loss of bone tissue, with thin, eggshell-like cortices and very little medullary cancellous bone. Many specimens demonstrate recent or healed fractures, with angulation and/or bowing (Fig. 6.16).

In general, the epiphyseal ends of the long bones, including the articular surfaces, retain a recognizable shape, although in proportion to the rest of the bone they appear larger and may show irregularity of the articular surface (Fig. 6.17). The secondary centers of ossification are often markedly distorted and may contain small cartilaginous nodules 1–4 mm in diameter (Fig. 6.18).

The appearance of the growth plate varies widely, ranging from normal, to exhibiting one or more indentations secondary to fracture, to total disruption of its regular outline. These latter changes correspond to the scalloped or popcorn lesions seen on radiographic examination. It is most probable that these epiphyseal changes are secondary to trauma. The fragmentation of the growth plate might be reasonably expected to interfere with normal growth.

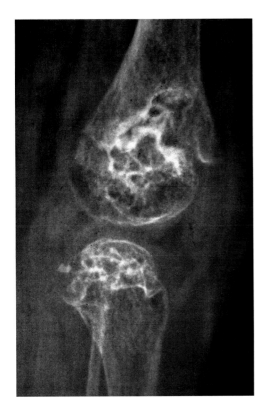

Figure 6.15 Lateral radiograph of the knee in a patient with OI congenita. There is irregularity and disruption of both the femoral and tibial growth plates, although less severe than that shown in Figure 6.14.

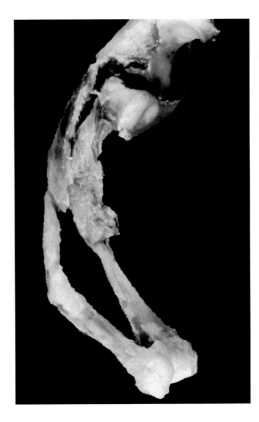

Figure 6.16 Dissected specimen of forearm bones shows multiple fractures, including fracture dislocation of the radial head.

Table 6.1   Summary of radiographic findings in osteogenesis imperfecta.

	Less severely affected 'Osteogenesis imperfecta (tarda)'	Severely affected 'Osteogenesis imperfecta'
Texture	Osteopenia	Proportional to the severity of the clinical disease
Fractures	Frequency 1–4 per year; generally seen during growth period; most frequent in lower limbs; fractures may be present at birth, but not commonly; deformities usually confined to lower limbs, most often the tibia and fibula	Fractures present at birth; many fractures each year; occur in all four limbs, but always associated with severe deformities
Long bones	Usually slender	May be widened during infancy due to telescoping; in older patients, usually very slender
Epiphyses	Usually normal in appearance, although irregularities may be present around the knee	Frequently irregular, with failure to recognize a normal growth plate, and replacement by bubbly calcified nodules; most frequently seen in lower femur, upper tibia, upper femur, and upper humerus
Spine	Osteopenia: platyspondyly; mild sclerosis	Severe osteopenia with biconcave vertebrae and frequently severe kyphoscoliosis
Ribs	Normal	Frequent deformities with thinning, malunited fractures
Pelvis	Normal	Triradiate

The large cartilage masses visible in the region of the metaphysis on both radiographic and gross examination result from fragmentation of the growth plate. On microscopic examination, the cartilage fragments show polarized maturation and columnization of the chondrocytes with peripheral ossification.

Microscopic examination of an intact growth plate from an OI patient may reveal some disorganization of the proliferative and hypertrophic zones, increased permeation of the cartilage by metaphyseal blood vessels, and decreased thickness of the calcified zone of the growth plate cartilage. The primary spongiosa

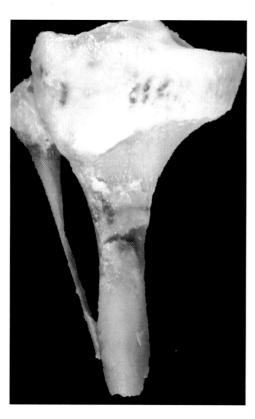

Figure 6.17 Upper end of tibia shows relative enlargement of the cartilaginous end of the bone and marked narrowing of the shaft of the fibula.

on the metaphyseal side is usually extremely scanty and of woven bone (Fig. 6.19).

Biopsy specimens from patients with the severe form of the disease are characterized by large areas of osseous tissue that are devoid of an organized trabecular pattern. Examination of the individual trabeculae reveals plump osteoblasts crowded along prominent osteoid seams, and large oval osteocytes surrounded by a small amount of matrix, which more often than not has a woven pattern (Fig. 6.20). Even in areas that display a lamellar pattern, the lamellae are thin. The osteoclasts appear to be morphologically normal, although both they and the resorptive surfaces are more numerous (Fig. 6.21).

Bone specimens from clinically less severely affected patients are characterized by a predominantly fine lamellar pattern, with only small areas of woven bone. Although osteoblasts are increased in number they appear smaller, more spherical, and less numerous than their counterparts in the severe group. Osteoid seams are prominent, probably due to an increased rate of bone formation. The osteocytes, although more mature in appearance than in severely affected patients, are still more numerous, larger, and less homogeneously arranged throughout the trabeculae than the osteocytes in age-matched controls (Fig. 6.22). Osteoclasts appear morphologically normal but are

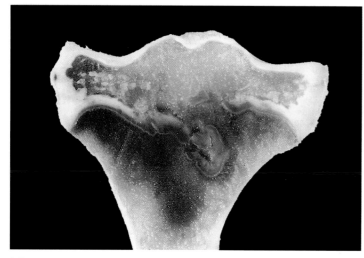

(a)

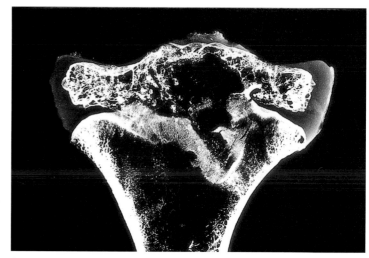

(b)

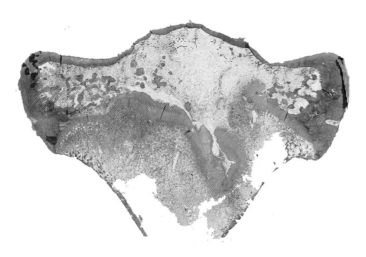

(c)

Figure 6.18   (a) Dissected specimen of the upper end of the tibia shows multiple cartilaginous nodules in the epiphysis and disruption of the growth plate. Radiograph of the specimen (b). Histologic section (c).

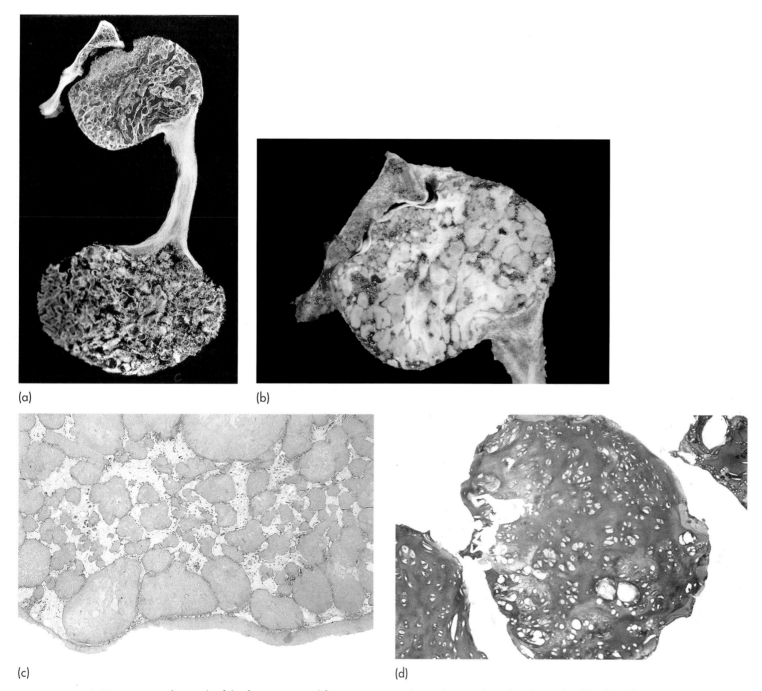

Figure 6.19   (a) Specimen radiograph of the femur removed from a patient with OI who was thought to have developed synchronous chondrosarcoma. However, these changes are compatible with fragmentation and continued growth of the epiphyseal cartilage plate (popcorn sign). (b) Photograph of a section through the upper end of the femur illustrated in (a), showing the large cartilage fragments. (c) Photomicrograph of a portion of the epiphysis shown in (b) (H&E, × 1 obj.). (d) Higher powered view of one of the cartilage nodules illustrated in (c) shows hypercellularity and disorganization. A thin rim of bone is present around each of the nodules, giving rise to the rim of radiodensity seen in the radiograph (H&E, × 10 obj.).

increased in number as compared with those in individuals not affected by OI.

A recent study found that 'bone from children with OI type I often appeared normal in microstructure and amount, but in some there was a dearth of bone and an abundance of osteocytes. Compared with age-matched controls, cortical and trabecular bone from children with OI types III and IV were markedly sparse and very cellular, and primary osteonal systems contin-

ued to be formed later than expected. A distinguishing feature of the bone from OI type V patients was the failure of patches of bone to mineralize, especially adjoining a reversal line. Packets of bone tissue exhibiting either considerably higher than normal or deficient mineralization would contribute to mechanical weakness.'

OI is not one disease; it is a collection of syndromes having in common decreased bone density and the propensity to fracture.

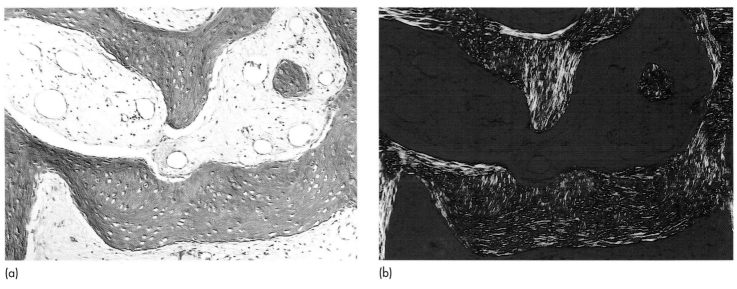

(a)

(b)

Figure 6.20   Photomicrograph of a biopsy of bone (**a**) obtained from a patient with severe OI showing irregular hypercellular bone which, on polarized light examination (**b**), is seen to have a poorly developed lamellar pattern (H&E, × 4 obj.).

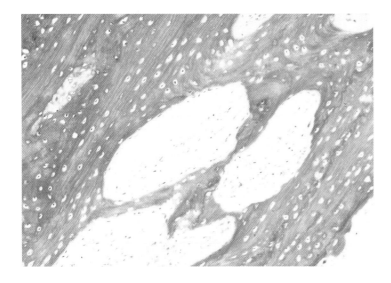

Figure 6.21   Bone biopsy from a severe case of OI showing marked hypercellularity of the bone with a fine lamellar pattern and extensively eroded resorptive surfaces (H&E, × 10 obj.).

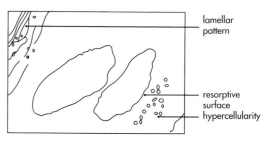

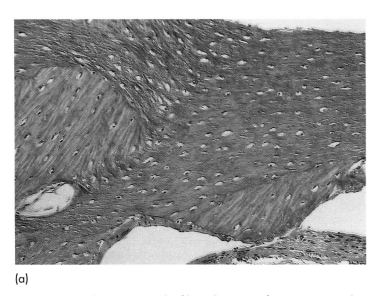

(a)

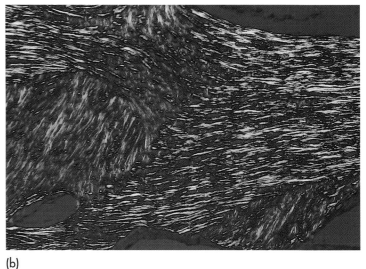

(b)

Figure 6.22   Photomicrograph of bone biopsy (**a**) from a patient with OI tarda, showing hypercellular bone. The fine and poorly developed lamellar pattern is more clearly seen in the polarized light picture (**b**) (H&E, × 10 obj.).

From an anatomic viewpoint, three levels of organization may be considered in patients with OI: genetic and cellular defects, tissue abnormalities, and structural skeletal abnormalities.

Although only scant information is available relating to cellular defects in OI, both genetic and biochemical evidence indicate that these diseases result from various disorders in collagen synthesis, quantitative and/or qualitative.

More information is available concerning tissue abnormalities. The increased number of osteoblasts and osteoclasts, the large size of the osteoblasts, and the greater amount of osteoid-covered surfaces all suggest an increase in bone turnover, and this is supported by microscopic studies including increased tetracycline labeling. One of the most characteristic histologic features in OI is the apparent abundance of osteocytes. The quantity of extracellular matrix separating the cells is reduced, and as a consequence the cells are much closer together. This finding is present in both woven and lamellar bone, suggesting a decrease in the amount of collagen matrix produced by each osteoblast before it becomes an osteocyte. The diminution in the size of the skeleton in OI can partly be attributed to this absolute decrease in extracellular matrix production, particularly of collagen. The fact that the lamellae appear unusually delicate and thin is in accordance with this interpretation.

Overall dwarfing results to some extent from decreased collagen matrix production by the connective tissue cells but other reasons for dwarfing must be considered. Sillence and co-workers have reported that patients with dominantly inherited OI develop a markedly short stature; nevertheless, at birth these same patients are of normal length. This suggests that it is only as the cartilaginous skeleton is replaced by bone that shortness becomes evident. Although some authors have reported that in cases of OI, the growth plate appears normal, others have noted scattered islands of cartilage in the metaphysis and that the epiphyseal plate might be broad and irregular, lacking the typical columnar arrangement in the hypertrophic and calcified zone.

In those patients the author has been able to study at necropsy, two processes were found to affect the epiphyseal ends of the bone. First, a failure in the normal development of the secondary center of ossification results in residual islands of cartilage in the epiphysis (this process was present in most of the epiphyses examined). Second, disruption of the epiphyseal growth plate which often leaves only irregular islands of growth-plate cartilage in the metaphyseal region. A radiographic survey showed that the most severe disruption and fragmentation of the growth plate occurred in the distal femur.

It seems likely that these epiphyseal changes are secondary to mechanical injury rather than being developmental in origin. This view is supported by the findings of progressive changes in the clinical radiographs. Since in these patients there is little or no supportive medullary cancellous bone, it seems likely that the delicate cartilaginous growth plate, rendered brittle by the zone of calcification, is extremely vulnerable to lateral compression. The resulting fragmentation of the growth plate might be expected to interfere with growth. In this regard, it is interesting to observe that in a number of patients with the moderately severe form of the disease, there is considerable disproportionate shortening of the femur as compared with the humerus. In such cases that the author has examined roentgenographically, fragmentation of the growth plate of the lower femoral condyles was generally apparent whereas the epiphysis of the proximal humerus appeared normal.

EHLERS–DANLOS SYNDROME

Like OI, Ehlers–Danlos syndrome, which gives rise to the 'India rubber man' of the circus, comprises a heterogeneous group of connective tissue disorders which have only recently been classified into a number of different types. The underlying biochemical defect in the pathway of collagen synthesis is unknown in most cases. However, some cases of Ehlers–Danlos syndrome type VI have demonstrated a hydroxylysine-deficient collagen, probably due to a lysyl hydroxylase deficiency which interferes with the formation of intramolecular cross-links in type I collagen. The type VII form of the disease is caused by a lack of procollagen peptidase. Thus, the conversion of procollagen to collagen is interfered with and the formation of collagen fibrils cannot proceed normally.

The characteristic clinical features of Ehlers–Danlos syndrome are hyperextensibility of the skin, easy bruisibility, hypermobile joints which are prone to dislocation and, in type IV disease, dissecting aortic aneurysm. Blue sclerae are not uncommon in Ehlers–Danlos syndrome, and their presence should not be taken as evidence of an associated OI.

In general, the bone is found on gross examination to be osteopenic (Fig. 6.23). Most patients exhibit a greater or lesser degree of kyphoscoliosis, which becomes worse during adolescence and may end in severe spinal curvature with pulmonary embarrassment (Fig. 6.24). Occasionally, severe spondylolisthesis is observed. No characteristic microscopic findings have been described in the bone.

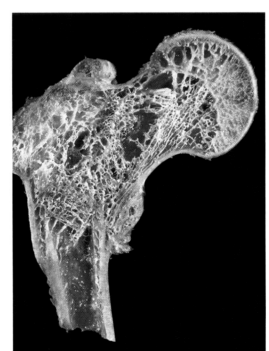

Figure 6.23 Photograph of an autopsy section through the femur of a young man with Ehlers–Danlos syndrome shows a healed intertrochanteric fracture and severe osteoporosis.

SCURVY

Scurvy is now an extremely rare condition, although an occasional case may arise as the result either of deprivation or of food faddism. In the past, when infantile scurvy was common, the disorder was frequently found to be associated with rickets.

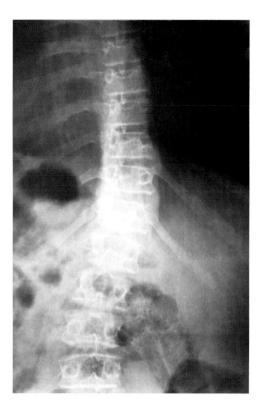

Figure 6.24 AP radiograph of a young adult with Ehlers–Danlos syndrome. The bone is markedly osteopenic and there is a mild scoliosis with some rotational deformity.

Scurvy is characterized clinically by hemorrhage secondary to capillary fragility. The hemorrhages occur in the skin, gums, muscle attachments, serosal membranes and, especially in children, subperiosteally in the bones (Fig. 6.25). Affected individuals may also exhibit anemia, osteoporosis, intra-articular hemorrhages, and poor wound healing.

The recognition that scurvy is a deficiency state occurred in the late eighteenth century, when it became understood that the disease resulted from a lack of vegetables and fruit in the diet and that citrus fruit could prevent its onset. It is now known to be caused by a deficiency of ascorbic acid (vitamin C), an essential cofactor for hydroxylation of the amino acids proline and lysine, which is an important step in the intracellular synthesis of collagen. In the absence of vitamin C, the conversion of proline and lysine to hydroxyproline and hydroxylysine cannot take place, with a resulting failure in the formation of intramolecular bonds and of a stable triple-helical collagen molecule (see Fig. 6.1).

In the vitamin-C-deficient state, microscopic examination reveals that recently formed areas of connective tissue (e.g. the metaphysis in a growing child) are markedly deficient in extracellular matrix formation. Indeed, the most prominent features in such areas are proliferating fibroblasts without significant collagen production and extravasated red blood cells as a result of failure to form new capillaries (Fig. 6.26).

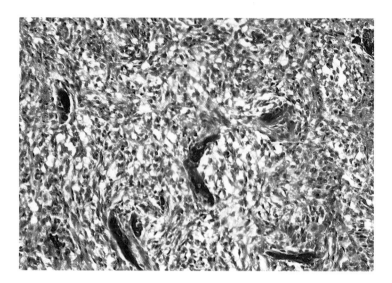

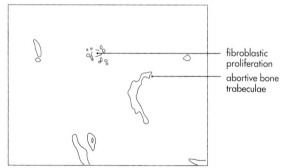

fibroblastic proliferation

abortive bone trabeculae

Figure 6.26 Photomicrograph shows extensive fibroblastic proliferation, with minimal bone and collagen production. Extravasation of red blood cells can be seen throughout the tissue (H&E, × 25 obj.).

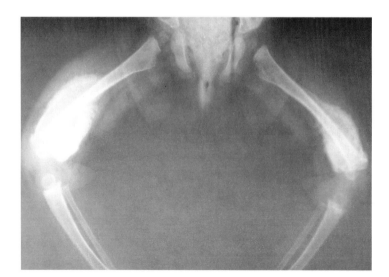

Figure 6.25 Radiograph of a young child shows extensive periosteal elevation in both femurs, with epiphyseal separation of the lower femoral epiphyses.

In young children with scurvy the bone lesions are characterized by subperiosteal hemorrhage that may be massive (Fig. 6.27). In addition, because the primary spongiosa fails to form adequately, a fracture through the metaphysis frequently occurs, with a resulting separation of the epiphysis (Fig. 6.28). These metaphyseal fractures are clinically manifested by marked costochondral tenderness and swelling around the major joints. (Because the periosteum is more securely attached to the bone in adults, subperiosteal hematomas are not a characteristic part of their clinical picture. However, adult patients may present with marked osteoporosis due to the defect in collagen synthesis.)

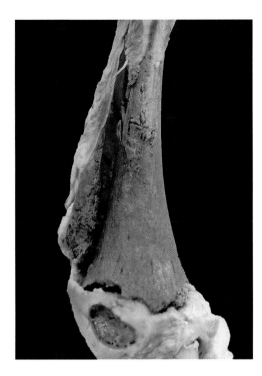

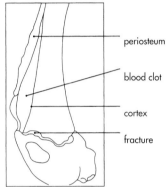

periosteum

blood clot

cortex

fracture

Figure 6.27   Photograph of a specimen from a case of scurvy showing periosteal elevation and subperiosteal hemorrhage. Separation of the lower femoral epiphysis has occurred.

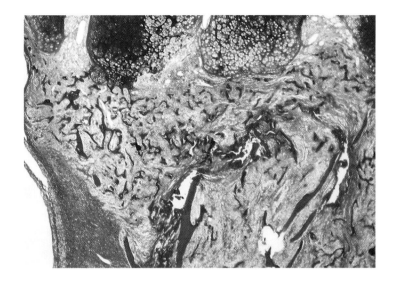

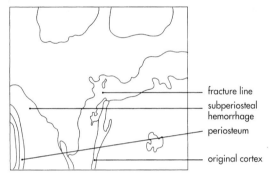

fracture line

subperiosteal hemorrhage

periosteum

original cortex

Figure 6.28   Photomicrograph of the region of the growth plate and metaphysis in a patient with scurvy. Subperiosteal hemorrhage and a fracture through the metaphysis are apparent (H&E, × 4 obj.).

VITAMIN A INTOXICATION

Although uncommon, the effects of vitamin A (retinoic acid) intoxication are occasionally seen in food faddists. Irritability, loss of appetite, scaly skin, and hair loss are the usual presenting symptoms. Hypercalcemia may result from increased osteoclastic activity and active bone resorption. Vitamin A has a role in the proliferation and differentiation of several tissues, and infants and young children with hypervitaminosis A may exhibit accelerated maturation of the growth plates, resulting in a slow-down of bone growth activity (Fig. 6.29).

MARFAN'S SYNDROME

Marfan's syndrome consists of a heterogeneous group of connective-tissue disorders characterized by an autosomal dominant pattern of inheritance. Affected individuals are usually tall and thin, with osteopenia, kyphoscoliosis, arachnodactyly, myopia,

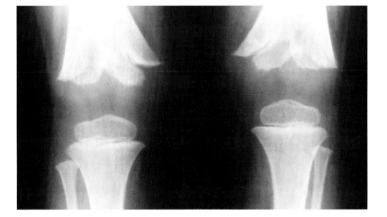

Figure 6.29   Radiograph of a young patient suffering from vitamin A intoxication, who developed fracture and displacement of the femoral epiphyses. An X-ray taken some years later (not shown) after correction of the intoxication showed complete restoration of normal anatomy.

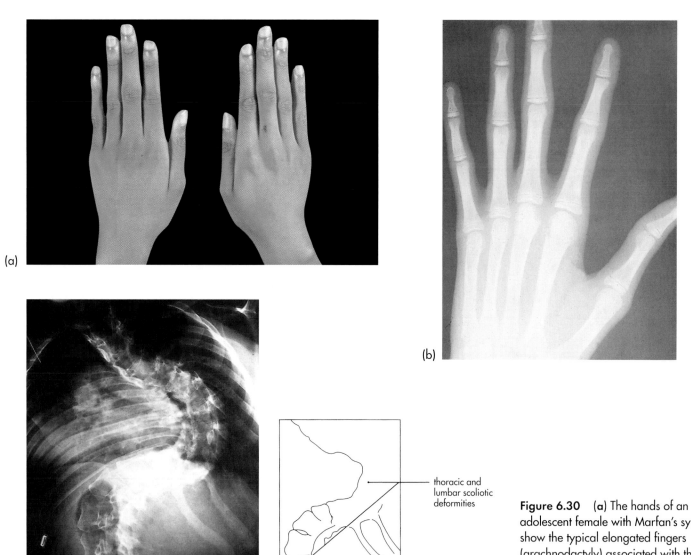

thoracic and lumbar scoliotic deformities

Figure 6.30   (a) The hands of an adolescent female with Marfan's syndrome show the typical elongated fingers (arachnodactyly) associated with the syndrome. (b) Radiograph of the hand. (c) Anteroposterior radiograph of the trunk of the same patient demonstrates the severity of the spinal deformity. (Courtesy of Dr David Levine.)

and often lens dislocation (Fig. 6.30). From a clinical standpoint, the most important aspects of the disease are cardiovascular abnormalities particularly affecting the heart valves and the aorta.

Microscopic examination of the heart valves and large arteries reveals a cystic necrosis of the media with pools of mucoid material that stains metachromatically with toluidine blue (Figs 6.31 and 6.32). Biochemical studies have shown that excessive amounts of hyaluronic acid are produced by the connective-tissue cells of these patients. In addition, in some cases of Marfan's syndrome a defect in the formation of cross-linkages in the type I collagen fibrils has been found.

HOMOCYSTINURIA

Homocystinuria is an extremely rare autosomal recessive disease, characterized biochemically by a deficiency in the enzyme cystathionine β-synthetase. The resulting elevated levels of homocysteine in the plasma affect the arterial walls, smooth-muscle proliferation, and possibly collagen synthesis. Clinical signs include tall stature, and arachnodactyly, similar to the changes seen in Marfan's syndrome. However, unlike Marfan's syndrome, patients with homocystinuria are often mentally retarded. Disturbances in collagen fibril formation lead to severe osteoporosis, with multiple compression fractures of the vertebral bodies and subsequent kyphoscoliosis.

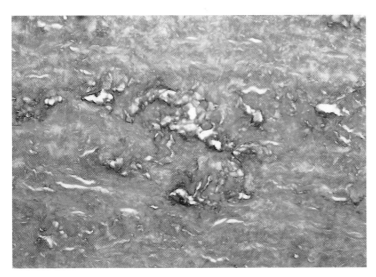

Figure 6.31 Photomicrograph of a portion of the wall of the aorta, demonstrating pools of mucoid material. The patient died of a dissecting aneurysm, a common complication in Marfan's syndrome (H&E, × 4 obj.).

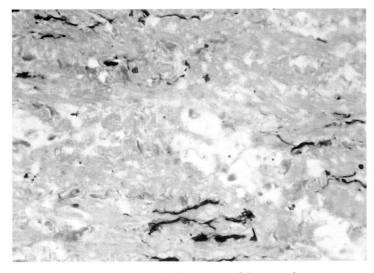

Figure 6.32 Photomicrograph of a section of the aorta from a patient with Marfan's syndrome stained to demonstrate the sparsity of elastic tissue (black), especially in the areas of mucoid degeneration contributing to weakness in the media and subsequent dissecting aneurysm (Verhoeff–van Gieson, × 4 obj.).

MUCOPOLYSACCHARIDOSES

The nonfibrillar amorphous component of the extracellular tissue matrix has been often referred to as the 'ground substance'. It is particularly prominent in cartilage and plays an important role in the mechanical properties of cartilage and bone, as well as in the development of the shape of the bones.

The ground substance is a mixture of many components, and its composition differs among different tissues. The principal ground substance constituents of cartilage are the acid mucopolysaccharides (glycosaminoglycans) which, combined with proteins, form the PG aggrecan (see Chapter 1, pp. 8 and 9).

The mucopolysaccharidoses, constitute a group of inborn errors of metabolism, which result from diminished activity of the lysosomal enzymes that degrade glycosaminoglycans (acid mucopolysaccharides). Mostly these conditions are autosomal recessive and characterized by defects in the metabolism, storage, and excretion of these glycosaminoglycans. The majority of these diseases are associated with marked skeletal abnormalities, probably because the mucopolysaccharides are so important in the formation of the cartilage and its subsequent endochondral ossification during development (Fig. 6.33).

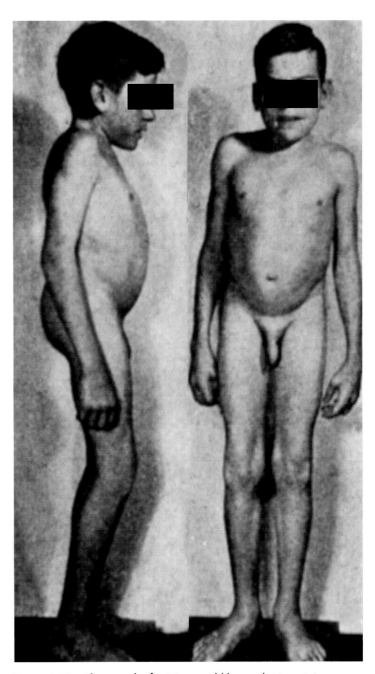

Figure 6.33 Photograph of a 15-year-old boy with Morquio's syndrome showing a typical disproportion in spine and limb lengths. The boy's grandfather was similarly affected.

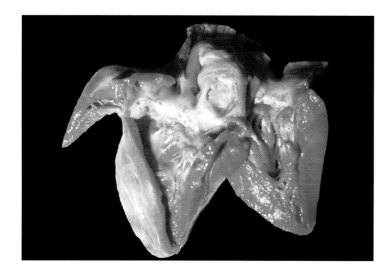

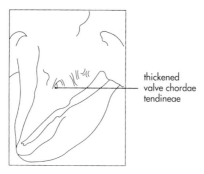

thickened
valve chordae
tendineae

Figure 6.34   The heart of a child with Hurler's syndrome. Note the thickening of the chordae tendineae cordis and opacity of the endothelial lining of the heart, both resulting from accumulation of macrophages filled with polysaccharides.

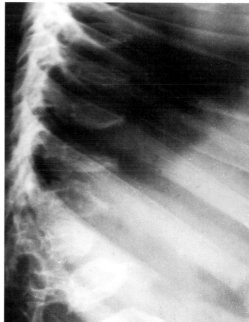

Figure 6.35
Lateral radiograph of the thoracolumbar spine in a 17-year-old girl with the clinical presentation of Morquio's disease. The vertebral bodies show an anterior beaking which is seen also in association with Hurler's syndrome. Note the associated mild kyphosis.

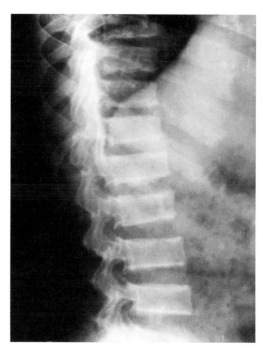

Figure 6.36
Lateral radiograph of the thoracolumbar spine in another patient with the clinical presentation of Morquio's disease. In this case there is a flattening of the vertebral bodies without obvious beaking.

At least seven distinct syndromes have been described, many of which are characterized by the storage of dermatan sulfate and heparan sulfate in various tissues. Strikingly affected are the reticuloendothelial system, the heart (Fig. 6.34), and the central nervous system, the latter often resulting in severe mental retardation. Because of the important role played by the glycosaminoglycans in the formation of the vitreous humor and other components of the eye, blindness is a common complication.

The two most common mucopolysaccharidoses associated with severe skeletal abnormalities are Morquio's syndrome (MPS IV) and Hurler's syndrome (MPS I).

MORQUIO'S SYNDROME

Morquio's syndrome (mucopolysaccharidosis IV) is characterized biochemically by excessive amounts of keratin sulfate and chondroitin sulfate in the urine. This condition appears to be phenotypically, genetically, and chemically distinctive, probably involving a defect in metabolism of the PGs of the cartilage. Affected patients are dwarfed, with characteristically flat vertebrae with some vertebral wedging, epiphyseal dysplasia, and generalized osteoporosis. There is usually marked shortening of the trunk with kyphosis and somewhat lesser shortening of the extremities (Figs 6.35–6.37).

HURLER'S SYNDROME

Hurler's syndrome (also known as gargoylism or MPS I) is caused by α-L-iduronidase deficiency. This condition may also involve some retardation of skeletal growth, although this is rarely severe. Although the vertebral bodies appear relatively normal, these patients frequently exhibit a kyphotic deformity resulting from the malformation of at least one vertebral body usually the twelfth thoracic or the first lumbar (Fig. 6.38). For unknown reasons, a portion of the anterior half of the affected body or bodies

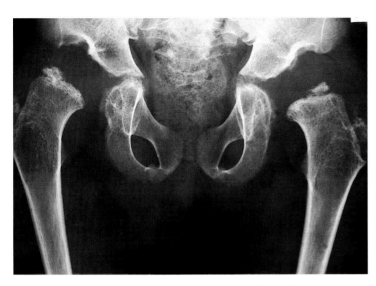

Figure 6.37 Radiograph of the hips of a boy suffering from Morquio's disease, demonstrating failure of development in the femoral heads as well as in the hip joints as a whole.

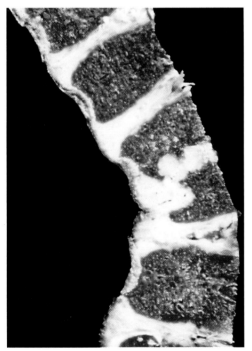

Figure 6.38
Photograph of a portion of the thoracolumbar spine in a patient with Hurler's syndrome, showing a hemivertebra at the level of T12. The vertebra above is also slightly deformed on its inferior surface, though the remaining vertebrae in this photograph appear to be within normal limits. (Courtesy of Dr James W. Milgram.)

fails to ossify, and the ensuing posterior displacement of one vertebral body on the other leads to kyphosis. However, in Hurler's syndrome the vertebral column does not show the general wedging of the vertebral bodies present in Morquio's syndrome. Unlike Morquio's syndrome, patients with Hurler's deteriorate rapidly and usually die within the first decade of life.

DISTURBANCES IN MINERAL FORMATION

HYPOPHOSPHATASIA

Hypophosphatasia is a rare, genetically transmitted error of metabolism in which there is a disturbance in the synthesis of the

enzyme alkaline phosphatase. Two forms of the disease have been described. The first, inherited as an autosomal recessive trait, manifests in children who are severely affected by a rickets-like syndrome. The second form is an autosomal dominant form, in which the disease is less severe, may become evident in childhood because of premature loss of the deciduous teeth or may never be detected clinically.

In infants, hypophosphatasia is manifested clinically as a failure to thrive with growth retardation, and is accompanied by a wide range of symptoms including irritability, fever, and vomiting. In general, infants diagnosed before 6 months of age follow a rapidly progressive fatal course. In older children or adults, the disease is less severe and usually asymptomatic. Hypophosphatasia is characterized by decreased levels of alkaline phosphatase in bones, intestines, liver, and kidneys. Levels of serum phosphorus and calcium are usually at the upper limits of normal. Increased amounts of phosphoethanolamine, which is believed to be a substrate of alkaline phosphatase, are present in the urine and in the serum, and levels of inorganic pyrophosphate are also elevated.

Radiographic manifestations of the disorder in children include poorly ossified and underdeveloped bones (Figs 6.39 and 6.40). Gross and microscopic examination of the affected tissue reveals increased osteoid and irregular epiphyseal cartilage with lengthened chondrocyte columns (Figs 6.41–6.45). The similarity to rickets is evident, and explains why this disease, for years, was named vitamin-D-resistant rickets (see Chapter 8, p. 215).

Hypophosphatasia may not present clinically until the fourth, fifth, or sixth decade of life, although there is often a childhood history of a rickets-like disorder. Edentia, short stature, and

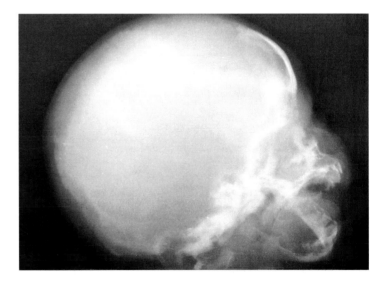

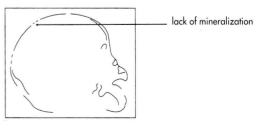

lack of mineralization

Figure 6.39 Hypophosphatasia: radiograph of the skull in a newborn baby shows poor mineralization of the vault of the skull.

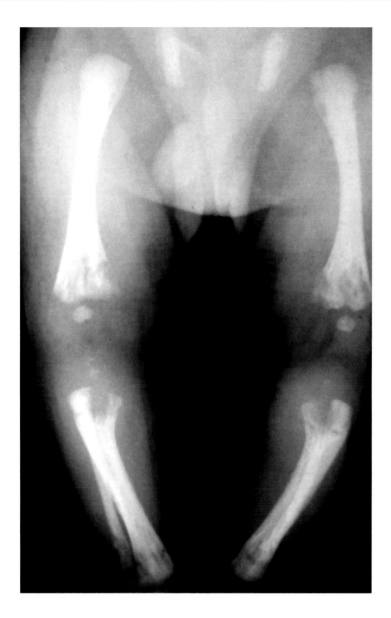

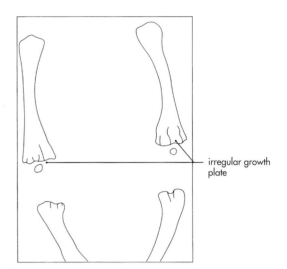

Figure 6.40   Hypophosphatasia: the lower limbs in a newborn child show marked irregularity of the growth plate, with streaks of radiolucency into the metaphysis. This appearance is indicative of poor endochondral ossification and mineralization.

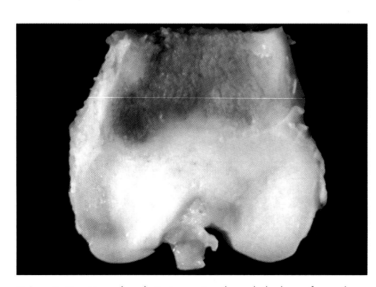

Figure 6.41   Hypophosphatasia: section through the lower femoral epiphysis and metaphysis shows the irregularity of the growth plate.

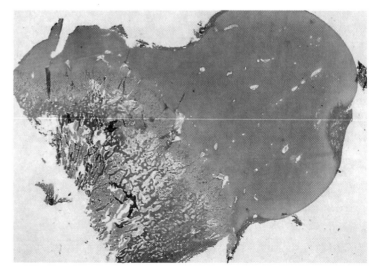

Figure 6.42   Hypophosphatasia: low-power photomicrograph of the upper femoral growth plate. The marked irregularity of the cartilage and the tongue of irregular cartilage extending to the metaphyseal region are evident (H&E, × 1 obj.).

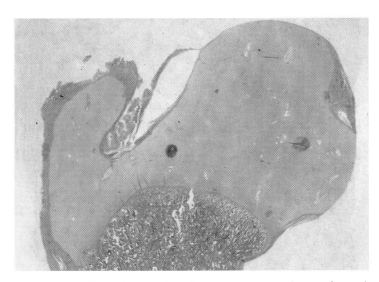

Figure 6.43 Photomicrograph to demonstrate a normal upper femoral epiphysis to show the difference in a patient of the same age as the subject of Figure 6.42 (H&E, × 1 obj.).

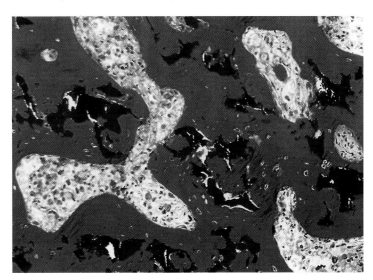

Figure 6.45 Photomicrograph shows the poor mineralization of the forming bone in hypophosphatasia. Only the areas stained black are mineralized (von Kossa's, × 25 obj.).

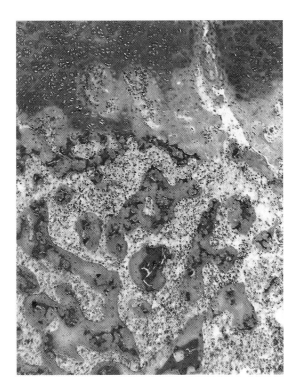

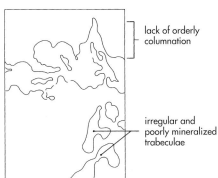

lack of orderly columnation

irregular and poorly mineralized trabeculae

Figure 6.44 Photomicrograph of a cross-section of a vertebral body demonstrates disturbed endochondral ossification (H&E, × 10 obj.).

deformity of the extremities, including bowing, are common clinical findings. Radiographic features include pseudofractures and osteopenia. Histopathologic examination of bone from these patients reveals an osteomalacic picture, with increased amounts of nonmineralized bone. Unlike osteomalacia due to vitamin D or calcium deficiency, hypophosphatasia is characterized by a paucity of osteoblasts.

HYPERPHOSPHATASIA

Primary hyperphosphatasia, also known as juvenile Paget's disease, is a rare congenital autosomal recessive disorder characterized clinically by short stature, a propensity to fracture, and marked subperiosteal bone formation which may be confused with Caffey's disease (see Chapter 5, p. 129). Patients with this condition have markedly elevated levels of serum alkaline phosphatase and acid phosphatase of bone origin, and an elevated level of urinary hydroxyproline.

On radiographic examination, a thickened skull with 'cotton ball' radiodensities may be seen. The long bones often exhibit an increase in width and loss of normal corticomedullary differentiation. These features are the result of the marked subperiosteal overgrowth. Bowing due to fractures may be present, and in infants the disease must be distinguished from a 'battered baby' syndrome.

Morphologic studies reveal that both the cortical and trabecular bone consist of immature or woven bone, with abundant osteoblasts and osteoclasts and prominent osteoid seams (Fig. 6.46). The marrow space is replaced by a well-vascularized fibrous connective tissue network. Using polarized light, a mosaic pattern of the bone matrix can be observed.

Hyperphosphatasia is distinguished clinically from Paget's disease by its early onset and the generalized symmetrical bone involvement.

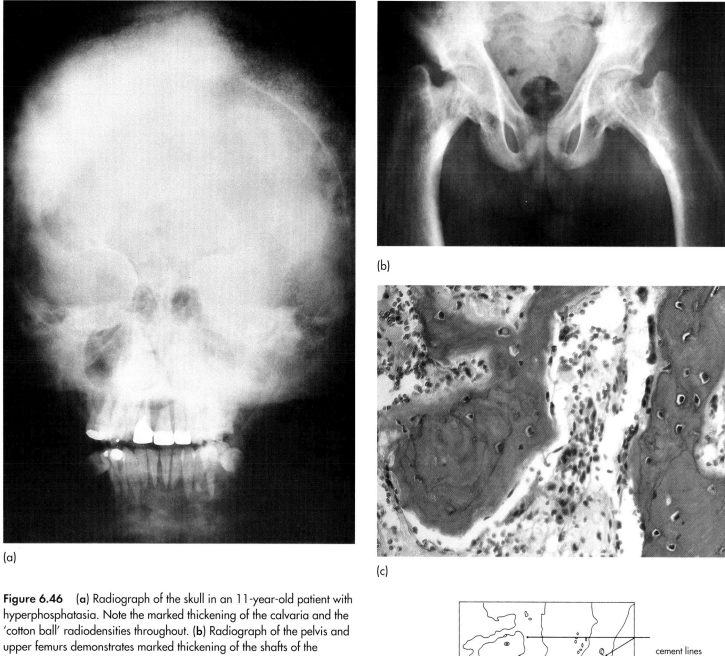

(a)

(b)

(c)

cement lines

prominent osteoblasts

Figure 6.46 (a) Radiograph of the skull in an 11-year-old patient with hyperphosphatasia. Note the marked thickening of the calvaria and the 'cotton ball' radiodensities throughout. (b) Radiograph of the pelvis and upper femurs demonstrates marked thickening of the shafts of the femurs, with bowing of the femur and a dense irregular cortex. (c) Photomicrograph of bone biopsy from the patient shown in (a and b). The bone is somewhat immature, with large irregular cells. Note prominent cement lines and many osteoblasts on the bone surface (H&E, × 25 obj.).

FLUOROSIS

Fluoride substitutes for some of the hydroxyl ion in hydroxyapatite to form a more stable crystal, fluorapatite, which is less soluble than hydroxyapatite.

Fluoride intoxication may result from either industrial or endemic exposure to fluoride. In populations exposed to a high fluoride content in water (in excess of 24 parts per 1,000,000), or in individuals exposed to high levels of industrial fluoride, the most dramatic radiographic change is marked coarsening and thickening of bone trabeculae, particularly involving the axial skeleton. Eventually, there is a significant increase in bone density, sometimes accompanied by periosteal new bone formation and marked spinal osteophytosis. There is a propensity for calcification and ossification of the muscles, ligaments, and tendons at the site of their attachment to the bone. Some patients in whom bone formation is particularly prominent in and around joints may develop debilitating arthrosis. Affected individuals may also exhibit mottled tooth enamel and anemia.

In recent years, fluoride has been used to stimulate bone

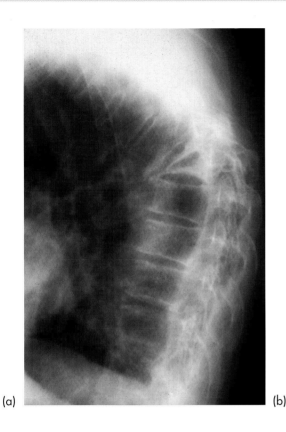 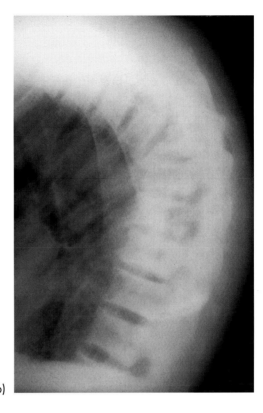

(a)   (b)

Figure 6.47 The effect of sodium fluoride on osteoporotic bone. Radiograph of an osteoporotic spine (**a**) shows collapse of thoracic vertebrae with marked osteopenia. After 3 years of treatment with sodium fluoride, calcium carbonate, and vitamin D (**b**), spinal radiograph shows increased radiodensity.

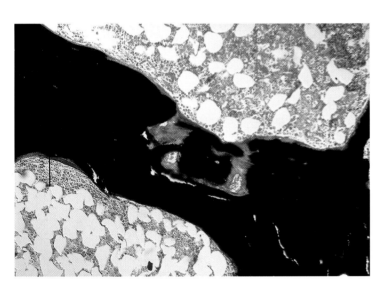 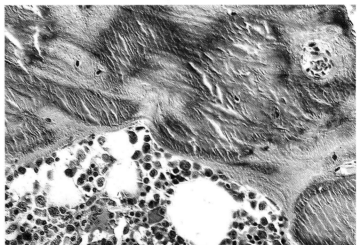

Figure 6.48 Photomicrograph of a section of undecalcified bone obtained from a patient treated with sodium fluoride, showing increased amounts of osteoid, both extensively along the bone surfaces and patchily within the bone trabeculae (von Kossa's, × 4 obj.).

Figure 6.49 Photomicrograph of a section of undecalcified bone obtained from a patient treated with sodium fluoride, showing the irregular appearance of the matrix which is seen in the newly formed bone (undecalcified specimen, H&E, × 10 obj.).

production in osteoporotic patients. Fluoride in doses of approximately 20–30 mg of elemental fluoride daily to achieve a serum level of approximately 10 μM may result in increased bone density in some subjects (Fig. 6.47). However, its usefulness as a mode of treatment has been questioned. (Normal adult serum fluoride ranges from 0.5–2.3 μM; lowest values are seen in young adults and levels progressively increase with age to reach peak values of 2 μM in the sixth to eighth decades.)

Microscopic examination of the sclerotic fluorotic bone in treated patients reveals it to be predominantly lamellar, though with increased osteocytes which themselves do not appear normal; the matrix frequently shows basophilic mottling around the osteocytic lacunae or enlargement of the lacunae themselves. An increased amount of osteoid as well as increased cement lines are also present (Figs 6.48–6.50). A marked increase in the diameter of the cortical haversian systems may give a spongy appearance to the cortex.

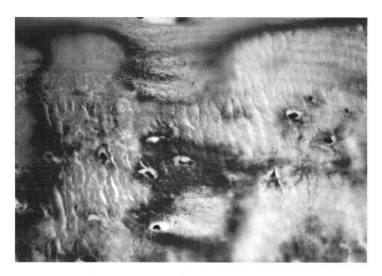

Figure 6.50 Photomicrograph of a section of undecalcified bone obtained from a patient treated with sodium fluoride, showing at a higher power patchy basophilia seen in the newly formed bone shown in Figure 6.49 (H&E, × 25 obj.).

DWARFISM (CHONDRO-OSSEOUS DYSPLASIA)

Many of the diseases discussed in this chapter result in a stunting of growth which is sometimes dramatic, as in OI and the various mucopolysaccharidoses, especially Morquio's syndrome. Dwarfism may also be caused by defects in the epiphysis or in the growth plate, either from a lack of an extrinsic factor necessary for cartilage growth, as occurs with deficiency of growth hormone (pituitary dwarfs), or from cellular deficiencies in the chondrocytes that might interfere with endochondral ossification, such as appears to be the case with achondroplasia (Figs 6.51–6.53). Although many different clinical syndromes have been described, mostly by radiologists, for the most part the underlying molecular defects remain unknown.

The radiographic classification is based either on the portion of the long bone (epiphysis, metaphysis, or diaphysis) most obvi-

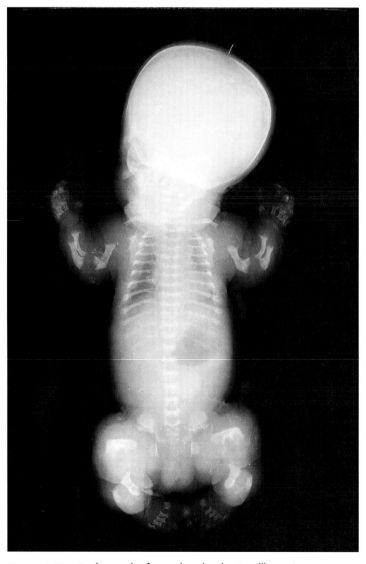

Figure 6.51 Radiograph of an achondroplastic stillborn.

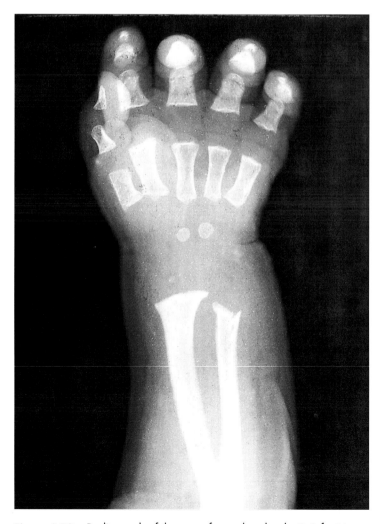

Figure 6.52 Radiograph of the arm of an achondroplastic infant to show the sharply defined sclerotic metaphysis indicating the absence of normal longitudinal growth and, consequently, the shortened diaphyses and flared metaphyses.

ously involved, and on the presence or absence of spinal involvement; or by the portion of the extremity involved (Fig. 6.54). Proximal shortening or disproportionate shortening of the humerus and femur is known as rhizomelic dwarfism; shortening of the bones of the leg or forearm is known as mesomelic dwarfism; and shortening of small distal parts is known as acromelic dwarfism.

The age of the patient at the time of presentation (e.g. newborn, infant, child, or adult) is important in categorizing and analyzing the abnormalities which result in dwarfism.

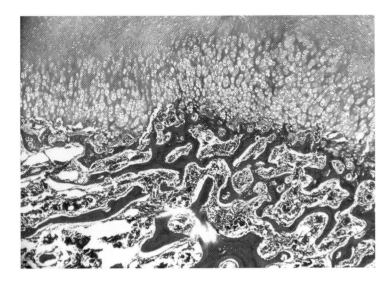

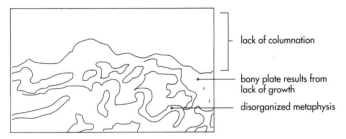

lack of columnation

bony plate results from lack of growth

disorganized metaphysis

Figure 6.53 Photomicrograph of the growth plate and metaphyseal bone from an achondroplastic dwarf to show the lack of normal maturation and columnation in the growth plate and the presence of a bony end-plate in the metaphysis (H&E, × 2.5 obj.).

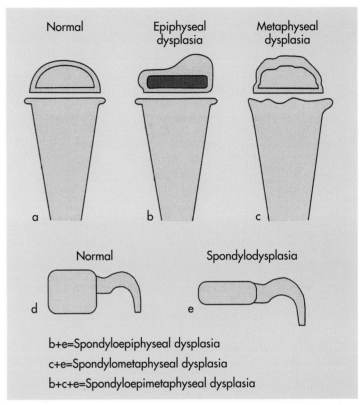

Figure 6.54 Radiologic classification of chondrodysplastic dwarfism.

Chapter 7

DISEASES RESULTING FROM DISTURBANCES IN CELL LINKAGE

Like almost all the tissues of the body, the bony skeleton is in a continuous state of formation and breakdown, enabling it to constantly adapt to the environment, especially the mechanical demands made upon it. For the amount of tissue to remain the same there must be a balance between formation of the extracellular matrix by the osteoblasts and its breakdown by the osteoclasts. Any disturbance in the linkage between these two processes will result in either a decrease in bone density (osteopenia) or an increase in bone density (osteosclerosis) (Fig. 7.1). These processes are regulated by both local and systemic factors (see Chapter 1, Tables 1.3 and 1.4), but in general disturbed skeletal homeostasis is not the result of disturbances of calcium homeostasis, and the blood calcium levels are essentially normal.

The first part of this chapter deals with conditions in which there is increased bone tissue formation, either localized or generalized. The second part discusses conditions characterized by osteopenia.

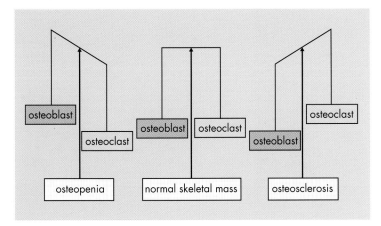

Figure 7.1 In each of these situations, it is the relative activity that matters, e.g. in osteopenia there may be increased osteoblastic activity but osteoclastic activity is even greater.

OSTEOSCLEROTIC CONDITIONS

Increased radiodensity is a common finding in the skeleton, and is usually associated with metastatic cancer (see Chapter 20). Much less commonly it may occur as a result of marrow disease, such as myelofibrosis (see Chapter 9, p. 235), or disturbed mineralization as occurs with fluorosis, as already discussed in Chapter 6, p. 168.

This section will focus on sclerosis due to disturbed cell linkage and mainly on osteopetrosis and Paget's disease, in both of which the primary defect appears to be a malfunction of the osteoclast.

OSTEOPETROSIS (MARBLE BONE DISEASE, ALBERS–SCHÖNBERG DISEASE)

Osteopetrosis is a rare heterogenous group of congenital disorders characterized by a marked increase in the density of the bones (Fig. 7.2). The bones are usually short and frequently exhibit a modeling defect characterized by loss of the normal metaphyseal flare, sometimes referred to as an Erlenmeyer flask deformity. This deformity is most prominent in the areas of rapid growth, i.e. the lower femur, upper tibia and upper humerus. (A similar deformity may also be seen with Gaucher's disease.) Osteopetrosis is often complicated by multiple fractures resulting from a disturbed microarchitecture (Fig. 7.3), and by anemia resulting from the marked reduction in the marrow space (Fig. 7.4).

Two clinical presentations have been recognized. In the severe (malignant) form that usually causes death in utero or in early childhood, it appears to be inherited as an autosomal recessive trait. In this form of the disease, marrow cavities fail to develop, leading to extramedullary hematopoiesis, anemia, leukoerythroblastosis and progressive hypersplenism. Obstruction of the cranial foramina results in increased intracranial pressure, optic atrophy, deafness and cranial nerve palsies. Development is progressively impaired in the majority of these children and death occurs during the first years of life from anemia, bleeding or infection. A less severe (benign) form in which the patients live into adult life, appears to be inherited as an autosomal dominant condition. In this latter form of the disease, diagnosis may be delayed until late middle age, where it is usually made because of a pathologic fracture or as an incidental radiologic finding. In such a case, the condition must be differentiated from other causes of increased bone density, such as widespread osteoblastic metastases or myelosclerosis.

In severely affected patients, radiologic examination of the skeleton may reveal a uniform opacity of the skeletal tissue, with complete loss of the corticomedullary demarcation (Fig. 7.5). However, in less severely affected patients it is not unusual to find, particularly in the pelvis and the peripheral bones, alternating

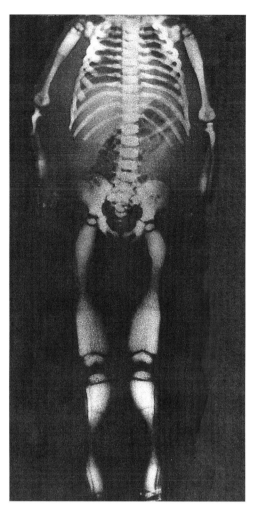

Figure 7.2 Whole-body radiograph of a young child with osteopetrosis showing a marked increase in the density of the bones. The normal demarcation of cancellous bone and cortical bone is lost. In addition, there is the typical metaphyseal flaring (Erlenmeyer flask deformity), which is particularly prominent around the knees, hips, and upper humerus.

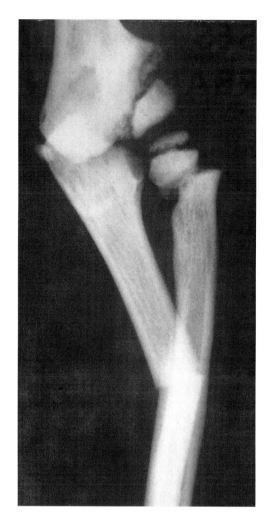

Figure 7.3 Multiple fractures of the forearm and elbow are demonstrated in this young patient with osteopetrosis. Although the bone is denser than normal it may be less strong because of a disturbed microarchitecture. Note the transverse direction of the fractures.

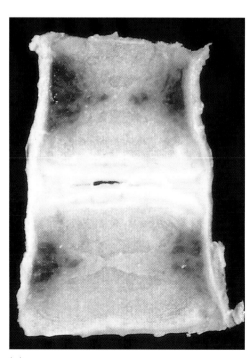

(a)

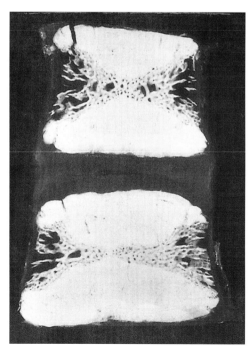

(b)

Figure 7.4 Osteopetrosis: gross appearance of two resected vertebral bodies in frontal section (**a**) and a radiograph of these vertebrae (**b**). The obliteration of the marrow space results in extramedullary hematopoiesis.

areas of affected and apparently normal bone, which give a peculiar striped appearance to the image (Fig. 7.6). In the vertebral bodies, a central, horizontal lytic stripe is often seen, which gives the vertebrae a sandwich-like appearance (Fig. 7.7). Occasionally, spinal involvement may give rise to a lumbar spondylolisthesis because of fractures through the pars interarticularis.

Gross examination of the bones obtained from fatal infantile cases has shown widening in the region of the metaphysis and diaphysis (the characteristic Erlenmeyer flask deformity) (Figs 7.8 and 7.9). The affected bones have increased density and may weigh two to three times more than normal bone, despite the fact that they are usually somewhat smaller than normal. On sectioning, the bone tissue is generally very hard and compact, with complete loss of the normal cancellous architecture.

Microscopic examination reveals extremely dense and irregular bone trabeculae, nearly all of which have a central core of cartilage (Fig. 7.10). (Compare with the primary spongiosa that normally forms in the metaphysis during development; which has a similar appearance but is rapidly remodeled to the adult form of bone. In patients with osteopetrosis, the mechanism by which this remodeling is effected appears to be deficient, and the primary spongiosa together with its cartilage core therefore persists.)

Although a paucity of osteoclasts has sometimes been reported in osteopetrosis, microscopic examination shows that in many cases osteoclasts are abundant. However, electron microscopic studies have demonstrated that, at least in some cases, these osteoclasts lack ruffled borders and that although the cells

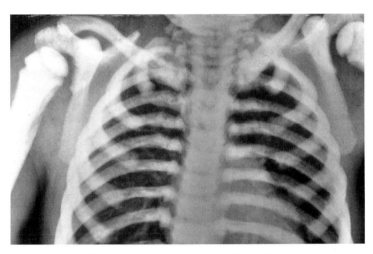

Figure 7.5   Radiograph of the upper body of a child with osteopetrosis. A marked increase in density of all the bones is apparent.

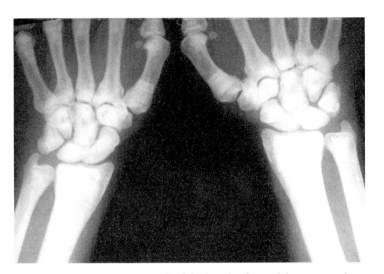

Figure 7.6   Clinical radiograph of the hands of an adult patient with osteopetrosis. The proximal end of the first metacarpal clearly shows alternating stripes of dense involved bone, with less dense and apparently normal bone distally.

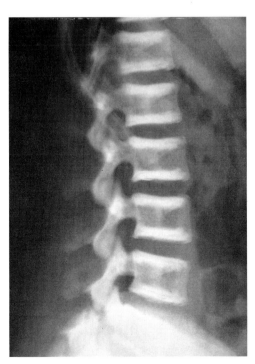

Figure 7.7   In this adult patient with osteopetrosis, a radiograph of the spine shows markedly increased density of the proximal and distal thirds of the vertebral bodies, giving a sandwich-like appearance.

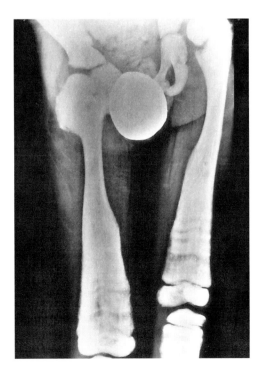

Figure. 7.8   Radiograph of the legs in a child with osteopetrosis shows a lack of metaphyseal remodeling, which gives rise to an Erlenmeyer flask deformity. Normal cortical medullary differentiation is not seen, and the bones are strikingly dense. Again a striped appearance is seen in the distal femoral metaphysis.

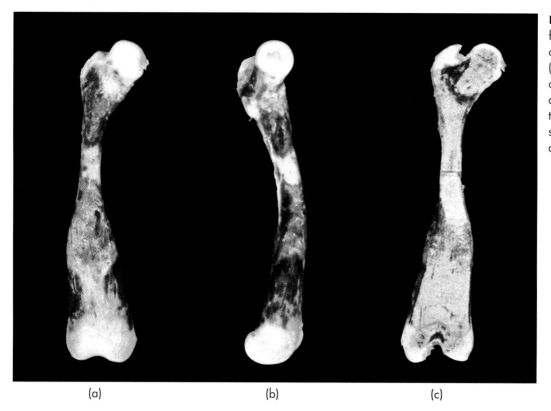

(a) (b) (c)

Figure 7.9 Gross appearances of a femur removed from a child with osteopetrosis seen in frontal (**a**), lateral (**b**), and cut section (**c**). Note the characteristic Erlenmeyer flask deformity of the distal end of the femur, the exaggerated anterior bowing, subperiosteal hemorrhage, and uniform density of the bone in the cut section.

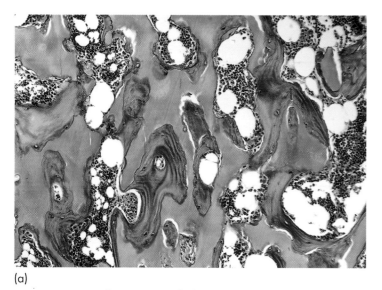

(a)

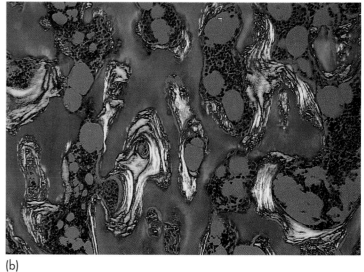

(b)

Figure 7.10 (**a**) Photomicrograph demonstrates residual cartilage in an adult patient with osteopetrosis. (**b**) The same field has been photographed using polarized light, which clearly differentiates the bone and calcified cartilage (H&E, × 4 obj.).

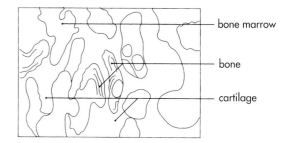

bone marrow

bone

cartilage

are in proximity to the bone and calcified cartilage, they do not show the cytologic features normally present in an active osteoclast (Fig. 7.11). In other words, although osteoclasts are present, they do not appear to be functioning normally. The most obvious defect is the failure to resorb calcified cartilage and it is perhaps here that the osteoclasts are most deficient.

In osteopetrotic mice, restoration of normal bone and cartilage resorption has followed the transplantation of normal bone marrow or spleen cells. This procedure has also been tried in humans with some promise of success.

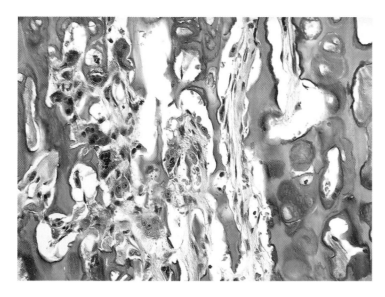

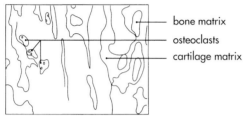

- bone matrix
- osteoclasts
- cartilage matrix

Figure 7.11 Histologic section taken from a young child with osteopetrosis, showing numerous osteoclasts in the tissue. However, these osteoclasts do not seem to be resorbing bone (H&E, × 10 obj.).

PAGET'S DISEASE (OSTEITIS DEFORMANS)

Paget's disease is in most instances a localized condition and clinically silent; generally it is discovered as an incidental finding on radiologic examination. The clinical disease, characterized by widespread bone involvement, as described by Sir James Paget in 1877, actually represents only a small portion of the total number of affected individuals.

Paget's disease is characterized microscopically by disordered bone architecture which results from an increased rate of bone tissue breakdown by osteoclasts. In response to the increased osteoclastic resorption, there is a compensatory increase in the rate of bone tissue formation by osteoblasts, and in the active phase the rate of bone turnover is markedly increased (Fig. 7.12).

Virtually any bone in the body may be involved, but the most common sites are the lumbar spine, pelvis, skull, femur, and tibia. Less commonly, the disease is multifocal or even generalized.

The incidence of the condition varies with ethnicity; although common in northern Europeans, it is very rare in blacks and Asians. In two large autopsy series in northern Europe, the incidence of Paget's disease was reported to be between 3% and 4% of all individuals over the age of 40 (this probably underestimates the true incidence, which in some localities may be much higher). In these autopsy studies the disease was most often limited to a part of the vertebral column and/or the pelvis (the only parts of the skeleton usually examined at autopsy) and in most the disease had not been diagnosed during life.

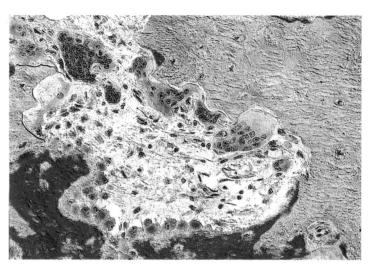

Figure 7.12 Photomicrograph of a histologic section obtained from a patient with Paget's disease demonstrates both bone resorption by large multinucleated giant cells and active bone deposition by swollen active osteoblasts, lower left (undecalcified section, Goldner stain, × 10 obj.).

Radiologic and gross features

The radiologic appearance of Paget's disease is variable. In the earliest stages, during which osteoclastic resorption predominates, there is a striking radiolucency without any thickening of the bone; in the skull this has been called osteoporosis circumscripta (Fig. 7.13). In the later stages of the disease, where resorption diminishes, the overall density of the bone increases (Fig. 7.14). The cancellous bone trabeculae can be seen to become thicker or coarser and more irregular. On the other hand, the cortical bone becomes radiographically less compact and there is loss of corticomedullary demarcation (Figs 7.15 and 7.16). The periosteal and endosteal surfaces become rough and

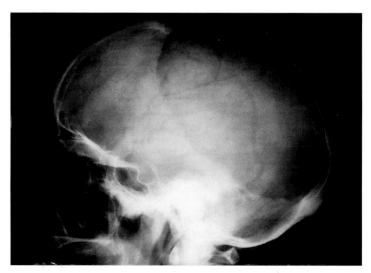

Figure 7.13 Clinical radiograph of a skull. Note the large, circular lytic defect involving the posterior half of the skull. Some patchy osteoblastic reaction in the bone around the defect can also be seen. This lesion, osteoporosis circumscripta, is a relatively common radiologic presentation of Paget's disease.

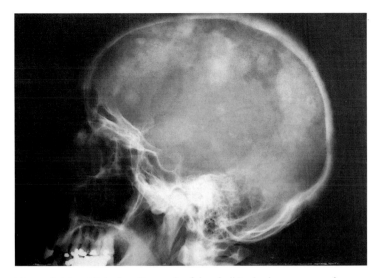

Figure 7.14 Clinical radiograph of the skull in the later stages of Paget's disease. Marked patchy sclerosis appears in the bone, the diploic architecture is lost, and the bone becomes extremely thick, on occasion several times thicker than normal.

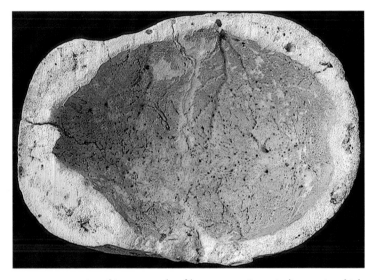

Figure 7.15 A striking example of late, severe Paget's disease in which the thickening of the skull, the loss of diploic architecture, and the granular pumice-like appearance of the bone can be seen.

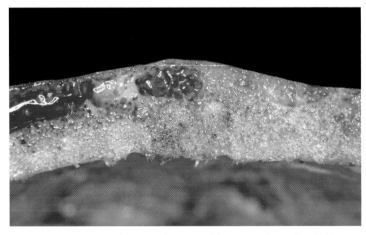

Figure 7.16 Paget's disease: close-up of the cut surface of a skull to show the loss of cortical bone and an overall spongy appearance. There are also large blood-filled lakes that may be present in pagetic bone.

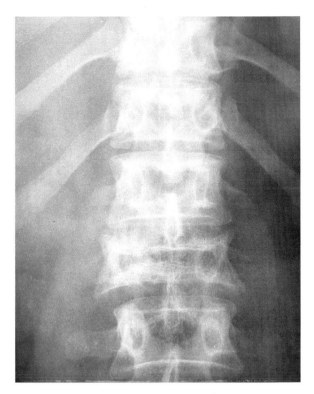

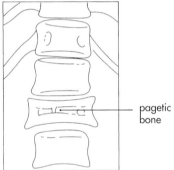

Figure 7.17 Clinical radiograph of the spine shows a solitary focus of pagetic bone. There is a loss of height of the vertebra, some increases in the width of the vertebra, and a typical 'picture-frame' appearance.

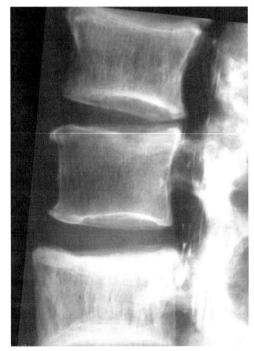

Figure 7.18 Radiograph of the lumbar spine in a 66-year-old male shows enlargement of L4 with coarsening of the trabecular pattern and a margin sclerosis – the so-called 'picture framing' characteristic of Paget's disease. (Courtesy of Dr Alex Norman.)

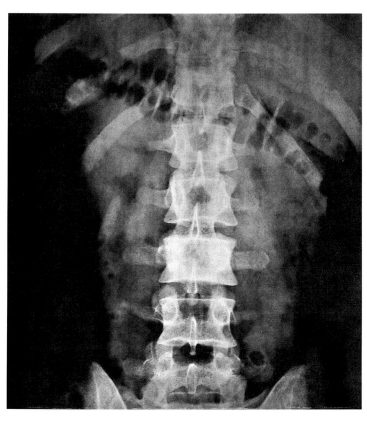

irregular rather than smooth, and there is usually an increase in the diameter of the affected bone (Fig. 7.17).

Radiologic examination of the vertebral bodies may reveal either uniformly increased radiodensity suggestive of lymphoma or metastatic tumor or, more commonly, a 'picture frame' appearance (Figs 7.18 and 7.19). In the pelvis, it is common to find combinations of increased density and lytic areas, as well as areas with a honeycombed, or striated appearance.

In long bones, the process usually starts at one end, occasionally both, and spreads towards the center. The junction between the normal and diseased bone is demarcated as an advancing wedge of rarefaction frequently described as 'flame-like' (Figs 7.20 and 7.21).

Figure 7.19 Clinical radiograph of a 38-year-old patient who presented with complaints of vague back pain. In this radiograph, a rather uniform sclerosis without evident enlargement is seen in the body of L3; the initial radiographic diagnosis was lymphoma. Because of the sclerosis a needle biopsy was obtained, with difficulty, which clearly demonstrated the mosaic pattern, marrow fibrosis and increased osteoclastic resorption typical of Paget's disease. This radiologic presentation is decidedly atypical. The more usual presentation is shown in Figures 7.17 and 7.18.

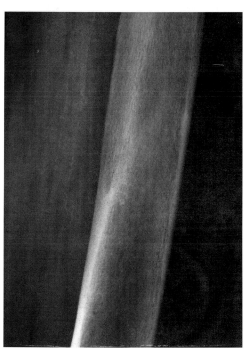

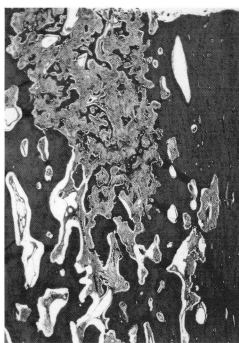

Figure 7.20 (a) Radiograph of femur involved by Paget's disease. The cortex of the posterior femur in the proximal portion is irregularly thickened and more porotic than that in the distal part. At the junction between the involved upper bone and the normal lower bone, note a flame-shaped advancing edge. (b) Histologic section of the advancing edge of involved bone – note the involved fibrotic and pagetic bone eroding the normal bone cortex (H&E, × 2.5 obj.).

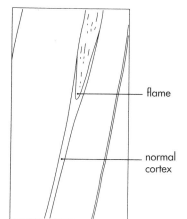

(a)

flame

normal cortex

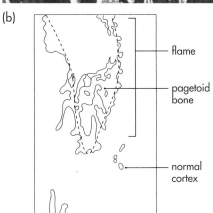

(b)

flame

pagetoid bone

normal cortex

In long bones the early phase of the disease may on occasion be mistaken for a tumor, especially when the diagnosis of Paget's is not considered as in the patient shown in Figure 7.22.

In scintigraphic studies, isotope uptake is increased at all stages of the disease (Fig. 7.23).

Microscopic appearance

Just as with the radiologic appearance, the microscopic appearance depends on the stage of the disease process. It has been divided into three phases. The osteolytic phase is characterized by an active osteoclastic resorption and an extremely vascular fibrous tissue that fills the marrow spaces. Inflammatory cells are absent (Fig. 7.24). In cancellous bone, the trabeculae are slender and sparse; in cortical bone, large resorption cavities are seen. Concurrent with the osteoclastic activity, appositional new bone formation by prominent osteoblasts may be found. The bone tissue being formed is often of woven type (Fig. 7.25). Both increased osteoclastic and increased osteoblastic activity are fre-

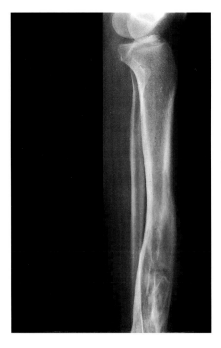

Figure 7.21   In this lateral radiograph of the leg of a 55-year-old female with Paget's disease of the distal tibia, an obvious junction is seen between the involved cortex and the noninvolved cortex, above which there is a flame-like or wedged outline. (Courtesy of Dr Alex Norman.)

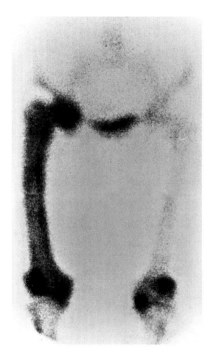

Figure 7.23   Scintigram shows increased ^{99}Tc uptake in a femur involved with Paget's disease. In this image, it is possible also to appreciate some bowing of the femur as well as varus deformity of the hip.

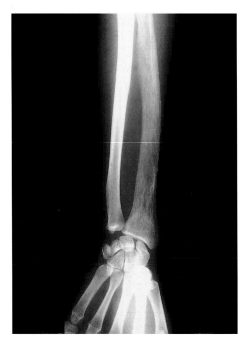

Figure 7.22 Radiograph of the forearm of a 25-year-old woman who suffered a fracture of the radius after lifting her 3-year-old son. The diffuse demineralization and altered trabecular pattern resulted in a differential diagnosis that included round-cell tumor, infection and adamantinoma. A biopsy showed this to be Paget's disease (< 4% of individuals with Paget's present under the age of 40). (Courtesy of Dr Howard Dorfman.)

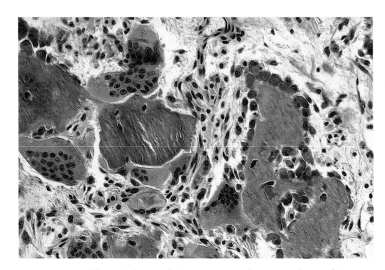

Figure 7.24   Photomicrograph demonstrates the acute phase of Paget's disease with very active osteoclastic resorption, marrow fibrosis, and formation of new bone. Note the huge multinucleate osteoclasts and the cytoplasmic clear areas in the osteoblast, which represent the prominent Golgi apparatus associated with increased bone matrix production (H&E, × 10 obj.).

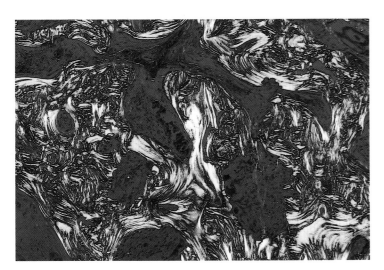

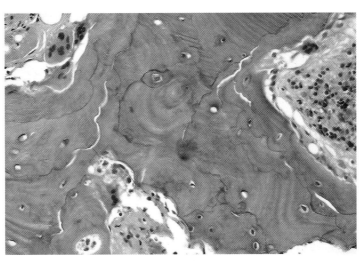

Figure 7.25 Photomicrograph taken using polarized light demonstrates both residual lamellar bone and extensive foci of woven bone in early active Paget's disease (polarized light, × 4 obj.).

Figure 7.26 Photomicrograph demonstrates the thick, irregular plates of bone formed in Paget's disease. In this section, the basophilic cement lines are clearly seen. Note the microcracks which occur at the site of the cement lines and result in structural weakness in pagetic bone (H&E, × 10 obj.).

quently observed on the same trabecula. The microscopic picture is one of frenetic cell activity, which may in some cases be impossible to differentiate from hyperparathyroidism. However in most cases they can be differentiated firstly because in Paget's disease, the osteoclasts are generally bigger with upward of 10–20 nuclei and in hyperparathyroidism there is tunneling resorption (see Chapter 8, p. 205 on hyperparathyroidism).

This initial, mainly destructive phase is followed by an osteoblastic phase in which new bone formation predominates over resorption. Massive trabecular plates are built up to a density

that is neither cortical nor cancellous in its architecture. The increased rate of bone formation and bone resorption results in an increased number of reversal fronts or cement lines, which in turn gives rise to the classic 'mosaic pattern' (Fig. 7.26).

The alteration in microarchitecture, together with the increased number of cement lines, leads to structural weakness in the tissue and facilitates the propagation of cracks. With the aid of polarized light microscopy, studies of the orientation of the collagen in bone reveal the discordant nature of the new structure, which may not be so apparent without it (Fig. 7.27).

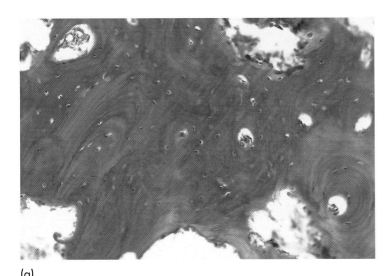

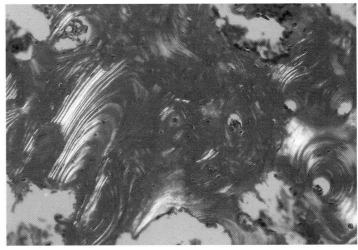

(a)   (b)

Figure 7.27 (a) Histologic features of the late stages of Paget's disease. The osteoblastic and osteoclastic activity is much less evident than in the early stages of the disease, furthermore it can be difficult to appreciate the mosaic pattern, either because the tissue has been over-decalcified or because the staining is not adequate to show the basophilic lines clearly (H&E, × 10 obj.). (b) When the same field is examined by polarized light using a first-order red filter, the disorganized pattern of the bone structure is clearly demonstrated.

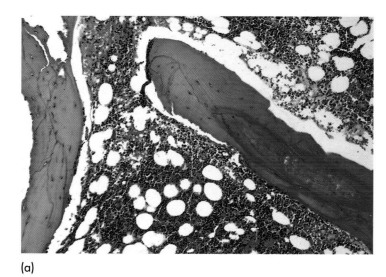

(a)

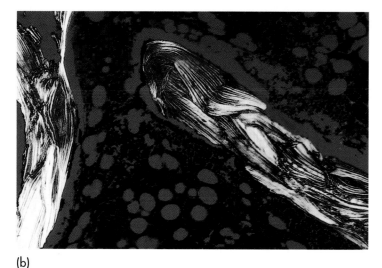

(b)

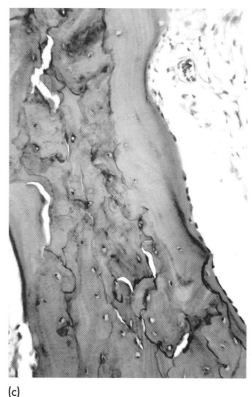

(c)

Figure 7.28 (a) Photomicrograph showing a fragment of cancellous bone and cellular bone marrow which at first sight might be passed over as normal. However, when examined using polarized light (b), the discordant arrangement of the collagen fibers should alert the pathologist to the possibility of Paget's disease (H&E, × 10 obj.). (c) A higher power to show disorganized pattern and irregular cement lines (H&E, × 25 obj.).

A final 'burnt out' phase is generally described, during which cell activity is less intense and vascularity diminished. The microscopic picture is that of heavily trabeculated bone showing a prominent mosaic pattern. However, the turnover rate of the diseased bone may not be much greater than that of normal bone. In this late stage the marrow may have a relatively normal appearance (Fig. 7.28).

The etiology of Paget's disease remains unknown. However, electron microscopic observations of the osteoclasts of patients with Paget's disease have demonstrated the presence of specific intranuclear inclusions composed of microcylinders. These inclusions have also been found in the giant cells of giant-cell tumors associated with Paget's disease and are illustrated in Figure 7.29. These structures suggest an analogy with the myxovirus of the measles group. Studies with indirect immunofluorescence and immunoperoxidase techniques have lent further support to the hypotheses of a viral etiology in Paget's disease of bone.

Clinical laboratory findings

An elevation of serum alkaline phosphatase activity (in association with the increased osteoblastic activity) to as much as 20–30 times the normal level has been recorded. The acid phosphatase level, too, tends to be at its upper limit or even slightly above normal.

The serum calcium and phosphorus levels are ordinarily within normal limits in Paget's disease. However, hypercalcuria and stone formation is an occasional complication following prolonged bed rest in a patient with extensive bone involvement. Elevated urinary hydroxyproline (or pyridinoline) levels can also be expected as a consequence of increased bone tissue breakdown. Regional blood flow studies have demonstrated increased vascularity, in some instances as much as 20 times the normal.

Clinical presentation

The complaints that bring the patient to the physician are pain in the affected parts of the skeleton or symptoms of the complica-

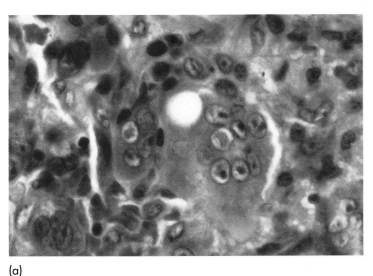

(a)

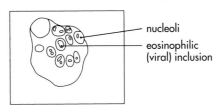

nucleoli
eosinophilic
(viral) inclusion

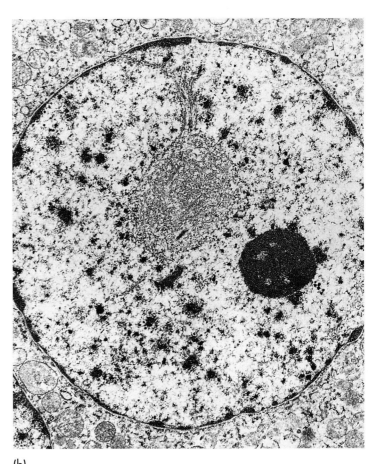

(b)

Figure 7.29 (a) Photomicrograph of a giant-cell tumor from a patient with Paget's disease. Note the intranuclear eosinophilic inclusions in addition to the more clearly defined basophilic nucleoli in the illustrated giant cell (H&E, × 50 obj.). (b) An electron photomicrograph of one of the nuclei containing an eosinophilic inclusion illustrated in (a) demonstrates microtubular structures – the image associated with the myxoma virus (original magnification × 20,000).

Table 7.1 Diagnosis of Paget's Disease.

Diagnosis of Paget's Disease
1. **History**
• duration
• symptoms
• family history
2. **Physical examination**
• warmth
• tenderness
• bone enlargement
• deformity
• decreased range of joint movement
3. **Laboratory tests**
• alkaline phosphatase
• urinary pyridinoline
• acid phosphatase
• serum calcium, phosphorus
4. **Bone scan**
• a sensitive indicator
• positive
5. **Radiographic studies**
• specific but sometimes unrecognized
• enlargement (characteristic)
• lytic, sclerotic, or both
• arthritis
• transverse fractures

tions of Paget's disease (fracture, arthritis, heart failure, or tumor) (Table 7.1). In patients with Paget's disease, small, incomplete cortical fractures may be numerous, particularly in weight-bearing bones. Progressive bowing of the femoral neck and wedging of the vertebrae are often the result of repeated microfractures, which may progress to complete transverse fractures. However as shown in Figure 7.30, bowing of the legs may result purely from bone overgrowth.

Clinical evaluation of patients with Paget's disease reveals a high incidence of arthritis in the joints adjacent to involved bones (Fig. 7.31). Clinical arthritis is commonly seen in the hip joint and is characterized on radiologic examination by concentric joint narrowing. This narrowing appears to result from an accelerated rate of endochondral ossification in the calcified zone of the articular cartilage (Fig. 7.32) (consequent to the increased vascularity and turnover of the subchondral bone; see Chapter 10, p. 242 for further discussion of this phenomenon). Overall bone deformity, resulting from accelerated bone modeling, also contributes to the arthritic process by altering the load distribution.

Sarcoma has been reported to develop in 1–2% of patients with widespread Paget's involvement (Fig. 7.33). However, considering that most cases of Paget's disease are undiagnosed, the true incidence of sarcoma in Paget's disease must be very low. However, sarcoma is a complication not only of widespread

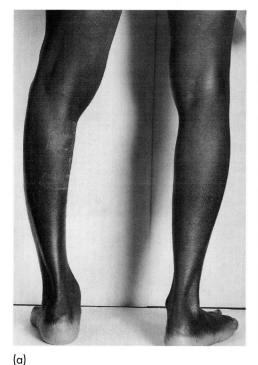
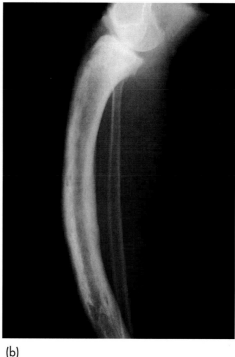

(a)

(b)

Figure 7.30 (a) Bowing of the leg is often seen in Paget's disease, and in the radiograph (b) of a patient with Paget's disease affecting the tibia – but not the fibula bone. Overgrowth has resulted in an increase in length of the tibia, associated with bowing. Irregularity of both periosteal and endosteal surfaces is clearly seen in this image.

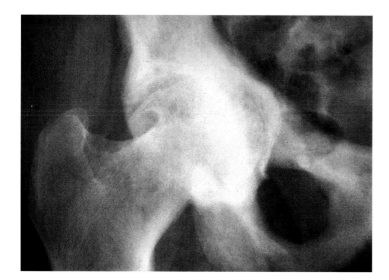

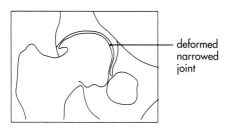

deformed narrowed joint

Figure 7.31 Clinical radiograph of a patient with Paget's disease. In the hip there is marked concentric narrowing of the joint space, indicative of degenerative joint disease. In addition note the irregular patchy bone sclerosis in the femoral head in particular.

disease; rarely it may be engrafted on monostotic Paget's disease (Fig. 7.34). The sarcoma that develops usually shows a mixed pattern of osteosarcoma, fibrosarcoma, chondrosarcoma, and malignant histiocytoma; i.e. a mixed mesenchymal pattern (Fig. 7.35). Occasionally a benign conventional giant-cell tumor pattern may be seen and in such cases the tumors may be multiple (Fig. 7.36).

Myeloma, lymphoma and metastatic cancer have all been reported in association with Paget's disease, and may on occasion need to be differentiated from Paget's sarcoma. Pseudo-sarcomatous lesions, in some cases characterized by florid new bone and abundant periosteal bone formation, have also been described (Fig. 7.37), further emphasizing the need for biopsy in cases where tumor is suspected, both for accurate diagnosis and so that treatment can be appropriate.

GENERALIZED OSTEOSCLEROSIS ASSOCIATED WITH INCREASED OSTEOBLASTIC ACTIVITY

Increased osteoblastic activity not associated with any increase in osteoclastic activity leads to increased skeletal density. Physiologically, such an increase in density results from increased physical activity and may be localized as for example in the bones of the forearm of tennis players (see Chapter 4, Fig. 4.5). Pathologic osteosclerosis may also result from a disturbance of normal cell linkage. Such cases are very rare. They are usually characterized by severe and unremitting bone pain, and their etiology is obscure.

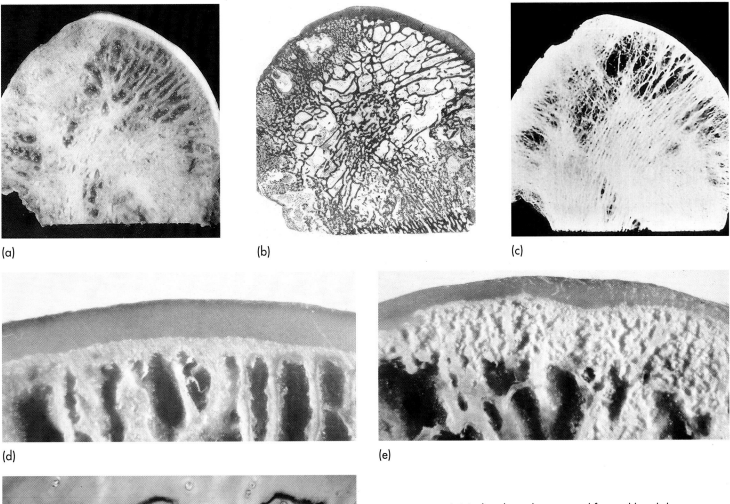

(a)

(b)

(c)

(d)

(e)

(f)

Figure 7.32   (a) A slice through a resected femoral head shows extensive involvement by Paget's disease and erosion of the cartilage on the medial side. Histologic section (b) of the femoral head (H&E, × 1.25 obj.) and a radiograph (c) of a slice of the specimen. The pagetic bone is seen to have a fine and disorganized trabecular pattern, which contrasts markedly with the normal cancellous bone that remains in some areas. Close-up of the articular surface. In (d) there is normal cancellous bone, subchondral end-plate, and articular cartilage. In (e), pagetic bone has resulted in an irregular subchondral bone end-plate with marked thinning of the overlying cartilage. It may be that the accelerated remodeling of the affected subchondral bone has resulted in accelerated endochondral ossification of the overlying cartilage, which produces the evident thinning. (f) Photomicrograph of the disordered Pagetic bone in the subchondral region. Note the thickening and irregularity of the tidemark (H&E, × 10 obj.).

Camurati–Engelmann disease (diaphyseal dysplasia)

The clinical features of Camurati–Engelmann disease are painful legs, a waddling gait, and wasting muscles. The disease is usually hereditary, with an autosomal dominant mode of transmission. The symptoms usually become manifest early in life, commonly before the age of 10 years. However, occasional cases have been reported in which the patient's age at diagnosis has been as late as the fifth decade.

The disease is diagnosed primarily on the basis of radiologic examination. Symmetric sclerosis is observed, and often a fusiform enlargement of the diaphysis of the long bones, especially the femur and tibia (Figs 7.38 and 7.39). The epiphyses are spared. There may also be changes in the skull, and rarely in the pelvis, mandible, clavicle, ribs, spine, metacarpals, and phalanges (Fig. 7.40).

The disorder is characterized histologically by a thickened cortex, which results mainly from increased endosteal new bone formation (Fig. 7.41). However, periosteal new bone formation is

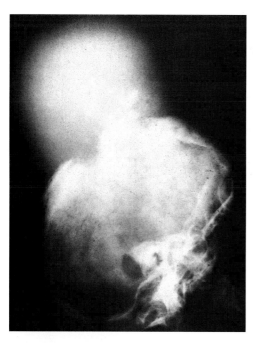

Figure 7.33 Radiograph of the skull of a patient with Paget's disease who had developed over the previous few months a large firm mass over the vault of the skull. Biopsy showed this to be a Paget's sarcoma.

sometimes observed. In children, the enlargement of the cortex of the bone produces a narrowed medullary cavity which, if the narrowing is severe enough, may lead to extramedullary hematopoiesis and eventual hepatosplenomegaly.

The serum chemistries in patients with Camurati–Engelmann disease are usually normal, although an increase in the level of alkaline phosphatase (of bone origin) is sometimes observed. The disorder is of obscure etiology. The pain may be relieved by the administration of steroids.

In 1962, van Buchem and associates reported seven cases of a disease that was similar in many ways to Camurati–Engelmann disease but different in that there was prominent skull involvement (hyperostosis corticalis generalisata).

Other obscure entities with diaphyseal cortical bone thickening include hyperostosis generalisata with pachyderma, in which the diaphysis, metaphysis and epiphysis are significantly involved.

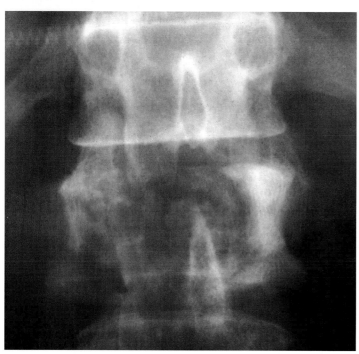

(a)

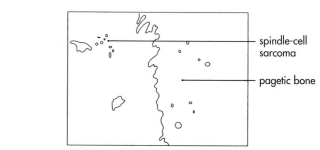

(b)

- spindle-cell sarcoma
- pagetic bone

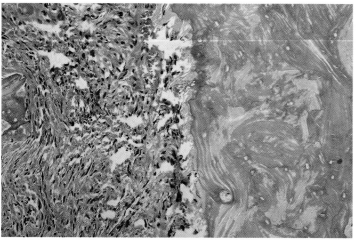

(c)

Figure 7.34 Spinal radiograph (a) of a 58-year-old female with a 2-month history of low back pain. She had undergone a hysterectomy for cervical carcinoma 14 years earlier. A patchy sclerotic and lytic appearance was noted, which was interpreted to be consistent with metastatic disease. However, there was some widening of the body, which is uncharacteristic of metastatic disease. Needle biopsy showed an anaplastic tumor with many giant cells, consistent with Paget's sarcoma; foci of bone obtained with this biopsy showed the typical mosaic pattern of Paget's. The patient died approximately 4 months later. Autopsy revealed local extension of the tumor, which involved T12 and L2, and compression and encasement of the vena cava. Extensive lung metastases had the pattern of a Paget's sarcoma. An H&E section (b) of a portion of bone adjacent to the tumor shows increased numbers of cement lines within the bone. In the polarized section (c) of the same field, the disorganized bony architecture is obvious (H&E, × 4 obj.). This case is significant because it demonstrates that, even in monostotic Paget's disease, a sarcoma may rarely occur as a complication.

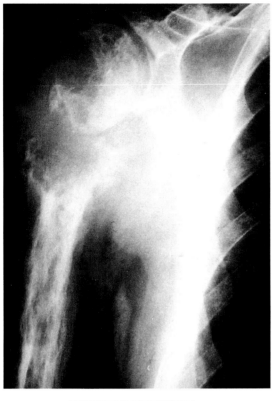

(a)

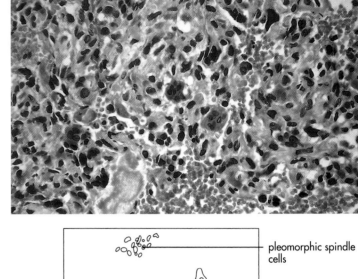

(b)

Figure 7.35   (a) Clinical radiograph of a patient with widespread Paget's disease of the skeleton showing, in addition, at the proximal end of the humerus, a destructive lytic lesion and a pathological fracture indicating sarcomatous degeneration. (b) High-power view of a biopsy from the patient in (a) shows a pleomorphic spindle-cell tumor with many giant cells, which is typical of the histologic appearance of Paget's sarcoma (H&E, × 25 obj.).

pathologic fracture with lytic destruction

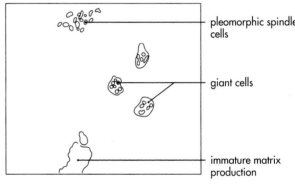

pleomorphic spindle cells

giant cells

immature matrix production

Figure 7.36   (a) Myelogram of the spine in a patient with Paget's disease (note the irregular coarse density of several vertebral bodies clearly seen in the pedicles). The myelogram shows an occlusion at the level of L1 with displacement of the dura by a soft-tissue mass. (b) Photomicrograph of tissue obtained from a biopsy of this mass reveals a conventional giant-cell tumor (H&E, × 10 obj.).

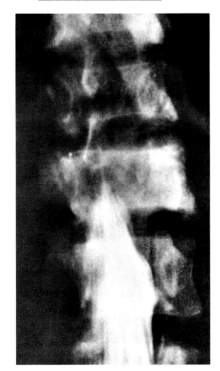

(a)

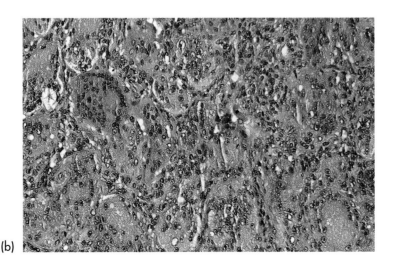

(b)

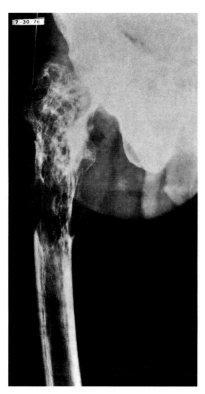

Figure 7.37 Radiograph of the femur from a patient with Paget's disease shows an expanded lytic area which seemed to indicate the development of a sarcoma; however, biopsy showed that this area was formed entirely of reactive tissue.

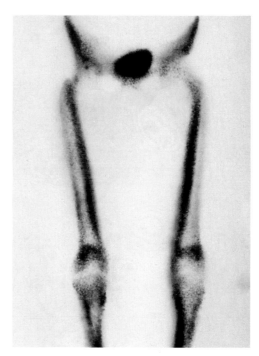

Figure 7.39 Bone scan demonstrates increased diaphyseal uptake over the femurs and tibias bilaterally in a case of hyperostosis generalisata.

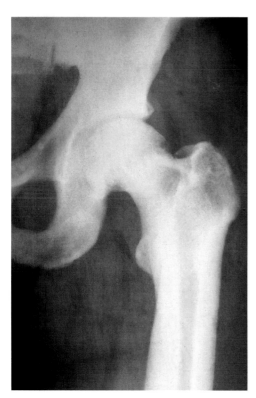

Figure 7.38 Radiograph of a 49-year-old man with a 3-year history of bone pain. Note the markedly thickened, dense cortex, which is more clearly defined than the thickened but sponge-like bone of Paget's disease. In this patient, the serum calcium and phosphate levels were within normal limits, although the alkaline phosphatase level was persistently elevated (up to 1600 mU/ml).

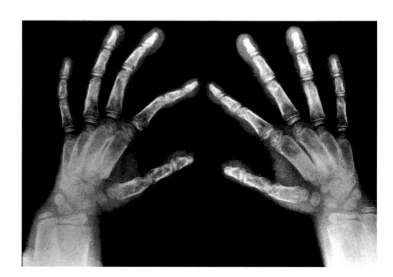

Figure 7.40 Radiograph of the hands of a child with Camurati–Engelmann disease illustrates the cortical sclerosis and fusiform enlargement of the metacarpals typical of this disease.

OSTEOPENIC CONDITIONS

GENERALIZED OSTEOPOROSIS

Decreased density of the skeleton (osteopenia) is a nonspecific condition that may result from any of a number of causes, including mineral and collagen disturbances, hematologic and endocrine abnormalities, neoplastic disorders, or immobilization (Table 7.2). The amount of bone tissue in the skeleton also decreases with age (Fig. 7.42). This decrease is more clinically significant in women than in men, and in whites and Asians than in blacks. This is because in general men and blacks start out with a higher bone density and also because of the association of osteopenia with the onset of menopause in women.

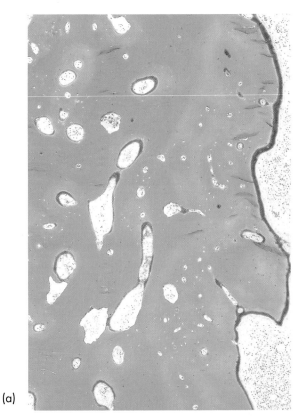

(a)

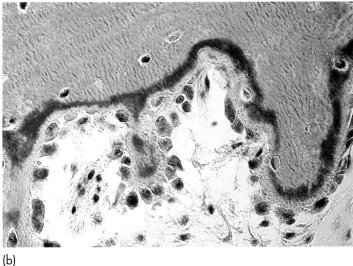

(b)

Figure 7.41 (a) Photomicrograph of a cortical biopsy from a patient with Camurati–Engelmann disease. Bone surfaces are covered by a thin layer of osteoid, indicating increased bone formation. The endosteal surface (right) appears hypercellular with respect to osteocytes. The bone is lamellar with no increase in cement lines, differentiating this from Paget's disease (undecalcified bone, Goldner stain, × 4 obj.).
(b) Photomicrograph taken at a higher power to demonstrate the prominent osteoblasts lining the endosteal surface of the bone together with a moderately thick layer of unmineralized osteoid (undecalcified section, Goldner stain, × 25 obj.).

Table 7.2 Causes of osteopenia.

Causes of osteopenia	
Disuse	Prolonged bed rest
	General inactivity
	Prolonged casting or splinting (localized osteoporosis)
	Angiodystrophy (localized osteoporosis)
	Paralysis
	paraplegia, quadriplegia, hemiplegia, lower motor neuron disease
	Space travel weightlessness
Diet	Deficiency of calcium, protein, vitamin C
	Anorexia nervosa
Drugs	Heparin
	Methotrexate
	Ethanol
	Glucocorticoids
Idiopathic	Adolescent (10–18 years)
	Middle-aged male
Genetic disorders	Osteogenesis imperfecta
	Homocystinuria
Chronic illness	Rheumatoid arthritis (juvenile, adult)
	Cirrhosis
	Sarcoidosis
	Renal tubular acidosis
Neoplasms	Metastatic cancer
	Bone marrow tumors
	myeloma
	lymphoma
	leukemia
	mastocytosis
Endocrine abnormalities	Pituitary hypersecretion tumor
	Adrenal cortex
	glucocorticoid excess (hyperplasia, tumor, iatrogenic)
	Ovary
	estrogen deficiency (postmenopausal, genetic, ovariectomy)
	Testis
	testosterone deficiency (genetic, castration)
	Parathyroid
	hyperparathyroidism (primary, secondary)
	Thyroid
	hyperthyroidism
Postmenopausal	Type I osteoporosis
Age-related	Type II osteoporosis (male or female)

Osteoporosis has been defined as characterized by low bone mass associated with microarchitectural deterioration of bone tissue leading to enhanced bone fragility and an increase in fracture risk.

Age-related osteopenia that results in fracture (usually vertebral crush fractures, Colles' fractures, or femoral neck fractures)

is generally referred to as senile osteoporosis, which is twice as common in females than in males. In about a third of women with osteoporosis, it is related to the menopause.

These two common types of osteoporosis, postmenopausal and senile, have been classified by Riggs and his colleagues on the basis of their different clinical findings as type I osteoporosis

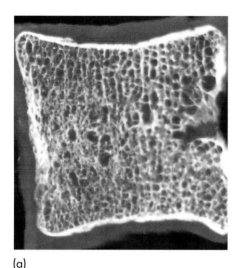
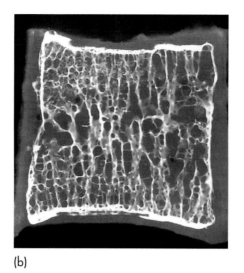
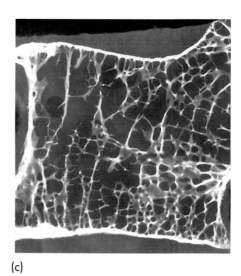

(a) (b) (c)

Figure 7.42 Specimen radiographs of 2 mm slices through the vertebral body of T2. **(a)** The first specimen represents normal bone texture, density, and pattern. **(b)** The second specimen shows a moderate degree of osteopenia, with accentuation of the vertical trabeculae and selective loss of the horizontal trabeculae. **(c)** The third specimen shows severe osteoporosis, with irregular thin trabeculae and partial central collapse of the superior end-plate.

(postmenopausal) and type II osteoporosis (senile or age related). In postmenopausal osteoporosis, bone loss is rapid and associated with increased osteoclastic activity. (It appears that estrogen normally acts as a block to a second messenger from the osteoblast to the osteoclast when the former is stimulated by parathormone. Thus estrogen deficiency may indirectly increase the sensitivity of the osteoclasts to parathyroid hormone.) In senile osteoporosis, bone loss is slow but relentless, and has been associated both with decreased synthesis of bone matrix by the osteoblasts as well as increased osteoclastic activity (Table 7.3).

It should be recognized that many factors affect bone tissue loss; particularly important are physical activity level and diet. The maintenance of skeletal mass is especially affected by activity level. Daily weight-bearing activity is essential to the health of the skeleton, and mechanical weight-bearing stress is perhaps the most important exogenous factor affecting bone development and bone modeling. An interesting example of this process has been observed in astronauts. The marked reduction in gravitational field that results in the weightless environment of space flight leads to profound and rapid loss of skeletal and muscle mass. In everyday experience, a sedentary person is more likely to become osteoporotic than a person who engages in some form of weight-bearing exercise.

An adequate and balanced diet is essential, and lack of it is an important contributor to disease. It has been said that the average American woman has a calcium intake of between only a third and a half of her total daily requirement. Chronic calcium deficiency in the diet leads to increased secretion of both parathyroid hormone and the hormonally active form of vitamin D, $1,25(OH)_2D$ (see Chapter 8, p. 200), both of which stimulate osteoclastic activity. Excessive alcohol consumption and smoking are also believed to contribute to osteoporosis.

The characteristic radiologic features in patients with osteoporosis are thinning of cortical bone and generalized rarefaction of the skeleton (Fig. 7.43). In postmenopausal osteoporosis, bone

loss is mainly of cancellous bone, with less cortical bone loss, whereas in senile, age-related osteoporosis both cancellous and cortical bone loss are present. As the cortex becomes thinner, the overall diameter of the bone tends to increase to maximize mechanical efficiency.

In the vertebral column, there is thinning and eventual disappearance of the transverse trabeculae and subsequent thickening of the vertical trabeculae followed later by the thinning of these trabeculae as well (Fig. 7.44). Compression fractures occur, giving rise to the widening of the intervertebral disc, the so-called 'fish-mouth' appearance (Fig. 7.45). In general, the lower thoracic and upper lumbar vertebrae are most affected. Radiological surveys have shown that about 20% of men and 30% of women over the age of 60 have compression fractures of the vertebral bodies. Therefore, back pain associated with loss of height due to vertebral compression and increased thoracic kyphosis are common manifestations.

Bone mass is one of the major determinants of strength and its quantification is predictive of future fracture risk. (In this regard, Carter and Hayes have shown that the compressive strength of trabecular bone is proportional to the square of its apparent density. Thus, if the density decreases by a factor of 2, the compressive strength decreases by a factor of 4.)

Because vertebral bone loss has to be approximately 30% before it can be radiologically detected, radiologists have long sought special techniques for the evaluation of bone mass, density, and calcium content. Three methods have been widely used for assessing the bone tissue mass based on measurements of bone mineral content:

1. Single-photon absorptiometry, performed for the assessment of cortical bone in the appendicular skeleton, uses the isotope iodine $125(^{125}I)$ as a source of photons, which are then passed through the forearm. The attenuation of the beam is measured by a scintillation counter.

Table 7.3   Involutional osteoporosis.

	Post menopausal (Type I)	Age-related (Type II)
Epidemiologic Factors		
Age	55–75 years	>70 years (F); >80 years (M)
Sex (F:M)	6:1	2:1
Bone physiology or metabolism		
Pathogenesis of uncoupling	Increased osteoclast activity; ↑ resorption	Decreased osteoblast activity; ↓ formation
Net bone loss	Mainly trabecular	Cortical and trabecular
Rate of bone loss	Rapid/short duration	Slow/long duration
Bone density	>2 standards deviations below normal	Low normal (adjusted for age and sex)
Clinical signs		
Fracture sites	Vertebrae (crush), distal forearm, hip (intracapsular)	Vertebrae (multiple wedge), proximal humerus and tibia, hip (extracapsular)
Other signs	Tooth loss	Dorsal kyphosis
Laboratory values		
Serum Ca^{++}	Normal	Normal
Serum P_i	Normal	Normal
Alkaline phosphatase	Normal (↑ with fracture)	Normal (↑ with fracture)
Urine Ca^{++}	Increased	Normal
PTH function	Decreased	Increased
Renal conversion of 25(OH)D to 1,25(OH)$_2$D	Secondary decrease due to ↓ PTH	Primary decrease due to decreased responsiveness of 1-α-OH$_{ase}$
Gastrointestinal calcium absorption	Decreased	Decreased
Prevention and treatment		
High-risk patients	Estrogen or calcitonin supplementation; calcium supplementation; adequate vitamin D; adequate weight-bearing activity; minimization of associated risk factors	Calcium supplementation; adequate vitamin D; adequate weight-bearing activity; minimization of associated risk factors

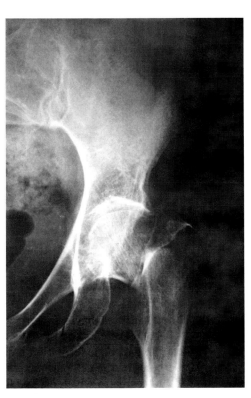

Figure 7.43
Radiograph of severe osteoporosis in the pelvis and femur. Note the thin cortices which outline the residual cancellous bone, in which its density is only slightly different from that of the surrounding soft tissues. There is a recent fracture of the femoral neck which, as is often the case, has drawn attention to the severe osteoporosis in this patient.

2. Dual X-ray absorptiometry (DXA) was introduced commercially in 1987, and at present is probably the most widely used system used for measuring skeletal mass. With this system, two distinct energy level beams are generated. The preferred anatomic sites for DXA measurement of bone mass include the lumbar spine, proximal femur, and the whole body, but other parts, such as the forearm and calcaneus, can also be scanned. When measuring the spine, it is important to realize that aortic calcification, degenerative arthritis of the spine, or both, may contribute to falsely high readings, as may vertebral compression fractures, where the porosity may be masked owing to compaction of the trabeculae and formation of fracture callus.

3. Quantitative CT scanning (QCT) allows densitometric measurements of cross-sections of a vertebral body, which are then compared with a phantom. Besides its usefulness in measurement of bone mineral density, QCT is an imaging technique that can provide structural information on the regions examined.

One of the problems with measuring local bone mass results from the lack of structural homogeneity, which is dramatically illustrated in a normal vertebral body from a healthy 19-year-old male in Fig. 7.46.

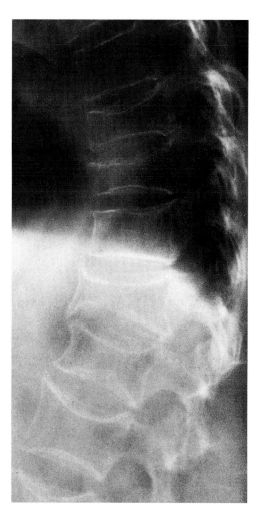

Figure 7.44
Biconcavity or 'codfish vertebrae', seen here on the lateral view of the thoracolumbar spine in an 80-year-old woman with osteoporosis. The deformities result from weakness of the vertebral end-plates and intravertebral expansion of nuclei pulposi.

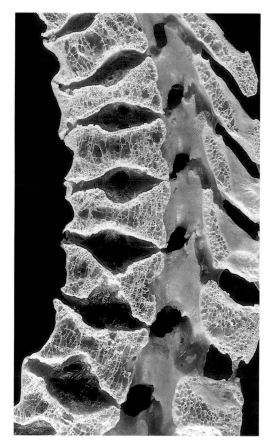

Figure 7.45
Photograph of a sagittal section of a macerated thoracic spine demonstrates the various patterns and degrees of collapse that may be seen within the vertebral bodies. In the upper part of the segment, there is flattening of the vertebral bodies with some anterior wedging. In the lower part, the more typical biconcave compression fractures of the central end-plates, which give rise to the so-called 'fish-mouth' vertebrae, are visible.

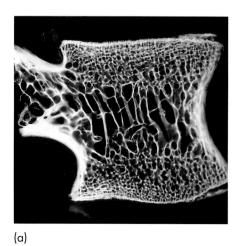

(a)

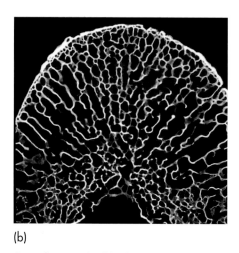

(b)

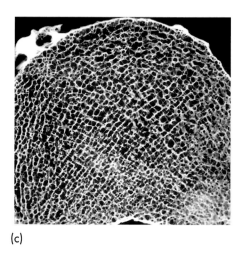

(c)

Figure 7.46 (a) A radiograph of a sagittal section through a vertebral body in a 19-year-old male. Note the variation in the cancellous bone mass. (b) A cross-section through the vertebral body may suggest osteoporosis when compared with the densely packed cancellous bone close to the vertebral end-plate (c).

Until recently only a bone biopsy could adequately evaluate the activities of osteoclasts and osteoblasts – factors that are critical in the assessment of osteoporosis and the determination of a suitable mode of treatment. However at present, there are excellent biochemical tools for measuring bone breakdown, especially the N-telopeptide level in the urine. In morphologic terms, osteo-

porosis is defined as a decrease in bone mass sufficient to result in spontaneous fracture, with the bone tissue itself having a normal biochemical make-up (Figs 7.47–7.49). Severe osteoporosis can develop only if there is a net uncoupling of bone formation and bone resorption. Morphometric analyses of the cell parameters, the amount of bone present, and the degree to which osteoid is

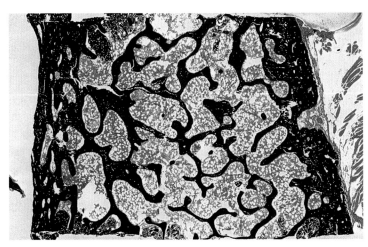

Figure 7.47   Transiliac biopsy of normal bone demonstrates a cortical bone volume of 20.3% and a trabecular bone volume of 37.2% (undecalcified bone, von Kossa's stain, × 1.5 obj.).

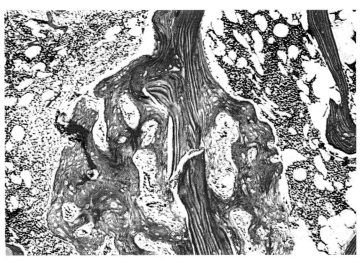

Figure 7.49   Photomicrograph taken from a vertebral body in a patient with osteoporosis shows a microfracture of one of the trabeculae. Surrounding the fractured trabecula is a small microcallus. In patients with osteoporosis such microfractures are abundant in the vertebral bodies (H&E, × 4 obj.).

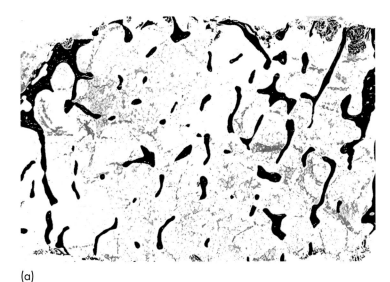

(a)

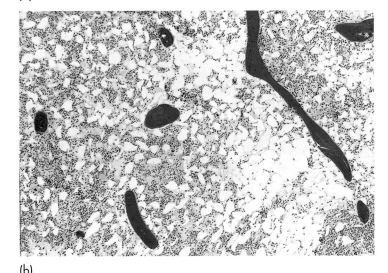

(b)

Figure 7.48   (a) Transiliac biopsy of a patient with moderate to severe osteoporosis. Morphometric analysis shows a cortical bone volume of 7% and a trabecular bone volume of 13% (undecalcified bone, von Kossa's stain, × 1.5 obj.). (b) In a higher power view of the same material, stained with hematoxylin–eosin, the disconnectedness of the trabeculae as well as attenuated appearance can be appreciated (H&E, × 4 obj.).

present on the surfaces of the trabecular and cortical bones have led to the characterization of some of the types of osteoporosis (Figs 7.50–7.52). Although cell activity, i.e. relative and absolute osteoblast and osteoclast counts, is usually low in senile osteoporosis, indicating a relatively 'inactive' state, it may sometimes be high. In more than 15% of patients this increased activity is associated with normocalcemic, normophosphatemic hyperparathyroidism. An additional subgroup of patients is noted to have increased osteoid surfaces. Since this increased osteoid does not seem to be associated with an increased rate of bone formation, it must be related to a mineralization defect, the nature of

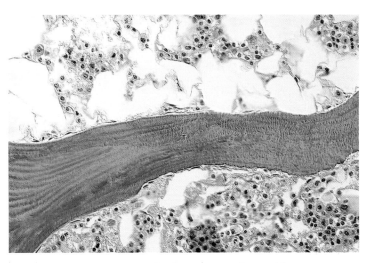

Figure 7.50   Photomicrograph of bone tissue obtained from a patient with inactive (senile) osteoporosis demonstrates the flat, inactive osteoblasts lining the bone, together with an inactive resorption surface (undecalcified section, Goldner stain, × 10 obj.).

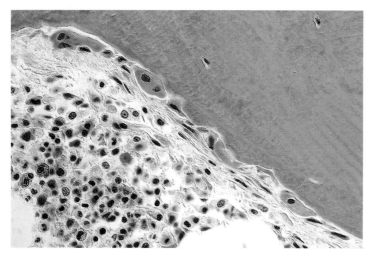

Figure 7.51   Photomicrograph of bone tissue obtained from a patient with active postmenopausal osteoporosis demonstrates active osteoclastic surface resorption (undecalcified section, Goldner stain, × 25 obj.).

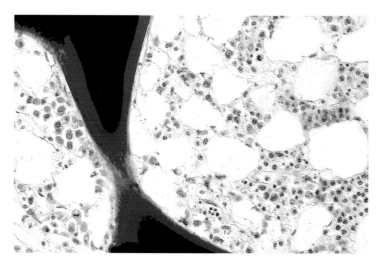

Figure 7.52   Photomicrograph to demonstrate increased osteoid in a case of inactive osteoporosis. Increased osteoid is sometimes present in osteoporotic bone and is usually not associated with any biochemical evidence of disturbed vitamin D metabolism (undecalcified section, von Kossa's stain, × 10 obj.).

which is at present unclear. In disuse osteoporosis, the most dramatic initial finding is an increase in the number of resorptive surfaces. In steroid-induced osteoporosis osteoclastic activity is high, with relatively normal bone formation.

The treatment of osteoporosis should, insofar as possible, be directed toward the underlying etiology. Long-term corticosteroid therapy, excessive alcohol intake, and endocrinopathies such as hyperthyroidism account for a significant number of cases of osteoporosis and should as far as possible be corrected medically. In patients with idiopathic osteoporosis, a number of therapeutic agents have been used with various degrees of success. Exercise is crucial in maintaining skeletal integrity. Calcium supplementation corrects the relative calcium deficiency in the postmenopausal state. At present, most emphasis is placed on the

suppression of osteoclastic activity (e.g. by the use of calcitonin and biphosphonates) and the stimulation of osteoblastic activity (e.g. by the use of oral phosphates or parathormone). Although estrogen-replacement therapy seems to be theoretically sound, its link with atypical endometrial changes has limited its use for the treatment of osteoporosis.

LOCALIZED (TRANSIENT) OSTEOPOROSIS

In 1900, Sudeck described a transient yet painful condition of the lower extremity associated with radiographic evidence of localized juxta-articular osteopenia. The disease occurred without obvious cause, though it was possibly related to trauma (Fig. 7.53). This syndrome, usually known as Sudeck's atrophy, has

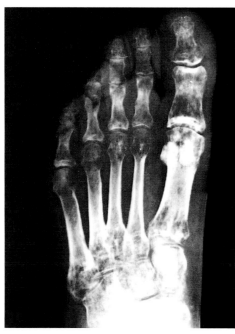

(a)

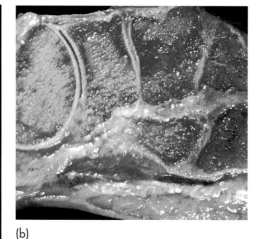

(b)

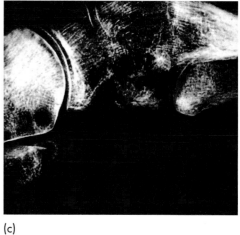

(c)

Figure 7.53   (a) Radiograph of a foot in a patient with complaints of severe pain localized to the foot and ankle following trauma. Note the patchy osteopenia, particularly in a juxta-articular location. (b) Gross specimen of a section through the foot shown in (a) reveals marked hyperemia in patches, but particularly juxta-articularly. Radiograph of a slice of the specimen is shown and demonstrates that the osteopenia corresponds to the hyperemic areas (c).

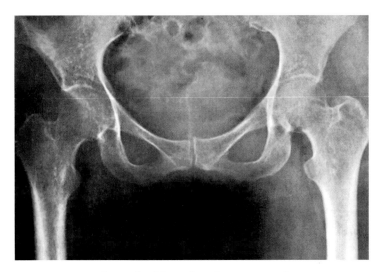

Figure 7.54 Radiograph of the pelvis of a woman with transient osteoporosis, who had complained for some months of severe pain and weakness in the right hip. Note the osteolysis affecting both sides of the hip joint.

hip joint of pregnant women. Since that time it has become apparent that this may occur without pregnancy and that middle-aged men are also sometimes affected by a similar condition (Fig. 7.54). A migratory form of transient osteoporosis has also been reported, which rather than being restricted to the hip may affect the knee as well as the foot and ankle (Fig. 7.55). This form, which is also associated with swelling of the affected part, has been called regional migratory osteoporosis. In all these syndromes, the radiographic lesions tend to be juxta-articular.

Laboratory findings are unremarkable. Magnetic resonance imaging (MRI) in these cases of transient osteoporosis reveals evidence of extensive bone marrow edema. The involved areas show an increased uptake of isotope on technetium bone scanning, and this increased uptake may predate the radiologic evidence of osteopenia by some months. Histopathologic findings have been only infrequently reported; however, microscopic examination of histologic sections has shown thinned-out bone trabeculae with evidence of osteoclastic bone resorption and hypervascularity of the marrow space (Figs 7.56 and 7.57). In some cases of transient osteoporosis, biopsy has demonstrated evidence of fat necrosis and fibrosis in the marrow, suggestive of an episodic ischemic etiology. If indeed the condition is related to episodic ischemia then the hyperemia and increased osteoclastic activity which has been observed may be regarded as secondary reparative phenomena. Recent reports have suggested that the condition is due to non-displaced intraosseous trabecular fractures similar to those seen in insufficiency fractures (see Chapter 11, p. 273) and this too would explain the reported microscopic findings.

been related to a reflex sympathetic dystrophy. The symptoms, often involving the entire extremity, include pain, hyperesthesia, and tenderness, and are frequently debilitating. The pain varies in severity and character and is associated with swelling and a decreased range of motion in neighboring joints. The skin may be clammy, cyanotic, and painful to the touch.

In 1959, Curtiss and Kincaid reported a number of cases of a painful localized and transient osteoporosis which involved the

Because the lesions usually remit spontaneously within a year or two, the importance of this disorder rests in recognizing its benign nature. It should not be confused with diseases such as

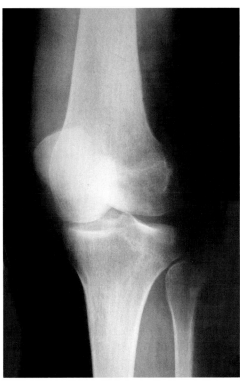

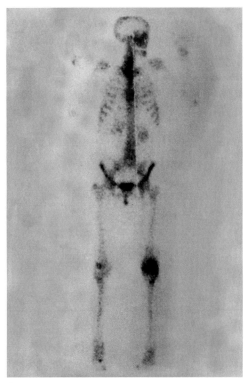

Figure 7.55 (a) Radiograph of the left knee of a 61-year-old female who developed severe pain of acute onset in the knee without any obvious local trauma, systemic disease or other antecedent event. The pain was aggravated by weight-bearing and disturbed normal sleep. An area of poorly defined lucency in the distal femur corresponded to increased uptake on a bone scan (b). The differential diagnosis at presentation was tumor or infection. Biopsy revealed a microscopic change in the bone most consistent with transient osteoporosis and over the following year the symptoms resolved.

(a)   (b)

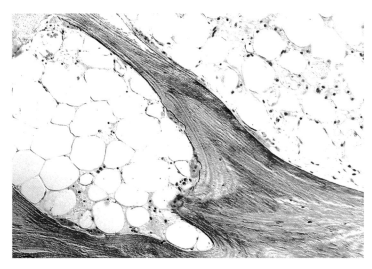

Figure 7.56 Photomicrograph showing early fat necrosis with foamy histiocytes in the marrow of a bone biopsy taken from a patient with transient osteoporosis. The adjacent bone trabeculae can be seen to be undergoing osteoclastic resorption (H&E, × 10 obj., Nomarski optics).

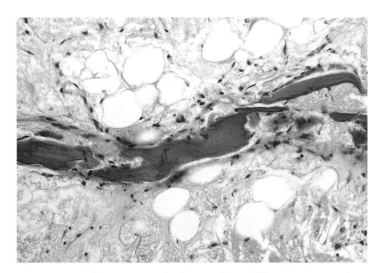

Figure 7.57 Photomicrograph of tissue obtained from a patient with transient osteoporosis. There is severe thinning of the bone due to increased osteoclastic resorption and the marrow shows ischemic changes with breakdown of the fat cells (H&E, × 10 obj.).

osteomyelitis or metastatic cancer, which it may mimic radiologically. Treatment with bisphosphonates or calcitonin have reported to be successful.

IDIOPATHIC OSTEOLYSIS

Primary idiopathic osteolysis is very rare. It is characterized by the spontaneous onset of bone resorption without any obvious cause. Bones that previously appeared normal begin to undergo partial or complete resorption. This process may continue for years, until eventually it ceases spontaneously. The end result is severe deformity and serious functional disability.

Torg et al. have classified the osteolyses into four types: hereditary multicentric osteolysis with dominant transmission; hereditary multicentric osteolysis with recessive transmission; idiopathic nonhereditary multicentric osteolysis with nephropathy; and Gorham's massive osteolysis.

Gorham's massive osteolysis

In 1955, Gorham and Stout reported 24 patients who presented with a monocentric, massive osteolysis. This disease, known as Gorham's osteolysis, disappearing bone disease, or vanishing bone disease, may start at any age and has no familial incidence.

Massive osteolysis is characterized radiographically by progressive and extensive reduction in bone density, and morphologically by the replacement of osseous tissue with fibrous tissue and thin-walled dilated vascular channels. Generally detected initially in children or young adults, the disorder usually affects the appendicular skeleton and is often confined to a single bone or to two or more bones centered around a joint. The shoulder and hip are the most common sites of involvement. The clinical course is protracted but rarely fatal, with eventual stabilization the most common outcome. Patients may complain of a dull aching pain or the insidious onset of progressive weakness. Radiologic examination reveals initial intramedullary and subcortical ill-defined lucent areas, with a subsequent loss of density extending from one end of the bone to the other. Reactive bone formation is not evident. Characteristic shrinkage or tapering of the long bones may occur (Fig. 7.58).

Reported descriptions of whole surgical specimens have featured thin, tapered, soft bone, and in specimens in which the mineralized bone has entirely disappeared, a fibrous band may be seen to replace the original bone. Biopsies of earlier lesions have revealed hypervascular fibrous connective tissue replacing bone; the proliferative vessels may be capillary, sinusoidal, or cavernous (Figs 7.59 and 7.60).

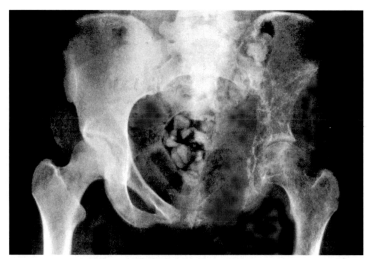

Figure 7.58 Radiograph of the pelvis of a young woman complaining of weakness of the hip. As can be seen from the radiograph, extensive bone loss involves most of the hemipelvis. The upper femur is also severely porotic.

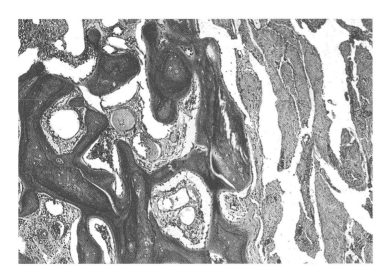

Figure 7.59   Bone biopsy from a patient with disappearing bone disease, adjacent to the site of involvement. Note the presence of large dilated vessels in the marrow spaces (H&E, × 4 obj.).

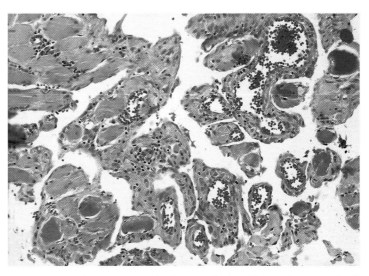

Figure 7.60   Photomicrograph of tissue obtained from a bone involved by Gorham's disease shows hypervascular tissue with an angiomatous appearance. No residual bone is present in this section (H&E, × 4 obj.).

Chapter 8

BONE DISEASE RESULTING FROM DISTURBANCES IN MINERAL HOMEOSTASIS

Calcium and phosphate play a crucial role in physiologic processes. About 85% of the body's phosphate and 99% of its calcium are contained within the skeleton as hydroxyapatite. Phosphate, especially in the form of intracellular phosphate esters, is important in the generation and transfer of cellular energy. Calcium is essential to neuromuscular function, cardiac function, and blood clotting. Calcium is an obligatory coenzyme in many processes, and contributes to the continuing integrity of cell membranes.

Calcium homeostasis is mainly under the control of the endocrine system, involving a combination of interactions among parathyroid hormone (PTH), vitamin D and calcitonin (CT); it also depends on the normal functioning of the target organs, i.e. the intestines, kidneys, and bone cells. Two principal patterns of bone disease associated with disturbed calcium homeostasis are recognized: 'osteitis fibrosa cystica' (von Recklinghausen's disease) (Fig. 8.1) and 'hyperosteoidosis' (osteomalacia and rickets) (Fig. 8.2).

Osteitis fibrosa cystica results either from over-production of parathormone by an adenoma, carcinoma or primary hyperplasia of the parathyroid glands, (primary hyperparathyroidism) or stimulation of the parathyroids by disease elsewhere (secondary hyperparathyroidism).

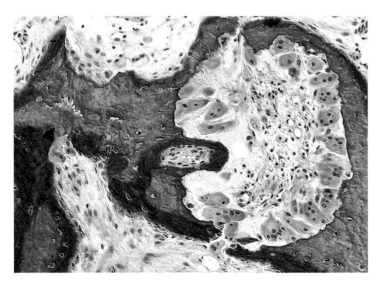

Figure 8.1   Photomicrograph of a bone biopsy from a patient with active hyperparathyroidism. The most characteristic histologic feature is the osteoclastic bone tunneling (also known as dissecting resorption). Note also the increased osteoblastic activity and marrow fibrosis (Goldner, × 10 obj.).

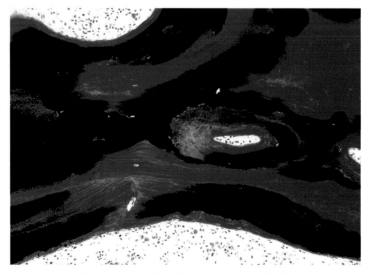

Figure 8.2   Photomicrograph to demonstrate the lack of bone mineralization that occurs in vitamin D deficiency. A thick band of unmineralized bone matrix (in this preparation stained red) covers all of the bony surfaces. The mineralized bone, stained black, has an irregular border with the unmineralized osteoid (von Kossa's stain, × 4 obj.).

The most important cause of secondary hyperparathyroidism is chronic renal disease (firstly because of the important role of glomerular filtration and renal tubule reabsorption in maintaining the levels of serum calcium and phosphorus as well as acid–base equilibrium; secondly because of the role the renal tubules play in the hydroxylation of vitamin D).

Rarely, secondary hyperparathyroidism may also result from phosphate deficiency or any disease that markedly stimulates bone formation (e.g. generalized Paget's disease) or retards mineralization of osteoid (e.g. aluminum-induced bone disease).

A common complication of disturbances in calcium and phosphorus homeostasis is soft-tissue calcification.

This chapter considers firstly normal calcium and phosphorus homeostasis and secondly hypercalcemia and hypocalcemia, especially with regard to abnormal parathyroid activity, disturbances in vitamin D metabolism, disturbed phosphate metabolism, and renal disease. Finally, the various forms of soft-tissue calcification are discussed.

CALCIUM AND PHOSPHORUS HOMEOSTASIS

Optimal neuromuscular function requires precise maintenance of the extracellular calcium ion concentration, even under conditions of dehydration, starvation or disease. (Most laboratory determinations of blood calcium levels measure total calcium, which includes both ionized calcium, protein-bound calcium, and calcium complexed to other organic ions. However, it is the ionized fraction of calcium that is physiologically most important. Changes in serum calcium that are associated with, for example, hypo- or hyperproteinemia, usually have no pathophysiologic significance.)

Figure 8.3 illustrates calcium and phosphorus homeostasis in a healthy adult with an adequate intake. The diagram shows that calcium and phosphorus are present in three principal pools: the bone tissue, the intracellular fluid, and the extracellular fluid. Calcium and phosphorus are added to the system from the gut, and lost from the system through the gut, the kidneys, and by

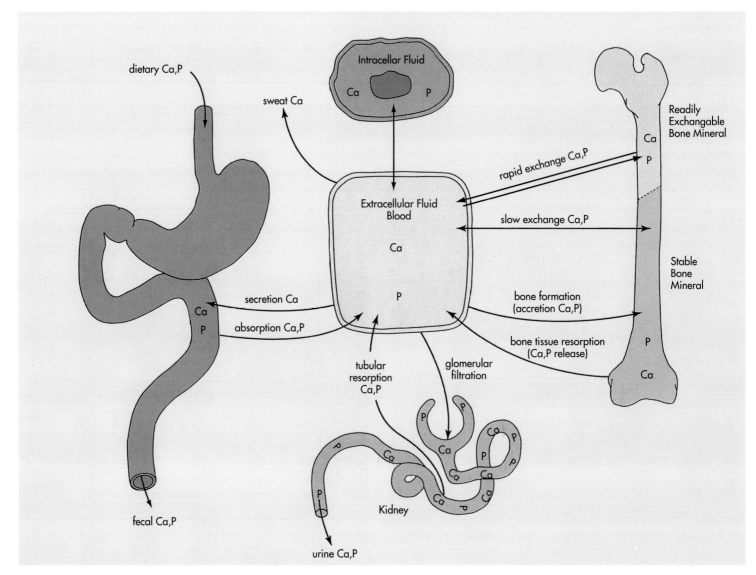

Figure 8.3   Schematic model of calcium and phosphorus metabolism.

sweating. (It should be noted that most of the blood calcium and phosphorus lost by glomerular filtration is reabsorbed through the renal tubular epithelium. Also that most of the bone mineral incorporated into the bone matrix is not available for rapid exchange with the extracellular fluid.)

The required daily calcium intake is 800 mg of elemental calcium. During adolescence and, for women, during pregnancy and lactation, this amount needs to be increased to 1200 mg per diem. Most calcium is obtained from dairy products and since 1 cup of milk is equal to 300 mg of calcium, it requires 3–4 cups of milk or equivalent cheese or yogurt per diem. Needless to say, many people have a diet which is deficient in calcium.

Figure 8.4 illustrates the interactive and interdependent endocrine control of calcium and phosphorus homeostasis. Parathyroid gland activity is largely regulated by the level of Ca^{++} in the extracellular fluid; an increase in serum Ca^{++} suppresses PTH release, and vice versa. Once in the circulation, biologically active PTH has a short half-life, probably on the order of

less than 5 minutes. It is degraded by enzymatic cleavage, mainly in the liver but also in the kidney and within the parathyroid gland itself. (Laboratory assays for measurement of PTH are focused primarily on biologically inactive fragments.)

PTH regulates the conversion of 25-hydroxy vitamin D (25-OH-D) in the kidney to its active form, 1,25-dihydroxyvitamin D (1,25(OH)$_2$D). Additionally PTH acts on the renal tubules to increase the tubular reabsorption of calcium while decreasing the reabsorption of phosphorus. PTH directly stimulates the osteoblasts to synthesize new bone and, through activation of a second messenger, stimulates osteoclastic resorption of bone, and hence the release of Ca^{++} into the extracellular fluid.

Figure 8.5 shows the pathway for vitamin D hormone. The principal natural source of vitamin D is the conversion of 7-dihydrocholesterol in the skin, through the action of ultraviolet irradiation, to vitamin D$_3$, which can then be stored in fat and muscle cells. (Vitamin D$_2$, commercially produced by ultraviolet irradiation of plant sterols, is biologically equipotent to D$_3$; in the USA it

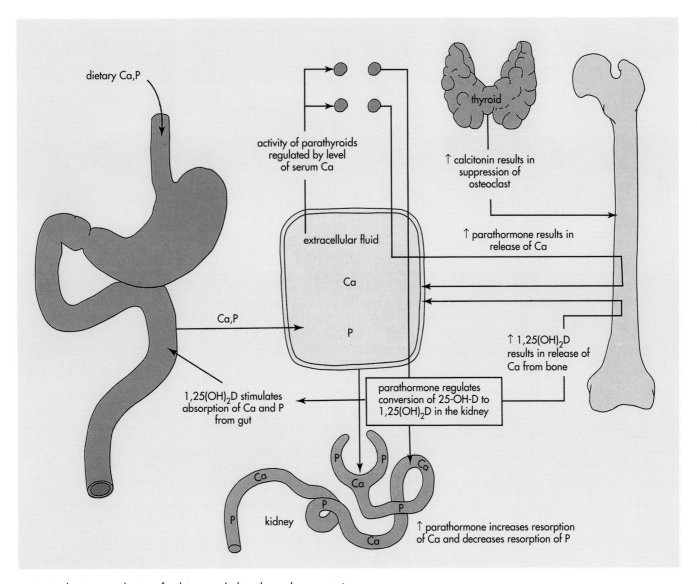

Figure 8.4   Endocrine regulation of calcium and phosphorus homeostasis.

is added extensively to milk, certain other foods, and vitamin supplements. Vitamins D_2 and D_3 circulate together in the body, are biologically interchangeable, and are usually referred to in the aggregate as vitamin D.)

Exposure to sunlight of no more than 10–15 minutes can provide the body with the amount of vitamin D required for the next 3 days. Only a small part of the skin needs to be exposed for adequate production of vitamin D. However, there is evidence that the chronic use of sunscreens, especially by the elderly, may occasionally cause frank vitamin D deficiency. Thus, generally speaking, dietary vitamin D supplements are probably unnecessary except in children, pregnant women, old people with poor nutrition who are confined indoors, and a few other exceptional instances.

Vitamin D is itself inactive and conversion to 25-OH-D takes place in the liver. The hepatic conversion of vitamin D to 25-OH-D can be disturbed by liver disease or by administration of anti-convulsant drugs, such as phenytoin. Although 25-OH-D has only minimal physiologic activity, nevertheless in pharmacologic dosage it can promote both gut absorption of calcium and bone mineralization.

There is a pathway for enterohepatic recirculation of 25-OH-D and its metabolites, which are excreted into the bile. For this reason, intestinal malabsorption or anatomic loss of intestinal absorptive area can interfere with the reabsorption of these substances and inexorably deplete the systemic pool of vitamin D. In this way, severe vitamin D deficiency can develop, even though exposure to sun and dietary sources of vitamin D is adequate.

In the kidney, under the control of specific alpha-hydroxylases, 25-OH-D is converted to either $24,25(OH)_2D$ or $1,25(OH)_2D$. Patients with advanced renal disease become deficient in both of these forms of the vitamin, which is probably the primary reason for the frequency and severity of bone disease associated with kidney failure.

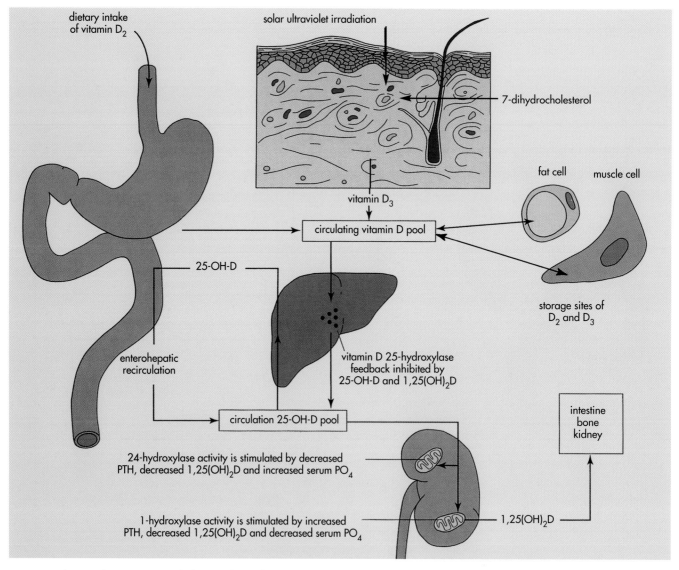

Figure 8.5   Regulation of vitamin D metabolism is shown from points of entry into the body pool: via solar irradiation of cutaneous 7-dihydrocholesterol, which produces vitamin D_3, and via ingestion of vitamin D_2. The major part of the vitamin D pool is stored in fat and muscle. A portion is continually converted in the liver to 25-hydroxyvitamin-D, the predominant circulating form; 25-OH-D is then converted in the kidney to the major active metabolite, $1,25(OH)_2D$.

The action of $24,25(OH)_2D$ on bone metabolism is largely unknown. Although it only weakly accelerates the absorption of calcium by the gut, some important role in bone cell differentiation is suspected. By contrast, $1,25(OH)_2D$ is the most biologically potent form of vitamin D known and has multiple and profound actions on osseus metabolism. It accelerates the gut absorption of calcium and phosphorus, promotes bone cell differentiation and the mineralization of osteoid, and enhances the sensitivity of bone to PTH-induced osteoclastic or osteocytic resorption to maintain serum calcium. Perhaps most importantly for patients on maintenance renal dialysis, it directly suppresses overactive parathyroid cells and enhances parathyroid suppression by ambient calcium levels.

In addition to its effects on bone metabolism, $1,25(OH)_2D$ also has other biologic actions, including inhibition of the production of interleukin-2 (IL-2) and immunoglobulins, and the stimulation of insulin and thyroid stimulating-hormone (TSH) secretion. With respect to its effect on cell proliferation and differentiation, it is of interest that $1,25(OH)_2D$ induces monocytes to become multinucleated giant cells which act in vitro as osteoclast-like cells.

The physiologic importance of human CT is unknown, but current theories are focused on the possibility that it is a regulator of skeletal homeostasis rather than calcium homeostasis. In pharmacologic doses, CT inhibits osteoclastic resorption of bone, suggesting that it might act in vivo to conserve skeletal mass. In this regard it has been reported that women have lower whole plasma immunoreactive CT (iCT) concentrations than men, and that peak calcium-stimulated iCT concentrations decline with age. Although the data are controversial, some investigators have suggested that CT secretion decreases at the time of menopause and can be stimulated by estrogen-replacement. It is possible,

therefore, that a relative, progressive deficiency of CT in postmenopausal women is a contributing cause of age- and sex-related bone loss.

HYPERCALCEMIA

Hypercalcemia is common; symptoms may arise in any organ system (Table 8.1) and its causes are numerous (Table 8.2). Mild hypercalcemia is common in patients with widespread lytic bone metastases and with multiple myeloma and on occasion, it may be seen in cases of sarcoidosis or vitamin D intoxication. However, its most important cause is hyperparathyroidism.

HYPERPARATHYROIDISM (OSTEITIS FIBROSA CYSTICA; VON RECKLINGHAUSEN'S BONE DISEASE)

Overproduction of parathyroid hormone occurs as either a primary or a secondary condition. Primary hyperparathyroidism (HPT) normally results from an adenoma, rarely from primary hyperplasia (of unknown etiology) or carcinoma (Figs 8.6 and 8.7). Blood chemistries usually reveal marked hypercalcemia, and usually hypophosphatemia. Patients with this disorder are in general between the third and fifth decades of life. Although many patients are asymptomatic, renal colic secondary to stone formation is the most common clinical presentation of primary hyperparathyroidism; bone pain is present in a small percentage of patients. Mild hyperparathyroidism in elderly individuals occasionally presents clinically as osteoporosis. As hypercalcemia becomes more pronounced, nausea, vomiting, weakness, and headaches may appear. On rare occasions a patient presents with a hypercalcemic crisis, leading to shock, kidney failure and death.

Table 8.1   Clinical features of hypercalcemia.

Clinical features of hypercalcemia
1 **Neuromuscular**
1. Headache
2. Muscle weakness
3. Altered states of consciousness (confusion, lethargy, stupor, coma)
4. Hyporeflexia
2 **Gastrointestinal**
1. Anorexia
2. Nausea
3. Vomiting
3 **Renal**
1. Nephrolithiasis
2. Polyuria
3. Polydipsia
4 **Others**
1. Bradycardia
2. Metastatic calcification
3. Dehydration

Table 8.2   Differential diagnosis of hypercalcemia.

Differential diagnosis of hypercalcemia
Primary hyperparathyroidism
Immobilization (especially with associated conditions, e.g., generalized Paget's)
Malignant disease
Multiple myeloma, breast carcinoma
Humoral peptide of malignancy (carcinoma of lung, esophagus, head and neck, renal cell, ovary, bladder)
Ectopic production of 1,25-dihydroxyvitamin D (lymphoma)
Thyrotoxicosis
Sarcoidosis and other granulomatous disease
Drug induced:
Vitamin D
Thiazide diuretics
Tamoxifen
Acute and chronic renal failure
Total parenteral nutrition
Familial hypocalciuric hypercalcemia

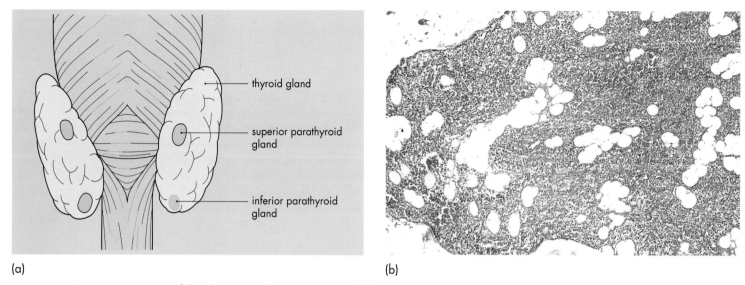

(a)

(b)

Figure 8.6 **(a)** Posterior aspect of the pharynx, and commencement of the esophagus and trachea. Note the usual position of the parathyroid glands. Normally measuring no more than 4–5 mm, they may be difficult to locate, especially when they are displaced. **(b)** Photomicrograph of normal parathyroid gland shows glandular tissue admixed with fat (H&E, × 2.5 obj.).

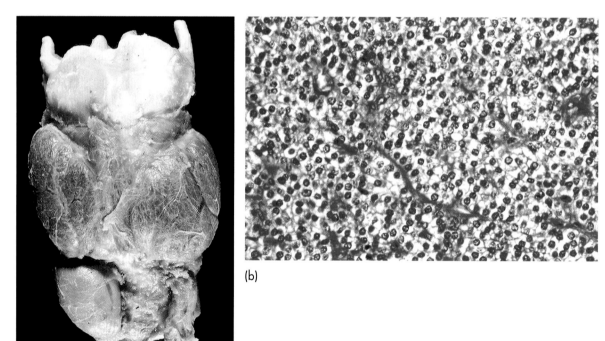

Figure 8.7 **(a)** Parathyroid adenoma: large tan nodule measuring approximately 2 cm on the left side of the lower pole of the thyroid. **(b)** Photomicrograph of parathyroid adenoma shown in **(a)**. The cells are of one type, chief cells, arranged in small acini and cords. Characteristically, no fat is visible in the adenomatous tissue (H&E, × 10 obj.).

(b)

(a)

When an adenoma is the cause of the condition, surgical removal of the neoplastic gland is the treatment of choice.

When hyperparathyroidism is the result of chronic renal failure, the inevitable consequence is further derangement of mineral and bone metabolism. Such derangements can be identified even in patients with mild reductions of glomerular filtration rate (GFR); they become progressively more severe, as renal function declines further.

Thus secondary hyperparathyroidism dominates the pathophysiology of metabolic bone disease in chronic renal failure. It results from:

- A fall in ionized calcium concentration as a consequence of phosphate retention

- Resistance of bone to the actions of PTH
- Malabsorption of calcium through the gut

Furthermore, in addition to the loss of 1-alpha hydroxylating capacity as renal cell mass declines, there is also an inhibition of $1,25(OH)_2D$ production by increased phosphate. Because $1,25(OH)_2D$ directly suppresses the parathyroid cells, loss of renal production of $1,25(OH)_2D$ encourages secondary hyperparathyroidism to develop more rapidly and severely.

Increased parathormone production promotes phosphaturia and thus tends to normalize plasma inorganic phosphate. In addition, by its direct effect on bone and kidney and its indirect effect on the intestine through $1,25(OH)_2D$, the increased level of PTH opposes the tendency of the serum calcium to fall. A new steady-state condition therefore develops, but only at the expense of the undesirable effects of secondary hyperparathyroidism. When PTH levels rise sufficiently, severe bone resorption gives rise to significant hypercalcemia, bone pain, and fractures. The combined effects of hypercalcemia and hyperphosphatemia lead to extensive metastatic calcification in blood vessels and at other sites. At this stage, subtotal parathyroidectomy may be necessary. [Biochemically, in addition to increased serum calcium, there are massive elevations in PTH and in serum alkaline phosphatase (the latter reflecting osteoblast stimulation).]

In chronic renal disease, phosphate restriction can reverse the above sequence of events to a certain extent. In children with stable chronic renal failure, phosphate-restricted diets have been shown to increase $1,25(OH)_2D$ concentrations and decrease PTH levels, thereby partially reversing the hormone imbalance.

Medical treatment of secondary HPT in dialysis patients consists of phosphate restriction, administration of phosphate binders, the use of a high-calcium dialysate, and of oral or i.v. supplementation with $1,25(OH)_2D$. When adequate, such therapy usually obviates the necessity for subtotal parathyroidectomy (which if it has to be done, may be followed by significant post-operative hypoparathyroidism). Therapeutic control of the hyper-parathyroidism, whether surgical or medical, is followed by a dramatic regression of the histologic changes, and subsequent improvement of the radiologic abnormalities. The serum alkaline phosphatase normalizes, and PTH may fall to levels seen in dial-ysis patients who do not have HPT.

In a minority of patients with chronic renal failure, the accumulation of aluminum (derived from aluminum-contaminated dialysate and/or aluminum-containing phosphate binders) at the mineralization front, results in osteomalacia with further disturbance of the skeletal function (Fig. 8.8).

Morphologic findings

The radiologic and pathologic features are similar in both primary and secondary hyperparathyroidism. Radiologic examination may reveal diffuse osteopenia and/or circumscribed lucent areas. However, the most characteristic changes include erosion of the tufts of the phalanges and subperiosteal cortical resorption, especially visible on the radial side of the middle phalanges (Fig. 8.9). Other sites at which erosive resorption may be seen are the symphysis pubis (Fig. 8.10), the distal clavicles (Fig. 8.11), and the end-plates of the vertebral bodies (Fig. 8.12), as well as the lamina dura (i.e. the layer of the dense bone at the roots of the teeth) (Fig. 8.13). The skull may show a granular demineralization, the so-called 'salt and pepper' appearance (Figs 8.14 and 8.15).

Microscopic examination demonstrates an increased number of osteoclasts on the bone surfaces (even on periosteal surfaces), and a characteristic 'tunneling' or 'dissecting' resorption of trabeculae (Figs 8.16–8.18) (See also Fig. 8.1). Other findings include resorption of pericellular bone by osteocytes (osteocytic osteolysis), increased amounts of woven bone, and marrow fibrosis, especially abutting trabecular surfaces (Fig. 8.19). [The finding of peritrabecular fibrosis should be distinguished microscopically from the more generalized fibrosis seen in association with myelofibrosis, which generally starts within the marrow and away from the bone surfaces (see Chapter 9, p. 235).]

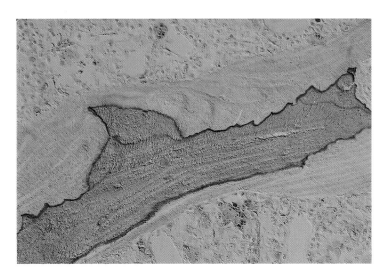

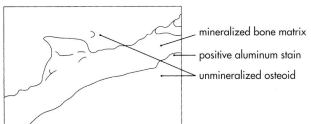

mineralized bone matrix

positive aluminum stain

unmineralized osteoid

Figure 8.8 Photomicrograph of a section of bone with increased osteoid, stained with aurin tricarboxylic acid stain, which stains aluminum bright red. The red stain is concentrated at the mineralization front; it has been proposed that the presence of aluminum at this site blocks further mineralization of the bone (Nomarski optics, × 10 obj.).

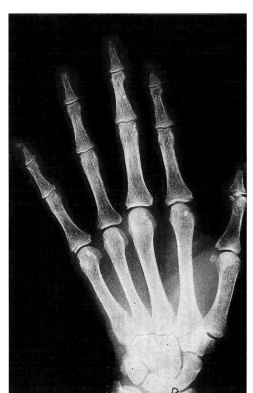

Figure 8.9 Clinical radiograph of the hand shows resorption of the tufts of the terminal phalanges. There is also characteristic subperiosteal resorption of the middle and proximal phalanges. This resorption is more marked on the radial side of the phalanges. (Courtesy of Dr Alex Norman.)

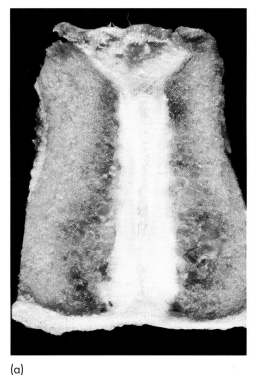

(a)

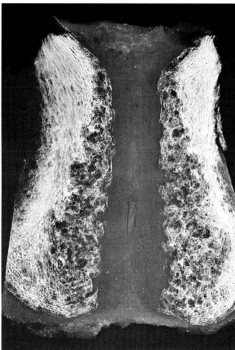

(b)

Figure 8.10 (a) Gross appearance of a symphysis pubis obtained at autopsy from a patient with hyperparathyroidism shows hyperemia, fibrosis, and resorption of the bone on each side of the symphysis. (b) Radiograph of the specimen.

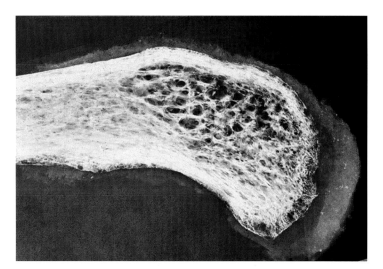

Figure 8.11 A characteristic anatomic site in which to observe erosion in hyperparathyroidism is the distal clavicle. In this specimen radiograph resorption is clearly seen, with loss of the smooth cortex and replacement by a lacy irregular outline.

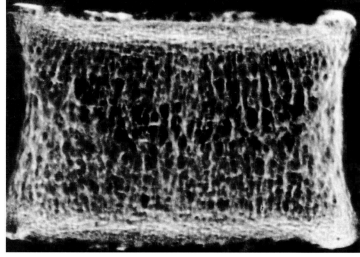

Figure 8.12 Specimen radiograph of a slice taken through a vertebra in a young person with hyperparathyroidism shows the irregularity and resorption of the cortical bone, particularly in the end-plates of the vertebral bodies.

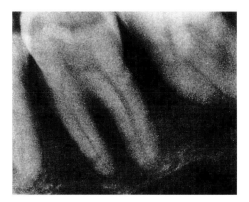

Figure 8.13 Radiograph of the lower second molar tooth in a patient with primary hyperparathyroidism shows loss of the lamina dura around the tooth socket.

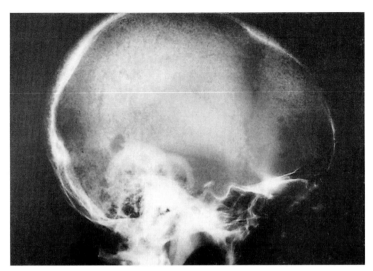

Figure 8.14 Hyperparathyroidism: clinical radiograph of a skull showing 'salt and pepper' appearance.

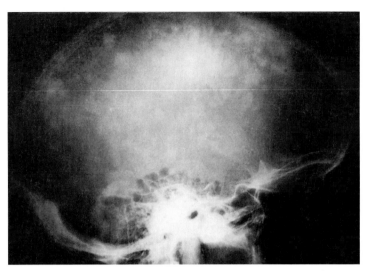

Figure 8.15 Radiograph showing blastic reparative changes after parathyroidectomy. This appearance could be mistaken for Paget's or metastatic disease. (Courtesy of Dr Alex Norman.)

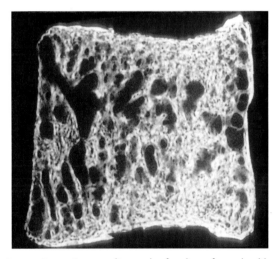

Figure 8.17 A specimen radiograph of a slice of vertebral body affected with primary hyperparathyroidism. The architecture of the cancellous bone is disturbed and the trabeculae contain lytic lines within them, due to the dissecting resorption characteristic of this condition. Note the partial resorption of the end-plates.

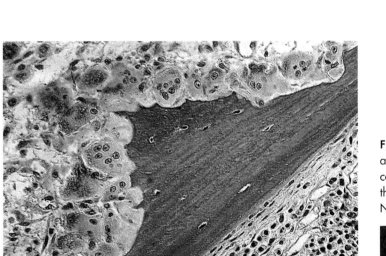

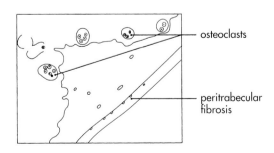

Figure 8.16 Photomicrograph to show severe osteoclastic bone resorption in a patient with primary hyperparathyroidism. Note the mild peritrabecular fibrosis, associated with bone formation, on the inferior bone surface (H&E, × 25 obj.).

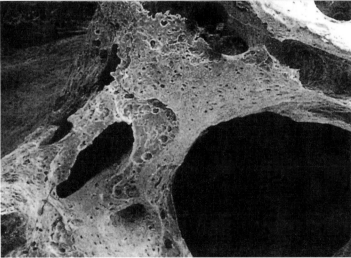

Figure 8.18 A scanning electron micrograph of the cancellous bone demonstrates numerous irregular erosions on the bone surface, due to osteoclastic resorption (× 750 magnification).

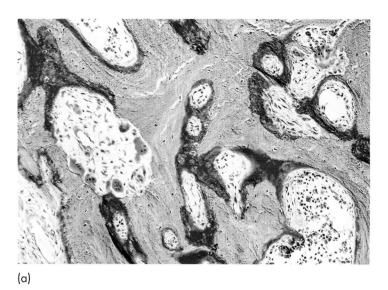

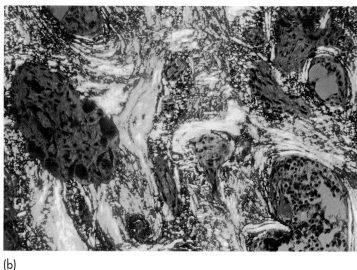

(a)   (b)

Figure 8.19   Photomicrograph of a biopsy from a patient with hyperparathyroidism (**a**) shows the overall pattern of marrow fibrosis, dissecting resorption and increased amounts of unmineralized bone (seen here in the Goldner stain as red seams at the bone surface) secondary to increased bone formation (Goldner, × 5 obj.). The polarized light picture (**b**) shows extensive woven bone present in this section.

Occasionally, patients who have undiagnosed hyperparathyroidism present on radiologic examination with a lytic lesion which suggests a tumor. Such lesions are particularly evident in the diaphysis of long bones, the jaw, or the skull. This entity is the so-called 'brown tumor' (brown because of old and recent hemorrhage). On microscopic examination it is composed of many clustered giant cells in a fibrous cellular stroma (Fig. 8.20). The 'brown tumor' of hyperparathyroidism must be differentiated histologically from a giant-cell tumor, giant-cell reparative granuloma and aneurysmal bone cyst (see Chapter 19, pp. 450, 454 and 465).

In many patients with chronic renal failure, increased density of the skeleton can be seen on radiographic examination. Histologically, this increased density appears as increased woven or immature bone superimposed on the usual characteristics of hyperparathyroidism (Fig. 8.21). Both the radiologic and histologic changes may occasionally be confused with those of Paget's disease.

HYPERCALCEMIA NOT ASSOCIATED WITH HYPERPARATHYROIDISM (PSEUDOHYPERPARATHYROIDISM)

Hypercalcemia may occur in association with certain rare tumors that secrete hormone-like substances referred to as parathyroid hormone-related protein (PTHrP) or 'osteoclast activating factor' (OAF). The tumors most commonly associated with this type of humoral hypercalcemia are squamous-cell lung cancer, other squamous-cell tumors, renal cell carcinoma, and urogenital tract carcinoma. When a small occult tumor is the cause of the hypercalcemia- and hyperparathyroid-like condition, the correct diagnosis may be delayed for some time. In these cases of 'humoral hypercalcemia of malignancy', the radiologic and microscopic appearance of skeletal tissue cannot be distinguished from that associated with primary hyperparathyroidism. The most important clue that the hypercalcemia is arising from a

malignancy in patients with this rare condition of pseudohyperparathyroidism is that because PTHrP and OAF are usually not detected by conventional assays for PTH, the measurable PTH levels are profoundly depressed.

HYPOCALCEMIA

With hypocalcemia the commonest symptom is neuromuscular irritability (Table 8.3), but it may be asymptomatic. Rarely, it is life-threatening. Like hypercalcemia its causes are numerous. The most common cause is vitamin D deficiency. Less common are hypothyroidism, hypophosphatemia (vitamin-D-resistant rickets) and hypomagnesemia (Table 8.4).

HYPEROSTEOIDOSIS

Hyperosteoidosis is a histologic term that describes an increase in the relative proportion of unmineralized to mineralized bone tissue. There are three basic causes of hyperosteoidosis.

Table 8.3   Clinical features of hypocalcemia.

Clinical features of hypocalcemia
Paresthesias
Neuromuscular irritability
Chvostek's sign
Trousseau's sign
Tetany
Seizures
Prolonged Q–T interval on EKG

Table 8.4 Common causes of hypocalcemia.

Common causes of hypocalcemia
Hypoparathyroidism
Postsurgical
Infiltrative conditions
Hemochromatosis
Metastatic carcinoma
Idiopathic
Vitamin D deficiency
Lack of sunlight exposure
Dietary lack
Malabsorption
Upper GI tract surgery
Liver disease
Renal disease
Anticonvulsants
Pseudohypoparathyroidism
Hypomagnesemia

1. A marked increase in the rate of bone formation, so that a prominent band of osteoid is present on the bone surface (Fig. 8.22). In this case, labeling with tetracycline reveals a thick, granular, and dense mineralization front.
2. Interference with calcium deposition at the mineralization front as happens in aluminum toxicity and, to a lesser extent, with iron overload. In this case, a wide osteoid seam is observed, usually with flat, inactive osteoblasts (Fig. 8.23). The mineralization front is sharply demarcated and often at a reversal line (Fig. 8.24). Tetracycline labeling fails to show any uptake at the mineralization front.
3. Most importantly, a lack of available calcium salts for mineralization of the bone. The clinical terms used to describe this are Rickets and osteomalacia. Rickets is a disorder of mineralization of the bone matrix in growing bone; it involves both the growth plate (epiphysis) and newly formed trabecular and cortical bone. Osteomalacia is a defect in bone matrix mineralization in adults and is the more common form of the disease seen nowadays.

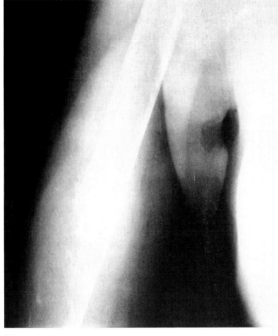

(a)

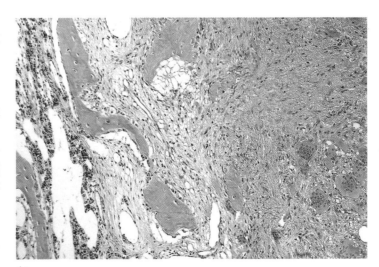

(b)

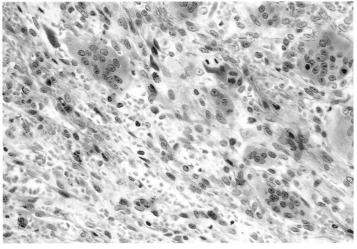

(c)

Figure 8.20 (a) Clinical radiograph shows a large destructive lesion in the lower half of the humerus. The patient presented initially with pain in the arm, and the radiologic examination suggested the presence of a neoplasm. Further investigation revealed hypercalcemia and other radiologic changes consistent with hyperparathyroidism. (b) Photomicrograph of the biopsy obtained from the lesion shows giant cells in a fibrous stroma (H&E, × 10 obj.). (c) Scattered hemosiderin-laden histiocytes and focal interstitial hemorrhage, and clustering of giant cells, are characteristic of a brown tumor (H&E, × 25 obj.).

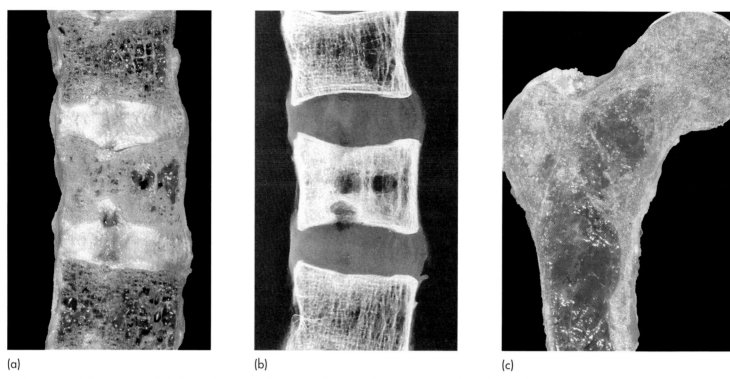

(a)   (b)   (c)

Figure 8.21   (a) A segment of the lower thoracic and upper lumbar spine from a patient with renal osteodystrophy shows loss of the normal trabecular appearance of the bone with increased sclerosis and some collapse. (b) Radiograph of the specimen. (c) Upper end of the femur from the same patient. Again, the disorganization of the bony architecture is apparent and the cortex is seen to be hyperemic and irregular. These gross changes, both in the vertebral bodies and in the femur may on imaging studies initially suggest Paget's disease.

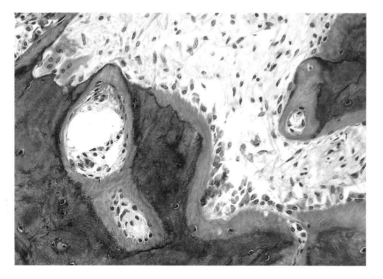

Figure 8.22   Photomicrograph of a bone biopsy from a patient with renal failure shows the stigmata of secondary hyperparathyroidism with bone resorption at the upper left. Note the markedly increased osteoblastic activity and widened osteoid seams (H&E, × 10 obj.).

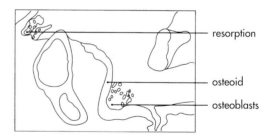

OSTEOMALACIA

Osteomalacia has a number of etiologies (Table 8.5). The availability of vitamin D may be decreased by poor nutritional intake, lack of sunlight, or by renal or hepatic disease. Calcium availability may also be disturbed by lack of calcium in the diet or by a malabsorption syndrome. Congenital defects in the renal tubules, leading to deficient reabsorption of phosphate and calcium into the blood, also result in rickets and osteomalacia (hypophosphatemic rickets; see later).

The most common symptom of osteomalacia in adults is bone pain, sometimes localized, more often bilateral and symmetrical; often initially vague but gradually becoming severe. There may also be proximal muscle weakness, which is often profound. The serum calcium level tends to be low normal, the phosphate very low, and the alkaline phosphatase very high (released from stimulated osteoblasts). Serum 25-OH-D levels are usually markedly depressed, while 1,25(OH)$_2$D levels may be initially normal, although they too eventually fall. PTH levels tend to rise considerably, resulting in relative preservation of the serum calcium.

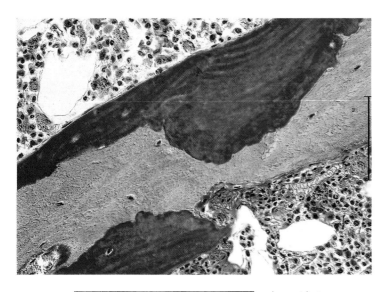

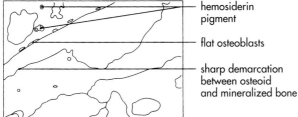

hemosiderin
pigment

flat osteoblasts

sharp demarcation
between osteoid
and mineralized bone

Figure 8.23   Photomicrograph of a bone biopsy from a patient with aluminum toxicity. The red staining is present where the bone is unmineralized. Note the sharp demarcation between the unmineralized (red) and the underlying mineralized bone (green). In contrast to other conditions where hyperosteoidosis is seen, here the overlying osteoblasts are flat and inconspicuous. Note the prominent hemosiderin deposition in the marrow, which is the result of repeated transfusions (undecalcified tissue, Goldner stain, × 10 obj.).

Table 8.5   Causes of osteomalacia.

Causes of osteomalacia
Vitamin-D disturbances
Inadequate endogenous production
Deficient exposure to sunlight
Dietary deficiency of vitamin D
Inadequate intestinal absorption of vitamin D
Malabsorption syndrome
Postgastrectomy
Celiac disease
Inflammatory bowel disease
Aberrant metabolism of vitamin D
Liver cirrhosis
Dilantin therapy
Renal disease
Kidney disease
Chronic renal failure
Renal tubular disorders
Acidosis
Hypophosphatemia
Familial errors in metabolism
Familial hypophosphatemia
Hypophosphatasia

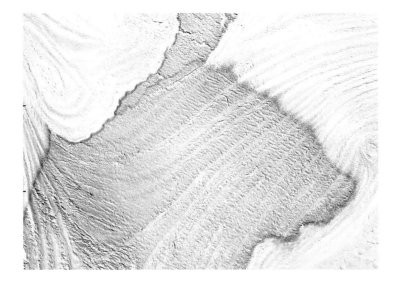

Figure 8.24   Photomicrograph of a section of a biopsy obtained from a patient with aluminum toxicity, which has been stained to show the localization of the aluminum. In this section the aluminum is seen at a reversal line, crossing the lamellar structure, and also at a mineralization front (aurintricarboxylic acid, × 10 obj.).

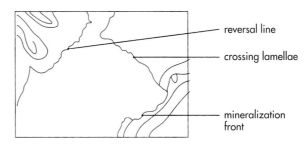

reversal line

crossing lamellae

mineralization
front

Radiologic examination may reveal generalized osteopenia as a result of the loss of calcified matrix, and classically, multiple bilateral and symmetrical cortical lucent areas in the ribs, scapula, pelvis and femoral neck. These lucent areas represent stress fractures and typically lie perpendicular to the long axis of the bone; they are sometimes referred to as Looser's zones, or Milkman's lines (Fig. 8.25). A radio-isotope scan is a most helpful examination in these patients (Fig. 8.26). In general, the axial skeleton, with its higher rate of turnover (e.g. the vertebrae, pelvis, ribs and sternum), is more often affected clinically than the peripheral skeleton.

Microscopic examination of undecalcified diseased bone

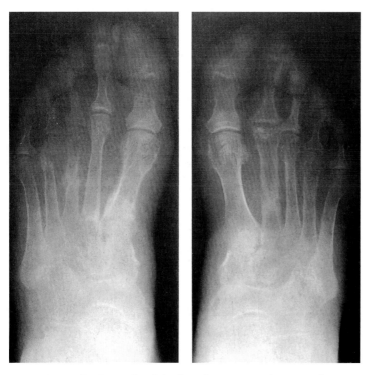

Figure 8.25   Radiographs of the feet of a patient with osteomalacia show bilateral fractures of the metatarsals.

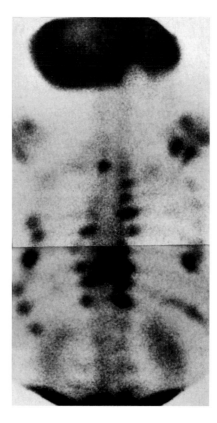

Figure 8.26   A gamma-camera image that shows the pattern of uptake of ^{99}Tc methylene diphosphonate in a patient with osteomalacia. There are multiple rib fractures as well as fractures at the neck of the scapula.

reveals a marked increase in the amount of nonmineralized matrix (osteoid) on the surfaces of the bone trabeculae and lining the haversian canals of the cortical bone (Fig. 8.27). Determination of the extent of osteomalacia requires quantitative histomorphometry (see Chapter 2), and this reveals that at least 10% and usually much more of the bone mass consists of

nonmineralized bone matrix. Tetracycline uptake studies show patchy, blurred uptake (Fig. 8.28). Resorptive changes typical of secondary hyperparathyroidism are also present in many cases. Microscopic examination of the stress fractures reveals poorly mineralized callus and fibrous tissue.

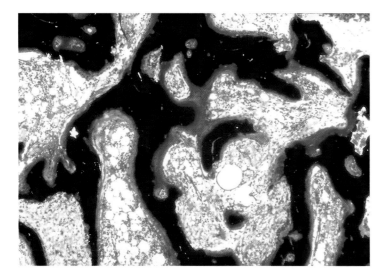

Figure 8.27   Low-power photomicrograph of a specimen from a patient with osteomalacia demonstrates that all the bone surfaces are covered by a thick layer of osteoid, which constitutes more than 15% of the total bone volume (von Kossa's, × 4 obj.).

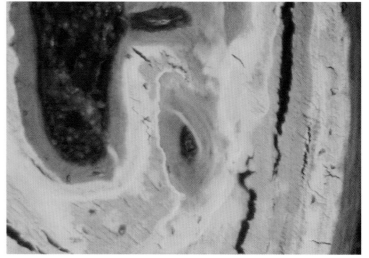

Figure 8.28   Photomicrograph taken using ultraviolet (UV) light shows fluorescence of a broad smudged band of tetracycline, which marks the irregular calcification front in a section of bone obtained from a patient with osteomalacia (tetracycline labeled, UV incident light, × 10 obj.).

RICKETS

In the early 19th century, as a result of the industrial revolution, the large northern European cities became increasingly crowded and polluted. Because of poor diet and little exposure to sun, the children commonly developed severe and debilitating rickets, which among the poor was almost universal. (Nowadays classic rickets, resulting from a deficiency of vitamin D, is only rarely seen and the most common cause of rickets in the USA is renal tubular dysfunction.)

Rickets is characterized by widespread skeletal deformities principally affecting the foci of most rapid growth. The disease may be recognized in patients as young as 6 months of age, at which time thinning and softening of the calvaria and bulging fontanelles may be evident. These cranial changes usually diminish by 2 years of age but are followed by other dramatic skeletal changes, including beading of the costochondral junctions of the ribs (the so-called rachitic rosary) (Fig. 8.29), a depression along the line of the rib–diaphragm attachment (Harrison's groove), and a chicken-breasted appearance. In particular, the wrists, knees, and ankles may be enlarged due to failure of the metaphyseal primary spongiosa to mineralize (Fig. 8.30). Eventually curvature of the long bones develops, especially anterior curvature of the tibia. Spinal abnormalities, including dorsal kyphosis, scoliosis, and lumbar lordosis may diminish height.

Radiologic examination reveals a widened and irregular growth plate, with a cup-shaped concavity and flaring of the metaphyseal end of the bone (Fig. 8.31). These changes correlate

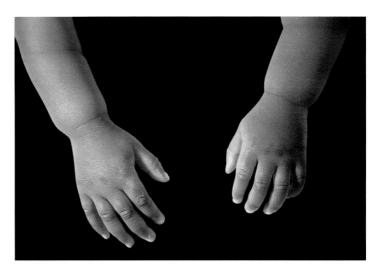

Figure 8.30 Rickets. Hand and forearm of a young child show prominence above the wrist, consequent upon the flaring and poor mineralization of the lower end of the radius and ulna.

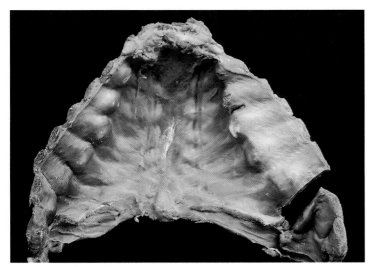

(a)

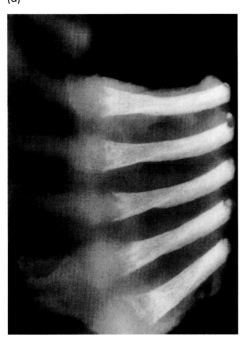

(b)

Figure 8.29 **(a)** Rickets: dissected specimen of the rib cage shows prominence of the costochondral junctions because of swelling. This gives rise to the so-called rachitic rosary. **(b)** Radiograph of a portion of this specimen demonstrates that the swelling results from irregularity and poor mineralization of the metaphysis with a characteristic 'cupping' at the junction of the cartilage and bone.

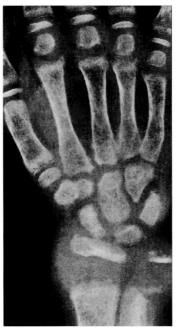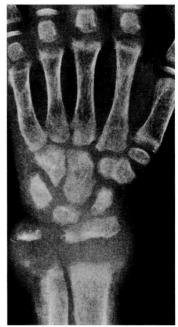

(a)   (b)

Figure 8.31 **(a and b)** Dorsovolar view of both hands of an 8-year-old boy from India with untreated dietary rickets shows osteopenia of the bones and widening of the growth plates of the distal metacarpals, with irregular mineralization and cupping. Note also the fracture subluxation which has occurred in the growth plates of the radius and ulna of the metaphyses – typical features of this condition.

microscopically with the presence of irregular, disorderly columns of proliferating cartilage in the growth plate and tongues of proliferating irregular cartilage extending into the adjacent bone (Figs 8.32 and 8.33). These findings are associated with absence of the calcified zone of the cartilage and a poorly formed primary spongiosa. The most striking histologic change is the presence of large amounts of nonmineralized bone throughout the skeleton. Stress fractures, similar to those seen in osteomalacia, are often present.

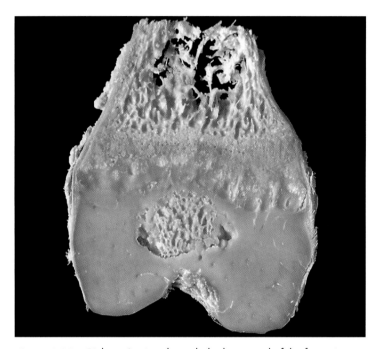

Figure 8.32   Rickets. Section through the lower end of the femur in a young child shows widening of the epiphyseal growth plate region, together with irregularity of the metaphysis with tongues of epiphyseal cartilage, penetrating into the metaphyseal bone.

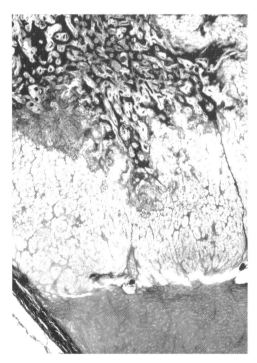

Figure 8.33
Photomicrograph of the costochondral junction in a patient with rickets shows widening of the growth cartilage region with irregularity at the cartilage-bone interface and poorly mineralized, disorganized primary spongiosa (H&E, × 4 obj.).

HYPOPARATHYROIDISM

Most commonly hypoparathyroidism follows extensive neck surgery, especially total thyroidectomy. Very rarely it is due to hypoplasia of the parathyroid glands. Treatment is aimed at restoration of serum calcium to a low normal level. Elemental calcium and vitamin D are the usual therapeutic agents used.

Pseudohypoparathyroidism refers to the rare condition, characterized by increased levels of circulating parathyroid hormone associated with glandular hyperplasia, which is paradoxically associated with hypocalcemia and hyperphosphatemia. This biochemical hypoparathyroidism results from resistance of the bone and kidneys (i.e. the target organs) to the biological actions of PTH, even in the face of elevated levels of PTH. In very rare cases patients with this condition demonstrate resistance to multiple hormones and demonstrate short stature, subcutaneus ossification and mental retardation, a condition known as Albright's hereditary osteodystrophy.

HYPOPHOSPHATEMIA

Phosphate is a significant physiologic buffer and also plays a major role in calcium homeostasis. The process by which phosphate retention leads to hyperphosphatemia and secondary hyperparathyroidism has already been discussed. Hypophosphatemia may result from any number of causes, either congenital or acquired. Among the latter are increased urinary phosphate loss caused by lowering of the renal tubule threshold for phosphate reabsorption (as seen in primary hyperparathyroidism) and therapeutic administration of diuretic agents. The condition may also be traced to decreased intestinal absorption, as seen in vitamin D deficiency, and malabsorption syndromes, or starvation, or it may be induced by the excessive use of phosphate-binding antacids. Acute hypophosphatemia also occurs after uptake of phosphorus from the serum into the cells, as seen after insulin administration, and in states of respiratory alkalosis, as in salicylate poisoning.

Disorders of phosphate metabolism, particularly those associated with severe hypophosphatemia, can cause cell damage with potentially serious clinical consequences; examples include erythrocyte hemolysis, leukocyte and platelet disorders, defects of the peripheral and central nervous system, myopathy and rhabdomyolysis.

In bone, the main consequence of hypophosphatemia is osteomalacia. This impaired mineralization appears to be a purely extracellular problem arising from changes in the calcium and phosphate concentration product (Ca × P), which reflect the extent of saturation of extracellular fluid with respect to these ions. Laboratory studies in patients with acquired hypophosphatemia reveal normal glomerular filtration rates, normal to high levels of serum calcium, a markedly lowered level of serum phosphorus, and elevated levels of alkaline phosphatase. PTH levels may be suppressed. $1,25(OH)_2D$ levels should be elevated but frequently are not, and may even be low. Bone biopsy specimens reveal characteristics of osteomalacia indistinguishable from those caused by vitamin D deficiency.

Most hypophosphatemic states can be corrected medically and do not progress to development of severe skeletal aberrations. However, uncorrected hypophosphatemia may lead to severe skeletal sequelae, especially in growing children.

Osteomalacia due to acquired hypophosphatemia is sometimes

seen in association with metastatic carcinoma, as well as a variety of benign or malignant mesenchymal tumors, including fibrous dysplasia, and vascular tumors, so-called oncogenic osteomalacia. The most outstanding feature of the disease is impaired renal tubule phosphate reabsorption, the mechanism of which is unclear. A marked reduction in serum $1,25(OH)_2D$ is usually observed. Complete excision of the tumor usually leads to resolution of the biochemical abnormalities and the osteomalacia. A recurrence of the tumor is usually made apparent by a reappearance of osteomalacia.

Familial hypophosphatemia (familial X-linked hypophosphatemic rickets; vitamin D-resistant rickets; refractory rickets)

Familial hypophosphatemic rickets is a genetic disease which is transmitted as an X-linked dominant trait and is usually manifested by the second year of life. Typically, the patient's urinary excretion of phosphorus is increased. The disorder is clinically characterized by childhood rickets with associated growth retardation and poor dental development (Fig. 8.34). The condition is unresponsive to physiological doses of vitamin D.

In middle age, other clinical problems begin to appear, with mineralization of the spinal ligaments and thickening of the neural arches. There is loss of mobility of the spine, shoulders, elbows, and hips. Reduction in the diameter of the spinal canal may lead to cord compression at more than one level.

The primary biochemical defect for this disorder of mineral metabolism remains unknown, although the site of the renal phosphate transport defect has been localized to the brush border membrane of the proximal convoluted tubule.

X-linked hypophosphatemic rickets has long been recognized as being different from any other form of rickets and osteomalacia in its clinical manifestations, pathogenesis, and difficulty of treatment. The disease is regarded primarily as a genetic defect of renal tubule phosphate transport, and this concept has led to treatment with phosphate supplements and large doses of vita-

min D. However, successful therapy, particularly full healing of the mineralization defects, usually requires that the phosphate therapy be combined with supraphysiologic dosages of $1,25(OH)_2D$.

FANCONI'S SYNDROME (RENAL GLYCOSURIC RICKETS)

Fanconi's syndrome is a recessively transmitted genetic disorder characterized by marked aminoaciduria, glycosuria, bicarbonaturia, and phosphaturia. The condition may be accompanied by an associated metabolic defect in cystine metabolism, the so-called Lignac-Fanconi disease. Patients with these disorders exhibit normal glomerular function, a decreased level of serum carbon dioxide, normal to low levels of serum calcium, low levels of serum phosphorus, and elevated levels of alkaline phosphatase.

Radiographic examination may reveal diffuse osteopenia and stress fractures. Irregular and widened epiphyseal cartilage zones are clearly seen in children, but the dramatic increase in nonmineralized bone observed in patients with rickets is not apparent. In patients with Fanconi's syndrome associated with cystinosis, cystine deposits are present in the bone and the visceral organs.

The osteomalacia is believed to result principally from the severe hypophosphatemia caused by the renal tubule dysfunction. Amino-acid deficiency may contribute to growth retardation.

HYPOMAGNESEMIA

Magnesium is the second most abundant cation in the intracellular fluids and essential to neurochemical transmissions and many enzyme activities. Magnesium deficiency is common and may be present in as many as 10% of patients admitted to general hospitals and more than half the patients in medical intensive care units. Hypocalcemia is commonly associated with chronic magnesium deficiency and under these circumstances is best treated by magnesium replacement. The hypocalcemia appears to be related to impaired PTH secretion in patients with chronic magnesium deficiency and in general patients with hypocalcemia of this type usually have normal or low normal PTH levels.

SOFT-TISSUE CALCIFICATION

METASTATIC CALCIFICATION

Metastatic calcification is caused by an increased calcium phosphate product in the blood, and therefore can result from hypercalcemia and/or hyperphosphatemia. It is commonly associated with secondary hyperparathyroidism, sarcoidosis, metastatic disease and myeloma (Fig. 8.35). Metastatic calcification is a particular problem in patients with hypermetabolic states who have undergone prolonged periods of bed rest.

The calcification is both intracellular and extracellular. Mineral deposition is particularly likely to occur in the kidneys (Fig. 8.36), alveolar walls of the lungs, cornea, conjunctiva, and gastric mucosa (i.e. those areas subject to the large pH changes), as well as in the media and intima of the peripheral arteries.

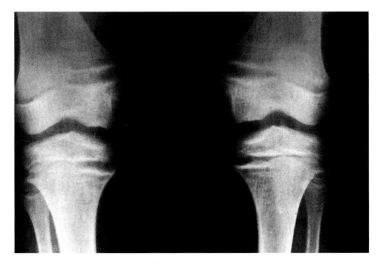

Figure 8.34   Radiograph of the legs of a young patient with hypophosphatemic rickets. Note the widening and cupping of the growth plates. Unlike the rickets secondary to vitamin D deficiency, which is illustrated in Figure 8.31, the metaphysis shows sclerosis.

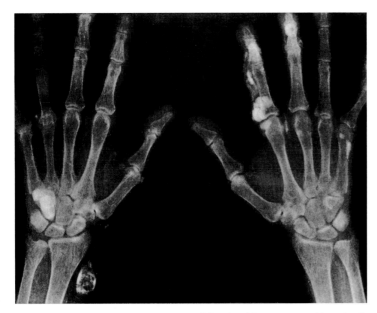

Figure 8.35   Postero-anterior view of the distal forearms and hands of a 48-year-old woman treated by long-term dialysis for chronic renal failure with resultant secondary hyperparathyroidism. There is soft-tissue and vascular calcification, characteristic findings in this condition. An arteriovenous fistula from hemodialysis has occluded and calcified, and is clearly seen in the soft tissue adjacent to the radial metaphysis.

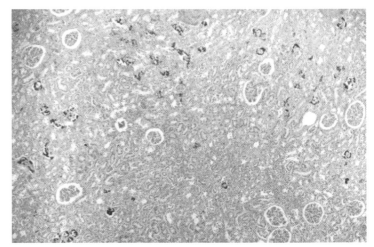

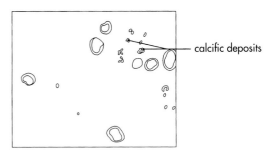

Figure 8.36   Photomicrograph of the kidney in a patient with prolonged hypercalcemia resulting from a parathyroid adenoma. Extensive calcium deposits are seen in relation to the proximal tubules (H&E, × 4 obj.).

TUMORAL CALCINOSIS

Tumoral calcinosis is a rare condition which primarily, but not exclusively, affects black people in otherwise good health. The disease usually presents in the second decade of life and is characterized by deposition of painless calcific masses around the hips, elbows, shoulders, and gluteal areas (i.e. areas subject to movement and/or pressure) (Figs 8.37 and 8.38). A familial incidence has been reported. In rare instances, intra-articular or intraosseous deposits may also occur (Figs 8.39 and 8.40).

The lesions may be massive, are often bilateral, and they affect multiple sites. The patient's serum phosphate level is usually elevated. Although the hyperphosphatemia should suppress $1,25(OH)_2D$ production, the serum levels tend to stay paradoxically normal. Surgical excision is the most successful form of treatment, although recurrences are common. Medical treatment to control the hyperphosphatemia (e.g. a low phosphate diet and oral administration of phosphate binders) is an important adjunct to surgical excision. (We have seen an instance of correction of hyperphosphatemia and radiologically documented disappearance of a large tumor mass achieved by the use of phosphaturic diuretics.)

Microscopic examination of tissues from these patients reveals calcific deposits which are surrounded by a mild infiltration of both histiocytes and chronic inflammatory cells. Some multinu-cleated giant cells may be present. X-ray diffraction studies have shown that the deposits are mainly formed of hydroxyapatite crystals.

CALCIFICATION IN INJURED TISSUE

Deposition of calcium hydroxyapatite in soft tissues may also occur as a complication of trauma and scleroderma. Dead tissue that does not undergo rapid absorption frequently becomes calcified. This type of calcification, which is not related to any disturbance in calcium homeostasis, is called dystrophic calcification. Calcification is common in areas of coagulation necrosis (e.g. in cases of infarction), in caseous necrosis seen in patients with tuberculosis, and in areas of fat necrosis (Fig. 8.41). Of particular interest to orthopaedic surgeons is the calcification that is common in tendons, ligaments, and bursae (Figs 8.42–8.44). A common clinical presentation for patients with dystrophic calcification is a painful shoulder that corresponds anatomically to the insertion of the supraspinatus muscle onto the humerus.

Gross examination reveals amorphous chalky white deposits or circumscribed gritty calcifications. These deposits have been shown by X-ray diffraction studies to be hydroxyapatite crystals. Microscopic studies reveal calcium in fibrous or fatty tissue sometimes with associated chronic inflammatory cells including, at times, multinucleated giant cells.

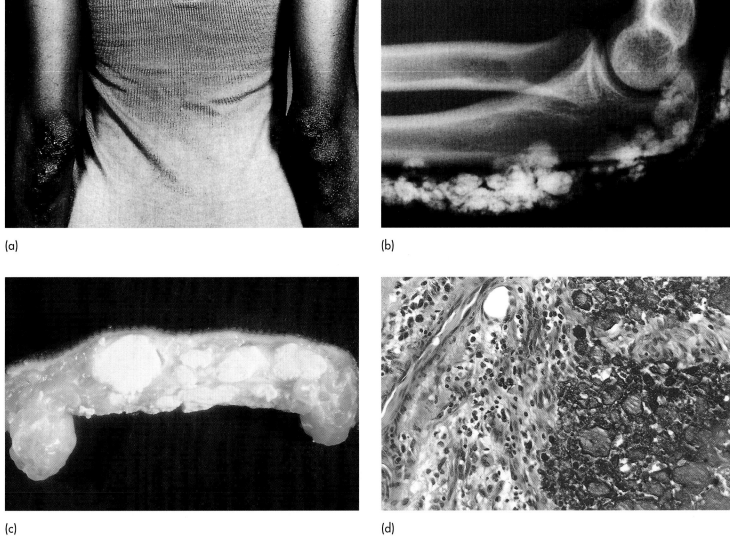

(a)

(b)

(c)

(d)

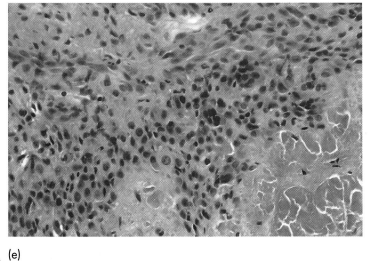

(e)

Figure 8.37 (a) Photograph of a young black woman with extensive subcutaneous calcium deposits (tumoral calcinosis) around the elbows and along the extensor surfaces of the forearm. (b) Radiograph of this patient's arm shows the extent of the calcified mass. (c) Cut surfaces of the excised specimen. (d) Photomicrograph of a calcium apatite deposit in tumoral calcinosis. Note the histiocytic and giant-cell response at the edge of the calcified deposit, which is seen here as a dark blue–purple area to the right of the picture (H&E, × 10 obj.). (e) Occasionally as seen in this photomicrograph, because of variations in processing the calcium apatite deposits appear pink rather than blue and in such a case their true nature may not be apparent to the examining histopathologist (H&E, × 10 obj.).

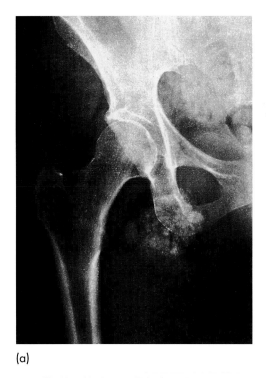

(a)

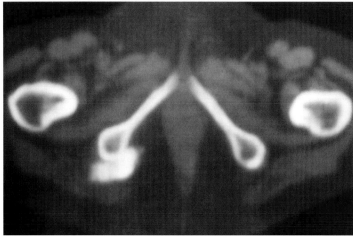

(b)

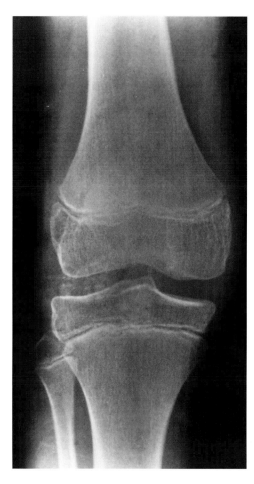

Figure 8.39
Radiograph of a 12-year-old boy seen for knee pain. A flocculent calcified mass is present mainly in the lateral compartment. There was no effusion noted. The child drank eight glasses of milk a day and had an elevated serum phosphate level which ranged between 7 and 8. Family history revealed chronic renal disease in the mother and renal calculi in the father. However, the boy was the only member of the family with hyper-phosphatemia; the condition was resolved with a phosphate-restricted diet and the use of phosphate binder.

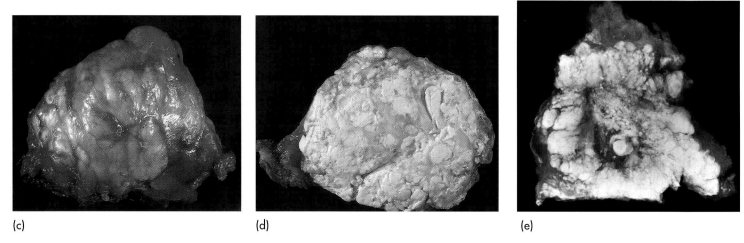

(c)   (d)   (e)

Figure 8.38 (a) Radiograph of a 56-year-old woman with tumoral calcinosis who presented with a mass in the buttock. (b) CT scan of the mass. (c) Photograph of the excised mass, which is well encapsulated. (d) Photograph of the cross-section. (e) Fine-grain radiograph of the specimen.

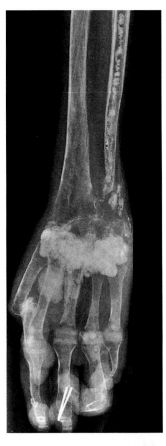

Figure 8.40   Radiograph of a 63-year-old woman with rheumatoid arthritis who, although normal with regard to CaPO₄ and vitamin D levels, nevertheless presented with both soft-tissue and intraosseous calcification as shown here. She was taking 1200 mg of CaCO₃ daily and 400 IU of vitamin D.

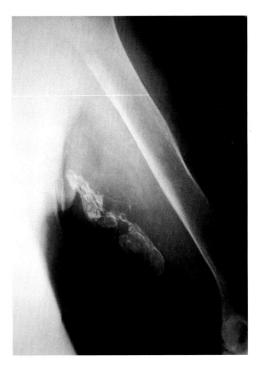

Figure 8.41 Radiograph of a middle-aged man who presented with swelling along the inner side of the left arm. The soft-tissue calcification seen on X-ray was shown at operation to be both calcification and ossification within a large lobulated lipoma which had undergone focal necrosis.

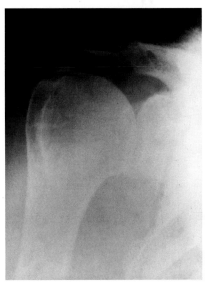

(a)

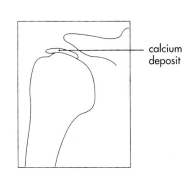

calcium deposit

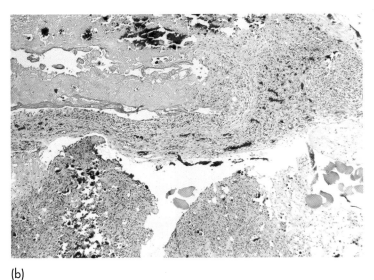

(b)

Figure 8.42   (a) Radiograph of an anteroposterior view of the shoulder demonstrating calcific tendinitis. (b) A low-power photomicrograph showing necrotic tissue with focal deposits of hydroxyapatite in the upper part of the image and mixed inflammatory tissue in the lower (H&E, × 4 obj.). (c) A higher-power reveals many giant cells, histiocytes and scattered lymphocytes with small and large foci of calcium deposition (H&E, × 25 obj.).

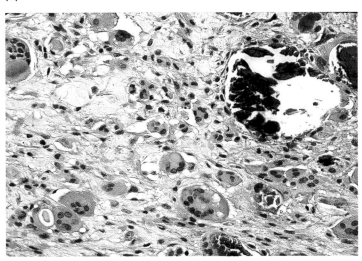

(c)

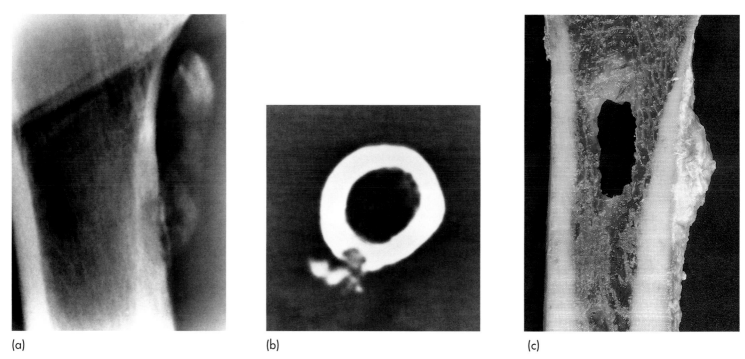

(a)　　　　　　　　　　　　　　　　(b)　　　　　　　　　　　　　　　　(c)

Figure 8.43 (a) Radiograph of the upper femur of a 58-year-old male who presented with a 1-year history of sharp, intermittent pain in the right thigh. The bone scan was hot. (b) CT scan shows bone erosion, which was misinterpreted as evidence of malignancy, and the upper femur was resected without biopsy being performed. (c) Photograph showing calcification occurring in the region of the linea aspera. Microscopically, the findings were similar to those found in association with tumoral calcinosis.

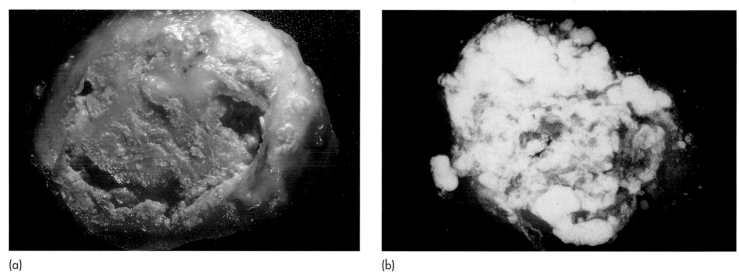

(a)　　　　　　　　　　　　　　　　　　　(b)

Figure 8.44 (a) The cut surface of a grossly thickened acromial bursa with extensive calcium deposits. (b) Radiograph of the specimen clearly reveals the extent of calcification. (c) Microscopic appearance of the calcified bursa shown. Note that although most of the tissue is necrotic and calcified, there is some viable fibrous connective tissue in the center of the field (H&E, × 10 obj.).

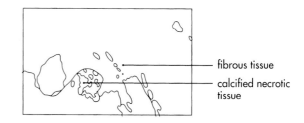

fibrous tissue

calcified necrotic tissue

(c)

Chapter 9

ACCUMULATION OF ABNORMAL METABOLIC PRODUCTS AND VARIOUS HEMATOLOGIC DISORDERS

Secondary oxalosis is more common. The setting is usually that of chronic renal failure and the degree of crystal deposition is generally less severe than in primary oxalosis. In affected individuals, blood levels of calcium oxalate are elevated and correlate significantly with the serum creatinine value. Oxalate deposits may be seen in many organs including the kidneys, heart, thyroid, lungs, bone, cartilage and synovium as well as in the synovial fluid.

Radiologic evidence of disease in the skeleton depends on the severity of the condition and therefore is more often seen in primary oxalosis. Radiodense areas in the metaphyseal region of the long bones are common; occasionally there is markedly increased density of the axial skeleton. In children, dense bands in the metaphysis may result from crystal deposition in growth arrest lines (Fig. 9.1).

Microscopic examination of skeletal tissue from both primary and secondary oxalosis reveals crystals in mineralized bone, artic-

Skeletal abnormalities characterized by the accumulation of metabolic products may complicate a number of systemic metabolic disturbances, some of which are discussed elsewhere. (Those in which the joint is most commonly affected, such as gout and calcium pyrophosphate deposition will be discussed in Chapter 12, p. 299, the mucopolysaccharidoses have been discussed in Chapter 6, p. 163.)

The first part of this chapter discusses oxalic acid deposition, amyloidosis, and various lipid disturbances; the second part covers the effects of various hematologic disorders.

DEPOSITION AND STORAGE DISEASES

OXALOSIS

Normally oxalic acid, an end-product of both amino acid and vitamin C metabolism, is excreted in the urine. However calcium oxalate crystals may be precipitated into various tissues, including bone, bone marrow and cartilage, in either primary or secondary oxalosis.

Primary (familial) oxalosis usually presents in childhood, although in a few cases its appearance may be delayed until adulthood. It is characterized by excessive biosynthesis of oxalate. The result is nephrolithiasis and secondary chronic renal failure. Deposition of calcium oxalate crystals in many tissues, including the bone and bone marrow, is a prominent feature.

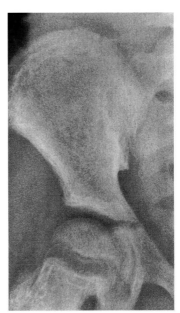
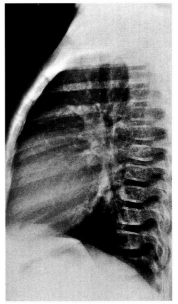

(a)　　　　　　　　(b)

Figure 9.1   (a) Radiograph of the right hip and pelvis from a child with primary oxalosis. There are dense lines in the metaphysis of the femur as well as paralleling the iliac crest. The widening of the growth plate is due to secondary rickets as a result of renal failure. (b) Radiograph of the thoracic spine in the same patient as (a) shows bony sclerosis in the metaphyseal region which gives a sandwich-like appearance to the vertebral bodies.

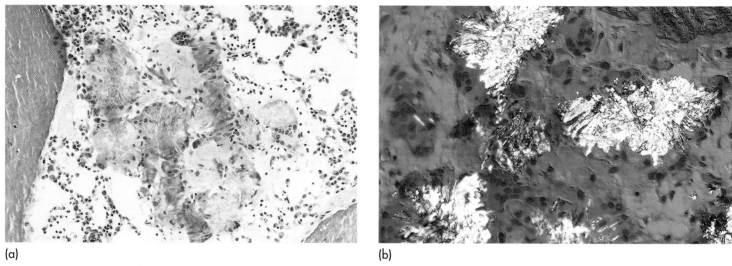

(a) (b)

Figure 9.2 (a) Photomicrograph of a section from a biopsy obtained from a patient with primary oxalosis. Faint greenish crystalline deposits can be seen in the marrow space (undecalcified section, H&E, × 10 obj.). (b) Photomicrograph of the crystalline material examined by polarized light at a higher magnification. The starburst clusters of sharp needles of high refractivity are typical of oxalosis. Around these crystalline deposits there is a histiocytic and giant-cell response (undecalcified section, Nomarski optics, polarized light, × 25 obj.).

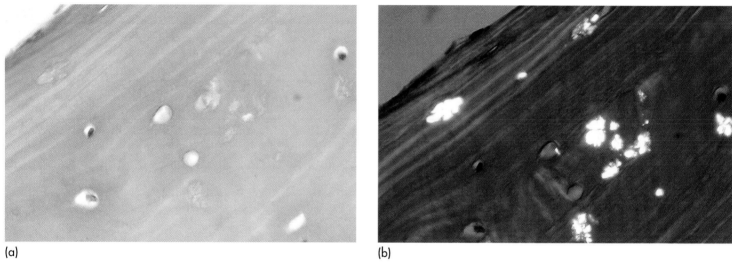

(a) (b)

Figure 9.3 (a) Oxalosis: photomicrographs of lamellar bone. Within the matrix of the bone and adjacent to and within the cellular lacunae can be seen some indistinct yellowish deposits. On examination with polarized light (b), these deposits become evident as brightly refractive star-like clusters of crystallized material (H&E, × 50 obj.).

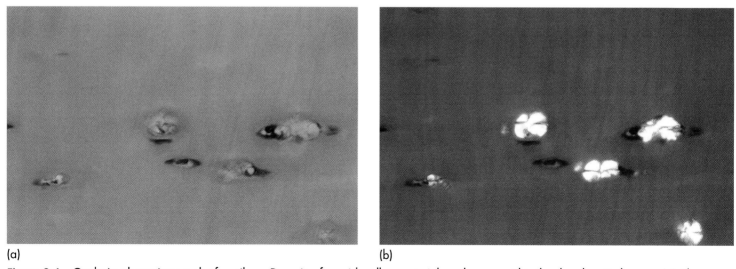

(a) (b)

Figure 9.4 Oxalosis: photomicrograph of cartilage. Deposits of grayish-yellow material can be seen within the chondrocytic lacunae (a). The same field photographed using polarized light (b) (H&E, × 50 obj.).

ular cartilage, and/or bone marrow. The crystals can be identified by polarized light microscopy, which reveals highly refractile needle-shaped crystals that form star-like clusters (Figs 9.2–9.4). Positive identification of the crystals can be achieved by chemical analysis, X-ray diffraction, or electron diffraction. (The latter technique offers a precise method for identification of extremely small quantities of calcium oxalate in bone biopsy specimens.)

Microscopic examination usually shows a lack of cellular response to the crystals, however, a mononuclear-cell reaction, or a giant-cell reaction similar to that seen in patients with other crystal deposition disorders may be present. (In the bone evidence of secondary hyperparathyroidism with increased osteoclastic resorption, as well as hyperosteoidosis, is also frequently seen and is to be expected in the setting of chronic renal failure.)

AMYLOIDOSIS

In both primary and secondary amyloidosis, deposits of a twisted β-pleated fibrillary protein may be seen in bone marrow and/or the juxta-articular synovial tissue. Although skeletal involvement is probably not that uncommon it is rarely recognized clinically. Some patients with amyloidosis may present with aching bone pain and pathologic fractures. Such patients are most likely to be diagnosed clinically as having a metastatic tumor and the true nature of the disease does not become apparent until histologic examination is performed (Fig. 9.5).

An increasing frequency of carpal tunnel syndrome (CTS) in patients on long-term hemodialysis has been reported, with a correlation between the length of time on dialysis and the devel-

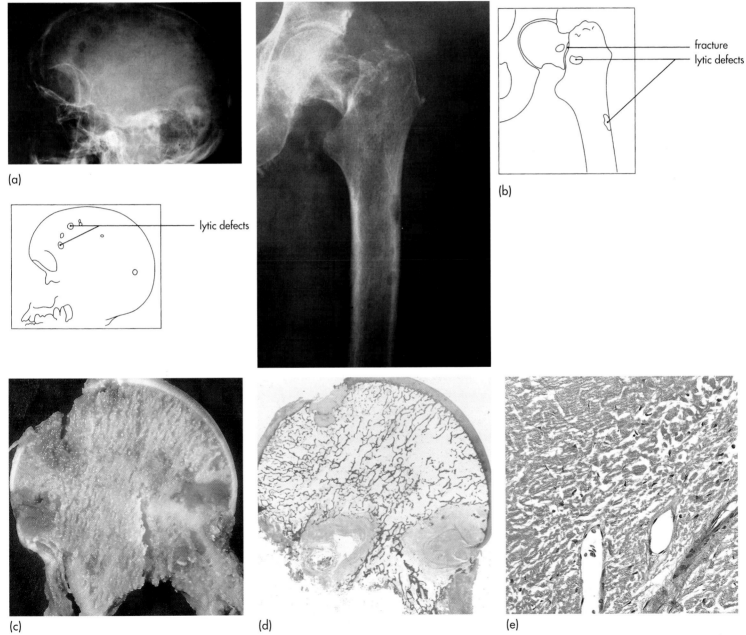

Figure 9.5 (a) Radiograph of the skull in a patient with generalized primary amyloidosis shows multiple lytic areas, which originally suggested the presence of a myeloma. (b) Radiograph of a portion of the pelvis and the right hip in the same patient illustrated in (a). Again multiple lytic lesions can be seen in the neck and shaft of the femur. In addition, a fracture has occurred through the femoral neck. (c) Cut surface of the femoral head removed from the patient with pathologic fracture shown in (b). The lytic areas are represented by sites of bone destruction filled by a glassy pink tissue. (d) Histologic section demonstrates that glassy areas are acellular deposits of amyloid (H&E, × 1 obj.). (e) A higher power view shows the dense eosinophilic amyloid deposits with admixed fibroblasts and vessels (H&E, × 10 obj.).

opment of CTS. In these patients amyloid deposits can usually be demonstrated in the synovial tissue. However, the amyloid may be difficult to distinguish microscopically from an excess of collagen tissue or hyalinized collagen (Fig. 9.6). In such patients, amyloid may also be seen as localized destructive bone lesions, in large joints as diffuse synovial deposits, or often with bilateral involvement of multiple joints. Radiologic examination may reveal juxta-articular osteoporosis, extensive swelling of the soft tissues, multiple well-defined subchondral cysts and pressure erosions from synovial hypertrophy. Despite these changes usually there is relative preservation of the joint space (Fig. 9.7).

Patients with diffuse marrow disease show a predominantly axial distribution of amyloid and may have painful compression fractures that may mimic those of myeloma. A localized lytic form of amyloidosis affecting the long bones, skull, or ribs, is usually manifest radiographically as one or more well-marginated lytic lesions.

Microscopic examination of sections stained with hematoxylin–eosin (H&E) will generally show irregular fragments of a

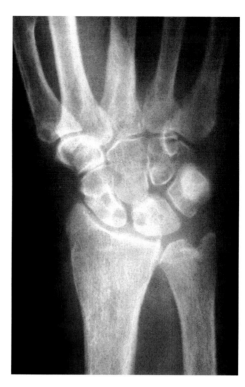

Figure 9.7
Radiograph of the wrist of a patient on long-term dialysis shows soft-tissue thickening and several lytic defects in the carpal bones due to pressure erosions from amyloid deposits in the synovial tissue.

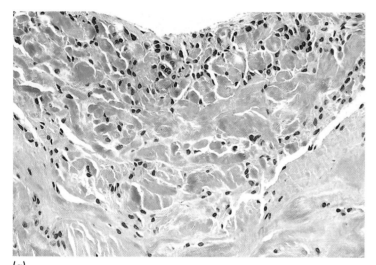

(a)

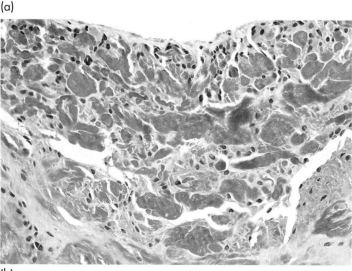

(b)

Figure 9.6 (a) Photomicrograph of a segment of synovial tissue stained with hematoxylin–eosin excised from the carpal tunnel of a patient with median nerve compression. Within the collagenous tissue are pink acellular areas which stain a positive red–orange color (b) when stained with Congo red stain (Congo red stain, × 10 obj.).

glassy eosinophilic material, sometimes with an adjacent histiocytic or even giant-cell response. Histologic sections of amyloid deposits stained with Congo red have a characteristic apple-green birefringence when examined under polarized light (Fig. 9.8). [It may be difficult to recognize amyloid deposits when they occur in connective tissue matrix, because collagen, especially denatured collagen, produces a similar apple-green color when examined under polarized light (Fig. 9.9).]

GAUCHER'S DISEASE

The so-called 'lipidoses' encompass a wide variety of disorders in which congenital enzyme deficiencies lead to the accumulation of complex lipid compounds. By far the commonest of these disorders, at least in New York City, is Gaucher's disease, where it is most common in Ashkenazic Jews. An autosomal recessively transmitted error of metabolism of the glucosyl ceramides (glucocerebrosides) results from a deficiency in the activity of glucosylceramide-α-glucosidase. The excess glucocerebrosides accumulate in cells of the reticuloendothelial system, including the liver, spleen (splenomegaly may be dramatic), lymph nodes, and bone marrow (Fig. 9.10).

Most patients have a chronic form of the disease that pursues a benign asymptomatic course and which often is not diagnosed until the patient is an adult. A few patients, however, develop complications much earlier. A common complication, especially in young people, is avascular necrosis of the femoral head (Fig. 9.11).

Although the clinical course varies, patients who present with the disease in infancy or childhood usually have a poor prognosis. In rare cases, an acute neuropathic form of the disease occurs in which most of those affected die before the age of 3 years.

Radiologically in more severely affected patients, the long bones show irregular thinning of the cortices, which gives

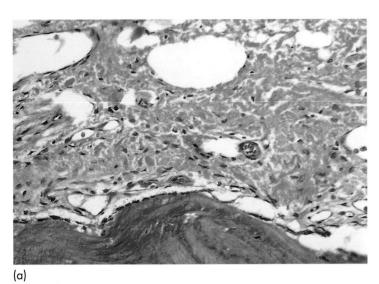
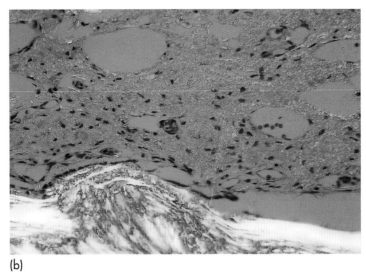

Figure 9.8 (a) Photomicrograph of extensive amyloid deposit in the bone marrow (H&E, × 10 obj.). (b) Photomicrograph of the same field under polarized light. The amyloid deposits are finely granulated, birefringent and apple-green as also is the bone collagen seen in the lower portion of the photograph (polarized light, × 10 obj.).

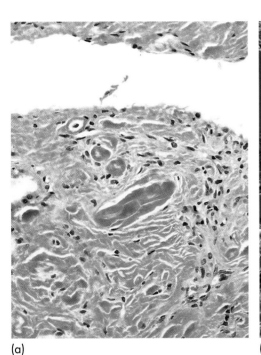
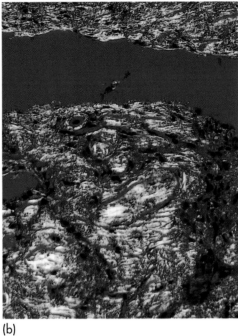

Figure 9.9 (a) Photomicrograph of a section of synovial tissue with a considerable amount of amyloid deposits (Congo red stain, × 10 obj.). (b) The same section polarized showing the difficulty of distinguishing amyloid from collagen by polarization.

(a)

(b)

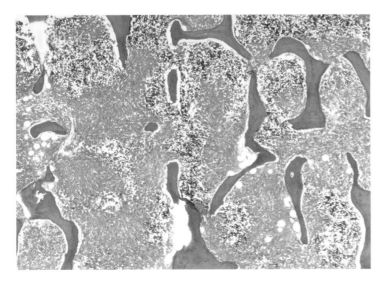

Figure 9.10 Gaucher's disease: photomicrograph shows widespread replacement of the bone marrow tissue by sheets of pink cellular tissue. Some residual normal marrow is seen at the top of the frame (H&E, × 4 obj.).

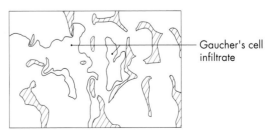

Gaucher's cell infiltrate

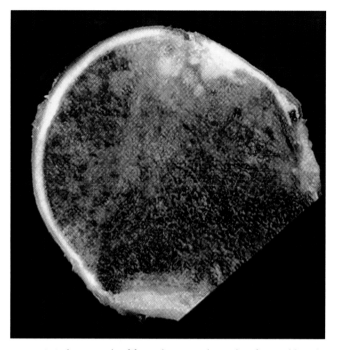

(a)

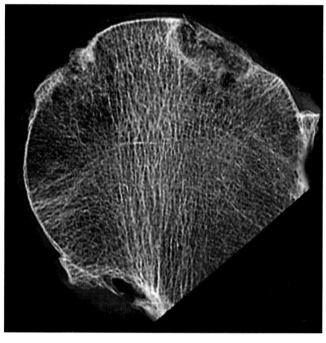

(b)

Figure 9.11 **(a)** Photograph of frontal section through a femoral head removed from a middle-aged female patient with Gaucher's disease. The marrow is dark red with a diffuse spotty infiltrate of grayish-yellow tissue. On the superior articular surface is a 1.5 cm wedge-shaped focus of scarring and necrosis. **(b)** A radiograph of the specimen slice; note the fractures which have occurred at the margins of the necrotic area.

them a trabeculated appearance. Frequently, the lower end of the femur, the upper end of the tibia, and the upper end of the humerus fail to remodel during development, leading to the 'Erlenmeyer flask' deformity (Fig. 9.12). The spine usually exhibits loss of density, and frequently one or more of the vertebrae show collapse with either a wedge-shaped deformity, platyspondyly, or occasionally fish-mouth deformities (Fig. 9.13). In less severely affected individuals a nonspecific osteopenia is the only skeletal finding. Occasionally in a few patients in addition to

osteopenia, some osteosclerotic lesions are also present. These areas of sclerosis probably result from infarction within the affected bone.

On microscopic examination the skeletal alterations in Gaucher's disease are seen to result from massive infiltration of the marrow space by large histiocytes that usually measure 40–80 μm in diameter. These histiocytes have a characteristic crumpled- or wrinkled-paper appearance of the cytoplasm (Figs 9.14 and 9.15).

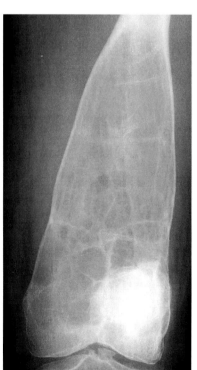

Figure 9.12 Radiograph of the lower femur of a patient with Gaucher's disease shows flaring of the metaphyseal region and distal diaphysis with a bubbly osteolysis of the affected bone.

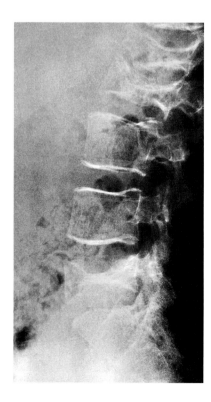

Figure 9.13 Later radiograph of a patient with Gaucher's disease, osteopenia and collapse of L1, L2, and L5.

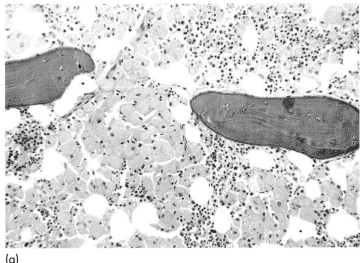

(a)

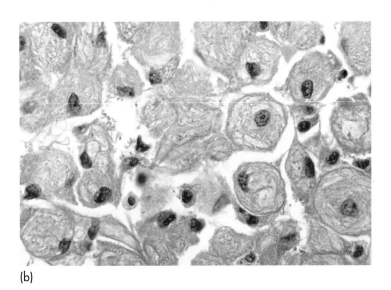

(b)

Figure 9.14 **(a)** A photomicrograph of an infiltrate of Gaucher's cells which are seen to be swollen histiocytes with a foamy cytoplasm and a crinkled appearance. The infiltrate is replacing the normal bone marrow (H&E, × 10 obj.). **(b)** A higher power image of the Gaucher's infiltrate (H&E, × 25 obj.). **(c)** Shows the size of the Gaucher's cells relative to those of the bone marrow (H&E, × 40 obj.).

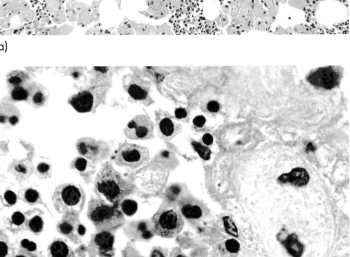

(c)

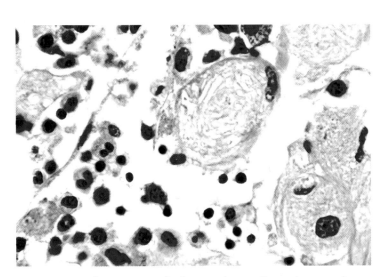

Figure 9.15 Photomicrograph of a Gaucher's cell seen here in a bone marrow aspirate. The cytoplasm of the Gaucher's cell has been likened to crumpled tissue paper (H&E, × 40 obj.).

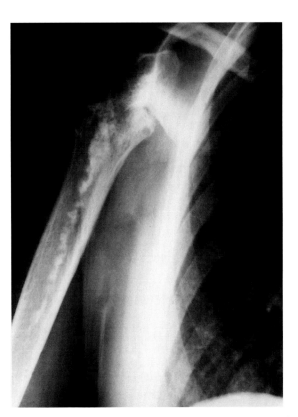

Figure 9.16 Radiograph of the humerus of a patient with Gaucher's disease complicated both by osteomyelitis and infarction. Note the linear marrow calcification so characteristic of infarction.

Because the infiltration of the marrow space tends to compromise the venous return, diagnostic biopsy may be complicated by secondary infarction and/or infection (Fig. 9.16).

NIEMANN–PICK DISEASE

Niemann–Pick disease is characterized by an accumulation of sphingomyelin in the reticuloendothelial system. Since there are at present no stains specific for sphingomyelin, chemical analyses are obligatory for the establishment of a diagnosis.

The classic presentation of Niemann–Pick disease is that of a child dying before the age of 4 years with clinical findings of massive hepatosplenomegaly, foam cells in the bone marrow, and irreparable disordering of the nervous system. Postmortem examination reveals many lipid-laden histiocytes in nearly every organ of the body. Very rarely some of these features have been

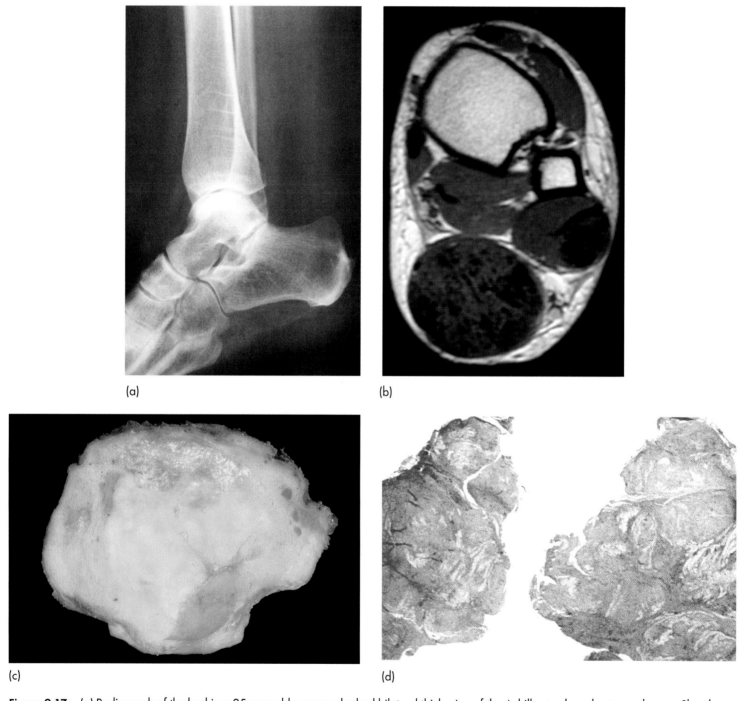

(a) (b) (c) (d)

Figure 9.17 (a) Radiograph of the heel in a 25-year-old woman who had bilateral thickening of the Achilles tendons due to xanthomas. She also had xanthomas of the patellar tendon and xanthelasmas of the skin. The patient had marked hypercholesterolemia. Several members of her family suffered from the same condition. (b) MRI shows extensive involvement of the Achilles tendon by xanthoma as well as involvement of the peroneus longus and brevis. (c) Tissue removed from the thickened heel cord shown in (a). The yellowish color results from the lipid accumulation. (d) Lower power photomicrograph of the removed tissue shows extensive cellular replacement of the normal collagenous tendinous tissue in which there are focal cleared areas which on closer examination were found to be due to cholesterol deposits (H&E, × 1.5 obj.).

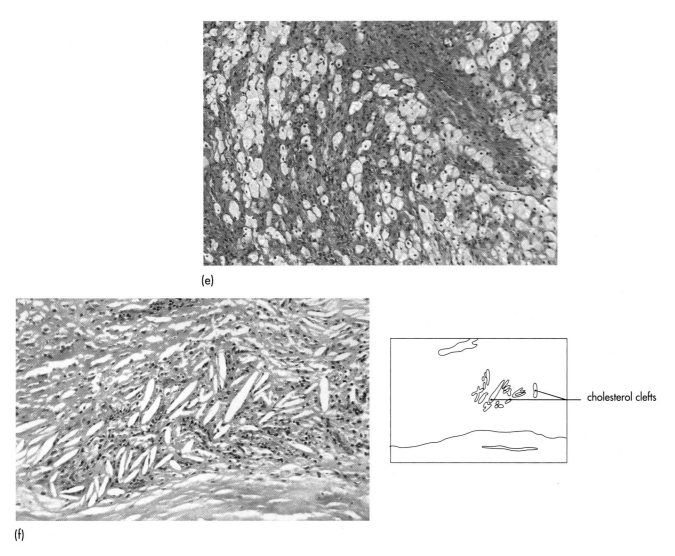

(e)

(f)

cholesterol clefts

Figure 9.17 (*contd*) (e) A higher power photomicrograph to demonstrate the packed fibrohistiocytic cells with many foamy lipid-laden cells (H&E, × 10 obj.). (f) Photomicrograph shows lipid-filled foamy histiocytes and focal cholesterol clefts (H&E, × 10 obj.).

observed in patients who live longer and may have no obvious clinical abnormality of the nervous system.

PRIMARY HYPERLIPIDEMIAS AND XANTHOMATOSIS

Patients with familial hypercholesterolemia and type III hyperlipoproteinemia as well as patients with biliary cirrhosis, or chronic pancreatitis are very likely to develop subcutaneus xanthomas as well as asymptomatic tendinous xanthomas. The most common sites for these tendinous xanthomas are the Achilles tendon (Fig. 9.17) and the extensor tendons of the fingers, where the lesions are likely to be bilateral and symmetrical. Occasionally the plantar fascia is found to be infiltrated with xanthoma cells.

The nontender masses in the tendons are generally only of cosmetic concern, though very occasionally associated tendinitis develops. Very rarely patients may complain of an acute transient arthritis of one or more joints.

Gross examination of tissue obtained from an affected site generally shows a bright yellow nodular lesion, which on microscopic examination reveals packed lipid-laden histiocytes, often with cholesterol clefts.

MEMBRANOUS LIPODYSTROPHY, LIPOMEMBRANOUS POLYCYSTIC OSTEODYSPLASIA (NASU–HAKOLA DISEASE)

A very rare disturbance in lipid metabolism, affecting both the skeleton and the central nervous system, has been described mainly in Japan and Finland, though the disease is not exclusively found in these races. The affected individuals are generally in their twenties or thirties and both sexes are affected.

The patients may initially present with bone pain or pathologic fracture, usually in the hands or feet or around major joints. Later neurologic symptoms occur such as ataxia, tremor or urinary incontinence, or psychiatric disease such as paranoia or even early onset Alzheimer's disease.

Radiographs show well-defined cystic lesions with sclerotic margins in the metaphysis of long bones and in carpal or tarsal bones. Radiographically the axial skeleton is generally not affected (Fig. 9.18).

Microscopically in the affected areas the fatty bone marrow is replaced by characteristic membranous lined cysts which have a markedly papillary and folded appearance. (Since occasionally

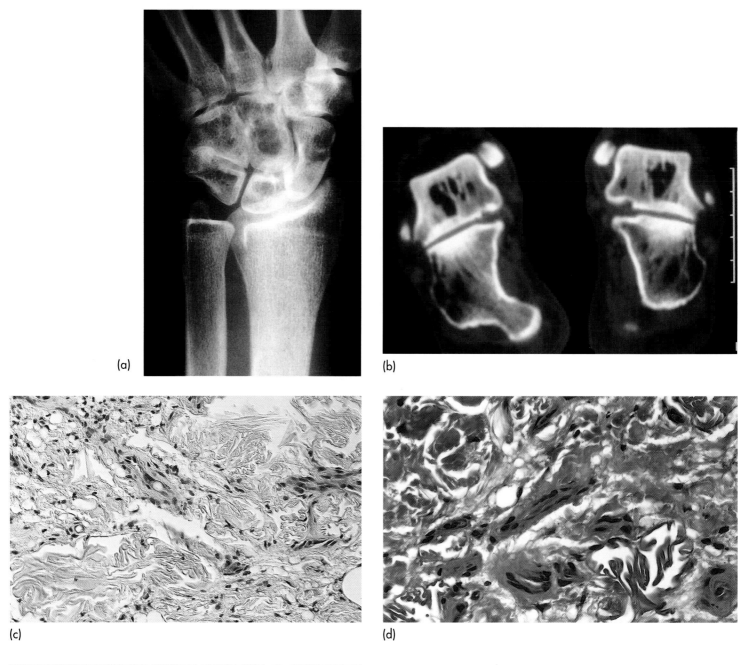

(a)

(b)

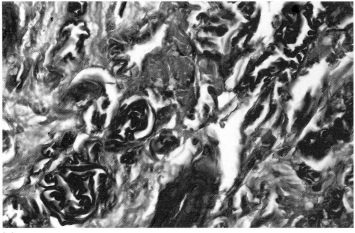

(c)

(d)

(e)

Figure 9.18 (a) Radiograph of the wrist in a patient affected by membranous lipodystrophy shows lytic defects in the carpal bones which would in the absence of clinical information most probably be interpreted as amyloid. (b) CT of the hind foot shows lytic lesions in both the calcaneus and talus. (c) Photomicrograph to demonstrate the characteristic cystic spaces with papillary lipid membranes seen in the affected areas of membranous lipodystrophy (H&E, × 25 obj.). (d) Photomicrograph of section stained with Luxol fast blue to demonstrate the lipid in the membranes (× 50 obj.). (e) Photomicrograph of section stained with PAS (× 50 obj.). (Radiographs and tissue sections, courtesy of Dr Gordon Harloe.)

similar membranous structures are seen in ischemic fat in association with other conditions, the diagnosis of Nasu–Hakola disease is therefore dependent not only on the histology but also on the clinical presentation.)

SKELETAL MANIFESTATIONS OF HEMATOLOGICAL DISEASES

Various hematologic conditions such as the hemolytic anemias, hemoglobinopathies, or bleeding diatheses often lead to bone disease and/or joint damage. (Joint destruction secondary to chronic bloody synovial effusions as seen in patients with hemophilia, will be considered in Chapter 12, p. 306.)

Changes in the cancellous bone are generally secondary to either erythroid hyperplasia, as seen in patients with thalassemia and the hemolytic anemias, or vascular thrombosis with subsequent infarction and infection, as seen in patients with sickle-cell disease.

The severity of disease seen radiographically depends, to a certain extent, on the age of the patient, with children often more dramatically affected.

Location also varies with age. In patients who manifest chronic hematologic disease during infancy, the hands and feet show marked skeletal alterations, whereas in slightly older children the skull may be the predominant site. In the mature skeleton of an adult the most dramatic changes usually affect the pelvis and the spine.

HEMOCHROMATOSIS

Primary hemochromatosis is an HLA-related inherited disease, most prevalent in northern Europe, in which increased iron absorption is associated with the accumulation of iron in various tissues. Early recognition and treatment of this condition can help prevent significant organ damage.

Excessive iron accumulation (especially of the visceral organs and in particular, the heart and liver) may also be caused by massive oral iron intake or by severe chronic hemolytic anemia that requires protracted courses of transfusion therapy. The resulting disease is known as secondary hemochromatosis and this is the commonest form of the condition.

Patients with hemochromatosis often first present when they are in their fifties with liver diseases. When younger patients present, the disease is usually more severe.

In general, the radiographic changes in the bones and joints in hemochromatosis are nonspecific and are best characterized as a noninflammatory arthropathy, classically with involvement of the metacarpophalangeal joints, especially the second and third (Fig. 9.19). Less commonly, large joints, such as the shoulder and elbows (a distribution that is atypical for classic osteoarthritis), are involved. There may be regional osteoporosis as well as peculiar cysts and erosions around the affected joints. Of interest is the associated high incidence of chondrocalcinosis in patients with hemochromatosis (15–30%), which is usually attributed to interference by iron with the enzymatic degradation of pyrophosphates (Fig. 9.20). Grossly the disease may be recognized by a

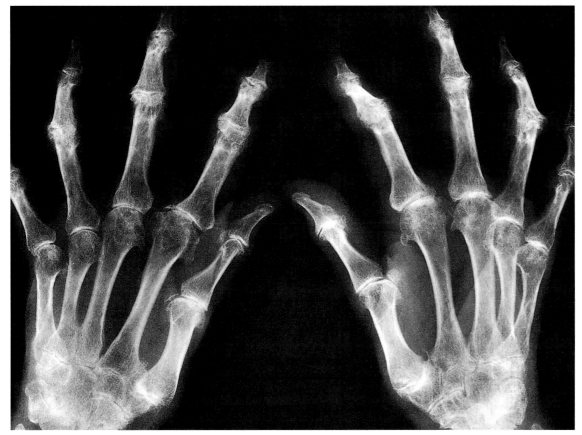

Figure 9.19 Dorsovolar radiograph of both hands of a 53-year-old woman with hemochromatosis. There is a generalized arthropathy which shows beak-like osteophytes arising from the heads of the second and third metacarpals on the radial aspect. The interphalangeal, metacarpophalangeal, and carpal articulations are also affected by severe narrowing, destructive changes and subluxation.

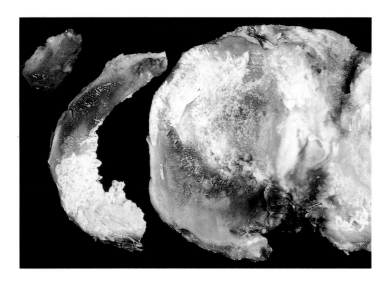

Figure 9.20   Photograph of the medial meniscus and a portion of the arthritic tibial plateau removed from a patient with hemochromatosis. In addition to a dark blue–black staining of residual cartilage, chalk white deposits of calcium pyrophosphate crystals are seen both on the meniscus and over much of the articular surface of the tibia.

generalized mahogany brown coloration of the tissues, which is reflected microscopically as an accumulation of hemosiderin pigment (Fig. 9.21). Treatment should be directed at the underlying disorder that is causing the accumulation of iron.

[The brown discoloration of the joint tissue classically seen in patients with this disorder may easily be confused with local iron deposition from extravasated blood, as seen in patients with traumatic arthropathy or hemophilic arthropathy. (See also Figs 12.62–12.64).]

SICKLE-CELL DISEASE

A number of hematologic diseases result from the formation of abnormal hemoglobin; these conditions are known collectively as the hemoglobinopathies. In sickle-cell disease, a substitution of one of the amino acids in the β-hemoglobin chain leads, under conditions of low oxygen tension, to crystallization of the hemoglobin molecule, which results in formation of abnormal sickle-shaped erythrocytes and to increased hemolysis. The hemolytic anemia in turn leads to bone marrow hyperplasia.

Sickle-cell disease is practically limited to Blacks. It is estimated that about 8–10% of Afro-Americans have the sickle-cell trait (the heterozygous form of sickle-cell hemoglobinopathy); however, only about 0.15% has sickle-cell anemia (the homozygous form of the disorder).

In those patients with sickle-cell anemia who survive into later childhood and adulthood, the clinical course is characterized by alternating exacerbations and remissions. During the remissions, there is persistent anemia, a slight icteric tint of the sclerae, and evidence of sickling of the red blood cells. At unpredictable intervals, there is exacerbation of the disease process (a 'crisis'), during which the anemia may become gradually or rapidly worse. This is characterized by rapid destruction of erythrocytes, with associated fever, increased icterus, nausea, vomiting, abdominal pain, and severe prostration. The crisis is often precipitated by an infection, especially in relation to the respiratory tract.

Other clinical features of the disorder include: enlargement of the liver, enlargement of the spleen (usually only in the younger patients – later the spleen shrinks due to repeated infarcts), cardiac hypertrophy, recurrent chronic ulcers of the legs (especially in the region of the ankles), and episodes of severe pain secondary to infarction in the chest, abdomen, and/or bones and joints.

Radiologic examination of the skeleton may reveal generalized osteoporosis in the spine, often associated with vertebral collapse, wedge-shaped deformities, and kyphoscoliosis (Fig. 9.22). Characteristic changes may also be observed in the phalangeal bones of the hands and feet following infarcts that develop in infancy and interfere with normal growth (Fig. 9.23).

A severe problem in sickle-cell disease is the development of infarcts which may occur in any organ but notably in the spleen. In the skeleton the infarcts may be located anywhere, although they are frequent in the hands and feet, as already discussed, as well as in the femoral head and spine (usually the lower spine). Infarction is often heralded by severe and sudden pain which may awaken the sleeping patient. Initial radiographs are normal, with infarct-related X-ray changes developing only after some months (see Chapter 15).

In addition to compression fractures and wedging fractures secondary to osteoporosis, the spines of affected children may also exhibit a double concavity resulting from collapse of the central portion of the vertebral body under the hyaline growth plate. Rather than being compression fractures caused by mechanical failure, it has been suggested that these lesions are the result of relative ischemia in this region of the vertebral body.

On macroscopic examination the bones show a congested, dusky red appearance, indicative of marked erythroid hyperplasia of the marrow (Figs 9.24 and 9.25). Microscopically the erythrocytes themselves are deformed and often crescent-shaped, which gives rise to the term sickle cell (Fig. 9.26). There may be profound osteoporosis because of marrow impingement on the adjacent trabecular bone structure.

Osteomyelitis is a well-recognized complication of sickle-cell disease, and is usually the result of infection with *Staphylococcus aureus*, however in some cases it is due to infection with the *Salmonella* organism (Fig. 9.27). In the past, this complication often necessitated amputation of the involved extremity (Fig. 9.28).

THALASSEMIA

The several types of thalassemia are characterized by anemia of varying degrees due to a hemoglobin deficiency resulting from suppression of the rate of synthesis of globin chains. Patients with homozygous β-thalassemia are usually severely anemic. Marked marrow hyperplasia (mainly due to erythroid hyperplasia) is associated with profound osteoporosis and the radiographic

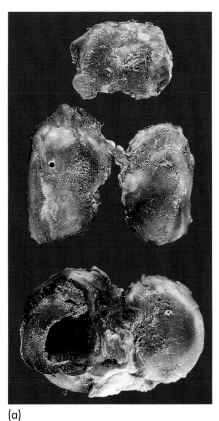

Figure 9.21 (a) Photograph of the articular surfaces of the knee joint of a patient with hemochromatosis. The black–green staining of the cartilage results from the accumulated blood pigment, which eventually interferes with chondrocyte function and hence cartilage matrix metabolism. (Note: the gross and microscopic changes in hemochromatosis are similar to those seen in hemosiderosis. See Figure 12.64.) (b) Photomicrograph demonstrating iron-containing particles within the chondrocytes of hemophilic cartilage (Gomori stain, × 50 obj.).

(a)

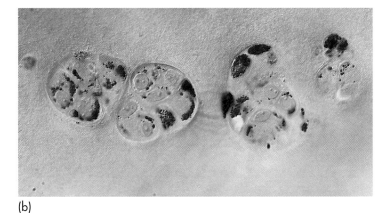

(b)

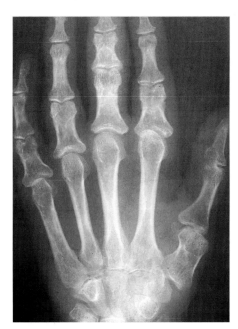

Figure 9.23 Radiograph of the hand of a patient with sickle-cell disease. The shortening of the first metacarpal and of some of the phalanges is secondary to growth disturbances following sickle-cell crises in infancy.

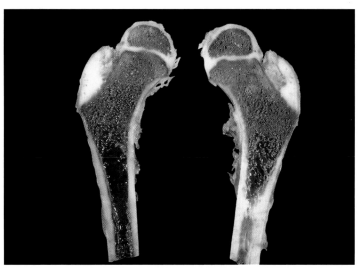

Figure 9.24 Photograph of a frontal section through the femur of a child who died from the complications of sickle-cell disease. Note the dusky reddish-brown appearance of the hyperplastic packed marrow.

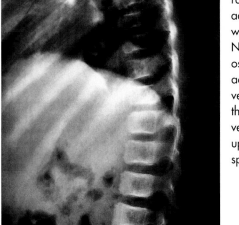

Figure 9.22 Lateral radiograph of an adolescent black male with sickle-cell disease. Note the mild osteopenia, with accentuation of the vertical trabeculae, and the central collapse of the vertebral bodies in the upper and midthoracic spine.

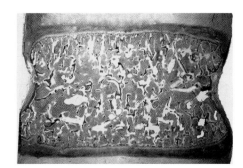

Figure 9.25 Histologic section of a vertebral body from a child with sickle-cell disease. The marrow space is entirely filled with hematopoietic tissue and there is very little fat evident. (Normally the marrow is 50% fat and 50% hematopoietic tissue. Many of the cleared areas seen in the bone marrow in this section are artefactual.) Osteoporosis is also present.

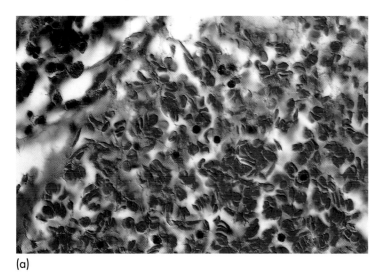

(a)

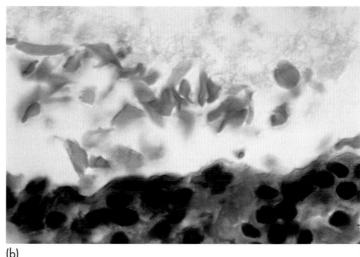

(b)

Figure 9.26   (a) Photomicrograph to demonstrate 'sickle' cells in blood clot (H&E, × 25 obj.). (b) 'Sickled' red cells within the lumen of a blood vessel. (Nomarski differential interference contrast microscopy, H&E, × 100 obj.)

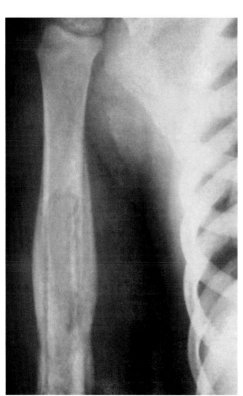

Figure 9.27 Radiograph of the right arm of a patient with sickle-cell disease who has developed a diaphyseal osteomyelitis due to infection with a *Salmonella* organism. Note the large sequestrum and extensive periosteal involucrum.

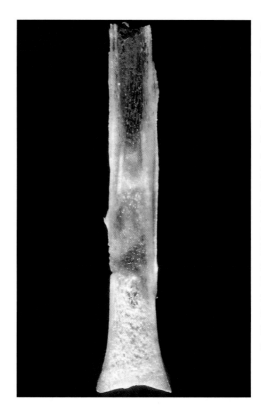

Figure 9.28   Section taken through the tibia from a patient with sickle-cell disease who developed osteomyelitis. The specimen shows extensive necrosis, seen as an opaque yellow coloration of the bone towards the ankle joint, and between the necrotic bone and the living bone above there is a focus of partly viable infected tissue. Surrounding the infected segment there is a periosteal reaction.

changes in children are evident mainly in the skull, long bones, and metacarpals and metatarsals; as the patient matures, there is less involvement of the peripheral skeleton.

In general the long bones show medullary widening with cortical thinning, often with development of 'saber shins'. Involvement of the spine is usually manifested as kyphosis or scoliosis, which results from vertebral collapse. There may be a dramatic widening of the diploic space of the skull, with thinning and displacement of the trabeculae, producing a 'hair-on-end' appearance (Figs 9.29 and 9.30). The hands and feet may exhibit medullary widening and cortical thinning of the metacarpals and metatarsals, which appear on radiographs as a honeycomb pattern (Fig. 9.31). Involvement of the maxillary bones and

sinuses may lead to a peculiar 'rodent' facies. Although osseous changes may be observed radiographically in patients with the mild forms of thalassemia, they are usually much less severe.

Grossly, the bones appear dusky red and are markedly osteopenic (Fig. 9.32). Microscopic examination of bone tissue from severely affected patients reveals dramatic hyperplasia of the marrow, especially of the erythroid components and marked osteopenia, Perl's Prussian blue staining demonstrates marked iron deposition in the bone marrow as well as in zones of mineralization and cement lines (Fig. 9.33).

Occasionally thalassemia is seen in association with sickle-cell disease, and in such cases infarcts may be superimposed on the other symptoms.

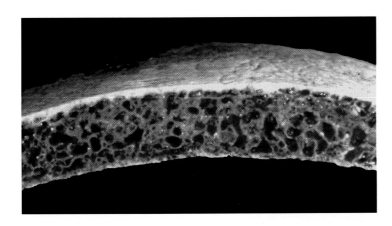

Figure 9.29   Thalassemia: section through the skull shows marked thinning of the inner and outer bone cortices and an open porotic cancellous bone. The mahogany brown color results from extensive iron deposition in the marrow.

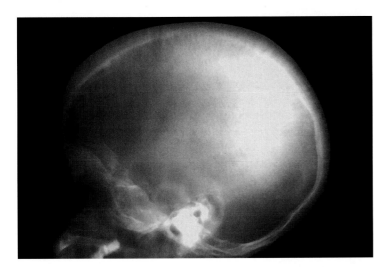

Figure 9.30   Radiograph of the skull of a patient with thalassemia major shows characteristic 'hair-on-end' appearance.

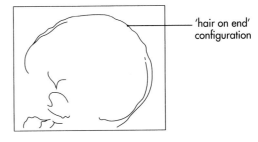

'hair on end' configuration

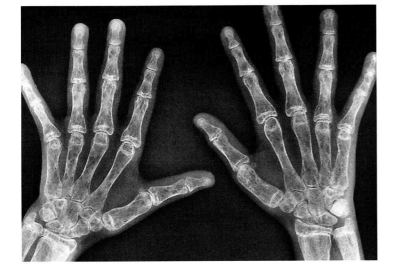

Figure 9.31   Radiograph of the hands in a patient with thalassemia shows severe osteoporosis with a 'honeycomb' and cystic pattern of the cancellous bone.

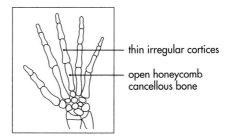

thin irregular cortices

open honeycomb cancellous bone

MYELOFIBROSIS (AGNOGENIC MYELOID METAPLASIA)

Myelofibrosis, a relatively uncommon disease, is characterized by marrow fibrosis with granulocytic hyperplasia of the hematopoietic elements and the slow development of extramedullary hematopoiesis. The disease occurs with about equal frequency in men and women, and is more common clinically among older individuals. The symptoms are progressive anemia and hepatosplenomegaly.

In approximately 50% of cases on radiographic examination,

the bones, particularly of the axial skeleton, show a diffuse but occasionally patchy sclerosis. The bony sclerosis, in combination with the marrow fibrosis, accounts for the frequency of 'dry taps' when marrow aspiration is attempted. Approximately half of all adult patients exhibit dramatic involvement of the spine, pelvis, ribs, sternum, proximal humerus, and femur (the common sites of adult hematopoiesis). The skull is rarely involved. The involved bones are not expanded and there is no change in their contour. The differential diagnosis is usually not difficult because of the diffuse sclerosis that occurs in this condition. Rarely, this disease may be closely mimicked by some cases of metastatic carcinoma

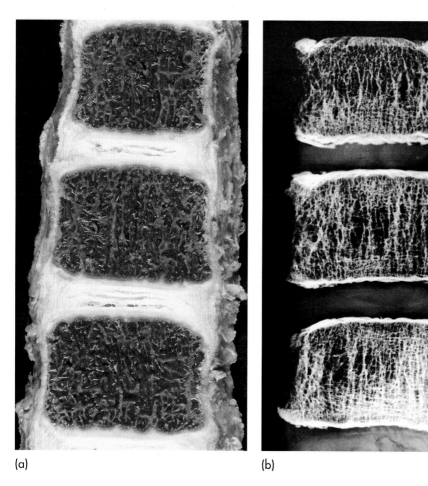

(a)   (b)

Figure 9.32 (a) Segment of the vertebral column from a young patient with thalassemia major. The bone marrow is mahogany brown in color. (b) Radiograph of the specimen reveals marked osteopenia.

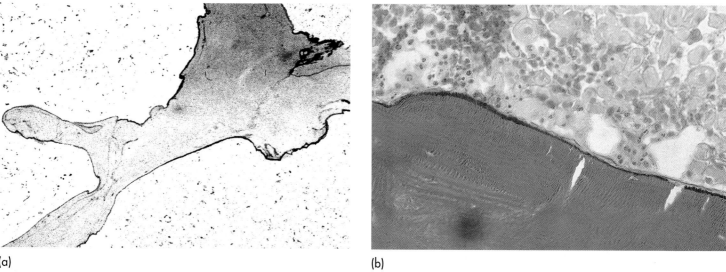

(a)   (b)

Figure 9.33 (a) Thalassemia: photomicrograph of a section of bone stained with Perls' stain, which stains iron a blue color. It can be appreciated that as well as extensive iron deposits throughout the bone marrow, the mineralization fronts and cement lines within the bone are also heavily stained (iron stain, × 4 obj.). (b) Higher power photomicrograph shows the location of iron at the mineralization front (× 25 obj.).

and the rare osteosclerotic form of myelomatosis. Rare cases of spinal cord compression resulting from an extradural mass of hematopoietic tissue have been reported. About 20% of patients with myelofibrosis eventually develop acute myelogenous leukemia.

Microscopic examination of the marrow shows obliterative fibrosis in the late stages. In early stages, marked marrow hyperplasia and bizarre cell types may be seen, as well as an increase in reticulum fiber production. When viewed with polarized light, the thickened bone may be found to have a largely woven appearance (Fig. 9.34).

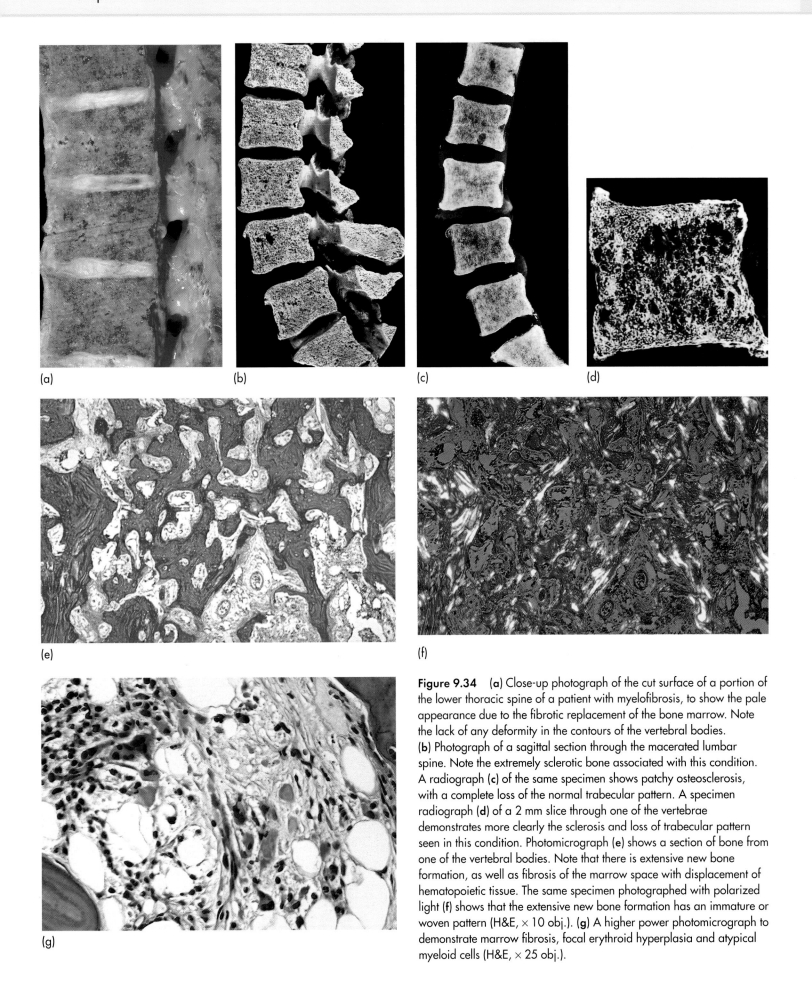

(a)　　　　(b)　　　　(c)　　　　(d)

(e)

(f)

(g)

Figure 9.34 (a) Close-up photograph of the cut surface of a portion of the lower thoracic spine of a patient with myelofibrosis, to show the pale appearance due to the fibrotic replacement of the bone marrow. Note the lack of any deformity in the contours of the vertebral bodies. (b) Photograph of a sagittal section through the macerated lumbar spine. Note the extremely sclerotic bone associated with this condition. A radiograph (c) of the same specimen shows patchy osteosclerosis, with a complete loss of the normal trabecular pattern. A specimen radiograph (d) of a 2 mm slice through one of the vertebrae demonstrates more clearly the sclerosis and loss of trabecular pattern seen in this condition. Photomicrograph (e) shows a section of bone from one of the vertebral bodies. Note that there is extensive new bone formation, as well as fibrosis of the marrow space with displacement of hematopoietic tissue. The same specimen photographed with polarized light (f) shows that the extensive new bone formation has an immature or woven pattern (H&E, × 10 obj.). (g) A higher power photomicrograph to demonstrate marrow fibrosis, focal erythroid hyperplasia and atypical myeloid cells (H&E, × 25 obj.).

ARTHRITIS

THE DYSFUNCTIONAL JOINT

'Norms are recognized as such only through infractions. Functions are revealed only by their breakdown'
Georges Canguilhelm, Le normal et le pathologique (Paris, 1966)

Joint dysfunction (arthritis) is characterized clinically by instability, loss of motion, maldistribution of load and associated pain. Normal joint function is characterized by: the maintenance of stability during use; freedom of the opposed articular surfaces to move painlessly over each other within the required range of motion; correct distribution of load across joint tissues, which might otherwise be damaged by overloading or become atrophied because of habitual underloading (disuse).

The function is fulfilled through the architecture of the joint and the mechanical properties of the matrices of the connective tissues of which the joint is constructed. The geometry of the articulating surfaces is particularly important and an intact neuromuscular system essential.

FUNCTION AND ANATOMY

The three interdependent aspects of joint function (stability, motion, and load distribution) depend on three features of joint design as will be discussed.

GEOMETRY OF OPPOSED ARTICULATING SURFACES OF THE JOINT

Perhaps the most obvious feature of any joint is its shape. In general, one joint surface is convex, whereas the other is concave. The convex or 'male' side of the joint usually has a larger articular surface than the concave or 'female' side. These complementary shapes of the joint surfaces are necessary to permit the normal range of motion, provide stability, and ensure the most equitable loading during use (Fig. 10.1).

In some joints (for example, the hip and the ankle) the articular surfaces appear at first sight to fit very exactly (i.e. they appear to be congruent). However, in other joints (e.g. knee and finger joints) it is readily apparent that the surfaces are incongruent. For a long time it was believed that congruence was a normal feature of a joint. However, the concept of congruence in all positions of the joint would imply that all joint surfaces were perfectly spherical, which they are not, and therefore no normal joint can be congruent in all positions, though it may be more congruent in one position than in others.

In many joints, of which the knee is a notable example, the gross incongruence of the opposed surfaces are partially compensated for by the interposed, pliable intra-articular fibrocartilaginous menisci. [These latter structures constitute an important component contributing to joint shape and function, and cannot be removed without significant consequences (Fig. 10.2).]

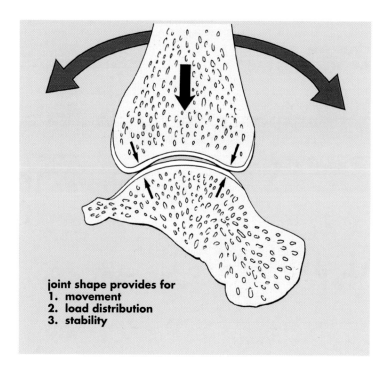

Figure 10.1   The physiologic incongruity between the articular surfaces also allows access for the synovial fluid, important for both nutrition and lubrication.

joint shape provides for
1. **movement**
2. **load distribution**
3. **stability**

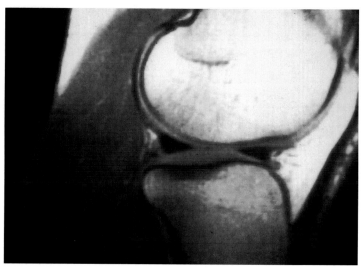

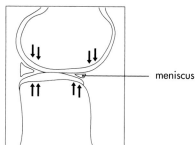

meniscus

Figure 10.2   A lateral MRI of a normal knee shows the gross incongruity of the cartilaginous surfaces partially corrected by the interposed menisci, which act as load-bearing structures.

Because the tissues of the joint undergo elastic deformation under load (particularly the cartilage but also the bone), as the load increases the surfaces of the joint come into increasing contact, thereby distributing the load more equitably (Fig. 10.3). Both the incongruence and the deformation of the joint space under loading conditions provide for the circulation and mixing of the synovial fluid essential to the metabolism of the chondrocytes.

MECHANICAL PROPERTIES OF EXTRACELLULAR MATRICES OF BONE, CARTILAGE, AND OTHER CONNECTIVE TISSUES

Most investigators since William Hunter have recognized the importance of the articular cartilage in the physiology of a joint. As Hunter noted in 1743, 'the articulating cartilages are most happily contrived to all purposes of motion in those parts. By

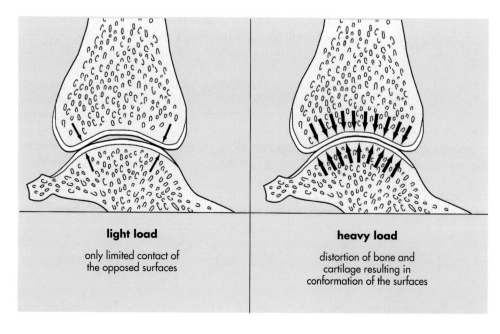

light load

only limited contact of the opposed surfaces

heavy load

distortion of bone and cartilage resulting in conformation of the surfaces

Figure 10.3   The dimensions of the interarticular space change with both load and position. These changes provide for circulation of the synovial fluid and also for the pumping of synovial fluid through the cartilage matrix.

their uniform surface, they move upon one another with ease; by their soft, smooth and slippery surface, mutual abrasion is prevented; by their flexibility, the contiguous surfaces are constantly adapted to each other and the friction diffused equally over the whole; by their elasticity, the violence of any shock, which may happen in running, jumping, etc. is broken and gradually spent; which must have been extremely pernicious, if the hard surfaces of bones had been immediately contiguous.' Hunter has in these few sentences perfectly summarized the function of cartilage. However, it needs to be recognized that the joint is an organ system that also includes the bone beneath the cartilage and the ligaments which conjoin the articular bone ends. Alterations in the mechanical properties of bone or disruption of the ligaments may have equally disastrous effects on joint function as alterations in cartilage properties.

The physical properties of connective tissues are determined by their extracellular matrices. In each of the different connective tissues, as well as in each particular structure, the matrices have a unique composition and organization which provide for mechanical function at that locus. Some of the details of this organization have already been discussed in Chapter 1.

The connective tissue matrices are both synthesized and broken down by their intrinsic cells (e.g. osteoblasts, osteocytes, osteoclasts, chondrocytes). In maintaining the physicochemical and mechanical properties of tissues, the function of these cells must be subject to highly sensitive feedback systems involving both local and systemic factors which are only now beginning to be studied (Fig. 10.4).

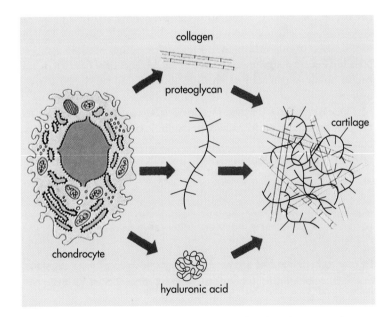

Figure 10.4 Diagrammatic representation of a chondrocyte to show some of its metabolic functions. In this diagram, the anabolic activity of the chondrocyte is stressed, but the chondrocyte also has a catabolic role, producing substances which break down the cartilage matrix.

INTEGRITY OF LIGAMENTS, MUSCLES, AND TENDONS SUPPORTING THE JOINT AND THEIR NEUROMUSCULAR CONTROLS

Functional joint anatomy must include a consideration of the ligamentous conjoining of the articulating surfaces as well as of the neuromuscular control of joint motion. Sensory feedback monitors our movements through the perception of touch, temperature, pain, and position. During childhood we explore, learn, practice, and perfect skills that will eventually become automatic. The fact that some of us develop better athletic skills than others is perhaps not as dependent on strength and endurance as it is on optimization of the sensory modulation of movement. Correct joint function is thus dependent on intact ligaments and neuromuscular coordination (Fig. 10.5). As recognized by Charcot in the nineteenth century, a breakdown of neuromuscular coordination can lead to profound arthritis.

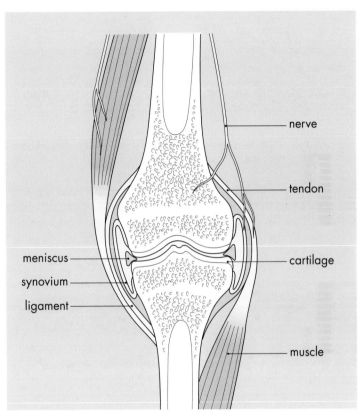

Figure 10.5 A joint should be thought of not only in terms of the articular cartilage and synovial lining, but also as a mechanical system which includes all the surrounding ligaments, tendons, sensory and motor nerves, and muscles.

NORMAL JOINT PHYSIOLOGY

Anatomy is concerned with the structure of living things, physiology with their normal dynamic phenomena. Wolff's law states that bone density and bone architecture correlate with the magnitude and direction of applied load. In the articular end of a bone, this implies that the subchondral bone trabeculae must also undergo a self-regulated modeling which maintains a joint shape capable of optimal load distribution. In other words, the shape of bones, including the articular ends, reflects a dynamic state that also incorporates a feedback dependent on mechanical stress.

One mechanism for both growth and bone modeling is endochondral ossification. This process is exemplified in the epiphyseal growth plate, where calcified cartilage is invaded by blood vessels from the metaphyseal bone and replaced by bone tissue synthesized by osteoblasts lying close to the invading blood vessels (see Chapter 1, p. 31). Studies of adult joints have shown that replacement of the calcified layer of articular cartilage by bone tissue involves a similar process.

Blood vessels from the subchondral bone penetrate the calcified zone of the articular cartilage and alongside the channels, which are created by this process, new bone is laid down; thus the calcified cartilage is slowly replaced by new subchondral bone (Figs 10.6 and 10.7). Replacement of the calcified zone of cartilage by bone might be expected to result in its eventual disappearance. However, histologic study of articular cartilage from subjects of various ages shows that this does not happen. The calcified zone of articular cartilage remains much the same

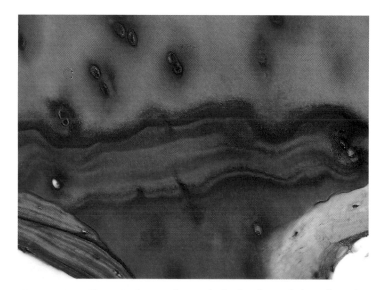

Figure 10.6   The articular cartilage is locked to the underlying bone by a layer of calcified cartilage. The edge of the calcified zone is marked by a basophilic line – the tidemark. With accelerated rates of calcification, many tidemarks may be present and unless ossification of the calcified zone takes place, the calcified layer will become thicker (H&E, × 25 obj.).

thickness throughout life because the calcification front (tidemark) continues to advance into the noncalcified cartilage at a slow rate which is in equilibrium with the rate of replacement from the subchondral bone. Therefore, it is postulated that articular cartilage is not a static tissue, as it was long believed to be. The extracellular matrix and the chondrocytes are replaced throughout life, and the joint undergoes continuous remodeling (see also Fig. 1.56).

Heterogeneity of cartilage tissue including both morphological and biochemical variations, can be observed within different regions of a normal weight-bearing joint. For example there is a variation in stiffness in different areas of the femoral head which has been related both to proteoglycan (PG) content and to the amount of water held by the tissue.

Another example of normal geographic variation can be observed in the tibial plateau of man as well as other animals, where there are distinct morphological differences between articular cartilage which is covered and that which is not covered by the meniscus. These differences consist of a rough surface and soft matrix in the uncovered area as compared to the smooth, firm areas covered by the menisci. We have examined adult human as well as dog knee joints at autopsy and found that articular cartilage not covered by meniscus always showed matrix softening and superficial fibrillation. The morphologic and biochemical findings in these two distinct articular areas as studies in the adult dog are summarized in Figure 10.8.

We hypothesize that these naturally occurring variations in matrix structure and mechanical properties are related to joint loading experienced in normal everyday use.

In the normally functioning knee, load is transmitted through the meniscus and onto the tibial cartilage underlying the meniscus, whereas the exposed cartilage that is not covered by the meniscus remains relatively underloaded. Other similar areas of possible disuse atrophy have been described around the rim of the radial head, in the roof of the acetabulum and on the perifoveal and inferomedial aspects of the femoral head.

The extracellular matrix of the cartilage and of the other connective tissues is synthesized by their intrinsic cells under the control of both local and systemic factors. Both in vivo and in vitro studies have demonstrated that changes in the immediate

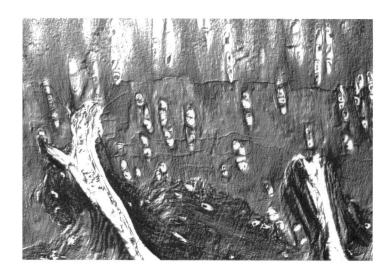

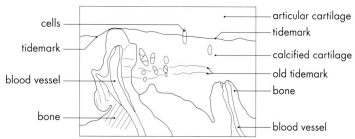

Figure 10.7   Photomicrograph to demonstrate vascular invasion of the calcified region of articular cartilage with subsequent bone formation (H&E, × 10 obj.).

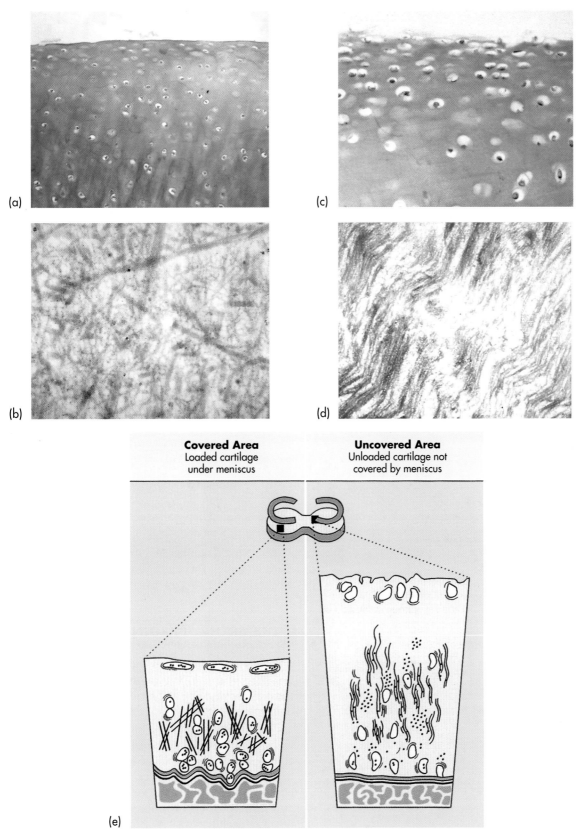

Figure 10.8 Summary of morphology and biochemistry. (**a**) In the covered area of the tibial plateau, the surface is smooth and covered by an amorphous electron-dense layer. The chondrocytes are flattened (H&E, × 4 obj.). With respect to lipid, there is an increased intracellular accumulation in all three layers, an increased extracellular matrix accumulation at the surface, and increased numbers of extracellular matrix vesicles in the deep zone. (**b**) Collagen appears in the electron microscope as randomly oriented fibers with thicker mean diameters; there is regular binding of PG to the collagen fibers, and the concentration of PG per wet weight is increased. (**c**) In the uncovered area, the surface is irregular, with a detached electron-dense layer. The cells are round (H&E, × 10 obj.). (**d**) Collagen appears in wavy aggregated bundles with thinner mean diameters (small range). An increased amount of PG can be extracted from the matrix. In both the covered and the uncovered areas, there is the same amount of DNA per dry weight of cartilage tissue. (**e**) Summary diagram of the differences in loaded and unloaded cartilage. Note that in the covered area the tidemark is irregular, whereas in the uncovered area the tidemark is smooth.

environment of the joint lead to alterations of the cartilage matrix. Thus, immobilization or unloading of a joint results in decreased synthesis of glycosaminoglycans (Fig. 10.9). Conversely, exercise appears to increase synthesis. These experimentally induced variations are in agreement with naturally observed topographic variations in joints which have been ascribed to normally occurring patterns of loading that affect the joints. In general, it seems that low levels of mechanical stress (i.e. below the physiologic range) are associated with enhanced catabolic activity, whereas stress within the physiologic range is associated with increased anabolic activity. Under conditions of supraphysiologic stress the chondrocytes are unable to adapt. In other words, there is a window of physiologic stress above or below which the chondrocytes cannot maintain an adequate functional matrix (Fig. 10.10).

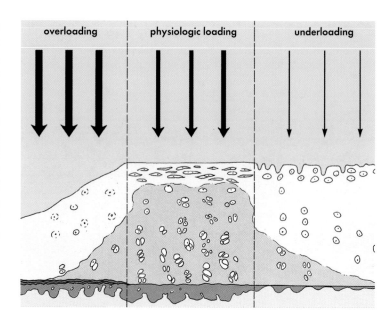

Figure 10.10 The continued optimal functional integrity of connective tissue depends on balanced rates of matrix production and breakdown by the cells. Healthy cartilage (center) results from a physiologic range of stress that maintains optimal chondrocyte activity. If this range of stress is exceeded (left), the result is cell injury and eventual necrosis (in cartilage, this is called chondrolysis). If the stress is inadequate (right), disuse atrophy, i.e. lack of adequate matrix production by the cells, may occur. In cartilage, this is associated with increased water content of the matrix and superficial fibrillation of the collagen as well as other changes (see Figure 10.8).

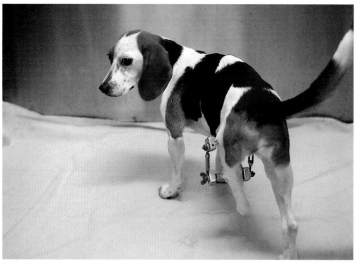

(a)

(b)

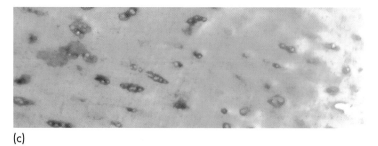

(c)

Figure 10.9 (a) This dog had a distraction device placed across the left knee joint to produce unloading of the joint. (b) Photomicrograph of articular cartilage harvested from the unloaded joint shown in (a), demonstrating diminished PG staining. In (c) a portion of normal control cartilage from the right knee is shown for comparison (Alcian blue stain, × 4 obj.).

Although a number of substances have been implicated in the transduction of mechanical stimuli to metabolic events, the exact mechanism remains unclear.

THE ARTHRITIC JOINT

Arthritis is a clinical term which describes the consequences of a breakdown in the joint's normal function. These dysfunctions include loss of capacity for the articulating surfaces to move over one another easily, loss of joint stability, and, almost always, pain.

The loss of freedom of motion with its associated instability and pain is associated with a change in joint shape and/or a change in the tissue matrices themselves, which in turn affects their mechanical properties. Instability may result from alterations in ligamentous support and neuromuscular control. Pain may have a variety of sources: it may originate in the bone, as a result of maldistribution of load; in the synovium, as a result of reactive synovitis; or in the muscle as a consequence of reflex spasm.

It follows therefore that malfunction of a joint can be caused by acute or chronic injuries that produce either:

- Anatomic alterations in the shape of the articulating surfaces, e.g. a fracture (Fig. 10.11)
- Loss of integrity of the cartilage matrix or support structures around the joint, e.g. by an inflammatory or traumatic destruction of ligaments, tendons or capsular tissue

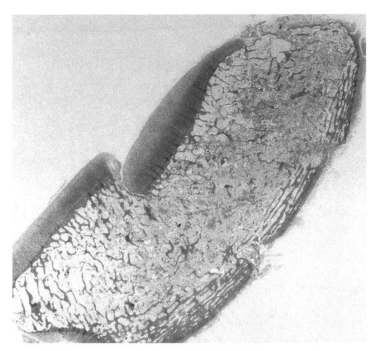

Figure 10.11 A section through a patella which has sustained a transarticular fracture. Such a change in the contour of an articular surface will lead rapidly to degenerative arthritic changes (H&E, × 1 obj.).

destruction. However, in OA, although bone and cartilage loss play an important part in the process, it is the addition of new bone and cartilage in the form of osteophytes, particularly at the joint periphery and sometimes beneath the articular surface, that forms one of the characteristic features of the disease (Fig. 10.12).

A change in joint shape, either sudden, as with a fracture, or gradual, resulting from altered rates of modeling, as in acromegaly or Paget's disease, may play an important role in the etiology of arthritis.

Tissue alterations

Before discussing the gross and microscopic findings in the cartilage, bone, and synovial tissues of arthritic joints, perhaps it is necessary to emphasize the following:

- Regardless of the cause, joint injury is characterized by certain basic cellular and tissue responses. There is usually macroscopic and microscopic evidence of both degeneration and repair and there are alterations both in the cells and in the extracellular matrix. (The changes in the extracellular matrix may result from direct physical injury, alteration in the cellular synthesis of the matrix, or its enzymatic breakdown.)

- Alterations in the mechanical properties of the tissue matrices making up the joint, due to disturbances affecting matrix synthesis (e.g. ochronosis) or enzymatic degradation of the matrix resulting from inflammation [e.g. rheumatoid arthritis (RA)].

During the past century on the basis of their characteristic individual clinical presentations and their morbid anatomy, several forms of arthritis have been well delineated. These include the infectious arthritides, both granulomatous and pyogenic; metabolic arthritis (e.g. gout and ochronosis); and the various 'rheumatic syndromes' that have been classified according to their clinical and immunologic characteristics. Histologically, these rheumatic inflammatory arthritides show a destructive pattern but are difficult to differentiate from each other solely by microscopic examination. However, even when these various etiologies have been considered, there remain an enormous number of cases of arthritis affecting especially certain small joints of the hands and feet and some larger joints, of which the hip and knee are particularly commonly involved. These cases, which run a chronic course, are essentially noninflammatory and usually occur in older individuals. The clinical presentation and morbid anatomy in these cases are similar enough for all of them to be classified under the general appellation of osteoarthritis (OA). In the majority of cases the etiology is poorly understood.

MORBID ANATOMY OF THE ARTHRITIC JOINT

Shape

A change in joint shape, resulting from cartilage and bone loss, is a characteristic result of most forms of arthritis. In the inflammatory arthritides the tissue loss results from inflammatory

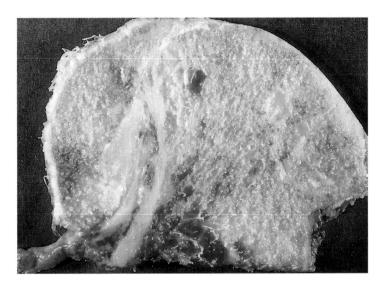

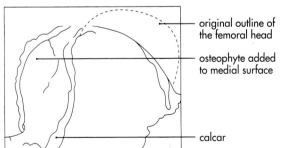

— original outline of the femoral head

— osteophyte added to medial surface

— calcar

Figure 10.12 Photograph of a slice through an arthritic femoral head in which, despite the loss of bone from the superior surface, the contour has been restored to something approaching sphericity by a large medial osteophyte, which is seen to extend well down the medial femoral neck. Note also the increase in transverse diameter of the head (almost 60% greater than the original diameter), a typical finding in OA of the hip as well as other joints.

- In vascularized tissues, injury is followed by an acute and then a chronic inflammatory response. As a result, the necrotic injured tissue is removed and replaced by proliferative vascular tissue (granulation tissue). The inflammatory response results in 'repair' of injured tissue by fibrous scar. Independently of scarring, a second mode of repair involves regeneration of tissue similar to that which was injured originally.

- In nonvascularized tissue, such as cartilage, an inflammatory response and subsequent scarring cannot occur, however this does not preclude tissue regeneration. (Note that cartilage injury always eventually invokes an inflammatory response, since some vascularized tissues, i.e. bone and/or synovium, are inevitably involved.)

Cartilage injury and repair

Macroscopic evidence of injury to cartilage is evident only in the extracellular matrix, mainly the collagenous component, and one of the earliest findings is a disruption of the surface which, instead of being smooth, becomes rough and/or eroded.

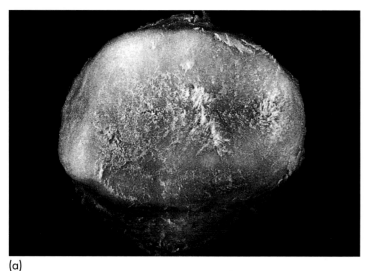

(a)

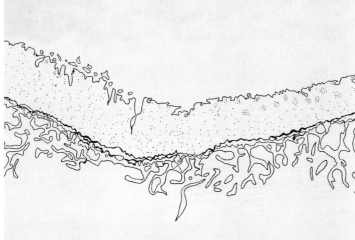

(b)

Figure 10.13 (a) Photograph of the articular surface of a patella obtained from a young individual at autopsy shows fibrillation of the superficial cartilage [photographed using ultraviolet (UV) light]. (b) Drawing to demonstrate the microscopic appearance of fibrillation.

Three patterns of collagenous injury can be identified: fibrillation, erosion (ulceration) and cracking.

The term fibrillation is used to describe replacement of the normally smooth, shiny surface by a surface similar to cut velvet (Fig. 10.13). This type of transformation can be observed both on very thick cartilage, such as the patella, and on very thin cartilage, such as that found in the interphalangeal joints. The 'pile' of the fibrillated area may be short or shaggy. The junction between the fibrillated area and the adjacent normal appearing cartilage is usually well defined and generally distinct.

There appear to be two patterns of fibrillation. Well-defined areas of fibrillation affect particular locations in certain joints and are present in everyone from an early age. It is suggested that these areas are related to underloading of the cartilage. In osteoarthritic joints there are areas of fibrillation which appear in different areas of the joint than those previously alluded to, and which appear to be secondary to mechanical erosion of the cartilage surface. The microscopic characterization of these two distinct types of fibrillation is incomplete, but perhaps the latter is distinguished by deeper clefts and when examined microscopically a greater tendency to form cartilage clones (see later).

Cartilage erosion, or solution of the surface, is characteristic of progressive degenerative changes in the joint. The base of the erosion appears initially to be either contoured or smooth. Tissue damage may eventually be so extensive as to completely denude the bone surface of its cartilage cover (eburnation) (Fig. 10.14).

The last form of structural lesion in this group, which is distinctly less common than either fibrillation or ulceration, is cracking of the cartilage. These cracks extend vertically deep into the cartilage and microscopically often have a deep horizontal component (Fig. 10.15).

In considering the pathogenesis of these three histologic types of cartilage matrix damage, it is important to recognize that in the early stages of OA, they may affect the opposed articular surfaces in different areas and to different degrees (Fig. 10.16). This is in marked contrast to eburnation, in which both of the opposed surfaces are affected. It therefore appears that in many cases fibrillation and other cartilage alteration cannot be solely ascribed as they usually are to 'wear and tear' as the opposed articular surfaces move over each other.

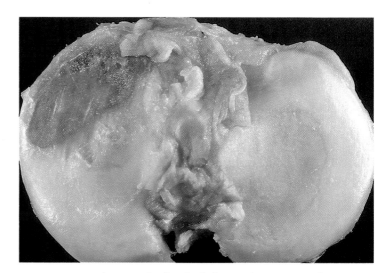

Figure 10.14 Photograph of a tibial plateau demonstrates deep cartilage erosion with exposed polished (eburnated) subchondral bone.

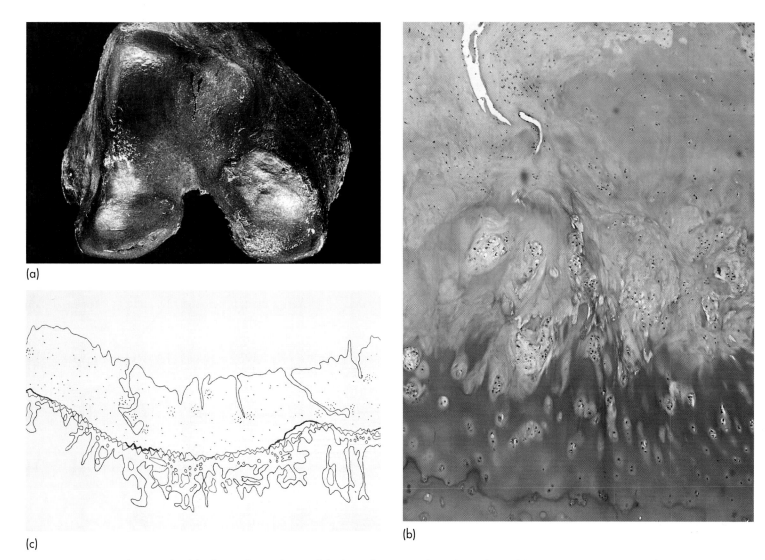

Figure 10.15   (a) Photograph of the femoral articulation of the knee shows a 'Y-shaped' cracking of the cartilage in the patello–femoral joint (photographed using UV light). (b) Photomicrograph of a section taken through a crack in the articular surface, showing the defect extending deep into the cartilage with focal degenerative changes in the surrounding tissue (H&E, × 4 obj.). (c) Drawing to illustrate the microscopic changes with deep cracks in the cartilage.

An increase in the ratio of water to PG in the cartilage matrix leads to softening of the cartilage (chondromalacia) (Figs 10.17 and 10.18). Chondromalacia and fibrillation usually occur together, but chondromalacia may be present before there is any obvious gross evidence of fibrillation.

Cellular injury is recognizable only under a microscope. Necrosis can be identified when only the ghost outlines of the chondrocytes remain. This ghosting, usually scattered but focal in distribution, is a common finding in arthritis (Fig. 10.19). Less often, all of the chondrocytes are seen to be necrotic (Fig. 10.20).

Just as the effect of injury to the articular cartilage is reflected by both the matrix and the cells, so too is the effect of subsequent cartilage regeneration. Within the pre-existing cartilage matrix there is focal cell proliferation with clumps, or clones, of chondrocytes (Fig. 10.21) and, when the tissue is stained with toluidine blue, there is often intense metachromasia of the matrix around these clumps of proliferating chondrocytes, evidence of increased PG synthesis. This process can be thought of as 'intrinsic' repair.

In a damaged joint, extrinsic repair by new cartilage may be initiated from either or both of two possible sites: either in the joint margin or in the subchondral bone. Extrinsic repair of cartilage, which develops from the joint margin, can be seen as a cellular layer of cartilage extending over, and sometimes dissecting into, the existing cartilage (Fig. 10.22). This extrinsically repaired cartilage is usually much more cellular than the pre-existing articular cartilage, and the chondrocytes are evenly distributed throughout the matrix (Figs 10.23 and 10.24).

On microscopic examination of H&E sections this type of repair cartilage can easily be overlooked. However, examination under polarized light will clearly demonstrate the discontinuity between the collagen network of the repair cartilage and that of the pre-existing cartilage (Fig. 10.25).

In arthritic joints in which loss of the articular cartilage has denuded the underlying bone, and especially in cases of OA, there are frequently small pits in the bone surface, from which protrude small nodules of firm, white tissue. On microscopic examination these nodules have the appearance of fibrocartilage and arise in

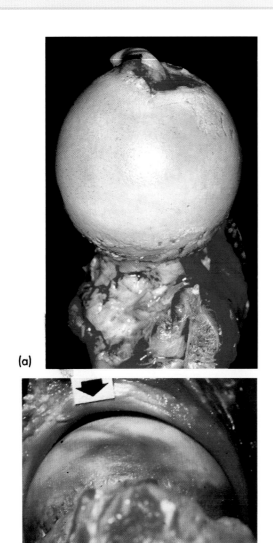

(a)

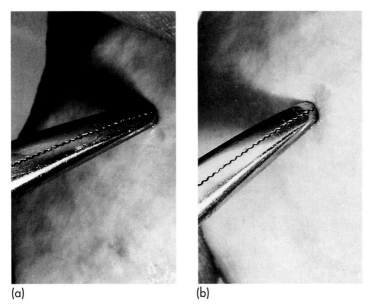

(c)

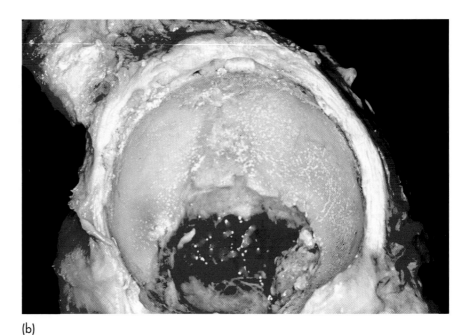

(b)

Figure 10.16 (a) Photograph of the superior surface of the right femoral head removed from an 86-year-old male. Note the generally smooth, intact articular surface. However, there is a superficial ulcer adjacent to the fovea and some roughening around the periphery of the femoral head. This photograph should be compared with (b). (b) The acetabulum of the hip joint shown in (a) demonstrates superficial erosion and fibrillation of the articular cartilage in the supero-lateral portion. Degenerative changes in this portion of the acetabulum are present in all adults, probably as a result of disuse atrophy, even though this area is often regarded as the 'weight-bearing area' of the hip joint. However, as is discussed in Chapter 1 and at the beginning of this chapter, joints are incongruent and the incongruence in the hip is at the dome of the acetabulum as shown in (c). (c) In the normal hip the femoral head articulates with the acetabulum with initial contact anteriorly and posteriorly. The roof of the acetabulum probably comes into contact with the femoral head only under certain load conditions.

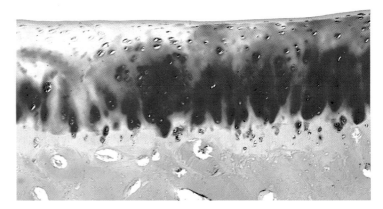

(a) (b)

Figure 10.17 (a) Normal cartilage is firm but resilient and can be compressed with some degree of pressure (exerted here by a hemostat). However, as the cartilage softens or becomes chondromalacic it also becomes palpably softer (b).

Figure 10.18 Intense staining of PG on the right is seen in this photomicrograph of normal cartilage. However, in soft chondromalacic cartilage (on the left), PG loss in the upper half of the cartilage matrix is seen by the decreased intensity of staining (safranin O, × 10 obj.).

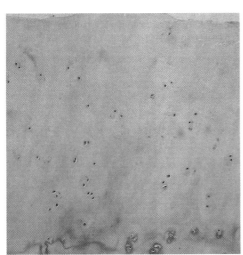

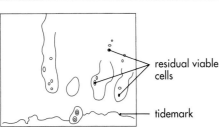

residual viable cells

tidemark

Figure 10.19
Photomicrograph demonstrates areas of the cartilage matrix with no visible chondrocytes, a consequence of focal cell necrosis (H&E, × 10 obj.).

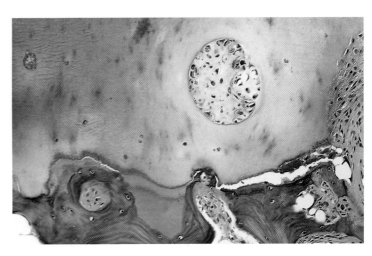

Figure 10.21 Photomicrograph of a portion of largely nonviable cartilage demonstrates a large nest of proliferating chondrocytes in the deep zone (H&E, × 10 obj.).

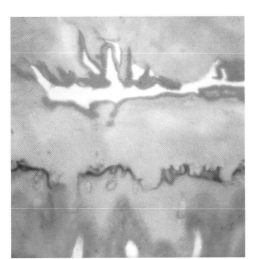

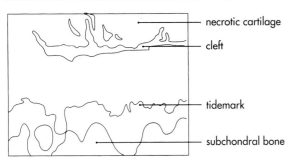

necrotic cartilage

cleft

tidemark

subchondral bone

Figure 10.20
Photomicrograph to demonstrate total cartilage necrosis. Note also the horizontal cleft resulting from failure of the cartilage matrix to resist shear forces within its substance (H&E, × 10 obj.).

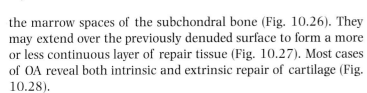

(a)

(b)

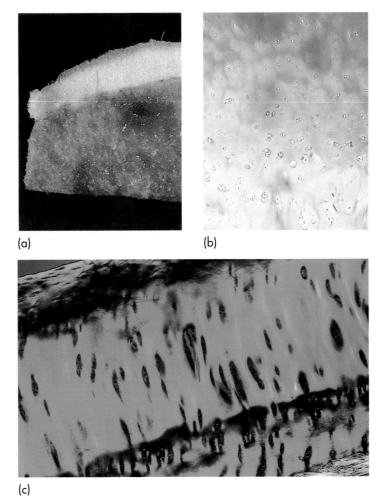

(c)

the marrow spaces of the subchondral bone (Fig. 10.26). They may extend over the previously denuded surface to form a more or less continuous layer of repair tissue (Fig. 10.27). Most cases of OA reveal both intrinsic and extrinsic repair of cartilage (Fig. 10.28).

The chondrocytes themselves are intimately involved in both the breakdown and synthesis of cartilage matrix and a wide

Figure 10.22 Gross specimen (**a**) demonstrates intrinsic cartilage repair, as evidenced by a white, wedge-shaped opaque area between the normal surface and the normal deeper cartilage. Photomicrograph of this area (**b**) shows proliferating cells, cell clumping, and disarrayed collagen. Under polarized light (**c**), one can more easily see the disarrayed collagen in the central area of the cartilage (× 4 obj.).

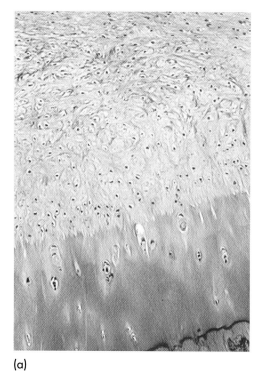 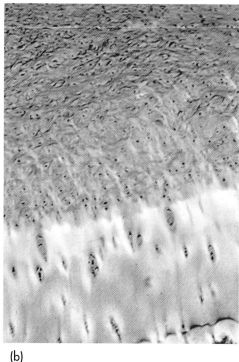

(a) (b)

Figure 10.23 After cartilage damage there may be regeneration of both normal cells and matrix. **(a)** The photomicrograph shows residual normal cartilage covered by a thick layer of reparative cartilage. **(b)** When viewed under polarized light, as here, one can appreciate the alteration in the collagen structure of the matrix.

The concept of articular cartilage repair is an important consideration in the management of patients with arthritis (H&E, ×10 obj.).

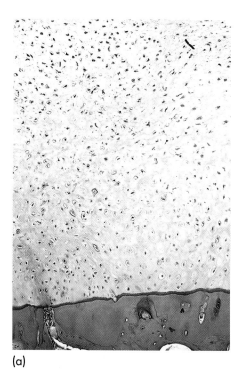 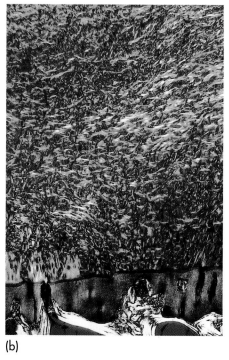

(a) (b)

Figure 10.24 **(a)** A section through the articular surface of an arthritic joint demonstrates extrinsic reparative fibrocartilage, which extends to the tidemark of the original articular hyaline cartilage (H&E, × 4 obj.). **(b)** The same field photographed with polarized light shows the coarse collagen fibers in the reparative cartilage and the discontinuity of the collagen between the calcified zone and the reparative cartilage above.

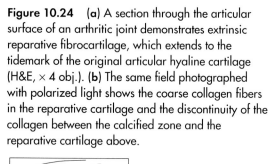
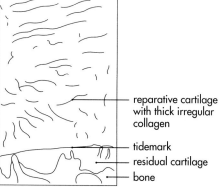

reparative cartilage
with thick irregular
collagen

tidemark
residual cartilage
bone

range of growth factors and cytokines are involved in these processes, both as part of the regulation of normal matrix and in the processes involved in the repair of osteoarthritic cartilage. The enzymes which break down collagen and PG, the metalloproteinases, are themselves regulated by proinflammatory cytokines such as tumor necrosis factor (TNF) and interleukin-1 (IL-1). Three main groups of metalloproteinases, the stromelysins, gelatinases and collagenases have been identified. The stromelysins degrade the PGs and basement membranes, and the collagenases the fibrillar proteins. It is probably important to realize that while the PGs are broken down and replaced rapidly, replacement of the fibrillar collagen is very slow. It might therefore be useful therapeutically to block collagenase activity in the early stages of the arthritic process.

Injury and repair of subchondral bone

Arthritis is a disease that affects not only the articular cartilage but also the underlying bone and the structures around the joint.

As the articular cartilage is eroded from the articular surface, the underlying bone is subjected to increasingly localized over-

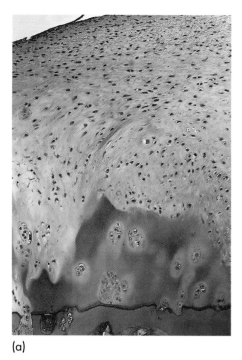
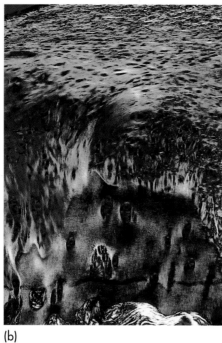

(a)

(b)

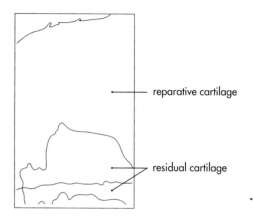

reparative cartilage

residual cartilage

Figure 10.25 (a) Photomicrograph of a section through the articular surface of an arthritic joint demonstrates extensive fibrocartilaginous repair overlying residual hyaline cartilage (H&E, × 4 obj.). (b) The same field photographed with polarized light.

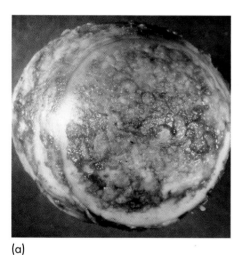
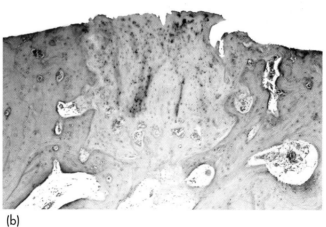

(a)

(b)

Figure 10.26 (a) Photograph of the femoral head removed from a patient with advanced OA. Most of the supero-lateral surface of the femoral head is covered with an irregular layer of tissue, which seems to be growing in the form of small tufts from the underlying bone. (b) Photomicrograph of one of the tufts shown in (a). The tuft is formed of fibrocartilaginous tissue extending from the marrow onto the joint surface. On either side of the fibrocartilaginous tuft is eburnated bone (H&E, × 10 obj.).

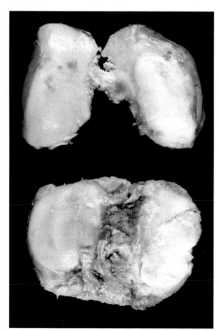
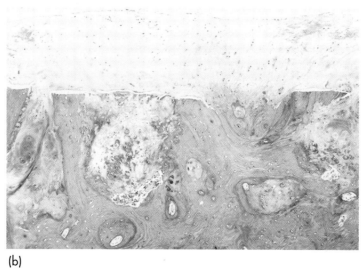

(b)

(a)

Figure 10.27 (a) Photograph of a knee joint showing a layer of reparative cartilage covering most of the femoral condyle and the opposed tibial plateau. In some cases of OA treated by osteotomy, and even in untreated cases, the damaged joint surfaces may be entirely recovered by a layer of fibrocartilaginous tissue, as seen in this example. (b) Photomicrograph of the fibrocartilage seen in (a) reveals extension of fibrocartilaginous tissue over the previously eburnated bone (H&E, × 4 obj.).

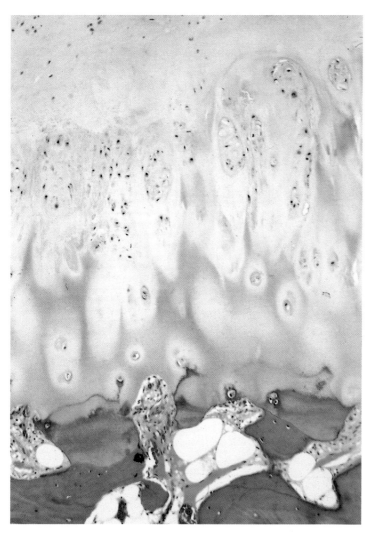

Figure 10.28   Microscopic examination of the articular cartilage covering of an osteoarthritic joint which frequently shows a heterogenous mix of extrinsic reparative cartilage, intensive repair and residual cartilage as shown in this photomicrograph (H&E, × 10 obj.).

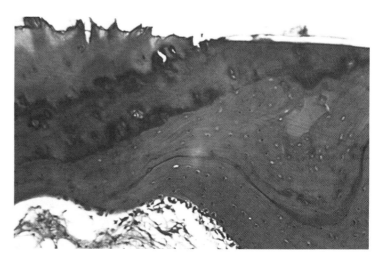

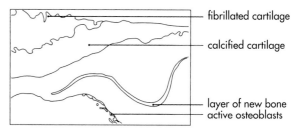

Figure 10.29   Photomicrograph shows increased osteoblastic activity and trabecular thickening underlying an area of cartilage erosion. (Section taken from the edge of a denuded and eburnated area) (H&E, × 10 obj.).

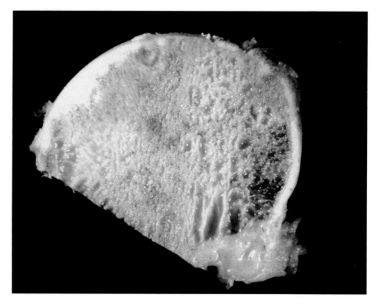

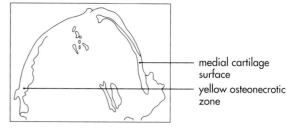

Figure 10.30   A portion of the eburnated surface of an osteoarthritic joint demonstrates focal superficial bone and bone marrow necrosis, which is seen macroscopically as an opaque yellow area.

loading. In subarticular bone that has been thus denuded, there is proliferation of osteoblasts and formation of new bone (Fig. 10.29), which occurs both on the surfaces of existing intact trabeculae and around microfractures. In X-rays of arthritic joints, this new bone may appear as increased density or sclerosis.

A further result of increased local stress is that the surface bone is likely to undergo focal pressure necrosis (Fig. 10.30). [This superficial necrosis is different both in its etiology and pathogenesis from that associated with 'primary' subchondral avascular necrosis, which itself leads to secondary OA. However, in clinical practice differentiation between the two may be difficult, especially in the late stages of primary subchondral avascular necrosis (see Chapter 15, p. 357).]

Subarticular cysts are usually seen only where the overlying cartilage is absent (Fig. 10.31). Such cysts are common in cases of OA and are believed to result from transmission of interarticular pressure through defects in the articulating bony surface into the marrow spaces of the subchondral bone (Fig. 10.32). The cysts increase in size until the pressure within them is equal to the intra-articular pressure. Cysts may also occur because of

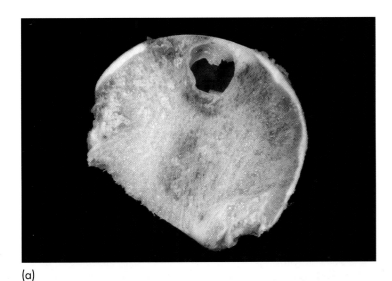

(a)

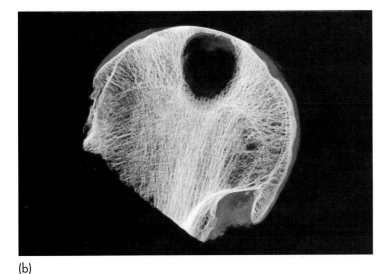

(b)

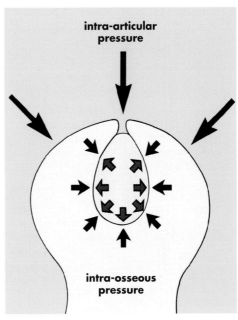

Figure 10.32
With the intrusion of synovial fluid into the subchondral bone, the bone becomes resorbed and a cyst is formed, which will increase in size until the intraosseous pressure is equal to the intra-articular pressure.

focal tissue necrosis. (In cases of arthritis due to rheumatoid disease or gout, periarticular radiologic 'cysts' may be associated with erosion of the marginal subchondral bone by the diseased synovium.)

Osteochondral loose bodies

Separated fragments of bone and cartilage from a damaged joint surface may become incorporated into the synovial membrane and digested, or may remain free as loose bodies in the joint cavity (Fig. 10.33). Under certain circumstances, proliferation of cartilage cells occurs on the surface of these loose bodies and consequently they grow larger (Fig. 10.34). As they grow, their centers become necrotic and calcified. In histologic sections it is possible to visualize periodic extension of this central calcification in the form of concentric rings which increase in number as the

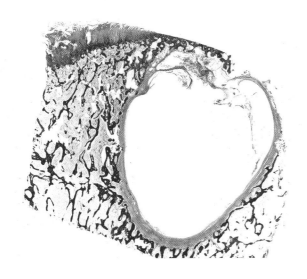

(c)

Figure 10.31 (a) An area of cystic degeneration in the subchondral bone of the superior surface of a femoral head. Such cysts are usually seen only in the absence of the overlying articular cartilage. Note also the large, flat osteophyte on the medial surface. (b) A radiograph of the specimen. (c) Photomicrograph of the subchondral bone cyst shown in (a) and (b). In this case the cyst was filled with a mucoid fluid and lined by a dense fibrous membrane. However, frequently the lytic area is entirely filled by loose fibrous tissue (H&E, × 2.5 obj.).

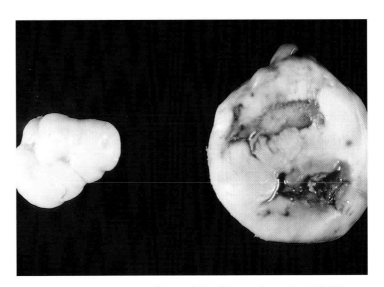

Figure 10.33 Traumatic arthritis of the elbow. A loose body (left) has arisen from the portion of the articular surface that is missing from the radial head (right).

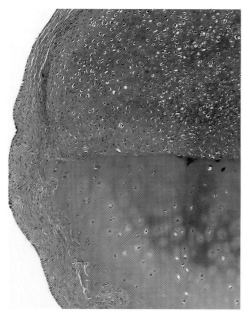

Figure 10.34 Photomicrograph shows the proliferation of immature cellular cartilage on the surface of a cartilaginous loose body; the original cartilage is seen in the lower part of the picture. Through this process of cartilage cell proliferation, loose bodies may grow to an enormous size (H&E, × 4 obj.).

loose body grows larger (Fig. 10.35). Sometimes the bodies reattach to the synovial membrane, in which case they are invaded by blood vessels. Endochondral ossification then occurs and the loose bodies become bony (Fig. 10.36).

There is some degree of loose body formation in many cases of arthritis. Occasionally, in cases of OA, the loose bodies are so numerous that they must be distinguished from those that occur in primary synovial chondromatosis (Fig. 10.37) (see Chapter 21, p. 490).

Ligaments

Microscopic evidence both of lacerations and of repair by scar tissue is common in the ligamentous and capsular tissue around an arthritic joint. Whether these preceded the arthritic process or whether they are a consequence of it cannot usually be determined by microscopic examination; however, there is abundant evidence from clinical studies that severe ligamentous injury is a significant cause of OA, especially in athletes and those engaged in heavy physical labor.

Injury of the synovial membrane

Even when cases of arthritis which have a primary synovial etiology have been excluded, microscopic examination of the synovium still demonstrates some degree of synovitis.

Injury and breakdown of cartilage and bone result in increased amounts of breakdown product and particulate debris within the joint cavity. This is removed from the synovial fluid by phagocytic cells (the 'A' cells) of the synovial membrane. In consequence, the membrane becomes both hypertrophic and hyperplastic (Figs 10.38–10.40). In addition, the breakdown products of cartilage and bone matrix evoke an inflammatory response.

For this reason some degree of chronic inflammation can be expected in the synovial membrane of arthritic joints, even when the injury has been purely mechanical. Inflammation is especially prominent where there has been rapid breakdown of the articular components as evidenced by the presence in the synovium of bone and cartilage detritus (Fig. 10.41).

Histologic studies have shown that there may be a similarity between the degree of inflammatory response as seen in some cases of severe OA and that of RA. However, in OA the synovial inflammation is likely to be the result of cartilage breakdown,

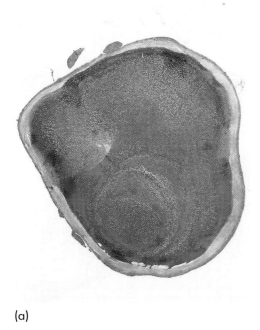

(a)

(b)

Figure 10.35 (a) Low-power photomicrograph of a cartilaginous loose body (H&E, × 1.25 obj.). (b) Photomicrograph of a section through a loose body. One can discern the concentric rings of growth. The tissue towards the center of the loose body is calcified (phloxine & tartrazine, × 4 obj.).

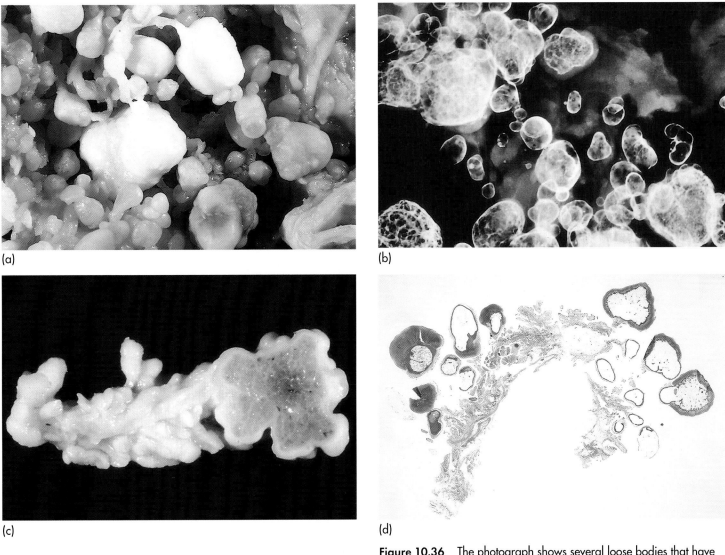

Figure 10.36   The photograph shows several loose bodies that have become attached to the synovium (**a**). In the specimen radiograph (**b**), many of the loose bodies can be seen to have an ossified center. One of the loose bodies (**c**) has been bisected and shows a viable osseus center which has resulted from vascular invasion and endochondral ossification of the cartilaginous loose body. (**d**) A low-power photomicrograph demonstrates numerous osteocartilagenous loose bodies attached to the synovium (H&E, × 1.25 obj.). (**e**) Photomicrograph of a portion of the loose body shown in (**d**) demonstrates formation of the osseous core by the process of endochondral ossification (phloxine & tartrazine, × 10 obj.).

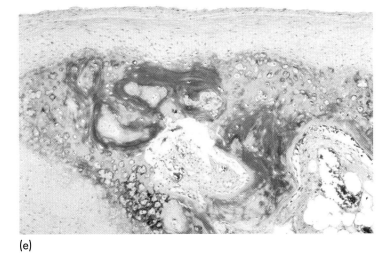

whereas in RA the synovial inflammation is the cause of the cartilage breakdown.

Extension of the hyperplastic synovium onto the articular surface of the joint (i.e. a pannus) is a common finding even in OA, particularly in the hip. However, the extent and the aggressiveness of this pannus with respect to underlying cartilage destruction is much less marked in OA than in RA (Fig. 10.42).

Under normal conditions, the synovial membrane is responsible for the nutrition of articular cartilage. In this regard, it might be expected that the chronically inflamed and scarred synovial membrane of an arthritic joint would function less effectively than that of a normal joint. Disturbance in synovial nutrient function, as well as increased enzymatic activity, may very well contribute to the chronicity of the arthritic process. The hyper-

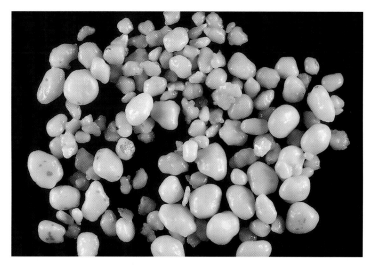

Figure 10.37 Photograph of multiple osteocartilaginous loose bodies removed from an osteoarthritic hip joint. This large number of loose bodies is uncommon and may be mistaken for synovial chondromatosis.

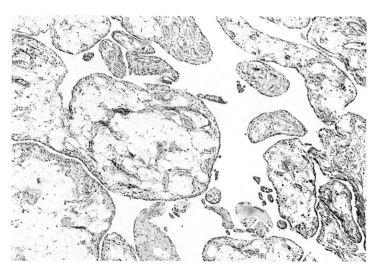

Figure 10.38 Photomicrograph of proliferative synovium from a patient with OA (H&E, × 4 obj.).

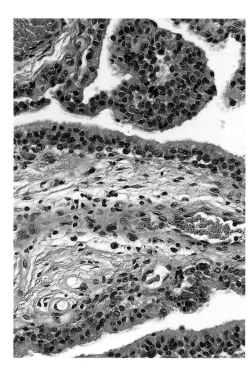

Figure 10.39 Photomicrograph to demonstrate a common pattern of synovial cell hypertrophy (H&E, × 10 obj.).

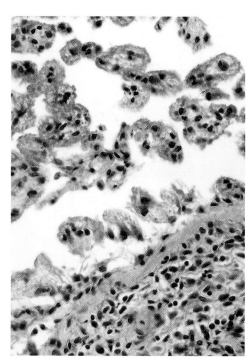

Figure 10.40 An uncommon pattern of synovial cell hypertrophy and hyperplasia with columnar and vacuolated cells resembling intestinal epithelium (H&E, × 10 obj.).

trophied and hyperplastic synovium is also likely to be traumatized as it extends into the joint cavity. Evidence of bleeding into the joint, with subsequent hemosiderin staining of the synovial membrane, is a common histologic finding and may occasionally be marked. When this is the case, and despite their similar color, the orange–brown staining of the fine villous synovium seen at operation should not be confused with the swollen papillary synovium of pigmented villonodular synovitis (Fig. 10.43).

Synovial fluid in an injured joint
Normal synovial fluid, a dialysate of plasma to which hyaluronic acid produced by the 'B' cells of the synovial lining is added, is viscous, pale yellow, and clear. Even in large joints the volume is small.

Examination of synovial fluid is extremely helpful in the diagnosis of arthritis for determining both the cause and the stage of the disease. Whatever the cause of arthritis, the synovial fluid is altered (Fig. 10.44, Tables 10.1 and 10.2). (For a discussion of the examination of synovial fluid for crystals, see Chapter 12, p. 305).

In cases of inflammatory arthritis there is an increased volume of synovial fluid while the amount of hyaluronic acid is markedly diminished. This leads to a typical decrease in viscosity. However, in degenerate forms of arthritis the amount of hyaluronic acid is increased, resulting in an extremely viscous fluid. Often there is also an increase in volume, although not to the same degree as that which is seen in the inflammatory arthritides.

Table 10.1 Normal synovial fluid.

Physical data	Normal synovial fluid	
	Average	Range
Amount in knee (ml)	1.1	0.13–3.5
Specific gravity (20°C)		1.0081–1.015
Viscosity (37°C) relative to water	235	5.7–1160
Cell count per mm^3	63	13–180
Differential %		
Lymphocytes	24.6	0–78
Polymorphonuclear leukocytes	6.5	0–25
Monocytes	47.9	0–71
Macrophages	10.1	0–26
Synovial lining cells	4.3	0–12
pH	7.434	7.31–7.74
Inorganic substances		
Electrolytes (Na, K, Cl, CO$_2$)	Approximately the same as plasma	
Calcium, phosphate, sulfate	Approximately the same as plasma	
Organic substances		
Hyaluronic acid (mg/ml)	4.0	
Nonprotein nitrogen		Approximately the same as plasma
Glucose		Approximately the same as plasma
Total lipid (mg/ml)	0.2	
Mucin nitrogen (mg/ml)	1.04	0.68–1.35
Mucin glucosamine (mg/ml)	0.74	0.12–1.32
Uric acid		Approximately the same as plasma

Source: Paget S, Bullough PG. **Synovium and synovial fluid**. In: Owen R *et al*, eds. *Scientific Foundation of Orthopaedics and Traumatology.* Philadelphia: Saunders, 1980.

Table 10.2 Examination of synovial fluid.

	Synovial fluid with disease			
	Normal	Noninflammatory	Chronic inflammatory	Septic
Clinical example		Osteoarthritis	Rheumatoid arthritis	Bacterial infection
Cartilage debris	0	+	0	0
Volume (ml) (knee)	<3.5	>3.5	>3.5	>3.5
Color	Clear	Clear yellow	Opalescent yellow	Turbid yellow to green
Viscosity	High	High	Low	Low
WBCs per mm^3	200	200–2000	2000–100,000	>100,000
Polymorphonuclear leukocytes (%)	<25	<25	50% or more	90% or more
Culture	Negative	Negative	Negative	Positive
Mucin clot	Firm	Firm	Friable	Friable
Fibrin clot	None	Small	Large	Large
Glucose (% blood glucose)	50–100	50–100	20–75	1–5
Total protein		Equal to normal joint	Elevated	Elevated

Source: Paget S, Bullough PG. **Synovium and synovial fluid**. In: Owen R *et al*, eds. *Scientific Foundation of Orthopaedics and Traumatology.* Philadelphia: Saunders, 1980.

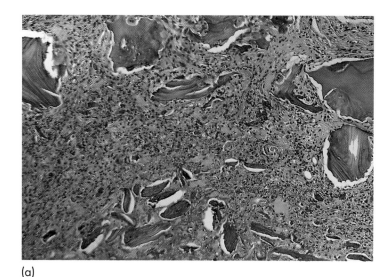

(a)

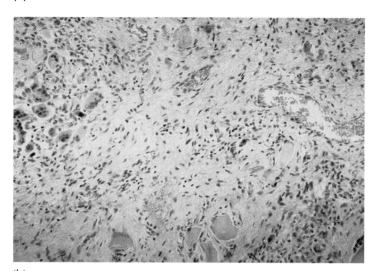

(b)

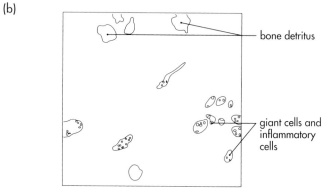

bone detritus

giant cells and inflammatory cells

Figure 10.41 (a) In association with rapid destruction of a joint, the synovium will often show a marked hyperplasia and chronic inflammation with pieces of detached bone and cartilage embedded within it, as seen here (H&E, × 4 obj.). (b) In a higher power view, fragments of bone and cartilage, as well as foci of histiocytes and phagocytic giant cells, are present (H&E, × 25 obj.).

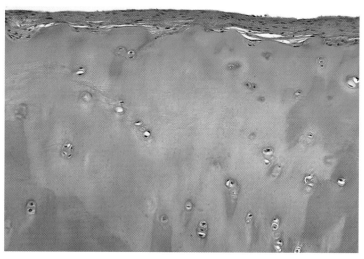

Figure 10.42 Fibrous pannus extending over the surface of the damaged articular cartilage in a case of OA (H&E, × 25 obj.).

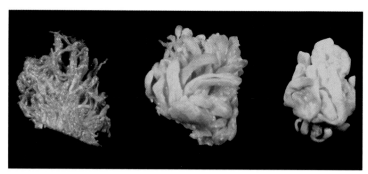

Figure 10.43 Hemophilia (left), pigmented villonodular synovitis (center), and RA (right). In this photograph the synovial membranes from individuals with three different conditions are compared. In patients with hemophilia, the hemosiderin staining of the synovium results from excessive bleeding into the joint, but in individuals affected by the other two conditions, the hemosiderin staining is probably secondary to trauma to the hypertrophic synovium. The plump papillary appearance of the synovium in pigmented vilonodular synovitis (PVNS) and RA, as opposed to the villous appearance of the synovium in hemophilia, reflects the considerable cellular infiltration of the subsynovium in patients with PVNS or RA.

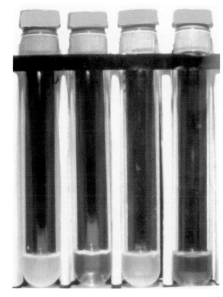

Figure 10.44 The examination of synovial fluid can provide valuable information concerning the etiology of a patient's condition. Samples of synovial fluid from four patients (from left to right): chondrocalcinosis – cloudy white fluid; normal – clear white/amber fluid; RA – cloudy yellow fluid; chronic traumatic arthritis – clear and xanthochromic fluid.

NONINFLAMMATORY ARTHRITIDES

The noninflammatory arthritides are certainly the most commonly encountered form of arthritis in the Western world, and osteoarthritis (OA) in its many and varied presentations is the most commonly encountered condition in orthopaedic practice. Primary OA is a degenerative disease which is clinically associated with age and obesity.

It affects 21 million patients in North America and a similar number in Europe, and presents clinically in three major forms that guide clinical decision making:

- Nodal OA results in Heberden and Bouchard nodes in the small joints of the hands, but it does not cause significant loss of hand function in contrast to rheumatoid arthritis (RA).
- Axial OA involves the neck and the low back, and will be discussed in detail in Chapter 13.
- OA occurs in weight-bearing joints and is the principle topic of this chapter.

Among the other types of noninflammatory arthritis discussed in this chapter, rapidly destructive OA following subchondral fracture either due to severe or repetitive trauma, in healthy individuals or bone insufficiency in older individuals, is also relatively common. (Arthritis secondary to bone necrosis will be discussed in Chapter 15).

OSTEOARTHRITIS (DEGENERATIVE JOINT DISEASE)

CLINICAL CONSIDERATIONS

Because the etiology of OA in most cases cannot be determined, there is as yet no generally accepted definition of the disease but for the purpose of this discussion the following is offered: 'Osteoarthritis is a functional disorder of joints characterized by altered joint anatomy, especially by the loss of articular cartilage and the formation of osteophytes. Unlike many forms of arthritis, it is essentially noninflammatory'.

Four patterns of disease are generally recognized:

1. OA presenting as disease limited to a single large joint, usually the knee or hip, sometimes with bilateral involvement (Fig. 11.1)
2. A generalized process involving the distal and proximal interphalangeal joints of the hand, the first carpometacarpal joint, and metatarsophalangeal joints (Fig. 11.2)
3. Extreme cases of OA known as Charcot's joints seen in association with a neurologic deficit. In these patients a characteristic rapidly destructive OA is observed, complicated by the production of multiple loose bodies, severe subluxation, and even dislocation of the joint (Figs 11.3–11.5). The underlying neurologic disorder associated with Charcot joint may be a peripheral neuropathy associated with pernicious anemia or diabetes mellitus, or spinal cord degeneration as in tabes dorsalis, or syringomyelia
4. A rare pattern, described clinically, is an erosive OA which radiographically has the features of an inflammatory process. This form of disease usually affects the distal or proximal interphalangeal joints of the hand (Fig. 11.6) but may occasionally involve large joints (Fig. 11.7).

A patient with OA typically presents with complaints of pain and usually stiffness. On examination, movement of the affected joint may be limited and the patient often lacks the capability for full flexion or extension.

The most characteristic radiologic finding is loss of the joint space. In the majority of cases bony osteophytes are also seen around the periphery of the joint, the bone on both sides of the joint exhibits increased density, and cystic lesions can frequently be noted in the subchondral bone.

PATHOLOGIC FINDINGS

The most obvious features of an osteoarthritic joint removed either at surgery or autopsy, are damaged cartilage and alterations in the shape of the articular surfaces. In the weight-bearing areas of the joint the cartilage may be entirely absent, and the exposed subchondral bone may have a dense polished appearance like that of marble (eburnation); when this area is sectioned, the bone usually is found to be markedly thickened (sclerotic) (Fig. 11.8).

Adjacent to the surface, cystic defects filled with loose fibromyxoid tissue (or sometimes with a thick mucoid fluid) may be found (Fig. 11.9). As already noted in Chapter 10, the superficial bone in the eburnated areas may be necrotic (see Fig. 10.30).

In areas of the joint that do not bear weight, and around its

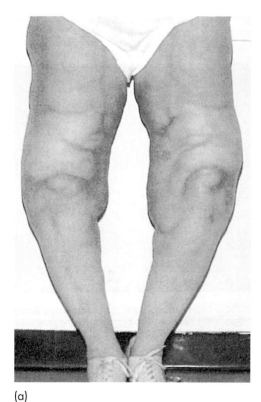

(a)

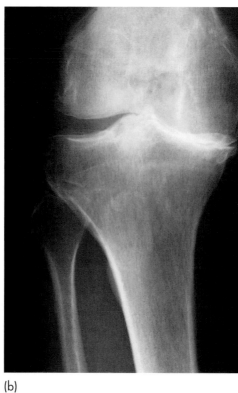

(b)

Figure 11.1   (a) This obese patient has a marked genu varus deformity of both knees associated with severe bilateral OA, predominantly in the medial compartment. (b) A standing radiograph shows the loss of the medial joint space. (Note a radiograph taken with the patient lying down as opposed to standing may fail to show this loss of joint space.)

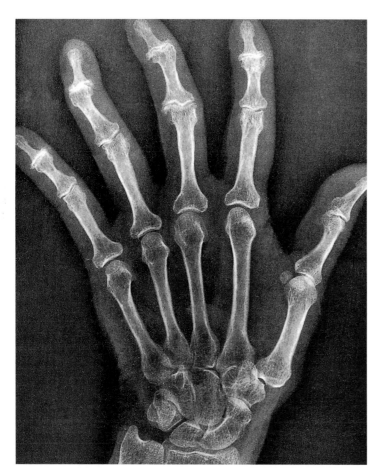

Figure 11.2   Radiograph of a patient with primary generalized OA shows the characteristic wavy deformity of the third and fourth digits. Irregular erosions at the articular surfaces usually affect the ulnar aspect of the joint.

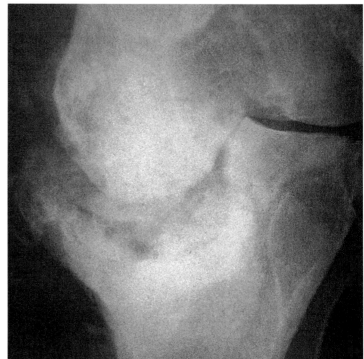

Figure 11.3   Radiograph of the knee in a patient with diabetes and a history of pernicious anemia. The patient presented with grossly deformed and unstable knees, however the condition was painless. Note extensive destruction of the medial compartment of the knee and the multiple loose bodies.

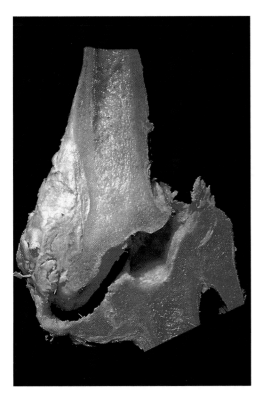

Figure 11.4
Coronal section
through a grossly
deranged knee joint
(Charcot's joint).
Subluxation and
severe destruction of
the joint surfaces are
evident. The
synovium is markedly
hypertrophic and
hyperplastic.

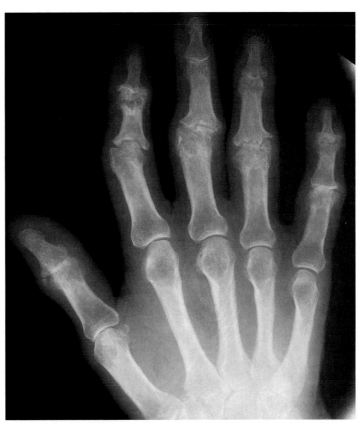

Figure 11.6 Radiograph of the hand of a 45-year-old woman with erosive OA, showing the typical involvement of the proximal and distal interphalangeal joints.

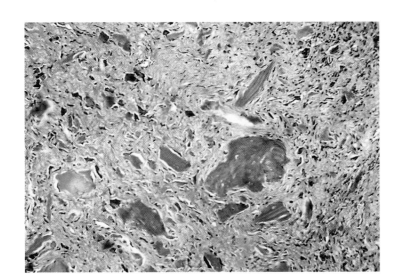

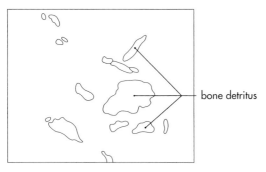

bone detritus

Figure 11.5 Photomicrograph of a portion of the synovium in a Charcot's joint. The scarred and chronically inflamed synovium is filled with multiple irregular fragments of bone and cartilage. The finding of bone and cartilage detritus in the synovial membrane usually denotes a rapid breakdown of the joint. In patients with OA it is rare to find any significant degree of detritus (phloxine and tartrazine, × 10 obj.).

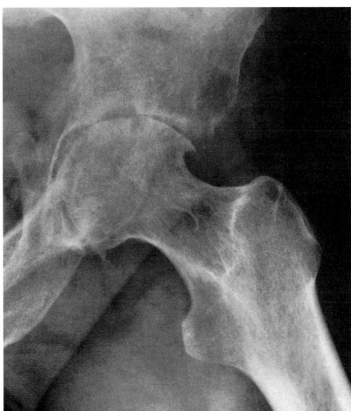

Figure 11.7 Radiograph of the hip of a 55-year-old woman with recent complaints of pain and stiffness, showing concentric narrowing of the joint space and erosive changes in both the femoral head and acetabulum. Testing for rheumatoid factor was negative in this case, which was clinically diagnosed as erosive OA.

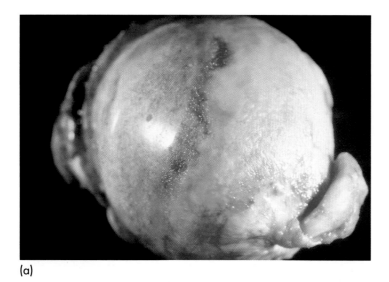

(a)

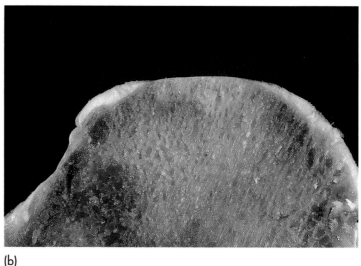

(b)

Figure 11.8 (a) Photograph of the femoral head removed from a patient with OA. Note the absence of the articular cartilage on the superior and lateral aspects of the femoral head, and the polished appearance of the exposed bone (eburnation). The remaining surrounding cartilage has a somewhat yellow color and a roughened surface. (b) In section the bone beneath the eburnated surface is much denser. (c) Microscopically the dense bone has an almost cortical appearance. Note the smoothness of the eburnated surface (H&E, partially polarized × 4 obj.).

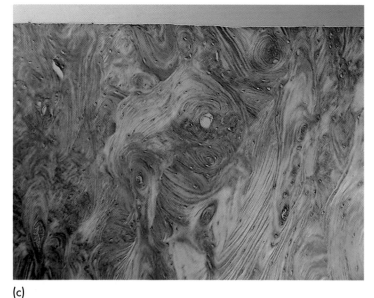

(c)

Figure 11.9 Photomicrograph of a portion of the articular surface in an osteoarthritic joint, showing focal absence of the articular cartilage. An underlying cyst connects via a short neck with the joint space (phloxine and tartrazine, × 2.5 obj.).

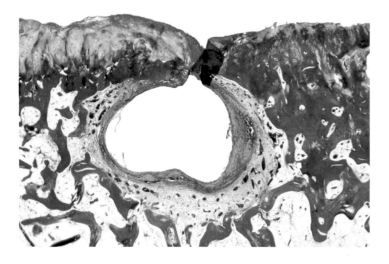

margins, bony and cartilaginous overgrowths (osteophytes or exostoses) develop. In different joints the location of the osteophytes is characteristic. In the distal interphalangeal joints the osteophytes (Heberden's nodes) are prominent on the dorsal and palmar aspects of both articulating surfaces. In the metatarsophalangeal joint of the big toe, the osteophyte is on the medial joint margin (hallux valgus) (Fig. 11.10). In the hip joint, although osteophytes are usually present around the entire joint margin, there is characteristically a large, flat osteophyte on the medial articular surface, extending to the fovea and this is associated with subluxation of the femoral head in the acetabulum (Fig. 11.11). Despite the loss of bone and cartilage in some parts

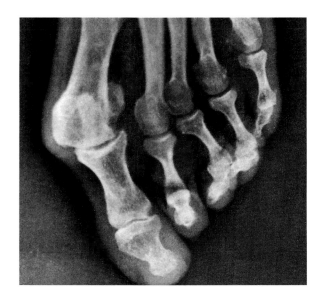

Figure 11.10   Hallux valgus deformity. Radiograph of the foot shows marked angulation of the first phalanx. Note the bone hypertrophy of the medial side of the head of the first metatarsal bone.

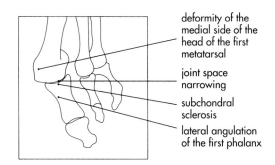

deformity of the medial side of the head of the first metatarsal

joint space narrowing

subchondral sclerosis

lateral angulation of the first phalanx

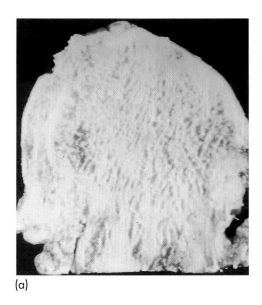

(a)

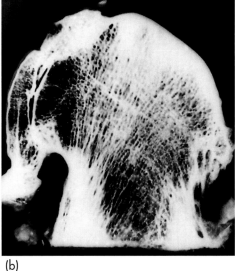

(b)

Figure 11.11   (a) A large, flat, medial osteophyte associated with subluxation of the femoral head in a patient with OA of the hip. The osteophyte extends from the joint margin to the region of the fovea. The residual cartilage of the medial surface of the femoral head can still be seen. (b) Radiograph of the tissue slice shown in (a) again illustrates the large medial osteophyte. Note that the loss of bone on the superior and lateral surfaces seems to equate with the gain of bone on the medial surface, so the sphericity of the femoral head is kept.

of the joint, assumed to be the result of overloading and mechanical abrasion, the net effect of reparative new bone and osteophyte formation is an overall increase in joint size. In general, an osteoarthritic joint is larger than its normal counterpart (see Fig. 10.12).

Osteophytes form through the process of endochondral ossification in one of two ways. The first involves vascular penetration into existing cartilage. In these areas the cartilage overlying the bone overgrowth is usually hypercellular, and the process histologically resembles the epiphyseal growth plate in the growing individual (Fig. 11.12). At the base of the osteophyte there are often remnants of the original tidemark and zone of calcified cartilage. In some cases these remnants are themselves undergoing ossification, not only from the region of the original subchondral bone but also from the osteophyte itself (Fig. 11.13). Osteophytes may also form from foci of cartilaginous metaplasia at the joint margins. [These foci of metaplasia often occur at the capsular and ligamentous insertions and may be the result of traction injuries (Fig. 11.14).]

In areas of residual cartilage on the articular surface of a dis-

eased joint there is often marked duplication and irregularity of the tidemark (Fig. 11.15). Evidence of increased endochondral ossification, which expands the periphery of the subchondral bone without actually forming an osteophyte, is recognized by irregularity of the bone cartilage junction, increased vascular penetration of the calcified cartilage, and the finding of woven (immature) bone at the bone-cartilage interface, indicating a rapid rate of bone formation at this site (Figs 11.16 and 11.17).

Microscopic examination of the cartilage that remains on the joint surface may reveal many clefts in its substance, most, but by no means all of which, are vertically oriented (Fig. 11.18). The cartilage cells far from the areas of eburnation may show considerable cell replication, with formation of prominent cell nests (Fig. 11.19). However, cell replication does not usually occur adjacent to the eburnated areas (Fig. 11.20). Proteoglycan (PG) staining of the matrix is usually diminished, although, as discussed in the previous chapter, there is evidence from radioactive SO_4 uptake studies that the amount of PG produced by the chondrocytes in OA may be increased, suggesting increased turnover with loss of glycoprotein residues into the synovial fluid.

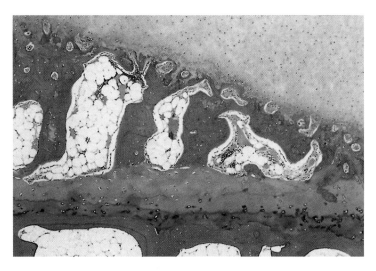

Figure 11.12 Photomicrograph of a section through a marginal osteophyte shows a wedge of bone formation dissecting into the cartilage. The cartilage on the articular side of the osteophyte is cellular, and there is more active endochondral ossification on this surface than on the lower surface that faces the bone (H&E, × 4 obj.).

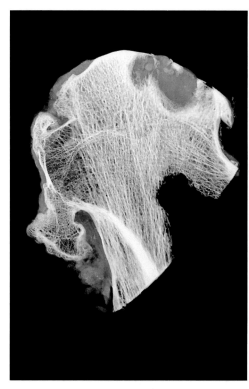

Figure 11.14 Specimen radiograph to demonstrate the various osteophytes which form around an osteoarthritic femoral head. Note especially the osteophyte on the medial neck of the femur which results from traction on the medial periosteum following lateral subluxation of the femoral head, note also the perifoveal osteophytes.

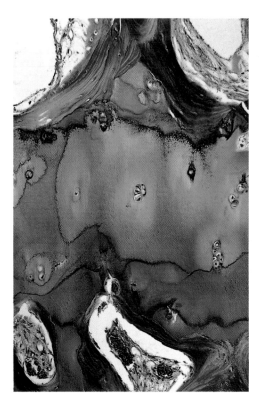

Figure 11.13 Photomicrograph of a portion of articular cartilage trapped under an osteophyte (H&E, × 10 obj.).

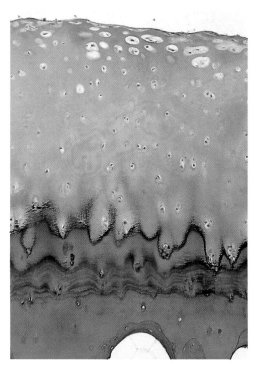

Figure 11.15 Photomicrograph of a portion of the articular cartilage in a patient with OA, showing irregularity and duplication of the tidemark (H&E, × 4 obj.).

The synovial membrane may show villous proliferation, slight hyperplasia of the lining cells, and mild chronic inflammation (Figs 11.21 and 11.22). Small osteochondral loose bodies are commonly found in the synovium and in the joint cavity. In some cases of degenerative arthritis of the knee, and occasionally in RA, a cystic herniation of the synovium may occur into the popliteal space, commonly referred to as Baker's cyst (Fig. 11.23).

NATURAL HISTORY

A wide variety of questions have been asked about OA. Is it a single disorder or a family of disorders? What is the role of acute and chronic trauma in its pathogenesis? Is OA an inevitable consequence of aging? How do the anatomic, physiologic, biochemical, and mechanical alterations in cartilage matrix interrelate in the pathogenesis of OA? What roles do extracartilaginous struc-

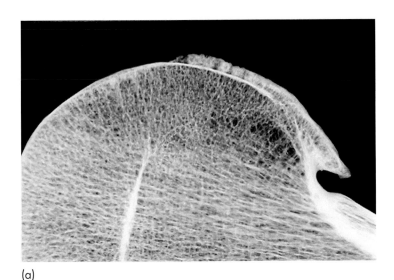

(a)

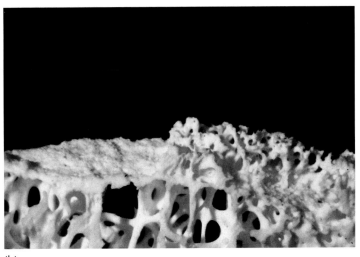

(b)

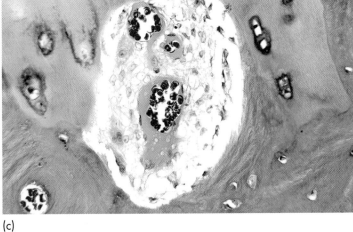

(c)

Figure 11.16 (a) A radiograph to demonstrate the formation of the medial osteophyte, a characteristic finding in OA of the hip. Note especially the hair-on-end appearance of the new bone lying on top of the subchondral plate of bone. (b) Photograph of the macerated specimen shown in (a) which demonstrates the new bone of the osteophyte in three dimensions. (c) These tongues of new bone are formed as the result of vascular canals breaking through the calcified articular cartilage and the tidemark (H&E, × 10 obj.).

tures play in OA? Under what circumstances does inflammation develop in OA? Does articular cartilage undergo repair in OA? Some of the answers to these questions have been addressed in the preceding chapter.

OA appears to comprise a family of disorders. In about one-fifth of the patients, it is evident to the clinician that an antecedent condition is causally related to the OA, which can therefore be considered secondary OA (Table 11.1). Individuals

Table 11.1 Conditions that may precede OA (secondary OA).

Hip dysplasia
Congenital dislocation or subluxation of the hip
Legg–Calvé–Perthes disease
Slipped capital femoral epiphysis
Intra-articular fracture; traumatic dislocation
Radiation damage
Infection
Metabolic diseases (e.g. gout, CPPD, ochronosis)
Unrecognized avascular disease
'Burnt-out' RA
Paget's disease

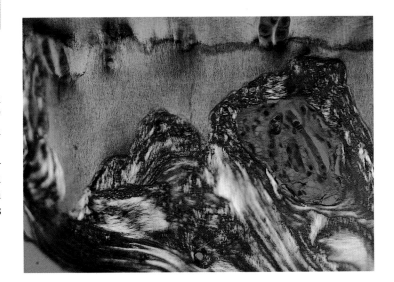

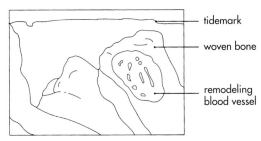

- tidemark
- woven bone
- remodeling blood vessel

Figure 11.17 Photomicrograph taken with polarized light shows woven bone formation in the subchondral region. This is an indication of accelerated modeling in a case of OA (× 25 obj.).

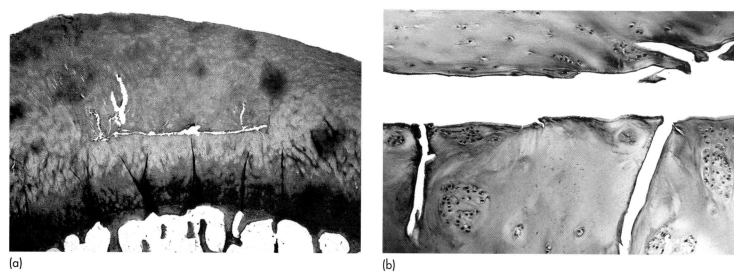

(a)   (b)

Figure 11.18   (a) Section through the articular cartilage of the patella demonstrates a horizontal failure with cleft formation in a patient with chondromalacia patellae. In patients with this condition, a soft blister on the articular surface may indicate structural shear failure within the substance of the cartilage (H&E, × 1.25 obj.). (b) A high-power view of the cleft shows marked cellular proliferation in the inferior cartilage as opposed to the cartilage on the side of the cleft closest to the surface (H&E, × 10 obj.).

affected by secondary OA are likely to be about 10 years younger than those with primary (idiopathic) OA, who are usually over 60 years of age. OA is not necessarily the consequence of aging per se, since many joints remain essentially normal even into extreme old age.

The pathogenesis of OA can be understood only in terms of the interdependence of anatomy, physiology, biochemistry, and mechanical function. All components of the joint play a role in the pathogenesis of the disease, not just cartilage. Tissue breakdown results in inflammation, which also plays its role in the disease processes.

A number of autopsy studies have demonstrated the incidence of degenerative changes in various joints, as well as its progres-

sion from mild to severe disease. As might be expected the incidence at autopsy is much more than the clinical incidence of disease (Table 11.2).

The availability of a large volume of tissue specimens from hip replacement arthroplasty, together with the availability of these patients' clinical radiographs and case histories, has made it possible for us to gain further insights into the natural history of OA of the hip.

One of the problems with most classifications of the radiographic changes in OA is that they tend to miss the dynamic progressive nature of the disease, which as already discussed, involves mechanical wear, cell injury, and repair. It has been possible for us to stage the disease radiographically not only on the

Table 11.2   Incidence of cartilage changes and OA at autopsy in joints at different ages (from *J. Heine*).

Age groups	Knee		Shoulder		Hip		Elbow		Great toe		Acromio-clavicular		Sterno-clavicular	
	A	B	A	B	A	B	A	B	A	B	A	B	A	B
(years)	%	%	%	%	%	%	%	%	%	%	%	%	%	%
15–19	3.1	0.0	0.0	0.0	0.0	0.0	0.0	0.0	0.0	0.0	0.0	0.0	0.0	0.0
20–29	9.2	0.0	0.8	0.0	0.8	0.0	1.7	0.0	9.6	0.0	4.4	0.0	0.0	0.0
30–39	48.1	1.0	2.0	0.0	7.8	0.0	18.0	0.0	27.0	0.0	20.0	0.0	2.0	0.0
40–49	74.0	0.8	4.7	0.0	16.7	0.8	26.9	0.0	35.7	0.0	35.9	0.8	6.2	0.0
50–59	87.1	2.6	14.3	0.7	44.8	0.7	61.7	1.3	60.5	7.9	73.0	1.3	16.1	0.0
60–69	92.6	12.0	22.1	2.6	60.0	2.7	73.7	5.2	72.6	13.7	91.0	9.6	36.3	1.1
70–79	97.5	33.3	44.1	9.7	76.1	12.2	87.4	10.5	78.1	18.2	100.0	12.3	40.0	1.5
80–95	100.0	39.4	60.0	15.7	89.4	16.7	95.8	15.5	84.6	24.6	95.7	11.4	62.0	7.0

Columns A: Joints showing naked-eye evidence of cartilage destruction to a lesser or greater degree.
Columns B: Joints showing naked-eye evidence of moderate to severe OA.

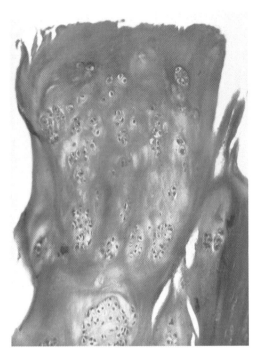

Figure 11.19 Photomicrograph of fibrillated cartilage away from the eburnated area shows a considerable proliferation of chondrocytes within the cartilage matrix. Many of the chondrocytes are seen to form cell nests or clones (H&E, × 10 obj.).

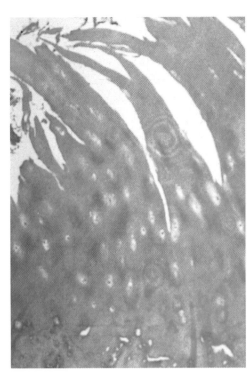

Figure 11.20 Low-power photomicrograph of the articular surface adjacent to an eburnated area. The articular cartilage contains vertical clefts resulting from fraying and splitting of the collagen fibers at the surface of the cartilage, but no obvious chondrocyte replication (H&E, × 10 obj.).

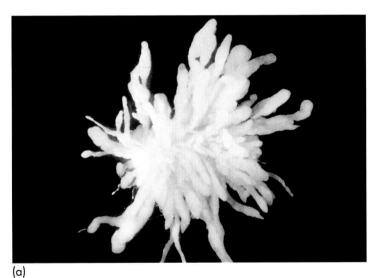

(a)

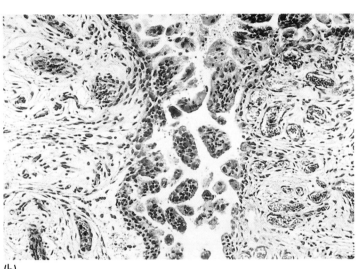

(b)

Figure 11.21 (a) The synovium from a patient with OA exhibits a marked villous pattern. The villi are fine and delicate, an appearance that grossly reflects the lack of any significant cell infiltrate in the subsynovium. (b) Photomicrograph of the specimen demonstrates the overgrowth of the synovial lining cells without significant inflammatory cell infiltration in the subsynovial tissue (H&E, × 10 obj.).

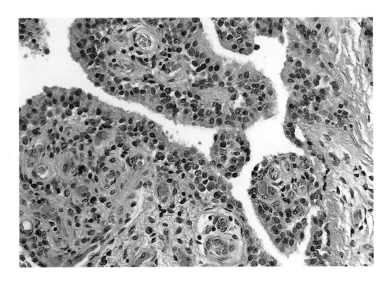

Figure 11.22 Photomicrograph of the synovial membrane in a patient with OA. The villous pattern of the synovium and hyperplasia of the synovial lining cells are evident. In this patient, as in many patients with OA, one may also note a mild chronic inflammatory infiltrate in the synovial tissue. (This inflammation can be quite severe in some individuals.) (H&E, x 4 obj.).

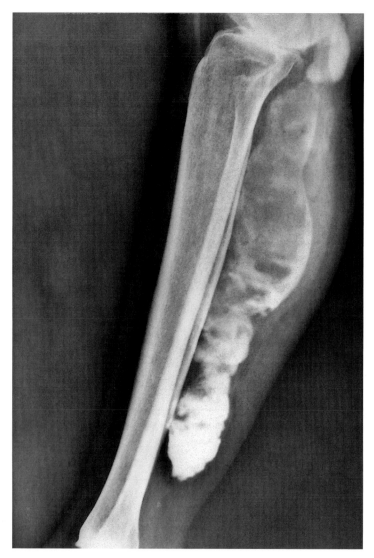

Figure 11.23   Radiograph of the leg of a young woman with a history of juvenile RA who complained of fullness in the calf. Injection of a radiopaque dye clearly demonstrates the extent of a Baker's cyst in the popliteal region.

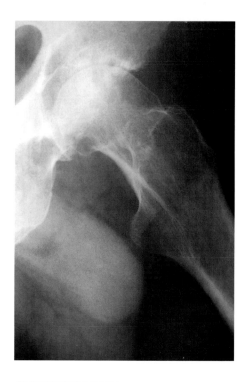

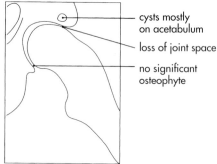

Figure 11.24   Radiograph demonstrating the characteristics of stage I OA. There is narrowing of the superior joint space, with some subchondral sclerosis and subchondral cyst formation in the acetabulum.

basis of horizontal comparisons of radiographs in different patient's hips but also in longitudinal studies of serial X-rays of the same patient:

- Stage I is characterized by narrowing or absence of the joint space, with preservation of the subchondral bone contours of the femoral head and of the acetabulum. In this early stage of the disease, migration of the femoral head has not occurred beyond the distance caused by the loss of the cartilage (Fig. 11.24).
- Stage II is characterized by complete absence of the superior joint space, with incomplete or complete loss of the subchondral bone contour. In this stage bone loss may be marked, and subchondral sclerosis and cystic changes in the bone on both sides of the joint are prominent. Migration of the joint, in most cases superiorly and laterally, also occurs relative to the bone loss (Fig. 11.25).

- Stage III is characterized by some reappearance of the joint space after maximal bone loss and migration have occurred. The bone contours again become relatively well defined. Sclerosis has diminished, and cysts have become indistinct (Fig. 11.26).

This radiologic staging corresponds well to the duration of symptoms.

A number of correlations can be made between this system of radiographic staging and the pathological appearance of the resected specimens. The most striking of these correlations is that reparative cartilage is much more prominent in radiographic stage III than in stage I (Figs 11.27–11.30). Subchondral cysts are most prevalent in stage II and tend to decrease in number in stage III.

When considering injury and repair within cartilage, bone, and synovium, it is important not to lose sight of the fact that

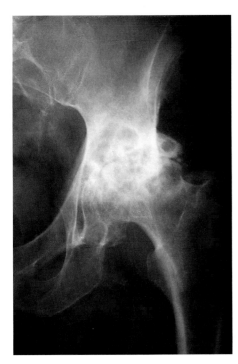

Figure 11.25
Radiograph
demonstrating the
features of stage II OA.
There is marked
subluxation of the joint,
with distortion of the
femoral head, and
severe sclerosis and cyst
formation on both sides
of the joint.

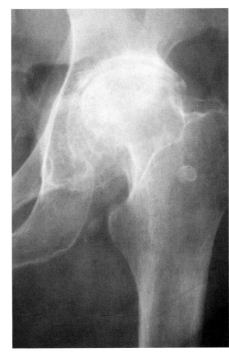

Figure 11.26
Radiograph showing the
features of stage III OA.
Maximal subluxation of
the joint is associated
with diminished sclerosis,
absence of subchondral
cyst, and reappearance
of the joint space.

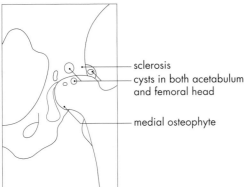

sclerosis
cysts in both acetabulum
and femoral head
medial osteophyte

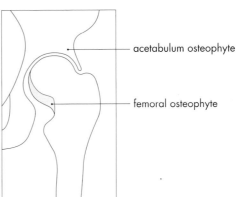

acetabulum osteophyte

femoral osteophyte

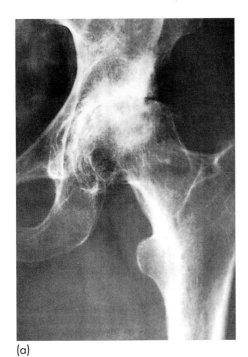

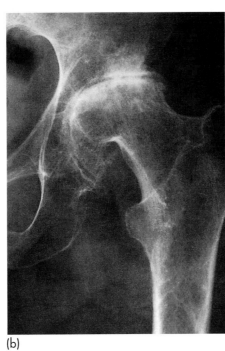

Figure 11.27 The radiograph shown in (**b**) was
taken 8 years after that in (**a**). It demonstrates the
improvement that may occur in the radiographic
appearance of a case of OA, even without
treatment.

(a)

(b)

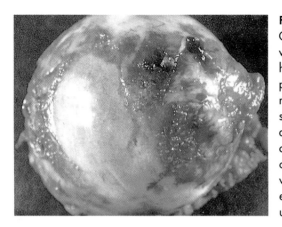

Figure 11.28 Gross superior view of a femoral head from a patient with radiographic stage I OA shows an area of complete cartilage loss, with polishing or eburnation of the underlying bone.

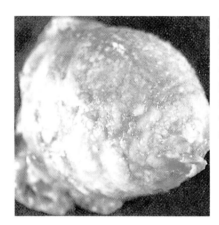

Figure 11.29 In this gross specimen of a deformed femoral head from a patient with radiologic stage III OA, the weight-bearing superior surface has been recovered with an irregular, cobble-stoned layer of cartilage.

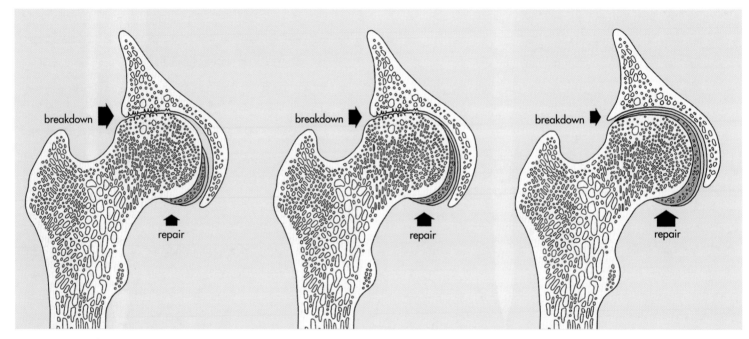

Figure 11.30 The radiographic and to some extent the clinical signs of arthritis depend on the balance between injury to the joint and repair of the joint (left). Deterioration is taking place because breakdown (i.e. loss of cartilage, bone, and bone shape, as well as bone necrosis) is proceeding more rapidly than repair (i.e. regeneration of cartilage and formation of new bone) (center). Both injury and repair are proceeding at about the same pace and the joint is stabilized (right). Repair is proceeding more rapidly than injury, leading to morphologic and perhaps clinical improvement.

joint function depends on the anatomy of the entire joint structure. If the repair processes, observed in the various tissues, are not directed towards restoration of the shape of the joint as well as restoration of stability and of an equitable loading pattern, then they serve no useful purpose.

The most easily recognized evidence of the attempt at functional restoration is the production of new bone, in the form of osteophytes, at various sites along the joint surface, particularly at the joint margins. Such remodeling of bone occurs early in the process of OA. The degree of remodeling by this process can be considerable and its efficiency is reflected clinically. The presence of osteophytes in the knee and hip by no means always heralds the development of symptomatic OA. Radiographic studies have

shown that two-thirds of knees that exhibit evidence of osteophyte formation, even when followed up for as long as 17 years, do not develop other degenerative changes.

The term osteoarthritis was first introduced by Archibald E. Garrod, in the 1890s. In 1909, Nichols and Richardson, on the basis of anatomic features, distinguished the two major categories of chronic arthritis by separating inflammatory arthritis from degenerative arthritis: 'These (various) joint lesions can be divided with great definiteness into two pathological groups: (1) those which arise from primary proliferative changes in the joints, chiefly in the synovial membrane and perichondrium, and (2) those which arise primarily as a degeneration of the joint cartilage. These two pathological groups are characterized by distinct gross and histological differences'. Nichols and Richardson went on to state that 'the earliest change to be observed in hypertrophic arthritis is a roughening of the cartilage, which begins near the center of the articular surface, i.e. at the point where pressure and friction between the ends of the bones is greatest'.

Since the time of that report, most authors on the subject have concluded that the earliest changes are found in 'those areas in which weight bearing is pre-eminently concentrated, and which are the most severely subjected to shearing and twisting types of stress'.

The wear-and-tear theory of causation, to which this author does not subscribe, has had a stultifying effect on medical opinion with regard to its views on prevention and treatment of the disease. It is more helpful to regard clinical arthritis as the consequence of a breakdown of normal physiologic pathways. Thus the etiology of arthritis can be defined, in general terms, as any condition that changes the shape of the articulating surface, changes the joint support, or alters the tissue matrices. It is not an inevitable disease resulting from wearing out of the joint by long use. Rather, OA is a disease of multiple etiologies, and searches for a single, all-encompassing cause of OA are fruitless. Although dysfunction may begin in any of the structures that make up the joint, by the time the disease comes to the attention of a clinician most structures of the joint are involved. Because of this overall involvement it is often impossible, especially in the later stages of disease, for the pathologist to determine the etiology.

OCHRONOSIS

The term ochronosis denotes a brownish-black pigmentation of connective tissue. Generalized degenerative joint disease or OA is often the presenting disease in ochronosis. The condition results from a rare hereditary disorder of tyrosine and phenylalanine degradation, in which the absence of the enzyme homogentisic acid oxidase leads to the accumulation of homogentisic acid in the body. The presence of excess homogentisic acid in the urine causes the condition known as alkaptonuria, characterized by darkening of the urine on exposure to air (this discoloration may be the only abnormality in children affected by ochronosis) (Fig. 11.31). However, in time, the widespread deposition of dark oxidative products occurs in virtually all collagen-containing structures in the body, including the sclerae and the skin. The predominant deposition of homogentisic acid in cartilage (including the intervertebral discs and articular cartilage) causes brittleness and consequent breakdown of the tissue, which in turn leads to spondylosis and arthropathy, in which the large joints are most severely involved (Fig. 11.32).

Radiographic examination of the spine of patients with ochronosis reveals calcification of the intervertebral discs, with narrowing of the disc spaces (Fig. 11.33). The changes seen in the large diarthrodial joints may be indistinguishable on radiographs from 'OA' with osteophytosis and subchondral bone sclerosis (Fig. 11.34).

Gross examination of the affected tissues reveals a brownish-black discoloration, often with degenerative changes (Fig. 11.35).

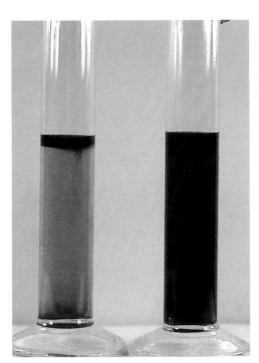

Figure 11.31 In the flask on the left is urine from a patient with ochronosis, which has been allowed to stand for 15 minutes. Some darkening, due to oxidation of homogentisic acid, is apparent at the surface. After 2 hours, with shaking, the specimen is entirely black (flask on the right).

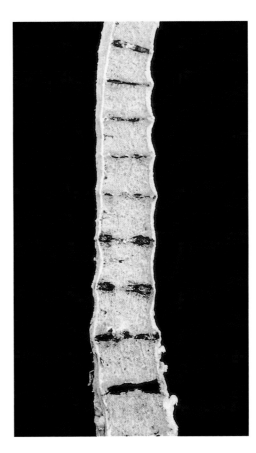

Figure 11.32 Section obtained at necropsy through the spine of a patient with ochronosis. Note the black discoloration of the intervertebral discs and the pronounced narrowing and irregularity of the disc spaces.

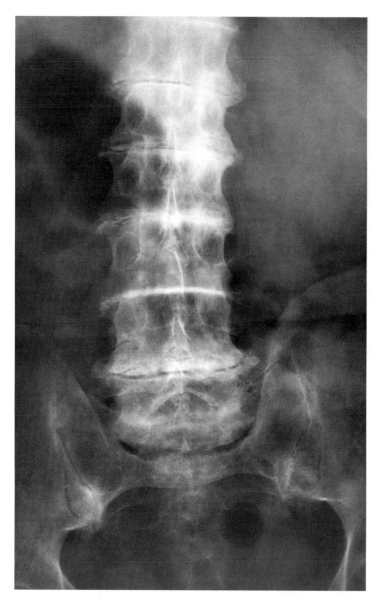

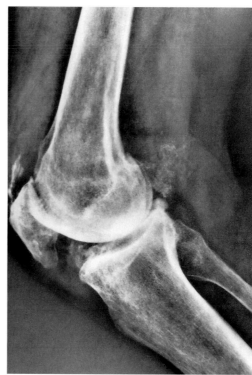

Figure 11.34 Radiograph of the lateral aspect of the knee in a patient with ochronosis. Note the joint space narrowing, together with irregular calcified material in the joint space.

Figure 11.33 Radiograph of the vertebral column in a patient with ochronosis. There is marked narrowing of the intervertebral disc spaces, together with some calcium deposition.

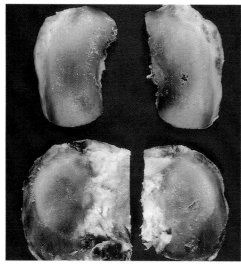

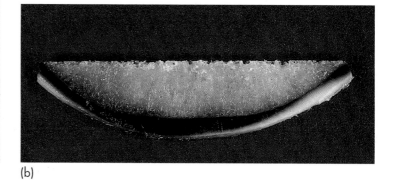

(a)

(b)

Figure 11.35 (a) Photograph of the articular surfaces of a knee joint from a patient with ochronosis, showing discoloration of the cartilage and mild degenerative changes. (b) Section through the femoral condyle illustrated in (a) shows that the pigmentation is mainly seen in the deep cartilage.

Histologic features of ochronosis include the intracellular accumulation of pigment and irregular fragments of pigmented cartilage that may be embedded in the synovium, a phenomenon that suggests a rapidly destructive arthropathy similar to that seen in a Charcot joint (Fig. 11.36). Ultrastructural study of the affected tissue has shown widening and fragmentation of collagen fibers in association with the deposition of the pigment in the matrix (Fig. 11.37).

The precise mechanism of the tissue injury is not fully understood, but the disruption of collagen cross-linking by metabolites of homogentisic acid is a probable explanation.

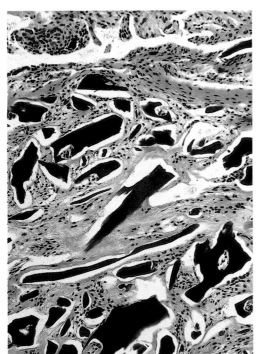

Figure 11.36 Photomicrograph of a portion of the synovial membrane from a patient with ochronosis demonstrates irregular fragments of pigmented cartilage, together with fibrosis and mild chronic inflammation in the subsynovial tissues (H&E, × 10 obj.).

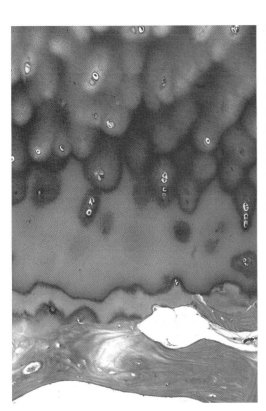

Figure 11.37 Photomicrograph of a portion of ochronotic articular cartilage shows the mahogany pigmentation of the cartilage matrix. Note the poor viability of the chondrocytes (H&E, × 10 obj.).

ARTHRITIS SECONDARY TO SUBCHONDRAL INSUFFICIENCY FRACTURE

Hip fractures are an increasingly important public health problem in the elderly. It has been estimated that in the USA more than 500,000 cases annually will occur by the year 2030. These estimates underline the importance of preventive measures to delay the onset of osteoporosis. The most commonly encountered fractures are through the femoral neck, either subcapital, intertrochanteric or subtrochanteric. Stress fractures of the femoral neck though much less common are also well recognized. Subchondral fracture is most commonly observed as a secondary phenomenon in cases with osteonecrosis of the femoral head.

Recent clinical reports of primary subchondral fractures in the femoral head include stress osteopathy of the femoral head in young military trainees, insufficiency fracture of the femoral head in renal transplant recipients, and most commonly in our experience elderly osteoporotic women. These reports have stressed the importance of its differentiation from osteonecrosis, especially when using magnetic resonance imaging (MRI), since the initial diagnosis will affect the treatment and management of the patient. Most of the clinically reported cases have resolved after conservative therapy without progressing to collapse or surgery. However, in our experience histologic evidence of subchondral fracture as the etiology of acute onset hip pain in elderly women has become increasingly commonplace.

Clinically, patients with subchondral insufficiency fracture are mostly elderly females who are osteopenic and overweight. These features distinguish this patient population from the majority of those with osteonecrosis. In the published cases of insufficiency fracture, shortly after the onset of hip pain, radiographic changes were reported to be unremarkable (which would seem inappropriate to the severity of the reported pain in these patients) (Fig. 11.38). However MRI has shown a bone marrow edema pattern which in about half the cases is associated with a focal low-intensity band on T_1 (Fig. 11.39). Although a low-intensity band is

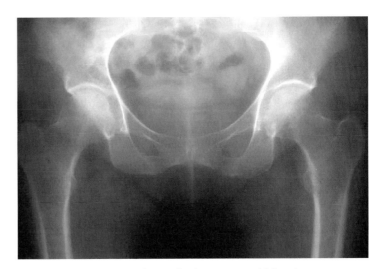

Figure 11.38 An AP radiograph of a 68-year-old female patient complaining of the sudden onset of severe and unremitting pain in the right hip which had persisted for 2 months.

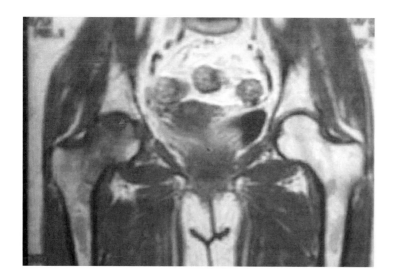

Figure 11.39 An MR image obtained in the patient shown in Figure 11.38 reveals a loss of signal intensity which was interpreted as evidence of osteonecrosis.

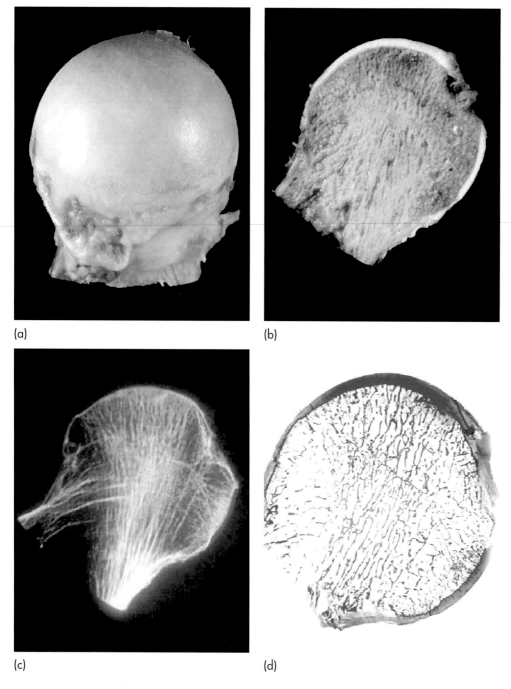

(a)

(b)

(c)

(d)

Figure 11.40 (a) Because of the unremitting pain a total joint replacement was done on the patient shown in Figures 11.38 and 11.39, but except for mild marginal osteophytes, no abnormality of the articular cartilage was seen. (b) Section taken through the femoral head showed no discernible abnormalities and in particular no evidence of osteonecrosis. (c) A radiograph of one of the slices shows subtle alterations in the architecture of the subchondral bone which were not immediately obvious to the prosector. (d) A microscopic section of the slice in (c). Slight thickening is focally present in the subchondral region (H&E, ×1 obj.).

also observed in primary osteonecrosis, it generally differs in two ways. First, in osteonecrosis the subchondral bone segment proximal to the low-intensity bands does not show high-intensity on fat suppression, while in subchondral fracture it usually does. Second, the shape of the low-intensity band in osteonecrosis is usually concave to the articular surface. In subchondral fracture the low-intensity band on T_1 may often parallel the articular surface and show a serpiginous shape (however, in our experience there is considerable variation, which makes the differentiation by MRI difficult).

A femoral head removed in the early stages of an insufficiency fracture is grossly unremarkable except for focal subchondral hemorrhage (Fig. 11.40).

Histopathologically the most characteristic finding in the cases reported was the presence of fracture callus and granulation tissue along both edges of the fracture line (Fig. 11.41). These cases had been previously diagnosed histopathologically as osteonecrosis, presumably because of the small foci of necrosis caused by the fracture (Fig. 11.42). [The failure to recognize the true etiology initially was most likely because the concept of primary subchrondral insufficiency fracture (SIF) was unknown to us.] However, we are now convinced that small foci of necrosis seen only around an area of fracture should not be considered as sufficient evidence for a diagnosis of primary osteonecrosis.

Subchondral fracture of the femoral head is a common complication in cases of osteonecrosis and is generally believed to be the cause of the symptoms. If a patient with a painful hip is shown by imaging studies to have a subchondral fracture, it has been generally assumed that it is a result of osteonecrosis.

The signs and symptoms of fracture secondary to osteonecrosis and of insufficiency fracture are probably similar. However, although most patients with osteonecrosis are in their early 40s, most insufficiency fractures are seen in patients over 60 who are radiologically osteoporotic.

First reported in the literature by Postel and Kerboull in 1970, rapidly destructive arthrosis (RDA) of the hip joint is a relatively uncommon form of arthritis that is seen mostly in elderly women. RDA is characterized by rapid joint destruction within 6–12 months, and disappearance of the joint space is the typical initial finding on radiographs, followed by rapid disappearance of the femoral head. In general, proliferative changes are minimal. The majority of cases are unilateral, without evidence of antecedent OA, osteonecrosis, neuropathy, infection, or inflammatory disease (Fig. 11.43).

Since we became aware of SIF, we have come to realize that this condition is relatively common in the elderly population, and that some cases of SIF show rapid disappearance of the hip joint space.

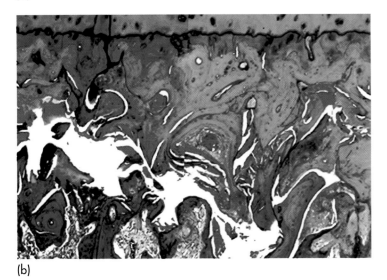

(a)

(b)

Figure 11.41 (a) A low-power microscopic view of the sclerotic area shown in Figure 11.40d reveals a linear fracture (H&E, × 1.5 obj.), which on higher power (b) reveals fracture callus on both sides of the fracture line (H&E, × 10 obj.).

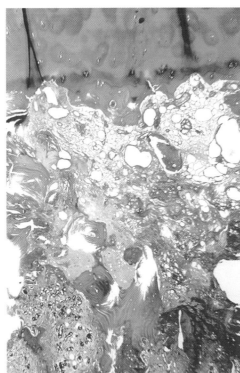

Figure 11.42 Focal necrosis between the fracture and the subchondral bone plate is a common finding in subarticular insufficiency fractures and should not be interpreted as evidence of primary osteonecrosis (H&E, × 10 obj.).

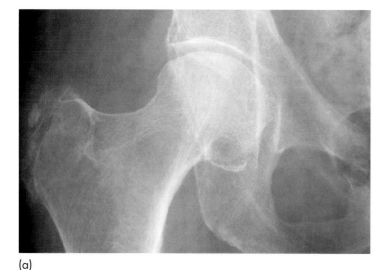

(a)

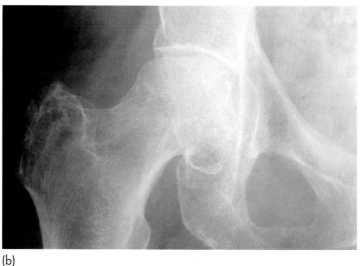

(b)

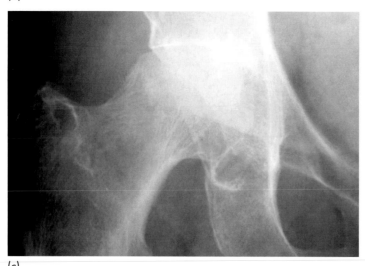

(c)

Figure 11.43 (a) An osteopenic 57-year-old woman complained of severe and intermitting pain in the right hip. (b) There is evident flattening of the superior surface of the femoral head 1 month later together with narrowing of the joint space. (c) There has been further loss of joint space as well as bone 4 months later. This pattern of events is typical of rapidly destructive osteoarthritis (RDA).

In most cases of RDA there is evidence of subchondral fracture histologically (Fig. 11.44). The articular cartilage at the superior portion of the femoral head may be thinned, detached from the subchondral bone or lost. In addition, in the superficial portion of the marrow space, round-to-oval foci of granulomatous tissue are usually observed, in which small fragments of bone and articular cartilage embedded in amorphous eosinophilic debris are found surrounded by aggregated epithelioid histiocytes and giant cells (Fig. 11.45). This type of granulomatous lesion has been observed to be prominent in the advanced stages of RDA, and we consider it pathognomonic of rapid joint destruction. No evidence of primary osteonecrosis was observed in these specimens.

Thin, disconnected bone trabeculae indicative of osteopenia may be observed throughout the femoral head. Although focal thinning and/or absence of the articular cartilage has been noted at the superior portion of the femoral head, it is relatively well preserved on the other areas of the femoral head, with viable chondrocytes, indicating that there is no evidence of chondrolysis morphologically. The synovial tissue generally shows mild hyperplasia and hypertrophy, with minimal inflammation and massive focal accumulation of eosinophilic amorphous debris, including small pieces of bone and articular cartilage detritus (Fig. 11.46).

The initial clinico-radiologic findings in individuals with RDA are similar to those seen in cases of SIF.

The mechanism of rapid joint destruction is almost certainly multifactorial, and no one factor is sufficient to explain it. Many factors seem to play an important role in the pathogenesis of rapid joint destruction, including increased levels of bone resorptive enzymes as well as use of anti-inflammatory drugs or corticosteroid injection into the joint after the fracture has occurred.

We consider the granulomatous lesion to be the result of the rapid rate of bone destruction, which does now allow for resorption in the usual way.

The presence of SIF resulting from osteopenia should be kept in mind when elderly patients have hip pain. Preventive treatment for osteoporosis and the early recognition of SIF may contribute to the elimination of RDA.

Spontaneous osteonecrosis of the knee has been recognized as a distinct form of osteonecrosis since it was first described in 1968. The lesion is clinically characterized by the sudden onset of severe knee-joint pain in older patients and is not usually associated with systemic disorders or previous corticosteroid therapy. In general, the lesion is immediately subarticular and is located in the medial femoral condyle. In the early period after the onset of pain, the radiographic findings are usually unremarkable (Fig. 11.47).

In our experience, spontaneous osteonecrosis of the knee is less common and has a very different morphology than classic

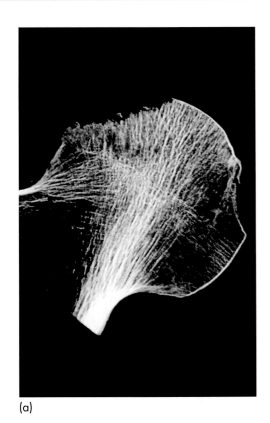

(a)

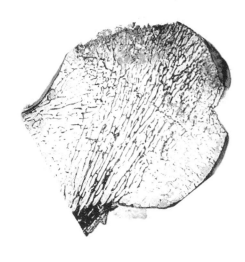

(b)

Figure 11.44 (**a**) A radiograph of a slice of the femoral head removed from the patient shown in Figure 11.43 demonstrates loss of tissue on the superior surface of the femoral head but no evidence of changes generally associated with OA. In particular there is a complete absence of osteophytes. (**b**) A microscopic section to show apparent crushing of the bone trabeculae superiorly (H&E, × 1 obj.), which on closer viewing (**c**) also reveals some immature fracture callus (H&E, × 4 obj.). (**d**) The attenuated trabeculae show focal resorption (H&E, × 10 obj.). (**e**) In other areas the marrow spaces are filled by immature cells (H&E, × 10 obj.).

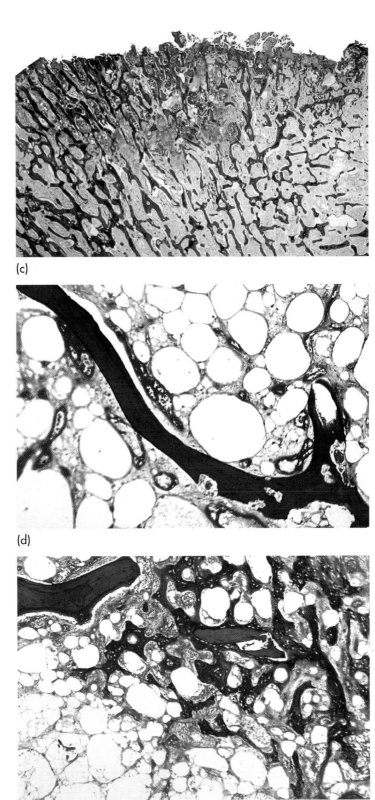

(c)

(d)

(e)

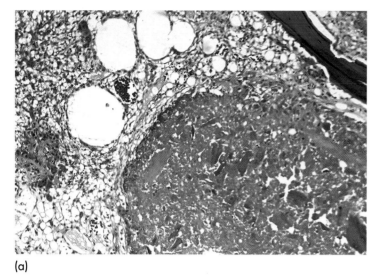

(a)

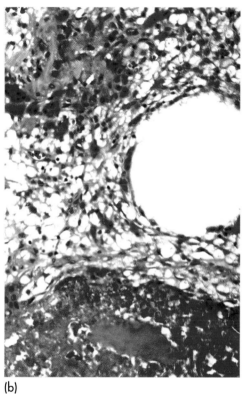

(b)

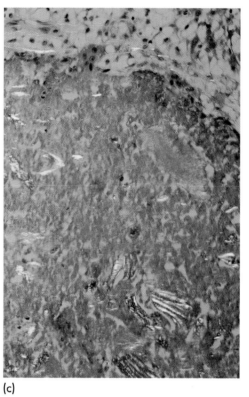

(c)

Figure 11.45 (a) In the deeper portion of the fracture shown in Figure 11.44, granulomas formed of an amorphous debris surrounded by histiocytes and giant cells are present (H&E, × 4 obj.). (b) A higher power view to demonstrate the histiocytes and giant cells (H&E, × 25 obj.). (c) Polarized light clearly demonstrates that within the amorphous debris there are crushed fragments of bone. These lesions are a characteristic finding in rapidly destructive arthritis and clearly reflect the clarity of the process (H&E, polarized light, × 25 obj.).

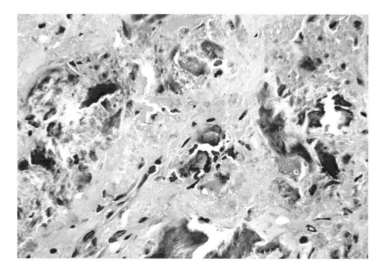

Figure 11.46 Another characteristic finding in rapidly destructive OA is abundant bone and cartilage debris within the synovial tissue (H&E, × 25 obj.).

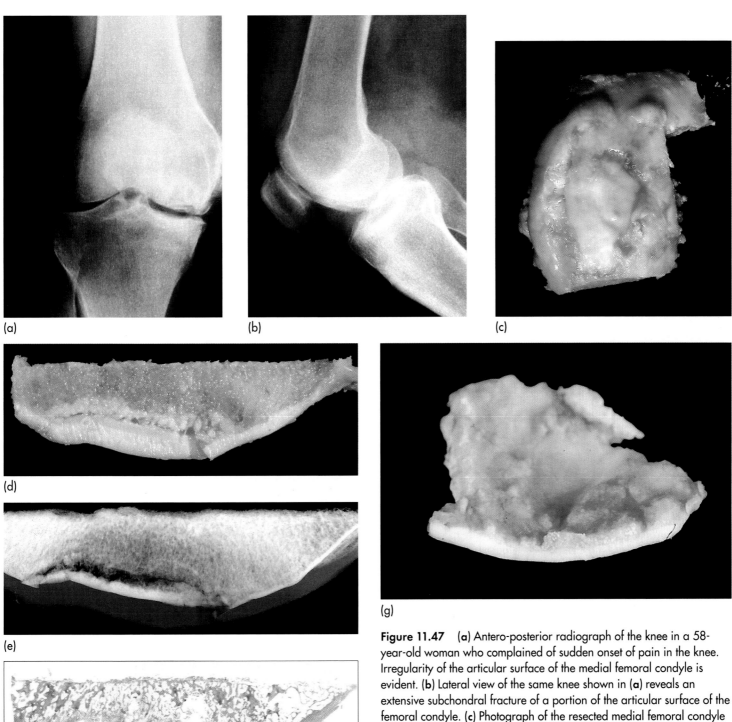

(a)

(b)

(c)

(d)

(e)

(f)

(g)

Figure 11.47 (**a**) Antero-posterior radiograph of the knee in a 58-year-old woman who complained of sudden onset of pain in the knee. Irregularity of the articular surface of the medial femoral condyle is evident. (**b**) Lateral view of the same knee shown in (**a**) reveals an extensive subchondral fracture of a portion of the articular surface of the femoral condyle. (**c**) Photograph of the resected medial femoral condyle to show fracturing of the articular cartilage around the infarcted area. (**d**) Frontal slice taken through the medial condyle. The zone of bone necrosis lies immediately under the articular surface and is characterized by an opaque yellow appearance. Immediately beyond the necrotic zone is a band of hyperemia. Separating the necrotic bone from the overlying cartilage is a gap created by collapse of the bone trabeculae in the necrotic segment. (**e**) Specimen radiograph to demonstrate the subchondral bone end-plate remains attached to the articular cartilage, and around the margin of the infarct the fracture extends through the bone end-plate, producing deformity of the articular surface. (**f**) Photomicrograph of a histologic section through the specimen (H&E, × 1 obj.). (**g**) Photograph of the undersurface of a detached piece of articular surface with visible fragments of attached necrotic subchondral bone.

osteonecrosis of the knee. The classic nontraumatic form of osteonecrosis of the knee has been associated with various factors, especially corticosteroid intake in patients with RA or lupus. It is often bilateral, frequently involves large portions of the epiphysis and metaphysis, and usually is apparent on plain radiographs at the time of the onset of symptoms.

The histopathological findings suggest that subchondral insufficiency fracture resulting from underlying osteoporosis is the etiology of spontaneous osteonecrosis of the knee.

OSTEOCHONDRITIS DISSECANS

Osteochondritis dissecans is a benign noninflammatory condition of diarthrodial joints which affects young adults. The most commonly affected joints are the knee, ankle, and elbow. The disorder

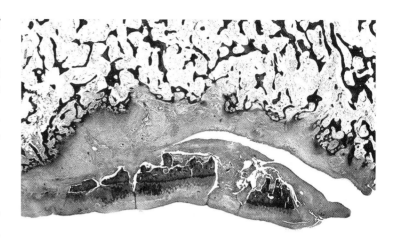

Figure 11.48 In traumatic osteochondritis the fragment may still be attached to the joint surface as illustrated in this photomicrograph (H&E, × 4 obj.).

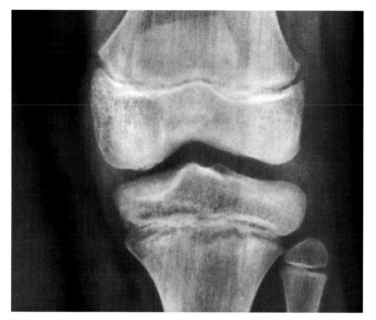

(a)

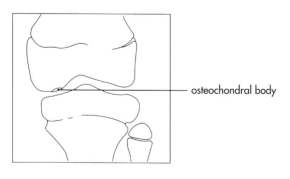

osteochondral body

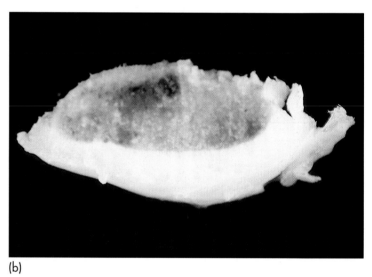

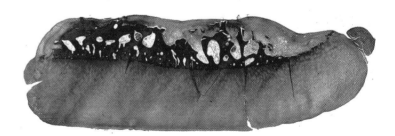

(b)

(c)

Figure 11.49 (a) Radiograph of the knee in a 12-year-old boy who complained of discomfort in the joint shows a well-demarcated defect on the articular surface of the medial femoral condyle. At this point the osteochondral body has not separated from the condyle and is still in situ. (b) Photograph of a section through a loose body removed from a patient with osteochondritis dissecans. There is a layer of intact articular cartilage on the lower surface with an overlying disc of attached bone which itself has a fibrous covering on its inferior surface. (c) Photomicrograph of the loose body. The bone may or may not be necrotic depending upon whether or not it is still attached to the affected epiphysis (H&E, × 1 obj.).

is characterized clinically by pain, limitation of motion, locking of the joint or effusion. Imaging studies reveal a well-demarcated fragment of bone and overlying articular cartilage, which may or may not be separated from the articular surface at the time of presentation (Fig. 11.48). The condition usually involves the lateral aspect of the medial femoral condyle, less commonly, the postero-medial aspect of the talus, or the antero-lateral aspect of the capitellum. Although osteochondritis dissecans is unilateral in most instances, rarely it may be bilateral and symmetrical.

Familial cases of osteochondritis have been reported, and in these the disorder is probably transmitted as an autosomal dominant trait. Affected children are often short in stature and may have an associated endocrine dysfunction. The underlying defect in osteochondritis dissecans may well be an accessory center of ossification, although trauma must play an important role in the initiation of clinical disease.

The gross appearance of a resected specimen is usually that of a flat, smooth nodule formed of avascular bone, with overlying viable articular cartilage. A layer of dense, fibrous connective tissue or fibrocartilage usually forms on the bone surface (Fig. 11.49).

Treatment consists of reattachment of the loose body (where feasible) or excision.

SLIPPED CAPITAL FEMORAL EPIPHYSIS (ADOLESCENT COXA VARA)

Slipped capital femoral epiphysis, a spontaneous fracture and disruption of the epiphyseal plate of the femoral head, usually occurs in overweight adolescent boys at the time of the growth spurt. The condition may be unilateral or bilateral. Early clinical complaints are of pain or limping, with eventual limitation of mobility.

On radiographs, early displacement may be evident only on lateral films, where it appears as a backward (or dorsal) displacement (Fig. 11.50). Eventually there is obvious separation of the femoral head and neck, with resultant coxa vara (Figs 11.51 and 11.52). Valgus presentation is rare.

The condition is very common in domestic pigs which have been bred for very rapid growth. In these animals the condition appears to result from the widening of the growth plate and the increase in vascularity that accompany the period of accelerated skeletal growth.

Microscopically, the epiphyseal growth plate in an affected individual may appear markedly irregular and thicker than normal. Hemorrhage is often present between the growth plate and the primary spongiosa, thus effectively blocking the ingrowth of the metaphyseal capillaries into the growth plate and preventing endochondral ossification (see Fig. 11.53). These circumstances would lead to an increased propensity for shear failure in the angulated growth plate of the femoral neck.

Treatment of a slipped epiphysis is generally by internal fixation of the femoral head.

In blacks, an increased incidence of chondrolysis has been noted in association with a slipped epiphysis. Patients with the combined disorder have elevated levels of immunoglobulins and the C3 component of complement. These findings suggest a localized antigen–antibody-mediated effect as part of a systemic disorder.

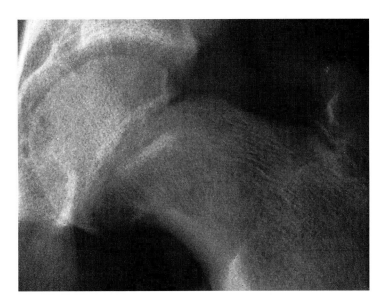

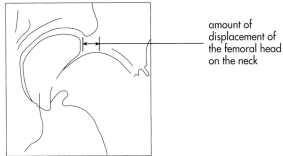

amount of displacement of the femoral head on the neck

Figure 11.50 Clinical radiograph of the hip joint in a patient with a significant slipped epiphysis. The inferior displacement of the capital femoral epiphysis on the neck of the femur can be readily appreciated.

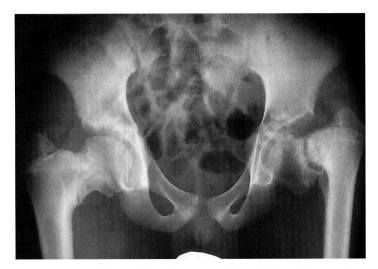

Figure 11.51 Radiograph to demonstrate bilateral slip of the capital femoral epiphysis. On the left side, the epiphysis is almost completely dislocated with respect to the metaphysis.

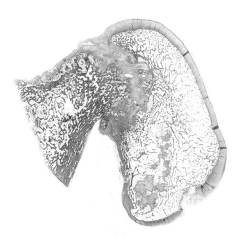

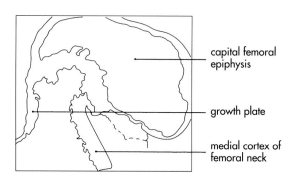

Figure 11.52 Photomicrograph of a section through the femoral head and neck of a case of slipped capital femoral epiphysis. The epiphyseal end of the bone has totally separated from the growth plate, a portion of which is seen on the outer surface of the lower left-hand side of the photograph (H&E, × 1 obj.).

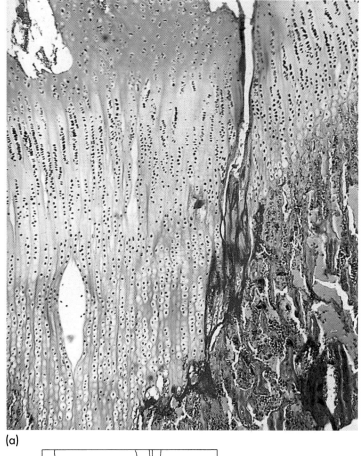

(a)

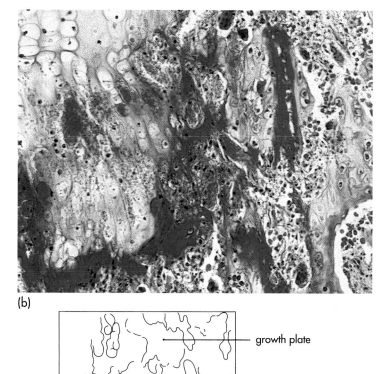

(b)

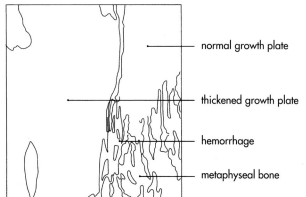

Figure 11.53 (a) Low-power photomicrograph taken during an early stage of a slipped epiphysis, before extensive displacement has occurred. On the left, focal thickening of the growth plate and separation of the growth plate from the underlying metaphysis by hemorrhagic tissue can be seen (Masson trichrome stain, × 4 obj.). (b) High-power photomicrograph of the tissue in (a) shows focal hemorrhage between the growth plate and the metaphysis. It is postulated that such hemorrhagic tissue serves to block continued endochondral ossification, and consequently the growth plate becomes thicker, due to the lack of endochondral ossification and conversion to bone (Masson trichrome stain, × 25 obj.).

CONGENITAL DISLOCATION OF THE HIP

Congenital dislocation of the hip (CDH) is a relatively common abnormality in which the femoral head is not properly positioned in the acetabular fossa at the time of birth (see Fig. 11.54). CDH is not a true congenital malformation, rather it results from either mechanical and/or physical factors that lead to instability of the hip in the newborn. These factors may include maternal hormones such as estrogen and relaxin (which affect fetal as well as maternal ligamentous laxity), tight maternal abdominal and uterine musculature, breech presentation, or forced hip extension following birth. The left hip is more often involved, but bilateral dislocation is present in more than 25% of patients.

Treatment consists of early detection and reduction, i.e. the return of the femoral head to its normal position as soon as possible after birth, and in those centers where this is routine practice the condition is vanishingly rare. However, in persistent dislocation resulting from delayed diagnosis, the bone and soft tissue adjacent to the joint undergo reactive changes which preclude easy reduction. Both the acetabulum and femoral head become irregularly contoured (see Fig. 11.55). Attempts at forcible reduction may compromise the blood supply and lead to avascular necrosis.

In untreated patients, secondary OA develops relatively early in life. Sometimes hip dysplasia (malformation of the joint) occurs without an obvious dislocation of the hip and in such a case there may be a subtle degree of subluxation (see Fig. 11.56). This type of congenital malformation also contributes to the early onset of secondary OA.

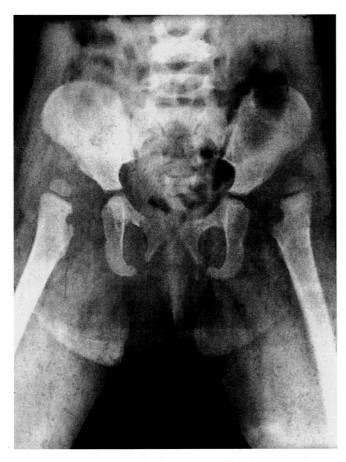

Figure 11.54 Radiograph of a young child with untreated congenital dislocation of the hips reveals that both hips are dislocated, and the roof of the acetabulum appears to be poorly formed. After reduction this patient developed avascular necrosis of the right hip, a common complication.

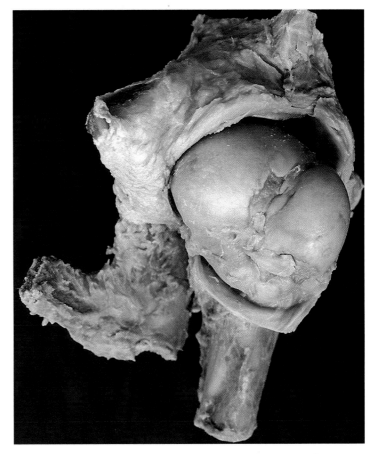

Figure 11.55 An anatomic dissection from a young child with congenital dislocation of the hip that was not reduced. Note the deformity of the femoral head, which has developed a saddle-shaped groove across its superior portion. On clinical radiographs this groove may give the appearance of a double head.

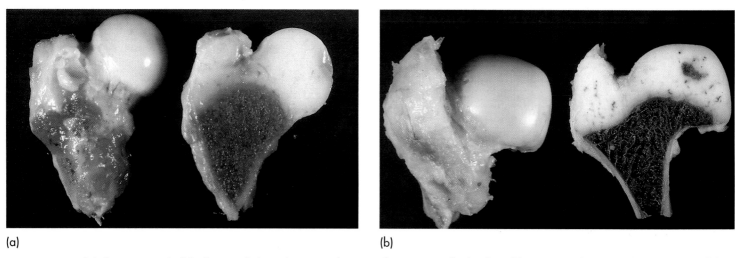

(a)   (b)

Figure 11.56   (a) The upper end of the femur, whole and in coronal section, from a normally developed hip in a newborn. (b) The upper end of the femur, whole and in coronal section, from an infant with hip dysplasia shows the abnormal configuration of the articular surface.

INFLAMMATORY ARTHRITIDES

Bacterial infections of the joint may lead to severe and rapid breakdown of the joint tissues, with resultant severe arthritis (see Chapter 5 under 'Joint infection'). The massive acute inflammatory infiltrate associated with pyogenic infection produces proteolytic enzymes which rapidly break down the articular cartilage and intra-articular structures (Figs 12.1 and 12.2). Aspiration of the joint in such cases reveals a predominance of polymorphonuclear leukocytes, with a count usually well over 100,000/mm³ (see Tables 10.1 and 10.2).

Since both acute gout and acute rheumatoid joint disease, two of the principal topics of this chapter, also may present with fever and hot tender joints, on occasion arriving at the correct diagnosis may be difficult. Rarely, infection may complicate pre-existing rheumatoid arthritis (RA), further adding to the clinical diagnostic difficulties.

INFLAMMATORY ARTHRITIS ASSOCIATED WITH DIFFUSE CONNECTIVE-TISSUE DISEASE

Generalized polyarticular arthritis (or rarely monarticular arthritis) is often the presenting symptom in patients with a variety of diffuse rheumatic connective-tissue diseases such as RA, systemic lupus erythematosus, and Sjögren's syndrome. However, RA is the most common of these conditions and is most typically characterized by arthritis.

Although the various rheumatic diseases differ markedly in clinical presentation, the histopathology of the associated joint disease tends to be similar. There are no specific qualitative microscopic findings in the synovium that distinguish RA from lupus erythematosus or from the arthritis associated with psoriasis or ulcerative colitis.

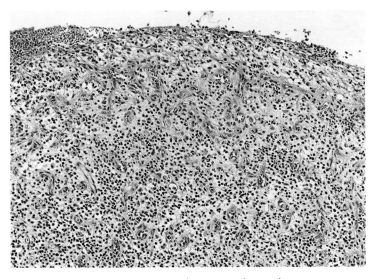

Figure 12.1 Acute synovitis in early septic arthritis. The synovium is heavily infiltrated by polymorphonuclear leukocytes, the hallmark of acute bacterial infection (H&E, × 4 obj.).

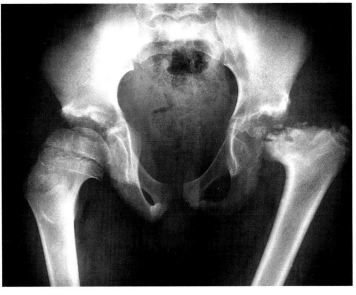

Figure 12.2 Radiograph showing destruction of both hip joints following infantile septic arthritis.

RHEUMATOID ARTHRITIS

RA is a chronic systemic disease of unknown etiology that most commonly involves the synovial lining of the peripheral joints; this inflammatory synovitis results in local destruction, ultimately leading to joint deformities (Fig. 12.3).

RA is characterized clinically by spontaneous remission and exacerbation, and is two to three times more common in women than in men. Although it may occur at any age, the peak age of onset in women is the period from the fourth to the sixth decades. Of all affected individuals, 70–80% test positive for the histocompatibility antigen DW4 and/or DR4, a finding that implies a

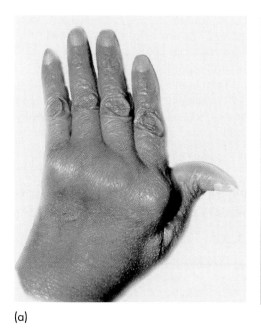

(a)

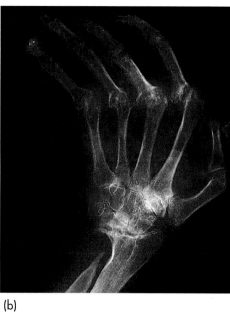

(b)

Figure 12.3 (a) In RA, the deformity is usually distinct. Swelling at the MCP joint has resulted in lateral slippage of the extensor tendon and ulnar deviation of the fingers. (b) Radiograph demonstrating the destructive joint changes associated with advanced RA. Note especially the marked bone destruction at the wrist, the subluxation and ulnar deviation at the MCP joints, and the dislocation of the IP joint of the thumb.

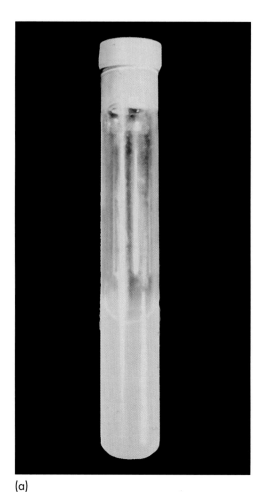

(a)

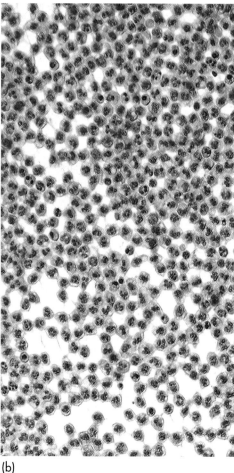

(b)

Figure 12.4 (a) Synovial fluid aspirate from a patient with RA. Note the turbidity of this specimen. (b) Microscopy reveals a majority of polymorphonuclear leukocytes (× 25 obj.).

strong hereditary component. Extra-articular features, such as arteritis, neuropathy, pericarditis, splenomegaly, lymphadenopathy, and rheumatoid nodules occur with considerable frequency, indicating the systemic nature of the disease.

The affected patient is likely to complain of symptoms of general malaise, as well as pain and stiffness in the joints, characteristically more pronounced in the morning. Although any joint can be involved, those most commonly affected are the small joints of the hands and feet. In general, the disease is polyarticular, bilateral, and symmetrical.

Clinical examination reveals the acutely affected joint to be hot, swollen, and tender. The aspirated synovial effusion is milky and turbid (Fig. 12.4). Compared with septic arthritis, in which the synovial fluid usually contains more than 100,000 white blood cells/mm³, at least 75% of which are polymorphonuclear leukocytes, the rheumatoid joint effusion usually contains 20,000–50,000 inflammatory cells/mm³, only about 50% of which are polymorphonuclear leukocytes. Cultures of the synovial fluid and synovial membrane for various organisms, including viruses, have generally been negative.

The principle macroscopic morphologic feature of rheumatoid disease, seen both on X-ray examination and at surgery, is joint destruction (Fig. 12.5). Unlike the noninflammatory arthritides, there is little reparative activity, and osteophytes and new bone formation are not prominent (Fig. 12.6).

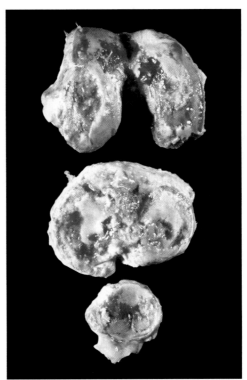

Figure 12.5 Gross photograph of the articular surfaces of a knee joint from a patient with RA. The articular cartilage is destroyed more at the periphery of the joint, whereas the central areas are spared. This finding is characteristic of the inflammatory arthritides, and should be contrasted with the findings in patients with OA, in whom the central cartilage is usually destroyed first and the periphery is spared.

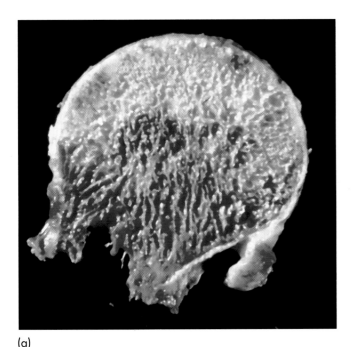

(a)

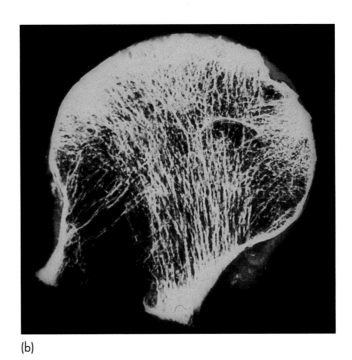

(b)

Figure 12.6 (a) Frontal section through the femoral head in a patient with RA. The joint surface is destroyed but there is no evidence of osteophyte formation or bone sclerosis. The absence of these two features is in marked contrast to the morphologic findings in patients with OA. (b) Specimen radiograph of (a).

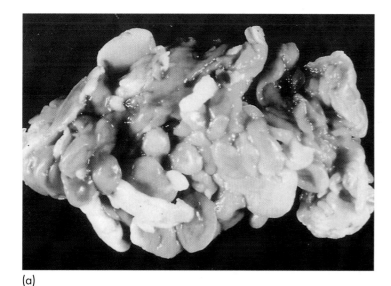

(a)

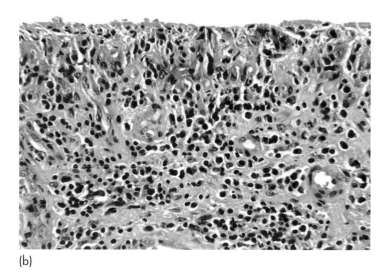

(b)

Microscopically nonsuppurative chronic inflammation of the synovium is accompanied by hypertrophy and hyperplasia of the synovial lining cells, resulting in a papillary pattern at the surface of the synovium (Fig. 12.7). Occasionally there are scattered giant cells among the synovial lining cells (Fig. 12.8). The inflammation is characterized by infiltration of the synovial membrane by lymphocytes, plasma cells, and some mast cells (Figs 12.9 and 12.10). The plasma cells often contain eosinophilic inclusions of immunoglobulin (Russell bodies), lym-

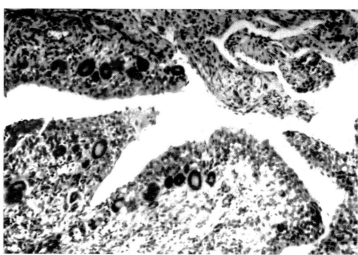

Figure 12.8   Photomicrograph of a section of synovial membrane from a patient with RA. The increased number of lining cells (hyperplasia) and their increased size (hypertrophy) are evident. Many giant cells are also present just below the surface. In the subintimal tissue there is a chronic inflammatory infiltrate (H&E, × 10 obj.).

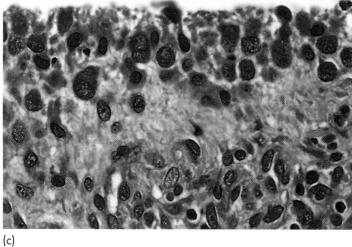

(c)

Figure 12.7   (a) Photograph of synovium from a patient with RA. The cinnamon color is caused by post-hemorrhagic hemosiderin deposits in the synovium. The plump papillae stem from the cellular overgrowth of the synovium, as well as from the lymphoid infiltration of the subintimal layer. The irregular white nodules on the surface are fibrin, the product of vascular exudation in the inflamed tissue. (b) Photomicrograph demonstrating the hyperplasia of the synovial lining (H&E, × 10 obj.). (c) A higher magnification of a section from (b) (H&E, × 40 obj.).

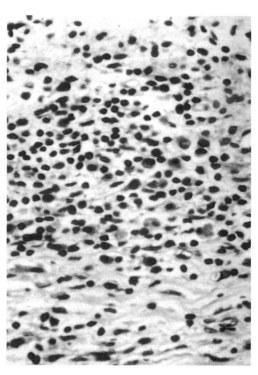

Figure 12.9
Photomicrograph of the subintimal region of the synovial membrane in a patient with RA shows infiltration of both lymphocytes and plasma cells (H&E, × 25 obj.).

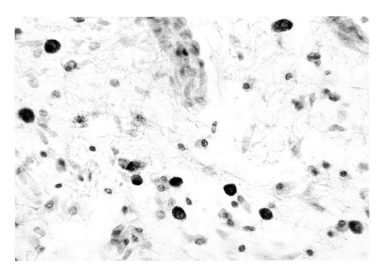

Figure 12.10 Photomicrograph to show mast cells within rheumatoid synovium (toluidine blue, × 25 obj.).

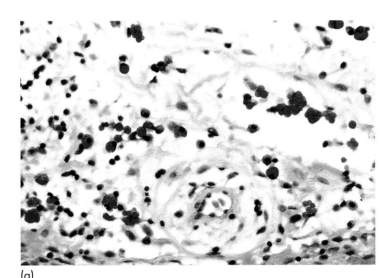

(a)

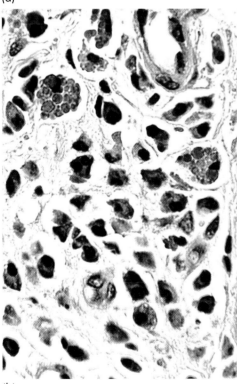

(b)

Figure 12.11
(a) Photomicrograph of inflammatory infiltrate in rheumatoid synovium reveals eosinophilic cytoplasmic inclusions (Russell bodies) in the plasma cells (H&E, × 10 obj.). (b) Higher magnification shows multiple accumulated Russell bodies in the cytoplasm of plasma cells (H&E, × 40 obj.).

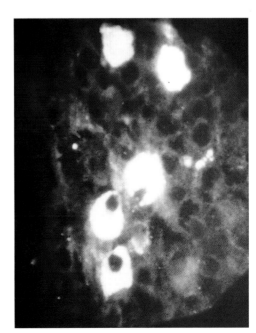

Figure 12.12
The plasma cells and Russell's bodies contain rheumatoid factor (immunoglobulin including IgM), demonstrated here by staining with fluorescein-labeled antibody to rheumatoid factor. This specimen is viewed with ultraviolet light.

phoid follicles, and fibrinous exudation. Admixed polymorphonuclear leukocytes, both at the surface of the synovium and within the synovial tissue, is a prominent feature in the acute phase (Figs 12.11–12.17). Vasculitis is a prominent feature in some patients (Fig. 12.18).

Later in the course of the disease the hypertrophied, inflamed synovium extends over the articular surface (pannus) and destroys the underlying cartilage by interfering with chondrocyte nutrition and by enzymatic degradation of the matrix (Figs 12.19 and 12.20). The end result of this inflammatory destruction of the articular surfaces may be fusion of the joint (ankylosis), either by fibrous granulation tissue or by bone (Figs 12.21 and 12.22). In addition to destroying the cartilaginous surface of the joint, the rheumatoid synovium usually invades and destroys the joint capsule and other periarticular supportive tissues. This process leads to marked instability of the joint, and frequently to subluxation or complete dislocation.

The inflamed synovium also invades the bone at the articular margins, a process that appears on radiographs as marginal erosion (Fig. 12.23). Extra-articular synovitis may lead to bursitis (Fig. 12.24), carpal tunnel syndrome or 'trigger finger', or tendinitis (Fig. 12.25), and in some cases these clinical syndromes are the herald to more generalized articular disease.

It is not always realized that joint destruction is not solely the result of synovial inflammation; in the subchondral bone not in contact with the articular margins, there may also be considerable chronic inflammation and formation of lymphoid follicles (Fig. 12.26). This inflammation is confined to the subchondral bone and does not extend far into the underlying cancellous bone. In some cases, the inflammatory tissue destroys the articular cartilage from below (Fig. 12.27) and in other cases it is possible to see both destruction from the synovial surface by pannus and from the subchondral bone (Fig. 12.28). Radiographs of

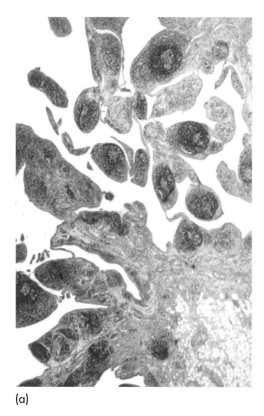
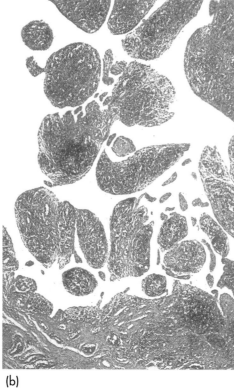

(a)

(b)

Figure 12.13 (a) Low-power photomicrograph of synovium from a patient with RA demonstrates the distribution of lymphoid follicles (Allison–Ghormley bodies) in the subintimal tissue (H&E, × 4 obj.). (b) A higher magnification photomicrograph shows the intensity of the inflammatory infiltrate (H&E, × 10 obj.). (c) Higher magnification shows a chronic inflammatory infiltrate of lymphocytes with focal plasma cell predominance (H&E, × 25 obj.). (d) At a higher magnification, microscopic exudation of fibrin is present in the synovial lining (H&E, × 40 obj.).

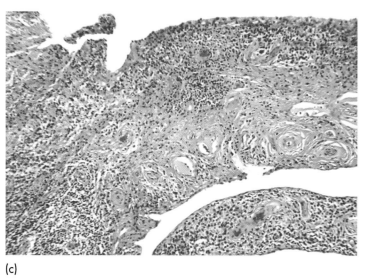
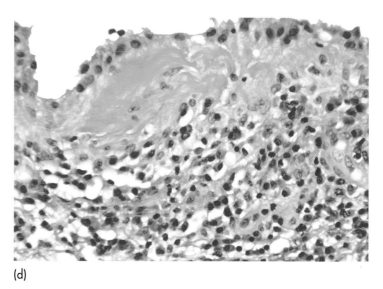

(c)

(d)

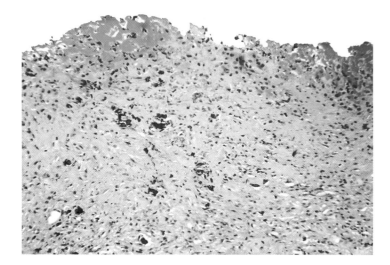

Figure 12.14 Photomicrograph of the synovium shows focal fibrinous exudate on the inflamed synovial surface. The dark irregular fragments represent bone detritus (H&E, × 10 obj.).

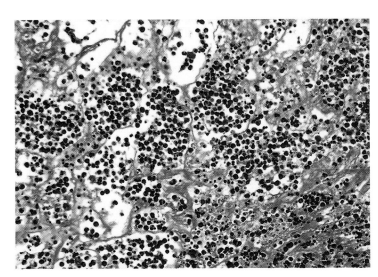

Figure 12.15 Photomicrograph showing polymorphonuclear leukocytes and nuclear debris in the fibrinous exudate of a patient with an acute rheumatoid joint. With this severity of acute inflammation, it is important to rule out an infection (H&E, × 10 obj.).

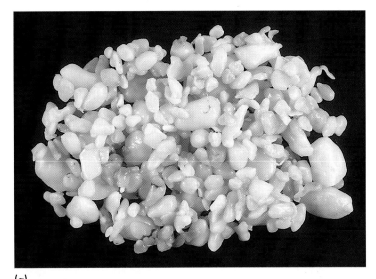

(a)

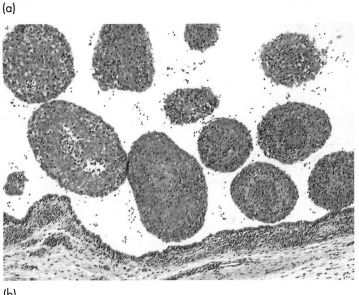

(b)

Figure 12.17 (a) Photograph of fibrinous loose bodies or 'rice bodies' recovered from the knee joint of a patient with RA. (b) Photomicrograph of fibrinous loose bodies with a portion of the synovial membrane in the lower part of the picture (H&E, × 4 obj.).

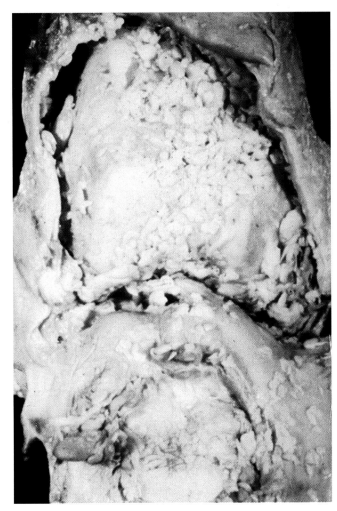

Figure 12.16 Gross photograph of the suprapatellar pouch and synovium of a knee joint demonstrates copious fibrinous exudate on the surface of the synovium.

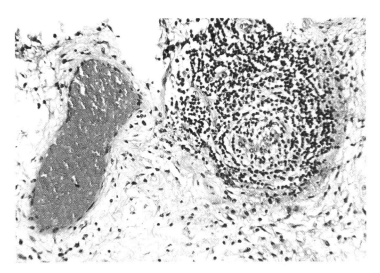

Figure 12.18 Photomicrograph showing a heavy chronic inflammatory infiltration in the wall of an arteriole (H&E, × 25 obj.).

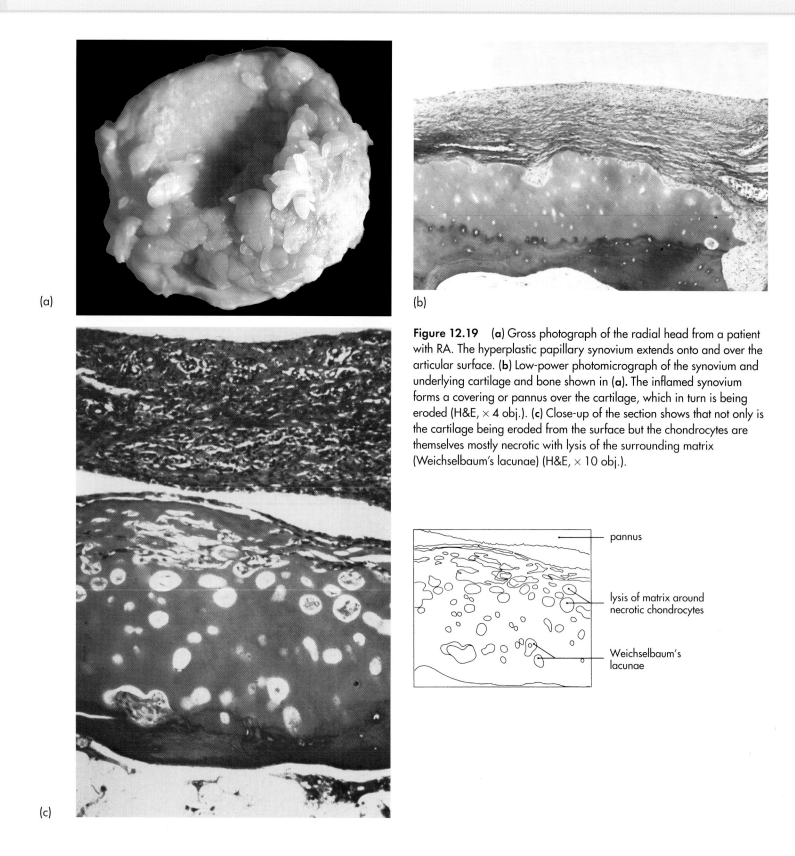

(a)

(b)

(c)

Figure 12.19 (a) Gross photograph of the radial head from a patient with RA. The hyperplastic papillary synovium extends onto and over the articular surface. (b) Low-power photomicrograph of the synovium and underlying cartilage and bone shown in (a). The inflamed synovium forms a covering or pannus over the cartilage, which in turn is being eroded (H&E, × 4 obj.). (c) Close-up of the section shows that not only is the cartilage being eroded from the surface but the chondrocytes are themselves mostly necrotic with lysis of the surrounding matrix (Weichselbaum's lacunae) (H&E, × 10 obj.).

affected joints usually reveal a juxta-articular osteopenia, which is caused by inflammation of the subchondral bone and/or by hyperemia secondary to the inflammation of the synovium (Fig. 12.29).

About 25% of patients with RA have subcutaneous nodules, most commonly over the extensor surfaces of the elbow and forearm (Fig. 12.30). Nodules may also occur in other subcutaneous

sites, as well as in the gastrointestinal tract, lungs, heart, and the synovial membrane itself (Fig. 12.31). The nodules can appear before any other signs of rheumatoid disease. The rheumatoid nodule is characterized histologically by its irregular shape and a central zone of necrotic fibrinoid material surrounded by histiocytes and some chronic inflammatory cells (Figs 12.32 and 12.33). The long axes of these histiocytes are frequently radially

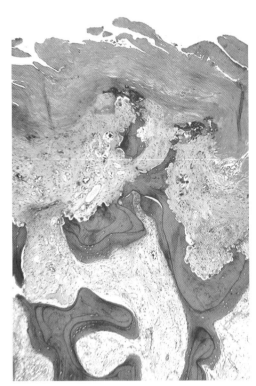

Figure 12.20 Photomicrograph of an articular surface in late RA, showing a destructive fibrous pannus with resorption of the underlying trabecular bone and chronic inflammation of the marrow space (H&E, × 4 obj.).

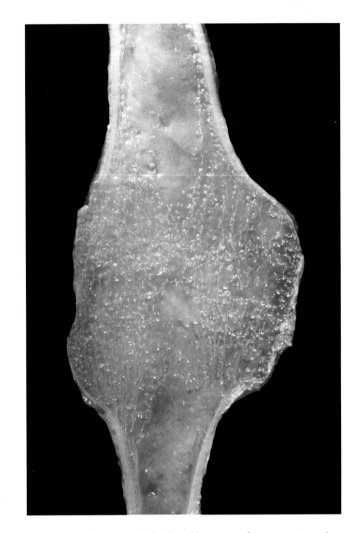

Figure 12.22 Photograph of a fused knee joint from a patient who had suffered from RA for many years.

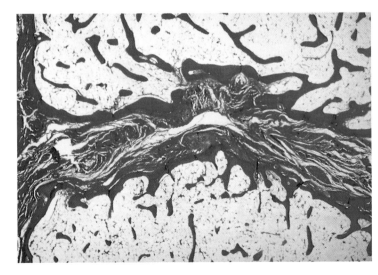

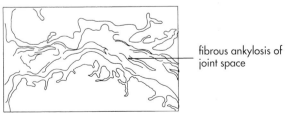

fibrous ankylosis of joint space

Figure 12.21 Low-power photomicrograph of an MCP joint with a fibrous ankylosis (H&E, × 2.5 obj.).

disposed or palisaded. The fact that generalized vasculitis is much more common in patients with rheumatoid nodules than in those without is consistent with the belief that the nodules are the result of vascular damage.

Although the etiology of RA is unknown, two important factors contribute to its pathogenesis: an immunologic reaction and an increased number of degradative enzymes. The serum and synovial fluid, of most patients with RA, contain a number of immunoglobulins in common the most frequent of which is immunoglobulin M (IgM). These immunoglobulins, known as rheumatoid factor, are produced by plasma cells both in the synovium and lymphoid system as antibodies to autologous immunoglobulin G (IgG), which in RA is believed to be altered in some way. These factors appear on microscopic examination, both within and in the vicinity of plasma cells, as dense, homogenous, eosinophilic globules (or Russell bodies). Approximately 70% of patients with RA have a positive rheumatoid factor, and high titers are usually associated with either acute disease or severe chronic disease.

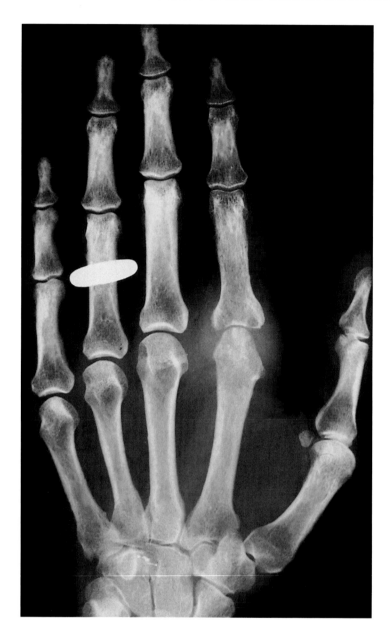

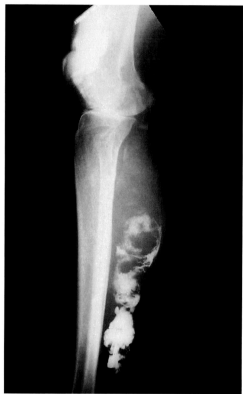

Figure 12.24
Lateral radiograph of the leg of a patient with RA which began as a juvenile disease. The patient had complained of swelling of the calf over many months. Radiocontrast material has been injected into the popliteal cyst to demonstrate its extent in this patient.

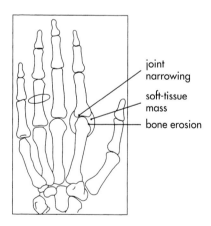

joint narrowing

soft-tissue mass

bone erosion

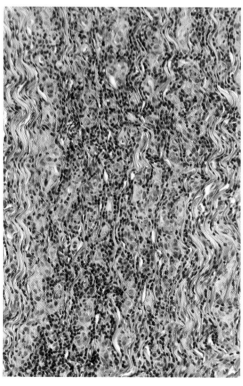

Figure 12.25
Photomicrograph of tissue obtained from an inflamed extensor tendon of the hand showing an inflammatory infiltrate between collagen fibers (H&E, × 25 obj.).

Figure 12.23   Radiograph of the hand in a patient with early RA. Note the soft-tissue swelling, reduction in the width of the joint space, and erosion that has taken place at the margin of the MCP joint of the index finger.

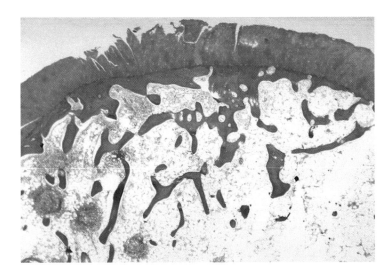

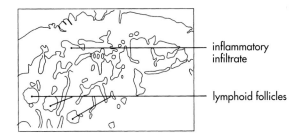

Figure 12.26 Low-power photomicrograph of a section through a joint in a patient with RA. Note the extensive chronic inflammatory infiltrate in the subarticular marrow space, as well as occasional lymphoid follicles (H&E, × 2.5 obj.).

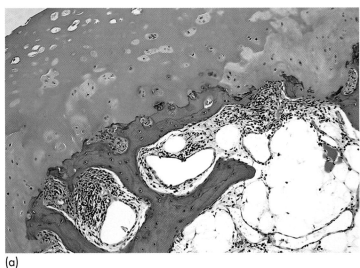

(a)

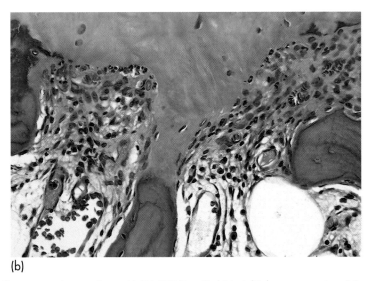

(b)

Figure 12.27 (a) Photomicrograph to demonstrate subchondral chronic inflammation in a patient with RA (H&E, × 5 obj.). A higher power view (b) to demonstrate the inflammatory destruction of the articular cartilage from its subchondral surface (H&E, × 25 obj.).

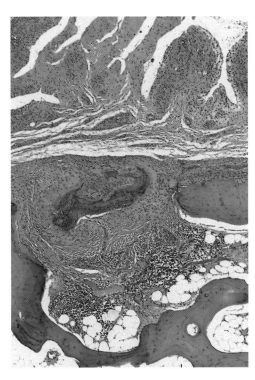

Figure 12.28 Photomicrograph to demonstrate destruction of the articular surface by both pannus and subchondral inflammation (H&E, × 5 obj.).

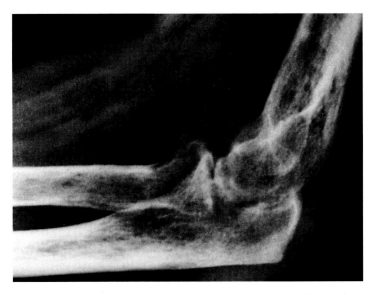

Figure 12.29 Radiograph of the elbow in a patient with polyarticular RA. Note the loss of joint space, resulting from destructive inflammatory synovitis. In this radiograph the soft tissue is clearly seen, making it apparent that there is considerable juxta-articular osteoporosis, a finding which is in marked contrast to the bony sclerosis associated with noninflammatory OA.

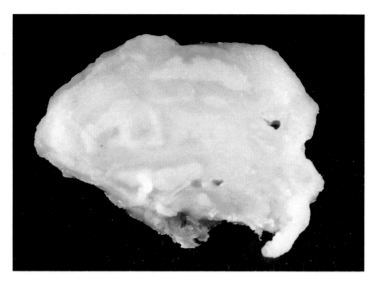

Figure 12.30 Photograph of the cut surface of a rheumatoid nodule. Note the well-defined, opaque yellow areas of necrosis with their irregular 'geographic' outlines.

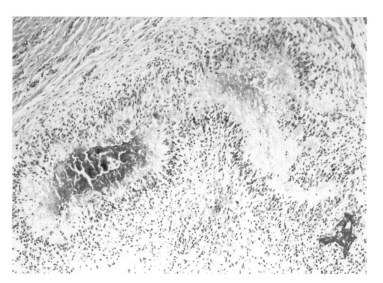

Figure 12.32 Photomicrograph of a rheumatoid nodule illustrates the serpiginous shape of the central geographic fibrinoid necrosis and the surrounding palisaded chronic inflammatory cells (H&E, × 2.5 obj.).

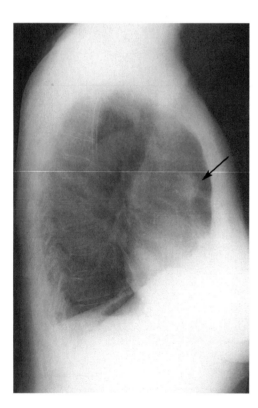

Figure 12.31 Radiograph of a lateral projection of the chest shows a well-defined opacity in the anterior lung field, which proved to be a rheumatoid nodule.

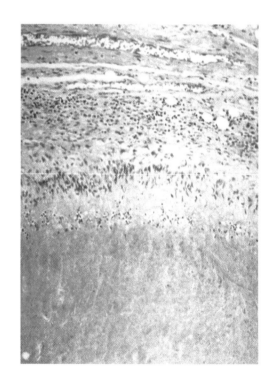

Figure 12.33 Photomicrograph of a portion of a rheumatoid nodule demonstrates well-defined zones of central fibrinoid necrosis surrounded by a layer of palisaded histiocytes, which in turn is surrounded by a layer of lymphocytes and dense fibrous connective tissue (H&E, × 25 obj.).

Rheumatoid factor complexes with IgG in a manner not unlike an antigen–antibody reaction. Leukocytes are attracted to the immune complexes which, along with fibrin, form deposits on the surface of the inflamed synovium. These leukocytes, filled with particles of ingested fibrin and immune complex, may be found in the synovial fluid and are called 'RA cells'. After destruction of the polymorphonuclear leukocytes, lysosomal enzymes are released into the extracellular space, where they further provoke an acute inflammatory response and tissue necrosis. These lyso-somal enzymes exist in large concentrations in both the synovial fluid and tissue of rheumatoid joints, and they play an important role in perpetuation of the tissue destruction that characterizes the disease.

In the late stages of RA with destruction of the articular cartilage, the affected joint may show very little inflammation though there may be some dystrophic calcification (Fig. 12.34). The end-stage disease may therefore become anatomically indistinguishable from osteoarthritis (OA).

Occasionally in histologic sections from patients with RA it is possible to find evidence of the therapies used in the course of the disease such as gold and local corticosteroid injections (Figs 12.35 and 12.36).

JUVENILE RHEUMATOID ARTHRITIS (JUVENILE CHRONIC POLYARTHRITIS; JUVENILE CHRONIC ARTHRITIS)

A chronic inflammatory arthritis may also occur in children. About 20% of cases are polyarthritic, presenting with systemic disease, 40% are polyarthritic without systemic disease, and 40% are pauciarticular, with few joints affected. Most of these children test negative for rheumatoid factor. The few patients who are positive tend to pursue a more severe course and are more likely to

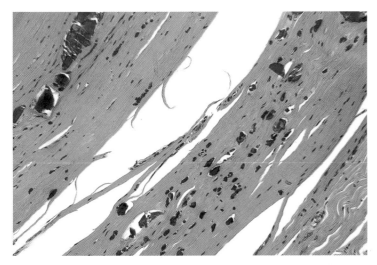

Figure 12.34   Photomicrograph demonstrating dystrophic calcification of the joint capsular tissue in late-stage RA (H&E, × 10 obj.).

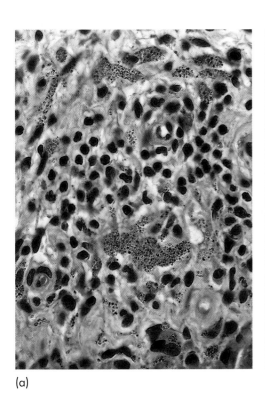

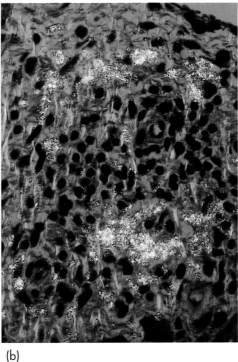

Figure 12.35   Photomicrograph of synovial tissue (**a**) obtained from a patient with RA reveals extensive fine deposits of a brown–black substance which is reflective when examined by polarized light (**b**). Analysis of this material by energy-dispersive analysis has shown it to contain gold (H&E, × 25 obj.).

(a)   (b)

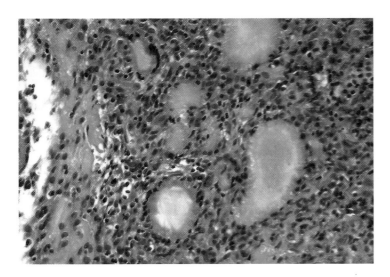

Figure 12.36   Photomicrograph to show deposits of an amorphous material within the synovial tissue taken from a patient with RA. This material can be seen to have evoked a giant-cell and histiocytic response. By history and by comparison with other patients these deposits are most likely to have resulted from the corticosteroid injections (H&E, × 10 obj.).

end with a crippling arthritis. However, the outlook for most children with juvenile rheumatoid arthritis (JRA) is good and although the disease is chronic, at least 75% of cases enter long remission with little or no residual disability.

Synovial biopsies in children affected by JRA usually show much less severe disease than the typical RA of adult onset (Fig. 12.37).

PSORIATIC ARTHRITIS

Perhaps just under 10% of patients with psoriasis have an associated inflammatory arthritis which, in general, is less severe than most cases of RA. Mostly it is the peripheral joints which are involved by the disease and most often the distal interphalangeal joints.

Subcutaneous nodules are not a feature in psoriatic arthritis, though they may on occasion be seen. These patients will usually be found to have rheumatoid factor and in these cases the two diseases are generally considered co-incidental.

The characteristic radiographic features in patients with psoriatic arthritis include a destructive arthritis affecting small joints with severe erosions resulting in a 'pencil-in-cup' appearance (Fig. 12.38). In a few cases there is a very severe mutilating process. Sometimes there may be periostitis along the shafts of the long bones and prominent syndesmophytes in the spine. Microscopically the synovium of psoriatic arthritis is similar to that of RA, though it may be somewhat more fibrotic.

BURSITIS

Bursitis is clinically characterized by pain, redness, and/or swelling of one of the many synovium-lined bursae that lie between muscles, tendons, and bone prominences, especially around the joints. Bursitis is usually caused by chronic trauma. It often occurs in the shoulders of professional athletes and in the prepatellar and infrapatellar bursae of those who frequently kneel (e.g. housewives and the religiously inclined). Bursitis is sometimes observed as a complication of RA.

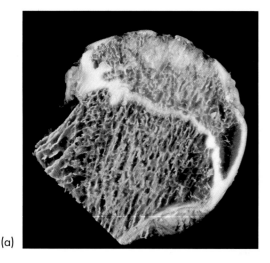

(a)

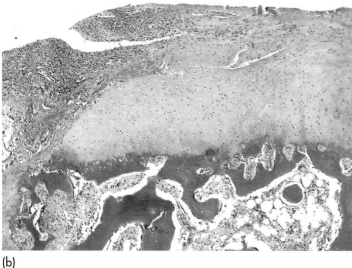

(b)

Figure 12.37 (a) Photograph of a frontal section taken through the femoral head of a child with JRA. Extensive destruction of the articular cartilage has occurred, with associated erosion of the subchondral bone. (b) Photomicrograph of a section taken at the articular margin of the specimen demonstrated in (a) shows a destructive inflammatory pannus extending onto the articular surface (H&E, × 4 obj.).

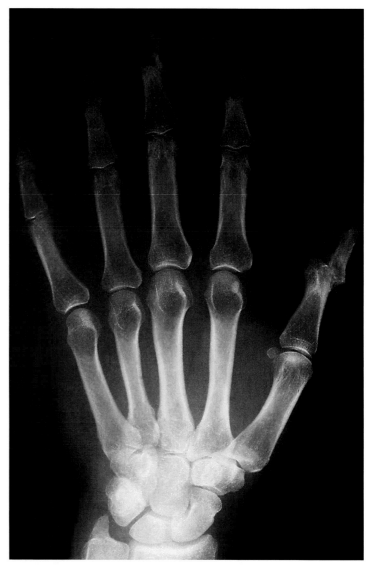

Figure 12.38 Radiograph of the right hand from a patient with psoriasis. Destructive lesions in the IP joint, particularly the distal joints. (Courtesy of Dr Robert Freiberger.)

In the past bursitis from infection was frequently due to tuberculosis.

A bursa may also be involved in other conditions that commonly affect the synovial membrane (e.g. gout, synovial chondromatosis, or pigmented villonodular synovitis).

On gross examination of an inflamed bursa, the wall of the bursal sac is usually markedly thickened and the lining often appears injected and shaggy due to fibrinous exudation into the cavity (Fig. 12.39). The microscopic findings depend on the etiology, and the various diseases that might affect the synovium, including infection, should be carefully sought. However, in most cases of post-traumatic origin, scarring and chronic inflammation predominate.

Sometimes extensive calcification may complicate a chronically inflamed bursa, which renders it visible on radiologic examination. Treatment depends on the etiology and the extent of the lesion.

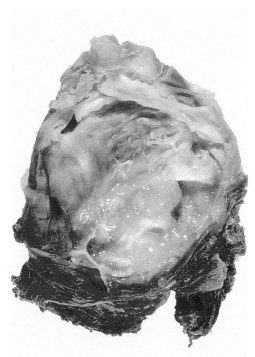

Figure 12.39
Gross photograph of an excised popliteal cyst, which was opened to demonstrate a thick fibrous wall with a roughened lining, and a fibrinous exudate.

DISEASES RESULTING FROM DEPOSITION OF METABOLIC PRODUCTS IN JOINT TISSUES

GOUT

Gout is characterized clinically by episodic acute attacks of inflammatory arthritis, usually monarticular, and by the development of deposits of sodium urate around affected joints.

Uric acid is the end-product of the catabolism of purines, and since humans lack the enzyme uricase, increased synthesis of uric acid or decreased secretion of uric acid by the kidneys leads to hyperuricemia. Uric acid is not very soluble and begins to precipitate as sodium urate at concentrations above 8.0 mg/dL, especially in a more acid environment such as in the kidneys and joints. Prolonged hyperuricemia eventually leads to the deposition of monosodium urate crystals in both the joints and visceral tissue, but especially in the kidneys, in which precipitates of urates and subsequent stone formation are seen in nearly all patients with gout. When crystals are precipitated in body cavities, such as a joint, they provoke an acute inflammatory response.

Primary hyperuricemia is an inherited error of metabolism that results from an enzymatic defect in purine synthesis and/or in the renal excretion of uric acid. However, hyperuricemia is most often secondary, and is due to disorders either that increase the production of uric acid by cell breakdown or that decrease the excretion of uric acid (as in various forms of chronic renal disease). The former group includes the myeloproliferative disorders, in which there is an increased turnover of nucleic acid, and cancer, in which there is increased cell breakdown.

Gout can be divided into three clinical stages: acute gouty arthritis, an intermediate stage called intercritical gout, and the chronic stage, in which diffuse deposits are seen (chronic tophaceous gout).

Acute gouty arthritis is usually monarticular and characterized by the rapid onset of severe pain and swelling, often accompanied by a low-grade fever and leukocytosis. It has a particular predilection for the lower extremities. The first metatarsophalangeal joint (the great toe) is the most common site of initial involvement. Acute attacks may be precipitated by trauma, intercurrent illness, or debauchery.

Between attacks of acute gout, the patient may have long clinically asymptomatic periods, even though the hyperuricemia persists. Eventually the state of chronic tophaceous gout occurs, in which deposition of monosodium urate crystals occurs throughout the body but particularly in the kidneys and para-articular regions (Fig. 12.40). Although the reason for the deposition of crystals is not completely understood, the process is known to be accelerated by the presence of a low pH, as is present in the joint spaces.

The radiographic features of gout include swelling of the periarticular soft tissues and subsequent erosion of the periarticular bone, giving rise to the classic punched-out lesion with overhanging edges, at the joint margin. Generally there is little reactive sclerosis and, in contrast to RA, there is no regional osteoporosis (Fig. 12.41).

In acute gouty synovitis microscopic examination, of the synovial fluid, reveals an inflammatory exudate which may be mistaken for evidence of infection. However, examination using polarized light and a first-order red filter will reveal crystals with a strong negative birefringence. Characteristically the crystals are found in polymorphonuclear leukocytes (Fig. 12.42) (For a discussion of the examination for crystals, see p. 305 of this chapter.)

The chalky white tophi associated with the chronic phase of gout consist of large deposits of crystals surrounded by fibrous tissue and rimmed by both mononuclear histiocytes and giant cells (Fig. 12.43). (It should be noted that preservation of the crystals for identification with polarized light microscopy requires the use of unstained sections since the aqueous dyes used in most staining techniques will dissolve the crystals. Crystal preservation is also improved by the use of alcohol rather than formalin fixative.)

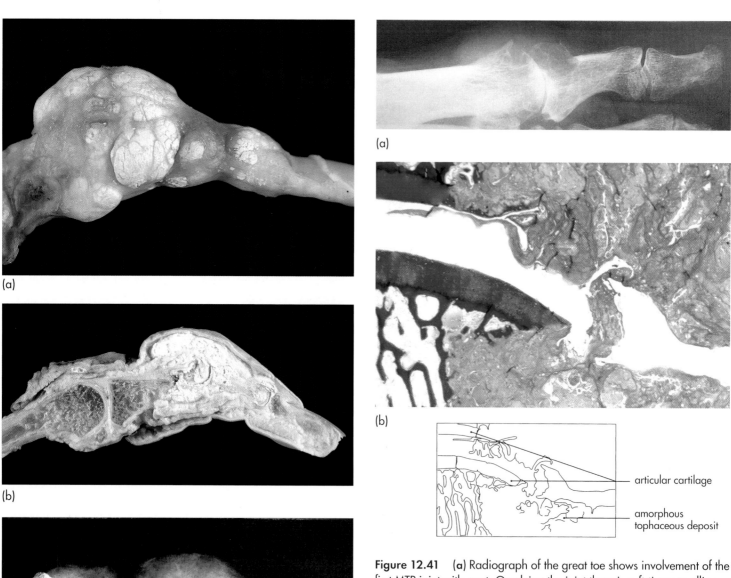

Figure 12.40 (**a**) Photograph of a partially dissected finger amputated from a patient with gout. The large, chalky white deposits are monosodium urate crystals. (**b**) Photograph of sagittal section through finger shows destruction of the PIP joint. (**c**) Specimen radiograph.

articular cartilage

amorphous
tophaceous deposit

Figure 12.41 (**a**) Radiograph of the great toe shows involvement of the first MTP joint with gout. Overlying the joint there is soft-tissue swelling, and at the joint margin a clear-cut bone erosion with a characteristic overhanging edge. There is no porosis of the surrounding bone, as would be seen in a patient with RA. (**b**) Low-power photomicrograph of a portion of the joint shows erosion of the bone and articular cartilage by nodular deposits of sodium urate with an associated histiocytic and giant-cell response (H&E, × 2.5 obj.).

CALCIUM PYROPHOSPHATE DIHYDRATE DEPOSITION DISEASE (CPPD) (PSEUDOGOUT, CHONDROCALCINOSIS)

As already discussed in Chapter 8, p. 215, most cases of calcium deposition seen radiologically in soft tissues are due to calcium hydroxyapatite and occur either as a complication of trauma with associated necrosis (e.g. fat necrosis), generalized connective-tissue diseases (e.g. scleroderma), or metabolic disturbances (e.g. hyperparathyroidism, familial hyperphosphatemia). These deposits are seen in many soft tissues including capsular tissue, ligaments, vessels, dermis, etc.

Disease resulting from the deposition of calcium pyrophosphate dihydrate was first identified in 1962 in the synovial fluid of patients who had gout-like symptoms without sodium urate crystals and consequently this entity was designated as pseudo-

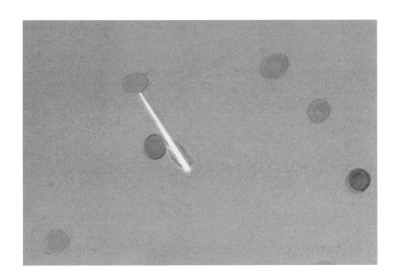

Figure 12.42 Needle-shaped crystal in a synovial fluid sample. When this crystal was aligned with the indicator on the compensating filter, it demonstrated negative birefringence (bright yellow), which is consistent with a sodium urate crystal (× 100 obj.).

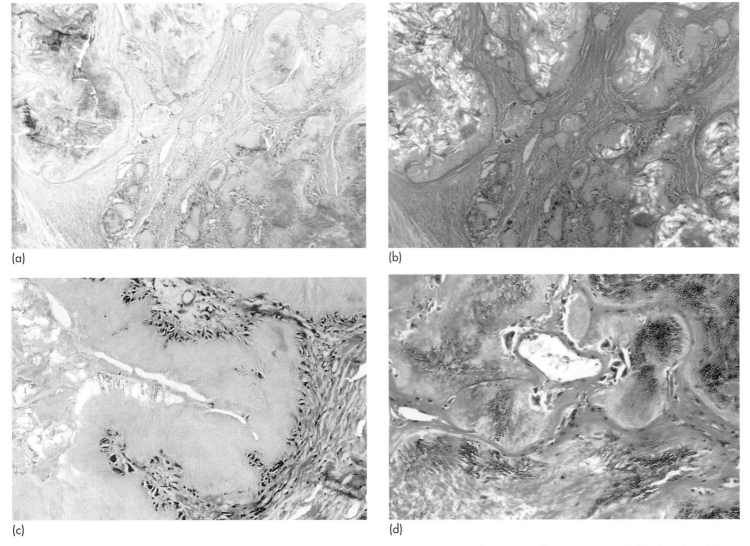

(a)

(b)

(c)

(d)

Figure 12.43 (a) Low-power photomicrograph of a tophaceous gouty deposit. A bluish amorphous material is seen surrounded by bundles of dense collagenized tissue and chronic inflammatory cells. (b) The same field examined by polarized light. The birefringence of the crystalline material is evident. (Preservation of the crystals is improved by fixation in alcohol) (H&E, × 4 obj.). (c) Photomicrograph shows a detail of the field shown in (b). Surrounding the amorphous crystalline deposit is a thin layer of mononuclear and giant cells (H&E, × 25 obj., polarized light). (d) Photomicrograph of another section that has been stained by de Galantha's method for demonstration of monosodium urate crystals (× 25 obj.).

gout by McCarty and his co-workers. The term chondrocalcinosis was introduced to describe a familial condition with typical radiologic evidence of calcification within the cartilage. Since the condition may clinically mimic many disease states, including gout, RA, OA, neuropathic arthritis, and ankylosing spondylitis, the term calcium pyrophosphate dihydrate deposition disease (CPPD) is perhaps more appropriate.

CPPD occurs either as a hereditary condition, or as a sporadic condition. In some cases it may be associated with some other metabolic dysfunction, such as hyperparathyroidism, hypothyroidism, gout, or hemochromatosis. Reports in the literature on the incidence of this disease vary considerably. However, because most affected individuals are asymptomatic, the incidence of CPPD found at autopsy or as an incidental finding in surgical specimens, is very much higher than that observed in clinical practice.

The initial manifestation of the disease is likely to occur in the patient's third or fourth decade. The most common clinical presentation of CPPD is similar to that of OA. About 50% of symp-tomatic patients present with a progressive degeneration that often affects several joints. In order of frequency of involvement, the joints most likely to be affected are the knees, ankles, wrists, elbows, hips, and shoulders. It is rare that the metacarpals or metatarsals are involved.

Patients with pseudogout account for less than 25% of those who clinically present with CPPD. Like gout, pseudogout has an acute onset with marked inflammatory changes and swelling. However, it is likely to be less severe than gout, and often there are cluster attacks – a single joint will first be affected, and then satellite joints around it will become involved. Pseudogout, like gout, may be provoked by an associated illness or by trauma (including surgery), and examination of the blood may on occasion show hyperuricemia, further complicating the diagnosis.

There are three other clinical presentations of CPPD that may occur, including multiple symmetrical involvement of the joints in a rheumatoid-like fashion, rapidly degenerating joint conditions similar to Charcot's joints, and stiffening of the spine (usually a familial condition).

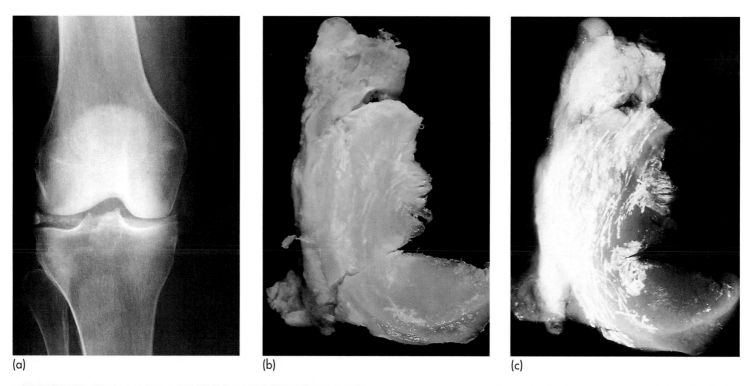

(a) (b) (c)

(d)

Figure 12.44 (a) Radiograph of a knee joint in an elderly individual with extensive calcification of the menisci. (b) Gross appearance of a meniscus with extensive calcium pyrophosphate dihydrate deposition. (c) A radiograph of this specimen. (d) Detail of the gross specimen.

On radiographic examination the deposits of CPPD are radio-dense and thus are generally easily distinguished from gouty deposits which are radiolucent. The calcium deposits are characteristically seen in fibrocartilage (Fig. 12.44), but may also be present in hyaline cartilage. The deposits are punctate or linear, and in hyaline cartilage they usually parallel the subchondral bone end-plate (Figs 12.45 and 12.46). Punctate calcification may also be seen in the synovial tissue (Fig. 12.47). In addition to the diarthrodial joints, the intervertebral discs and symphysis pubis are often affected. Chondrocalcinosis may be associated radiographically with joint space narrowing and bony sclerosis similar to that seen in patients with degenerative joint disease, but differing in location. The radiocarpal compartment of the wrist and the glenohumeral joint are commonly involved.

On microscopic examination the chalky white deposits appear either crystalline or amorphous. In vascularized tissue they may be surrounded by a chronic inflammatory and giant-cell reaction (Fig. 12.48). In nonvascularized tissue no inflammatory reaction is present (Fig. 12.49). The crystals are distinguished from gout crystals by their shape (rhomboidal) and by their weakly positive birefringence (Figs 12.50 and 12.51). As is the case with gouty deposits, the crystals may not show up with polarized light in stained sections but are perfectly visible in unstained sections (Fig. 12.52).

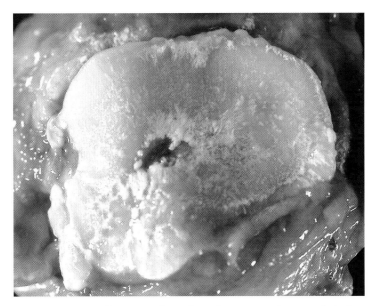

Figure 12.45 A degenerated patella with extensive deposits of chalky white material identified as calcium pyrophosphate both on the surface of the cartilage, as well as in the synovium.

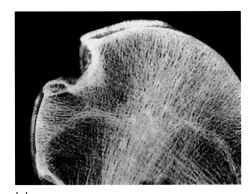

(a)

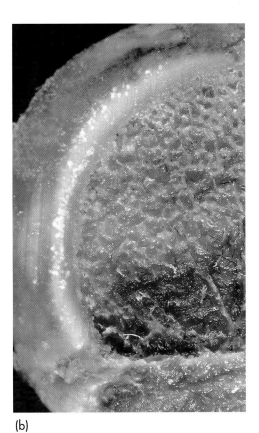

(b)

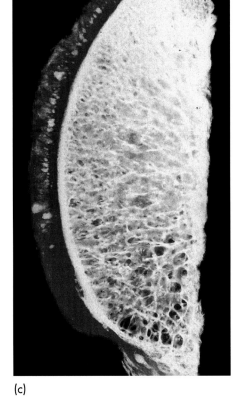

(c)

Figure 12.46 (a) Radiograph of a slice taken through the femoral head of a patient with hemochromatosis shows extensive calcification of the articular cartilage. (b) In this cut surface of the femoral head, chalky white deposits of calcium pyrophosphate dihydrate can be seen in the depths of the cartilage. (c) Specimen radiograph shows radio-opaque calcium deposits.

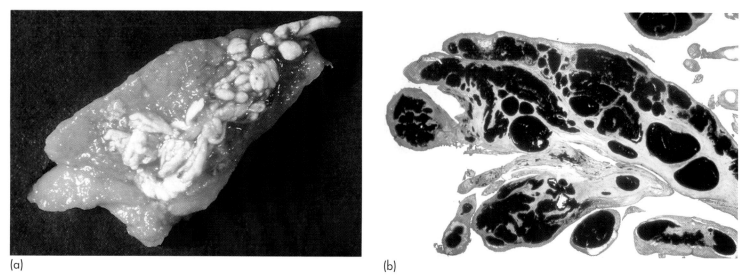

(a)   (b)

Figure 12.47   (a) Synovial tissue in a patient with CPPD, with extensive calcific deposits immediately at the surface. (b) Histologic preparation of the tissue which has been stained with a von Kossa stain to demonstrate the calcium deposits (von Kossa, × 1 obj.).

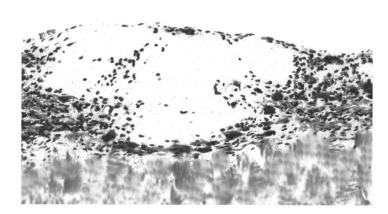

Figure 12.48   This photomicrograph shows a deposit of calcium pyrophosphate dihydrate on an articular surface. The deposit is surrounded by mononuclear histiocytes and giant cells, which gives the lesion an appearance very similar to that seen in patients with gout (H&E, × 10 obj.).

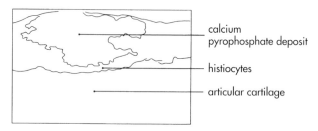

calcium pyrophosphate deposit

histiocytes

articular cartilage

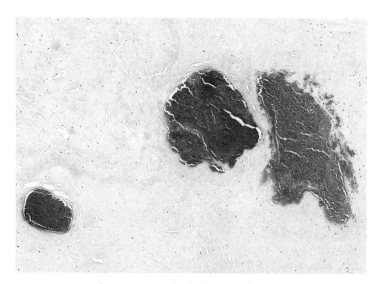

Figure 12.49   Photomicrograph of a deposit of CPPD in the meniscus. Note the absence of any inflammatory response (H&E, × 10 obj.).

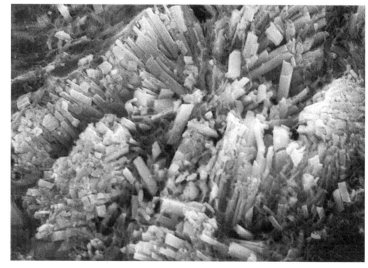

Figure 12.50   Scanning electron photomicrograph of a deposit of CPPD, showing the characteristic rhomboidal crystals (× 2,400).

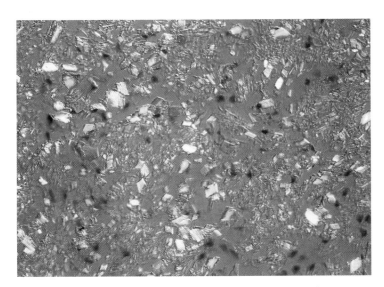

Figure 12.51 Photomicrograph of a deposit of CPPD crystals examined using polarized light and a first-order red compensating filter. When aligned with the compensating filter, the crystals are faintly refractive and blue (weak positive birefringence) (× 50 obj.).

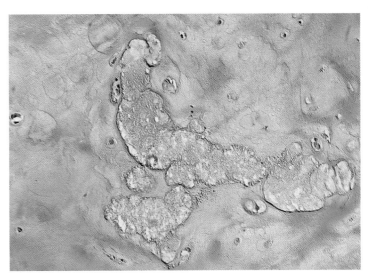

Figure 12.53 Photomicrograph of a portion of articular cartilage demonstrates the appearance of the mucoid pools around the chondrocytes associated with the deposition of CPPD (H&E, × 25 obj.).

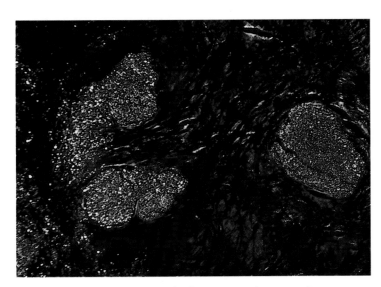

Figure 12.52 Photomicrograph of an unstained section taken using polarized light, showing the refractive properties of the CPPD crystals (× 10 obj.).

Most investigators who have studied chondrocalcinosis believe that the crystal deposition has a chondrocytic origin, at least in the articular form. The earliest changes involve the cartilage lacunae, which become enlarged and coalescent. The adjacent matrix is replaced by chondromucoid material from which the cells ultimately disappear (Fig. 12.53). The characteristic calcified punctate lesions come about through the deposition of crystals in these chondromucoid pools. It is thought that the deposits are finally released into the joint, where they produce an inflammatory reaction.

There have been occasional reported cases of massive focal CPPD crystal deposition disease (tophaceous pseudogout) in atyp-ical locations for CPPD, such as the temporomandibular joint and finger. Most commonly the patients were older females who presented with a periarticular mass or swelling with or without pain. In these cases of tophaceous pseudogout, clinical and radiographic evidence of CPPD crystal deposition disease in any other joints is usually not present. Radiographs have shown calcified lesions with a granular or fluffy pattern. Histologically, the lesions have shown small or large deposits of intensely basophilic calcified material containing needle-shaped and rhomboid crystals with weakly positive birefringence characteristic of CPPD. Foreign body granulomatous reaction to the CPPD deposition was constantly found. Chondroid metaplasia in and around the areas of CPPD deposition has been commonly observed, sometimes with cellular atypia in chondrocytes, suggestive of a malignant cartilage tumor. It is important to recognize this rare form of CPPD crystal deposition disease and to identify the CPPD crystals in the calcified deposits and thereby avoid the misdiagnosis of soft-tissue chondrosarcoma (Fig. 12.54).

EXAMINATION OF SYNOVIAL FLUID FOR CRYSTALS

An important diagnostic procedure for the clinical diagnosis of crystal synovitis is examination of synovial fluid for crystals and identification of these crystals by polarized light microscopy. This examination requires a polarizing microscope with a compensating first-order red filter. With the red filter in position, the crystals in the synovial fluid should be aligned so that their long axis is parallel to the line that is drawn on the compensating filter, which is the axis of slow vibration (Fig. 12.55).

Sodium urate crystals are usually needle shaped and exhibit strong negative birefringence, that is, they appear bright yellow when aligned parallel with the line on the compensating filter. CPPD crystals are usually rhomboidal and they exhibit weakly positive birefringence, i.e. when their long axis is aligned with the line on the compensating filter, they appear blue and much less

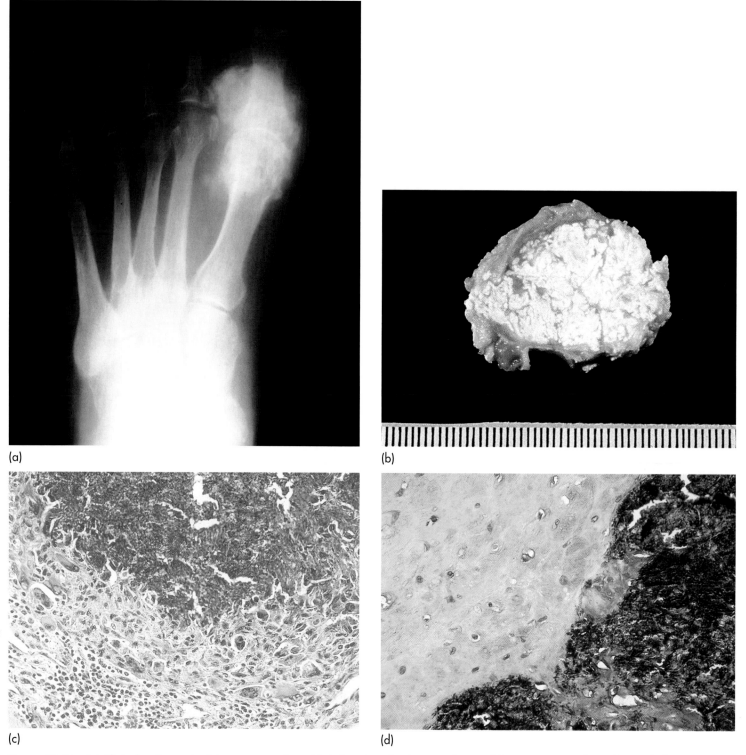

(a)

(b)

(c)

(d)

Figure 12.54 (a) Clinical radiograph of the great toe of an elderly female with a history of a painful mass over a prolonged period of time. This was initially diagnosed as a soft-tissue chondroma or calcified bursa. Grossly (b) it was found to be formed mostly of a chalky white material. On microscopic examination (c) deposits of calcium pyrophosphate with a histiocytic and giant-cell reaction were present (H&E, × 10 obj.). In many areas (d) there was a cartilaginous matrix associated with the lesion (H&E, × 25 obj.).

bright than urate crystals (Fig. 12.56). It is important to remember that when a crystal is oriented at 90° to the line on the compensating filter, it will appear the opposite color to which it appears when parallel. Furthermore, the shape of the crystal may be misleading, since pyrophosphate crystals are occasionally needle shaped, and urate crystals may be broken up into short, squared-off fragments (Figs 12.57 and 12.58).

HEMOPHILIA

Hemorrhage into a joint space, resulting in a hot, painful, and swollen joint, is one of the commonly observed clinical complications of hemophilia. These bloody joint effusions can be precipitated by even minor trauma or stress, and typically involve the knees, elbows, and ankles. Chronic, even subclinical, bloody

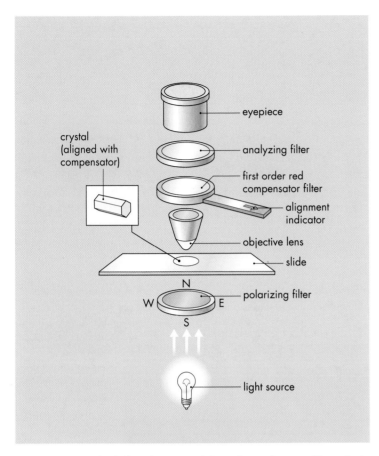

Figure 12.55 The light is first passed through a polarizing filter, which is usually oriented east-west. The polarizing filter will lie somewhere between the light source and the object being examined. The analyzing filter will lie between the object being examined and the observer, and usually the analyzer is oriented north-south. A refractile body will usually show maximum refraction when the axis of the body is oriented at 45° to the axis of the polarizing filter and the analyzing filter. When the axis of the body being examined is either parallel to or at right angles to the orientation marks on the polarizing filter, it does not refract, and these points are called the extinction points. The use of a first-order red compensator filter enables the observer to distinguish between positive and negative birefringence.

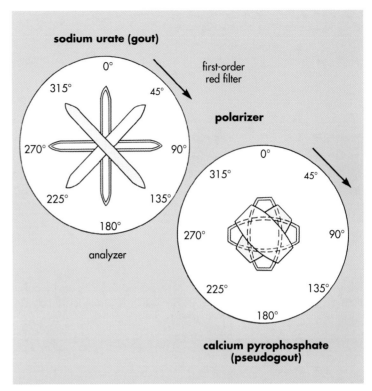

Figure 12.56 This illustration shows the effect of rotating a crystal of calcium pyrophosphate dihydrate or sodium urate through 90°. With the crystal lying at 45° to the orientation line on the polarizing filter, and parallel to the orientation line on the first-order red compensator filter, the calcium pyrophosphate dihydrate crystal appears faintly blue. This appearance is described as weakly positive birefringence. However, when the crystal is observed perpendicular to the orientation line, rather than parallel to the orientation line, it appears pale yellow. In the case of sodium urate, when the crystal is parallel to the orientation line it appears bright yellow, and this appearance will be called strong negative birefringence. When the crystal is perpendicular to the orientation line of the first-order compensator filter, it appears bright blue.

effusions into the joint spaces may lead to a destructive arthropathy, which is characterized on radiographic studies by a narrow joint space, cartilage destruction, bone erosion, multiple juxta-articular cysts and, if the lesion has progressed over a long period of time, osteophytes (Fig. 12.59). Radiographs may also reveal a peculiar juxta-epiphyseal osteoporosis (Fig. 12.60). Bleeding into the periosteum sometimes gives rise to a large, eccentric pseudotumor (Fig. 12.61).

Chronic hemarthrosis due to hemophilia or other bleeding diatheses is characterized by copious iron deposition and a markedly hyperplastic synovium (Fig. 12.62). The hyperplasia and hemosiderin deposition are usually limited to the synovial lining cells, although proliferative changes in the subsynovial capillary bed may be dramatic. On the basis of gross examination of the synovium, the differential diagnosis may include RA and

pigmented villonodular synovitis. However, microscopic examination of the synovium in hemophilia-related destructive joint disease does not reveal the striking lymphoplasmacytic infiltrate that characterizes RA, nor is there the nodular proliferation of mononuclear and giant cells characteristic of pigmented villonodular synovitis (though on occasion these two conditions may be confused, even microscopically) (Fig. 12.63).

A characteristic finding in joints affected by chronic hemorrhage is a greenish-black discoloration of the articular cartilage, which may be mistaken at surgery for ochronosis. Microscopic examination of the cartilage often reveals widespread necrosis of the chondrocytes, as well as hemosiderin deposits in the chondrocytic lacunae (Fig. 12.64). However, no iron pigment is seen in the extracellular matrix with the use of conventional light microscopy.

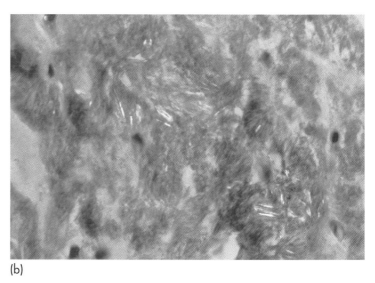

(a)
(b)

Figure 12.57 (a) Tissue removed from a patient with calcium pyrophosphate dihydrate deposition disease. The crystals are needle shaped rather than rhomboidal; however, they are only weakly birefringent (× 100 obj.). (b) Same field viewed under polarized light (× 100 obj.).

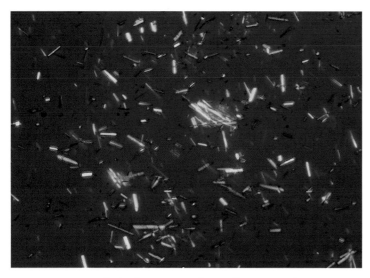

Figure 12.58 Multiple short pieces of crystalline material are seen in aspirated fluid. Despite their shape, these are sodium urate crystals (× 100 obj.).

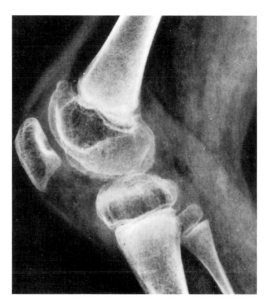

Figure 12.60 Radiograph of a young patient with hemophilia. Note the osteoporosis of the epiphyses, irregularity of the articular margins, and squaring-off of the patella.

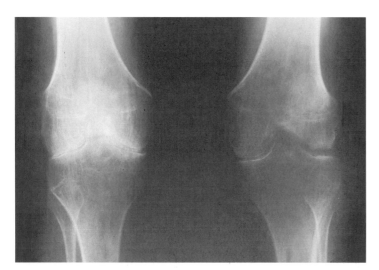

Figure 12.59 Radiograph of the knees of a hemophilic patient shows destructive arthritis of both knees, with marked juxta-articular osteopenia.

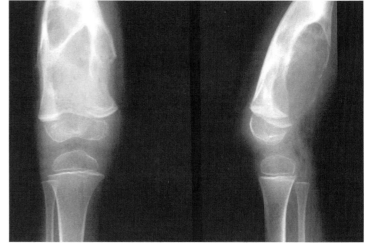

Figure 12.61 Radiograph of a large pseudotumor secondary to a subperiosteal hemorrhage in the distal femur of a hemophiliac.

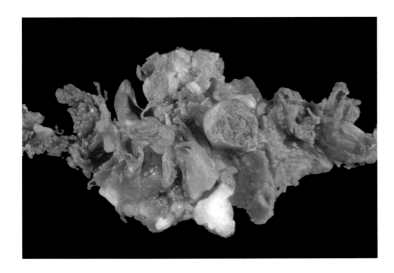

Figure 12.62 Photograph of synovium removed from the knee of a patient suffering from hemophilia. The staining with hemosiderin is apparent as a mahogany color. Also apparent is the papillary proliferation of the synovial lining.

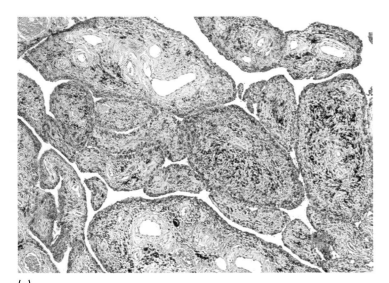

(a)

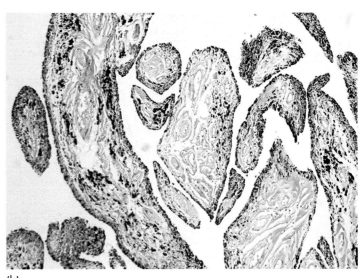

(b)

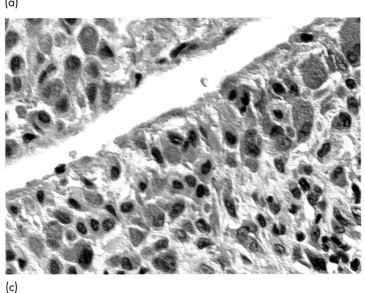

(c)

Figure 12.63 (a) Photomicrograph of hemophilic synovium demonstrates hemosiderin deposition both within the synovial lining cells and in the chronically inflamed and fibrotic subsynovial tissue (H&E, × 10 obj.). (b) Photomicrograph of another field stained by the Gomori iron stain to demonstrate the distribution of iron in the tissue (× 10 obj.). (c) Higher magnification shows marked hypertrophy and hyperplasia of the synovial lining cells (H&E, × 40 obj.).

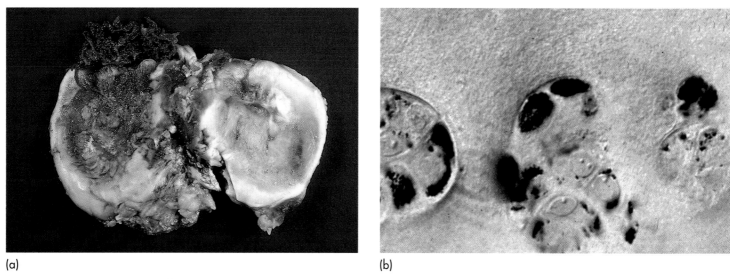

(a)   (b)

Figure 12.64   (**a**) Photograph of the articular surface of the tibial plateau excised from a patient with hemophilia. Attached to the joint margin is a heavily pigmented papillary synovium. The articular cartilage has a greenish-black discoloration. (**b**) Photomicrograph of the articular cartilage to show hemosiderin deposition within the chondrocytes of hemophilic cartilage (Gomori iron stain, × 50 obj.).

Chapter 13

SPINAL ARTHRITIS AND DEGENERATIVE DISC DISEASE

The vertebral column plays a central role in both static and dynamic motor functions, supporting the head, shoulders, arms, as well as the thoracic and abdominal contents, and transmitting their weight to the pelvis. In addition the vertebral column protects the spinal cord and nerves, provides sensory orientation, and participates in the locomotion of the entire body. Each component of the vertebral column – vertebrae, intervertebral discs, muscles, and ligaments – contributes in different ways to its biomechanical function.

Because the spinal column contains over 130 articulations, including both the solid intervertebral discs and the synovial joints of both the posterior articular processes and the vertebral articulations of the ribs, many pathological conditions that affect the spine are arthritic. Some processes initially affect the discs, whereas others, such as rheumatoid arthritis (RA), affect the diarthrodial joints. In general however, both the joints of the vertebral bodies and those of the arches are eventually involved.

This chapter discusses the different types of disc-tissue displacement, and degenerative arthritis of the spinal column (facet joint arthrosis, spondylosis, degenerative spondylolisthesis, and Charcot spine). Finally, the effects of inflammatory arthritis and the ankylosing spondyloarthropathies will be discussed.

DISPLACEMENT OF DISC TISSUE

The intervertebral disc comprises a nucleus pulposus consisting mainly of water and proteoglycan (PG) confined within an annulus of obliquely oriented collagen fibers (see Chapter 1, p. 8). Because water is incompressible, loads are transmitted hydrodynamically from one vertebra to the next through the cartilage and bony end-plates, while radial forces are absorbed through the tension in the fibers of the annulus (Fig. 13.1).

The appearance of the disc alters with age. The disc of the young adult, with its bulging mucoid nucleus pulposus, dense collagenous annulus fibrosus, and well-defined cartilaginous end-plates, can be clearly differentiated from that of the elderly person, with its shrunken, yellowed, and dehydrated nucleus pulposus (Figs 13.2 and 13.3).

If it is assumed that 'normal' intradisc pressure exists in the standing position, then a 5% tilt of the spine increases it by about 25%. Sitting increases it by about 40%, but lying supine reduces it by about half. Forward flexion of the spine, however, may increase the intradiscal pressure by as much as 400%, demonstrating the importance of lifting with bent knees and a straight back (Fig. 13.4).

In general, acute displacement of the disc tissue is a disease of young people in their third and fourth decades. It is less likely to occur or to cause significant compromise of the neural canal or foramen in an older individual, in whom disc tissue, especially

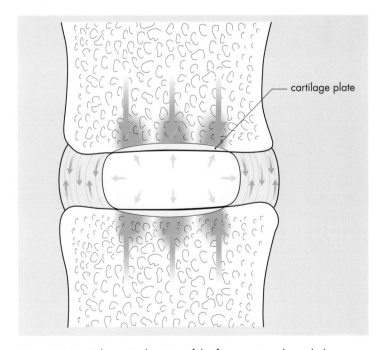

cartilage plate

Figure 13.1   Schematic drawing of the forces acting through the vertebral body and intervertebral disc. Compressive forces are transmitted through a central layer of hyaline cartilage interposed between the nucleus and bone, whereas tensional forces generated in the annulus are transmitted to the bone through Sharpey's fibers attached around the periphery.

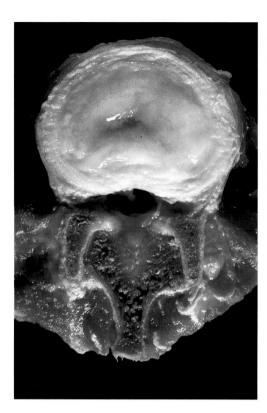

Figure 13.2 Transverse section through the L1–2 disc from an adolescent. Note the clear demarcation between the bulging mucoid nucleus pulposus and the laminated annulus fibrosus.

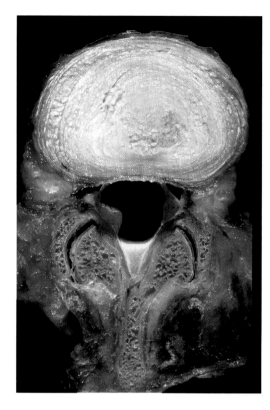

Figure 13.3 Transverse section through the lumbar disc of a 70-year-old. There is no clear distinction between the annulus and the shrunken, dehydrated nucleus.

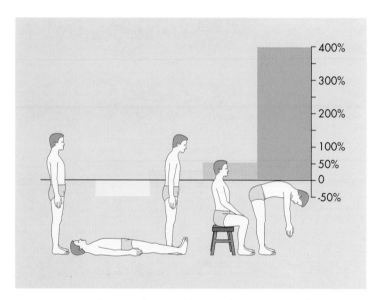

Figure 13.4 Schematic drawing showing the percentage change in load on the lower lumbar discs according to body position. The standing position is taken as the reference point (based in part on the original work of Dr Alf Nachemson).

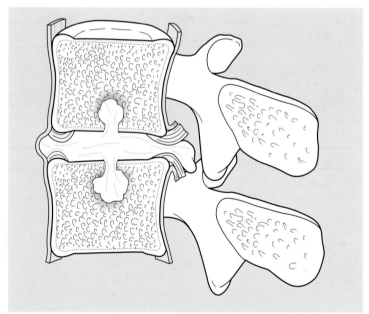

Figure 13.5 Schematic drawing showing the several directions in which disc-tissue displacement may occur: anteriorly, posteriorly, superiorly, or inferiorly.

the nucleus pulposus, is shrunken and dehydrated. Displacement of disc tissue (usually the nucleus pulposus) from the intervertebral disc space may occur anteriorly, postero-laterally, superiorly, or inferiorly (Fig. 13.5). (Posterior displacement is generally postero-lateral because of the firm attachment of the posterior longitudinal ligament to the annulus of the disc. This is in contradiction to the anterior longitudinal ligament, which is firmly attached to the vertebral body and only loosely attached to the disc.) Displacement of disc tissue anteriorly produces spondylosis deformans, whereas displacement postero-laterally produces pressure on the nerve roots or encroachment on the contents of the spinal canal. Displacement superiorly or inferiorly, into the adjacent vertebral bodies, will lead to the development of Schmorl's nodes.

The different forms of displacement include protrusion, prolapse, extrusion, and sequestration (Fig. 13.6). Protrusion is a bulging of the nucleus pulposus through a weakened annulus fibrosus, usually in a posterior or postero-lateral direction. Prolapse is a rupture of the nucleus pulposus through the annulus but not through the posterior or anterior longitudinal ligament; extrusion is a rupture of the nucleus pulposus through both the annulus and the ligament, usually the posterior longitudinal ligament. Sequestration is a fragmentation of the extruded segment, occasionally with displacement of the free fragment into the spinal canal and often to a site removed from the point of rupture. The general term disc herniation is used to describe either prolapse, protrusion, or extrusion. For displacement of the nuclear tissue to occur, there must be prior traumatic laceration of the annular fibers. Such tears are usually associated with torsion and compression injuries resulting from the sudden application of force, frequently the result of incorrect lifting of a heavy weight.

Anterior protrusion (spondylosis deformans) is one of the most common forms of spinal disease seen both radiographically and at autopsy. By the age of 50 it is present in at least 50% of women and more than 60% of men. The disease appears to occur more frequently in people engaged in occupations that require heavy physical labor. The lumbar spine is the site most commonly affected. Spondylosis deformans is initiated by tears that occur anteriorly in the periphery of the annulus, where the collagen bundles attach to the vertebral bodies by Sharpey's fibers (Fig. 13.7). This leads to anterior herniation of nuclear disc tissue and is potentiated by weight-bearing and by spinal motion. Because the anterior longitudinal ligament has only weak attachments to the annulus, continuous tearing of these attachments by prolapsed disc material stimulates the development of beak-like bony outgrowths or spurs from the adjacent vertebral bodies (Fig. 13.8).

Postero-lateral displacement is found at autopsy in approximately 50% of older individuals, mostly in the lumbar region of the spine. The basis for posterior disc displacement is small tears that accumulate in the annulus of the disc as a result of the injuries resulting from daily activities. These clefts, especially the radial ones, pave the way for displacement of the nucleus pulposus after acute trauma (Fig. 13.9). Disc material removed at the time of surgery usually displays evidence of degeneration, fraying of the collagen tissue and cellular necrosis, along with regenerative clones of chondrocytes, occasional granulation tissue and reparative fibrocartilage (Fig. 13.10). (In general it seems that chondrocyte proliferation is much more prominent in the younger subject.)

Displacement of disc tissue posteriorly and postero-laterally often causes clinical symptoms, depending on the amount of disc tissue displaced and its proximity to neural structures. The typical clinical presentation is that of nerve root compression with

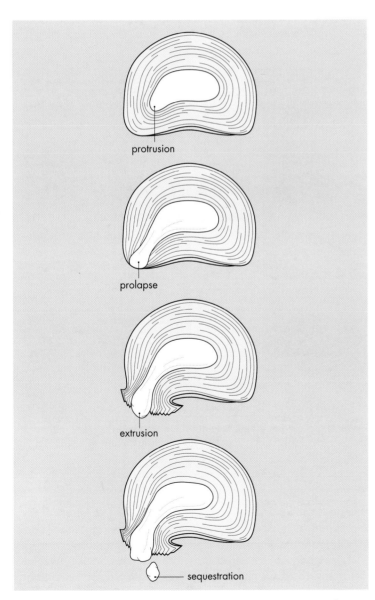

Figure 13.6 Schematic drawing illustrating the different types of disc-tissue displacement: protrusion, prolapse, extrusion, and sequestration.

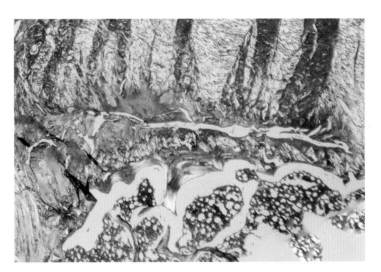

Figure 13.7 Polarized photomicrograph showing the early development of spondylosis deformans, taken at the junction of the annulus fibrosus, subchondral bone, and anterior longitudinal ligament. At the insertion of the annulus into the bone is a linear tear through Sharpey's fibers, providing a route for the herniation of nuclear material. The defect is partially filled with reparative fibrocartilage (polarized light, × 1.5 obj.).

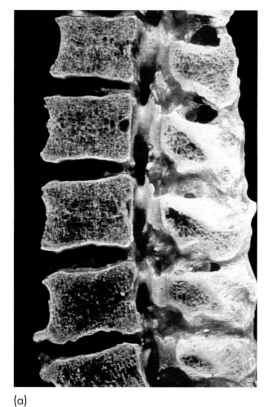

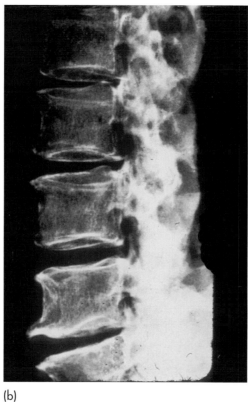

(a)   (b)

Figure 13.8   (a) Photograph of a macerated sagittal section of a lumbar spine with spondylosis deformans. Note the narrowing at the L4–5 disc space, compared with the levels above, and an anterior traction osteophyte. (b) A specimen radiograph.

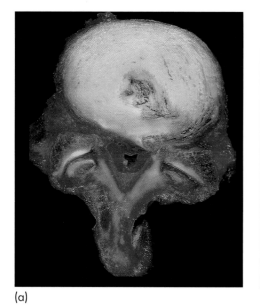

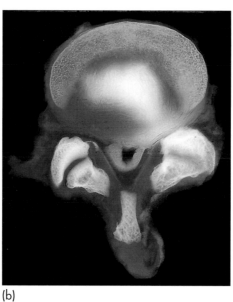

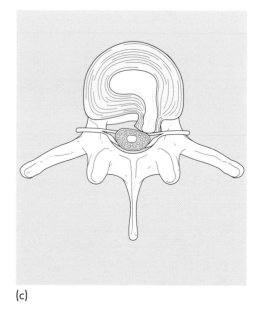

(a)   (b)   (c)

Figure 13.9   (a) Photograph of the L4–5 disc in cross-section after injection of contrast medium into the nucleus pulposus. Note extension of the dye postero-laterally. It is dissecting between the disc and the posterior longitudinal ligament, which appears to be intact. There is a bulging that results in an impression upon the dura, with narrowing of the intervertebral foramen (lateral recess). (b) A CT scan of the same specimen demonstrates the postero-lateral bulging. (c) Schematic drawing.

radiating pain, resulting from an immediate acute inflammatory response to the displaced tissue. After a period of bed-rest there is regression of edema and inflammation, and the pain usually subsides. Later recurrence of pain may result from further displacement of disc tissue or from scarring, which is sometimes accompanied by calcification and ossification. (The relative infrequency of osteophyte formation in the posterior aspect of the ver-

tebral body is due to the firm attachment of the disc to the posterior longitudinal ligament.)

Herniation of disc substance through the cartilaginous endplate into the adjacent vertebral body leads to the formation of Schmorl's nodes. These herniations, which are in most people probably traumatic in origin, extend for variable distances into the cancellous bone of the adjacent vertebral body. When they

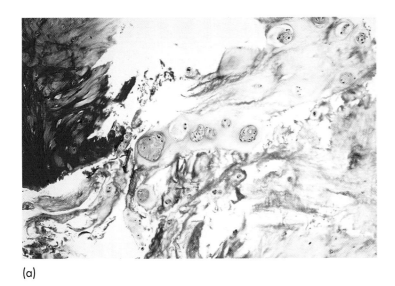

(a)

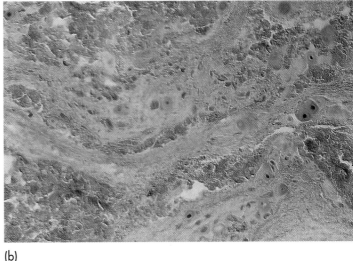

(b)

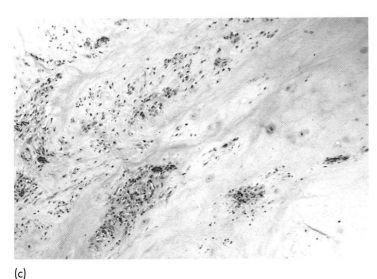

(c)

Figure 13.10 (**a**) Photomicrograph of tissue removed at surgery from a herniated intervertebral disc. Note the irregular fibrillated matrix of the nucleus pulposus, which appears to be largely necrotic but has foci of proliferating cartilage cells (H&E, × 4 obj.). (**b**) Shows a focus of granular, largely necrotic tissue (H&E, × 10 obj.). (**c**) With extended disc tissue there is often an inflammatory response as shown in this photomicrograph. The inflammatory granulation tissue will contribute to the nerve root compression (H&E, × 10 obj.).

are large and symptomatic, Schmorl's nodes may be misdiagnosed radiologically as tumors. Biopsy can lead to a histologic misdiagnosis of chordoma or a cartilaginous tumor (Fig. 13.11). The clinical significance of Schmorl's nodes is that as disc tissue escapes into the vertebral bodies, the intervertebral disc becomes degenerated and thinned, thus placing strain on the facet joints and leading to osteoarthritis (OA) in those joints.

OSTEOCHONDROSIS

The term osteochondrosis describes the pathologic changes that occur in the intervertebral disc and adjacent bone of the vertebral bodies as a result of disruption in the region of the end-plate of the disc. After disruption of the cartilaginous end-plate, the other disc components exhibit rapidly progressive degeneration, with focal necrosis, fissuring, radial or circumferential tearing in the anulus fibrosus, and replacement of normal disc tissue by fibrous tissue. Large horizontal clefts develop in the central part of the disc tissue and can be seen on clinical radiographs, where they are often referred to, incorrectly, as the 'vacuum phenomenon' (Fig. 13.12).

Calcification is common. However, apatite crystal deposits can be easily overlooked in sections prepared with hematoxylin–eosin staining (Fig. 13.13), and are clearly revealed only with the von Kossa stain. Calcium pyrophosphate dihydrate deposition disease (CPPD) is also not an infrequent finding in surgical specimens, being found in both disc tissue and the ligamentum flavum (Fig. 13.14).

As disc tissue degeneration progresses, with subsequent narrowing of the disc space, formation of new bone takes place around the periphery of the disc, at the junction of the annulus and the vertebral body, resulting in marginal osteophytes. New bone formation also occurs as a result of endochondral ossification of the cartilaginous end-plate, which contributes to narrowing of the disc space (Fig. 13.15). After vascular invasion, progressive breakdown of the disc tissue contents will lead to their resorption. Frequently, the final stage of the resorption process is a spontaneous fusion of adjacent vertebral bodies.

SCHEUERMANN'S DISEASE

Scheuermann's disease, also known as juvenile kyphosis, has its clinical onset in adolescence. It is characterized clinically by an abnormal increase in the dorsal convexity of the thoracic spine

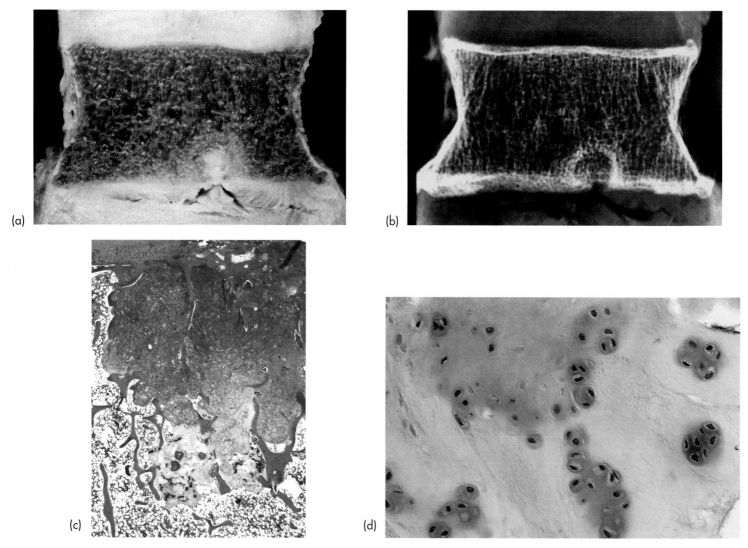

(a)

(b)

(c)

(d)

Figure 13.11 (a) Photograph of a segment of spine removed at autopsy demonstrates herniation of the intervertebral disc into the adjacent vertebral body. Such herniations are commonly found at autopsy and are known as Schmorl's nodules. (b) Specimen radiograph of (a). (c) Photomicrograph of Schmorl's node (H&E, × 4 obj.). (Courtesy of Dr Howard Dorfman.) (d) At a higher magnification the cellularity of the cartilage could, in a clinical setting in which a tumor was suggested, be misinterpreted as chondrosarcoma (H&E, × 25 obj.).

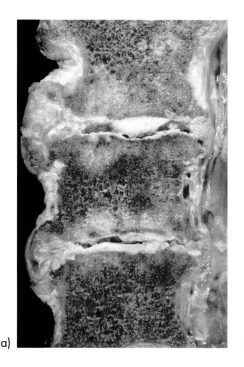

(a)

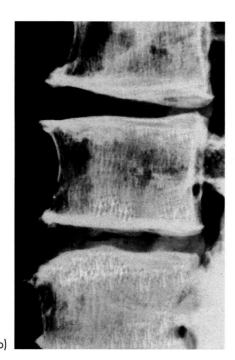

(b)

Figure 13.12 (a) Photograph of a sagittal section through L3–5 of a 72-year-old male. Note severe disc degeneration, along with irregularity of the end-plates and adjacent sclerosis of the bone. (b) Specimen radiograph of the portion of spine illustrated in (a). Note the radiolucent line within the disc, which corresponds to the cleft seen in the gross photograph. This line is usually referred to by radiologists as the 'vacuum phenomenon'.

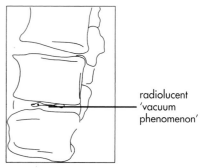

radiolucent 'vacuum phenomenon'

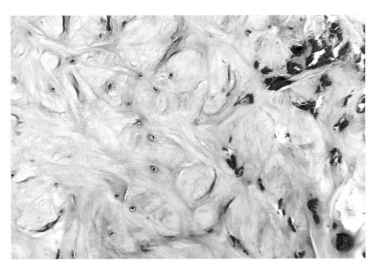

Figure 13.13 Photomicrograph showing focal pericellular calcium apatite deposits in the right-hand third of the field (H&E, × 10 obj.).

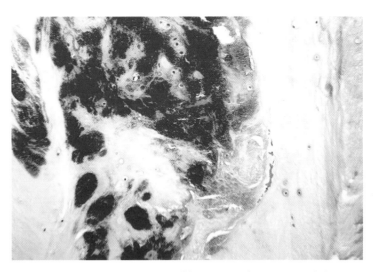

Figure 13.14 Photomicrograph of fragments of intervertebral disc tissue obtained at surgery, demonstrating islands of calcium pyrophosphate crystal deposition (H&E, × 4 obj.).

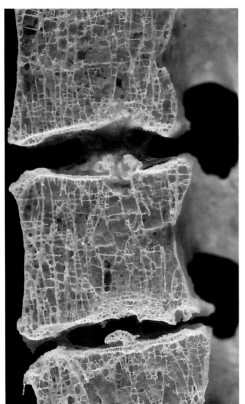

Figure 13.15 Photograph of a sagittal section through a portion of the macerated osteoporotic spine of an 83-year-old female. Ossification extends into the disc space. Such ossification may eventually occlude the space entirely. In addition, note fractures through the end-plate and the associated bony sclerosis.

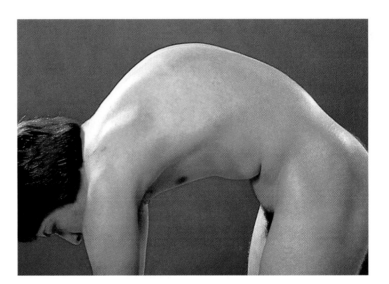

Figure 13.16 Clinical photograph of a 16-year-old boy with adolescent kyphosis. In this case, significant thoracic kyphosis has occurred as a result of Scheuermann's disease. (Courtesy of Dr David S. Bradford.)

(Fig. 13.16). Although the etiology of the disease is unknown, it is generally believed to be caused by an abnormality in the cartilaginous end-plate. Lateral radiographs are most helpful in clinical diagnosis and classification. Anterior wedging of the thoracic vertebrae is characteristic, and irregularities of the vertebral endplates constitute a prominent feature (Fig. 13.17). Schmorl's nodes are characteristic, and narrowing of the intervertebral disc space occurs in the late stage of the disease. Concomitant with the earlier mentioned changes is an increase in the thoracic

kyphosis (beyond 40°). The apex of the curve is usually around T7–T9. Characteristic anatomic findings in Scheuermann's disease include intervertebral disc narrowing and irregularly thinned cartilaginous end-plates, with focal attenuations through which herniations of the intervertebral disc tissue extend into the adjacent vertebral body (Fig. 13.18). Narrowing of the disc is usually more pronounced anteriorly than posteriorly, possibly resulting in interference with growth of the vertebral ring epiphysis.

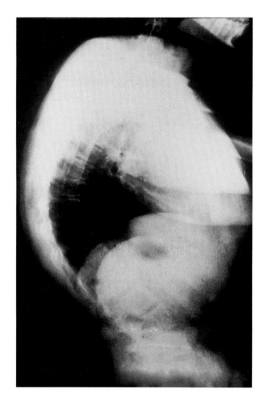

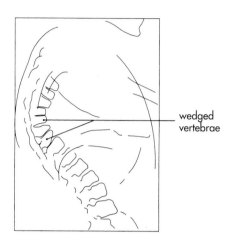

Figure 13.17 Lateral radiograph of a 13-year-old female with Scheuermann's kyphosis. Note the wedging of the vertebrae at the apex of the curve and the irregularities of the end-plates.

wedged vertebrae

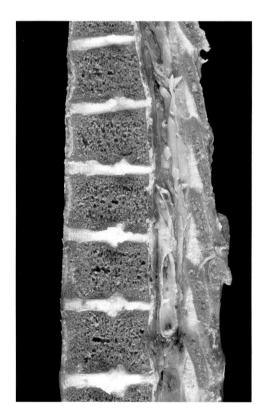

Figure 13.18 Photograph of a sagittal section through the thoracic spine removed from a patient with Scheuermann's disease. Note the multiple end-plate irregularities as well as herniation of the disc tissue into the adjacent vertebral bodies.

SPONDYLOSIS (OSTEOARTHRITIS OF THE SPINE)

Anatomic evidence of OA of the spinal articulations is rare before the age of 30. However, after the age of 45 OA becomes more common, and is found at autopsy in more than 80% of spines from older individuals. The term spondylosis embraces the clini-cal disease resulting from degenerative disc disease (osteochondrosis), together with the associated vertebral osteophytosis, ligamentous disease, facet joint disease, and accompanying neurologic complications. In the older population, this condition is almost universally present and even amongst the middle aged it is one of the greatest single causes of morbidity, particularly among those who do heavy manual labor.

In the normal intact spine, the facet joints carry between 12% and 25% of the combined load. However, in the presence of disc narrowing from osteochondrosis, the load on the facet joints may increase to as high as 70%. Such excessive loads lead to the initiation of degenerative joint disease in the facet joints. The morphologic features of OA that are seen in other diarthrodial joints (i.e. capsule laxity, synovitis, cartilage fibrillation, cartilage loss with eburnation of the exposed bone, and marginal osteophyte formation) are all present in facet joint disease (Fig. 13.19). It is likely that facet joint disease of itself is a significant cause of low back pain.

Degenerative spondylolisthesis, the displacement of a vertebral body on the one directly below it, results from degeneration of the facet joints, which in turn is caused by narrowing of the intervertebral disc space. The end result of degenerative spondylolisthesis is stenosis of the spinal canal (Fig. 13.20). Although spondylosis can occur in any spinal segment, it most often affects the more mobile segments of the spine (the cervical and lumbar segments).

The cervical portion of the vertebral column possesses the greatest mobility and thus has the greatest susceptibility to functional stress and trauma. Therefore, cervical spondylosis is very common and is often debilitating (Fig. 13.21). Degenerative arthritis of the zygapophysial (or facet) joints of the cervical spine is usually progressive, leading to the formation of osteophytes, which may protrude into the intervertebral foramina, causing vascular congestion and subsequent irritation of the spinal nerve roots (Fig. 13.22). Vertebral artery insufficiency is yet another potential complication, as a result of osteophytes impinging on the vertebral artery within the transverse foramina of C2–C6. This complication is usually compounded by the presence of atherosclerotic vascular disease.

Lumbar spondylosis, which occurs most often in males, particularly affects the lower lumbar spine, where it represents one of the most common causes of low back and leg pain. Lumbar disc degeneration follows a chronic course, with repeated injury playing a precipitating role. These degenerative changes cause

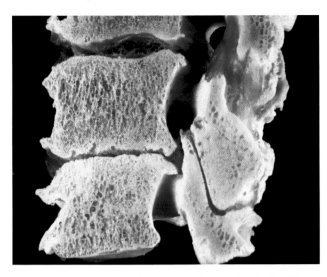

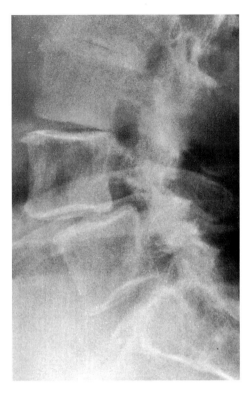

Figure 13.20 Lateral radiograph of the lumbar spine of a 58-year-old woman with back pain and pseudoclaudication. At L4–5, there is spondylolisthesis secondary to degenerative disc diseases. Note the narrowing of the spinal canal at that level.

Figure 13.19 Macerated sagittal section through L4–5 of a 79-year-old male shows severe narrowing of the facet joint, with associated subchondral sclerosis and osteophyte formation. Note the associated disc narrowing, posterior vertebral osteophytes, and lateral recess stenosis.

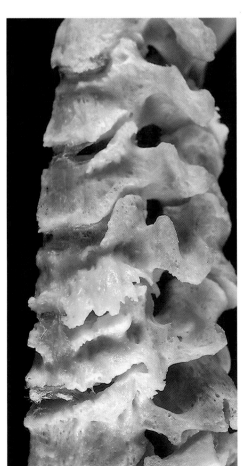

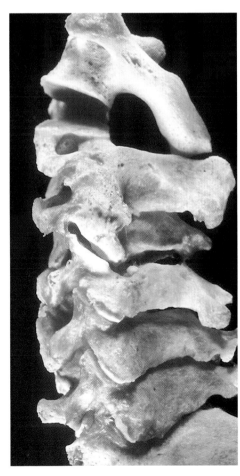

Figure 13.21 Photograph of the anterior oblique view of the macerated cervical spine of a 77-year-old female. There is marked osteophyte formation of the uncovertebral joints, particularly in the lower cervical region. Note encroachment of the osteophytes on the intervertebral foramina, particularly at C5–7.

Figure 13.22 A macerated preparation of the cervical spine in a 74-year-old female is shown externally in lateral view. Note the marginal osteophytes, which affect all of the facet joints.

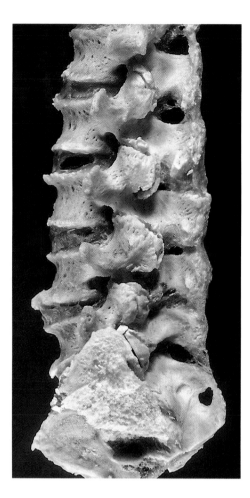

Figure 13.23 Posterior oblique view of the lumbar spine of an elderly male, revealing severe facet joint arthritis. Note the exuberant marginal vertebral osteophytes with their irregular, serrated margins.

NEUROPATHIC (CHARCOT) SPINE

Trauma to the articulations, with their ultimate destruction, may occur as the result of impaired perception of pain or of proprioception, and is generally referred to as neuropathic arthropathy. Tabes dorsalis (neurosyphilis), diabetes, syringomyelia, paraplegia, peripheral neuropathy, and congenital indifference to pain, as well as intra-articular steroid injections, are considered etiologic factors in the development of neuropathic arthropathy. Of patients with tabetic arthropathy of the peripheral joints, 10–15% also have involvement of the lumbar spine (Fig. 13.24). In advanced cases, the spine may exhibit extensive disc destruction, with sclerosis and fragmentation of the vertebral bodies and massive osteophytosis. Histologic features include marked joint destruction, with bone debris in the synovial tissue and many loose bodies – changes similar to those seen in Charcot joints elsewhere (Fig. 13.25).

INFLAMMATORY SPONDYLITIS

Approximately 60–70% of all RA patients develop symptoms and signs relating to the cervical spine. Pain is the most common symptom. Vertebrobasilar artery insufficiency may also occur, leading to transient blindness, vertigo, loss of consciousness and occasionally, sudden death. Radiographically, bone erosion and apophysial joint space narrowing are common, and may be followed by fibrous ankylosis and occasionally by bony ankylosis (Fig. 13.26). Erosions of the odontoid process secondary to inflammation of the transverse ligament occur in one-third of patients with RA. As a result of such erosions, three major complications may occur: fracture of the odontoid after minimal trauma, disappearance of the odontoid if the erosion is severe enough, or atlantoaxial subluxation and/or basilar invagination (Figs 13.27 and 13.28). In the rheumatoid patient it is important to recognize that secondary infections are also common,

alterations in the size and shape of the vertebral canal and its lateral recesses, with the development of spinal stenosis and subsequent nerve root compression (Fig. 13.23). The clinical manifestations include sciatica and/or ischemia of the cauda equina, with pseudo-(neurogenic) claudication.

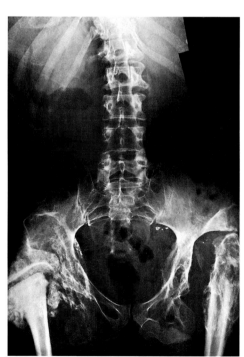

(a)

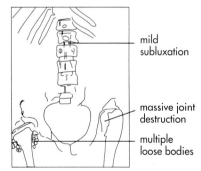

mild subluxation

massive joint destruction

multiple loose bodies

Figure 13.24 (a) Radiograph of the pelvis and thoracolumbar spine in a 30-year-old male with congenital syphilis and severe bilateral hip disease. In the lumbar spine, at the level of L2–3, there is mild lateral subluxation. (b) The lumbar spine and pelvis in the same patient seen 11 years later. At L2–3, there is severe destruction and collapse of the bony elements, with large productive osteophyte, characteristic of a Charcot joint.

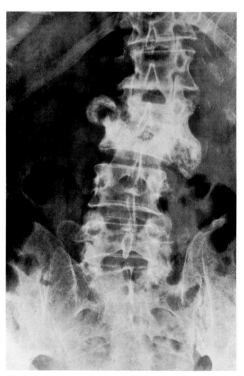

(b)

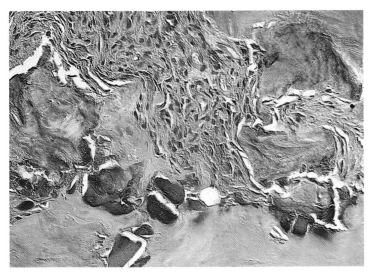

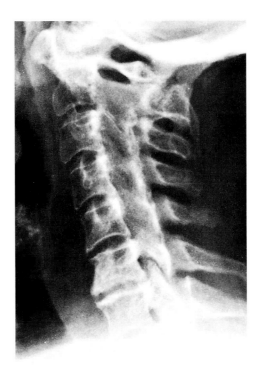

Figure 13.25   Photomicrograph of tissue obtained from around a Charcot joint. Fragmented bone and fibrocartilage is embedded in chronically inflamed granulation tissue (H&E, × 10 obj.).

Figure 13.26
Lateral radiograph of the cervical spine of a 50-year-old woman with RA. Note the fusion of the facet joints in C2 through C6. There is narrowing of the spinal canal at the level of C1–2 due to anterior displacement of the atlas. The entire spine is osteopenic.

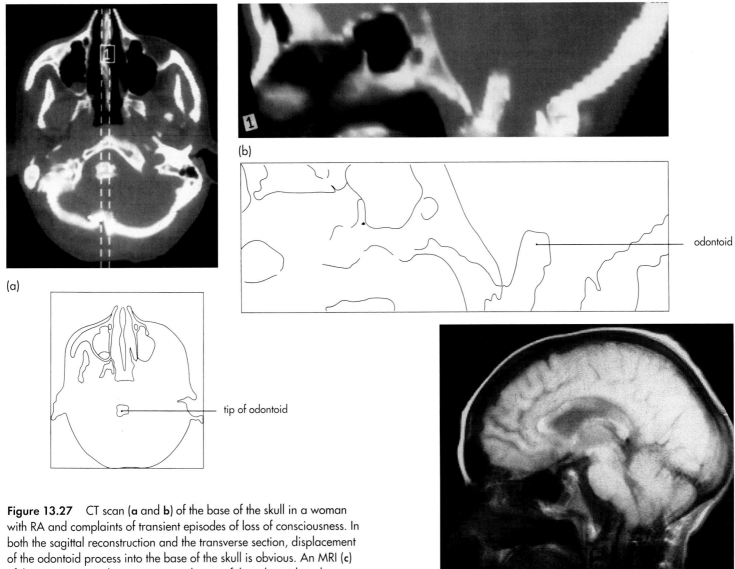

Figure 13.27   CT scan (**a** and **b**) of the base of the skull in a woman with RA and complaints of transient episodes of loss of consciousness. In both the sagittal reconstruction and the transverse section, displacement of the odontoid process into the base of the skull is obvious. An MRI (**c**) of the same patient shows an encroachment of the odontoid on the medulla oblongata.

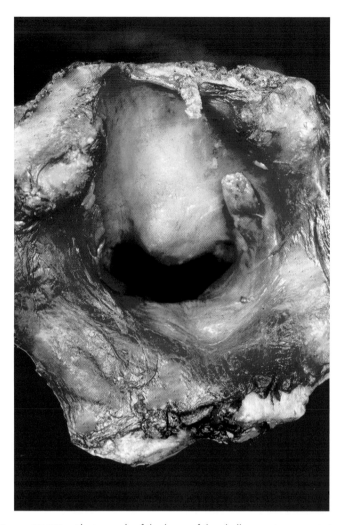

Figure 13.28 Photograph of the base of the skull, superior aspect, in a patient with RA who died suddenly in a minor automobile accident. The odontoid process protrudes through and narrows the exit of the foramen magnum.

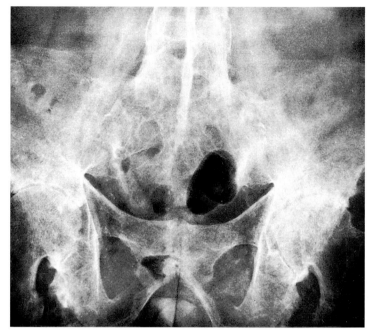

Figure 13.29 Antero-posterior radiograph of the lower lumbar spine, pelvis, and hips of a man with advanced ankylosing spondylitis. Note generalized osteoporosis with fusion of the spinous process, intervertebral discs, sacroiliac joints, and symphysis pubis, and severe concentric degeneration with partial fusion in both hips. Thus, the entire skeletal unit has been transformed into one continuous osseous mass.

especially with the use of steroids and other immunosuppressive agents and it is not unusual for such infections to be clinically silent.

Inflammatory spondylitis is also seen in patients who have tested negative for rheumatoid factor. Many of these patients have systemic disorders such as psoriasis or inflammatory bowel disease. Characteristically, the distribution and morphology of spinal articular lesions in these conditions are different from those of RA. Whereas in rheumatoid disease the lesions are most obvious in the cervical region, in the seronegative spondylitidies, sacroiliitis and involvement of the lumbar and lower thoracic spine are more common. Osteoporosis is not usually seen, and in marked contrast to rheumatoid disease, there is bony proliferation and occasionally intra-articular osseous fusion.

ANKYLOSING SPONDYLITIS

Ankylosing spondylitis is a systemic ankylosing arthropathy which primarily affects Caucasian men in their late adolescent or young adult years. Although the onset of the disease is usually insidious, its manifestations may evolve clinically in one of three patterns: in the axial skeleton, chiefly in the lumbar and sacroil-

iac joints; in the peripheral large joints, predominantly in the hips, knees, and heels, especially among adolescents; or as recurrent iritis, aortic valvular disease, fatigue, and other systemic features, without obvious arthritis (Fig. 13.29). The spinal disease may eventually progress in an ascending fashion to involve the thoracic and cervical vertebrae, along with other axial articulations such as the ribs, resulting in a marked restriction of chest expansion. Either transient or chronic involvement of the peripheral joints has been reported in 50% of cases, especially in the hips and knees, but the small joints of the hands and feet are not commonly affected. The natural course of the disease is usually characterized by slow progression without periods of remission. The histocompatibility antigen HLA B27 is present in 90–95% of patients with ankylosing spondylitis, compared to an incidence of 6–9% in the general population. Other laboratory findings characteristic of the disease may include an elevated ESR and mild hypochromic anemia (in less than one-third of cases). Elevated levels of serum creatinine phosphokinase (CPK) of muscular origin are seen in about one-third of patients. Examination of the spine at autopsy of a patient with end-stage ankylosing spondylitis reveals fusion of the apophysial joints and intervertebral discs, resulting in a rigid, immobile vertebral column with accentuated kyphosis. However, unlike ankylosing hyperostosis or diffuse idiopathic skeletal hyperostosis (DISH) (see later), ossification of the paravertebral ligaments is not a prominent feature (Fig. 13.30).

ANKYLOSING HYPEROSTOSIS OF THE SPINE

Ankylosing hyperostosis of the spine, also known as Forestier's disease or DISH, is an ankylosis of the vertebral column resulting

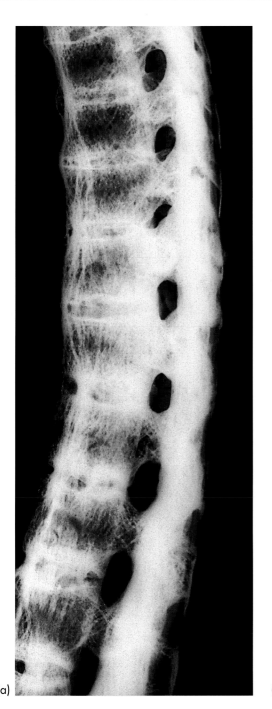

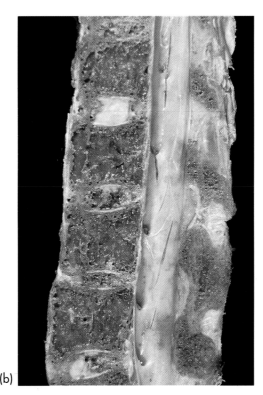

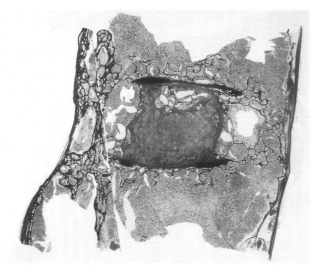

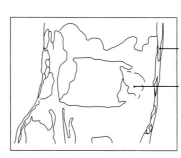

Figure 13.30   Radiograph of a sagittal section through the vertebral column of a patient with ankylosing spondylitis. There is complete fusion of the spine, and there was accentuated kyphosis with loss of lumbar and cervical lordosis. Complete fusion of the apophyseal joints, as well as fusion across the intervertebral disc spaces, is obvious. **(b)** Photograph of a sagittal section through the lumbar spine of the patient in **(a)**. Fusion of the intervertebral disc spaces is apparent. The paravertebral ligaments are spared, both anteriorly and posteriorly. (This is in marked contrast to ankylosing hyperostosis of the spine seen in Figure 13.31.) **(c)** Photomicrograph of a lumbar disc and adjacent vertebral bodies shows absence of ossification in the anterior and posterior longitudinal ligaments, with severe osteoporosis of the vertebral bodies. Fusion is mainly confined to the intervertebral disc, mainly in the region of the annulus (H&E, × 1 obj.).

posterior longitudinal ligament

osseous fusion across the disc

(a)

(b)

(c)

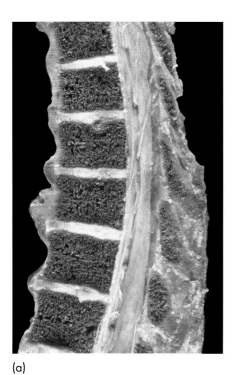

(a)

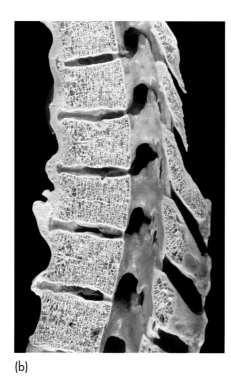

(b)

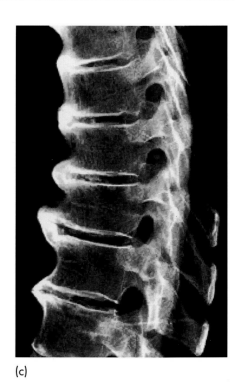

(c)

Figure 13.31 (a) Photograph of a sagittal section through a segment of midthoracic and lower thoracic spine demonstrates ossification of the anterior longitudinal ligament, with consequent ankylosis of the anterior segment. Note that the disc spaces are relatively normal. (b) In the same specimen, macerated, a thick plate of bone is seen lying along the anterior cortices of the vertebral bodies and extending in front of the intervertebral discs, like a layer of armor plating. (c) Radiograph of the macerated specimen shows ossification of the anterior longitudinal ligament with intact vertebral end-plates.

from ligamentous ossification without significant disc disease. It usually is found in older men who are usually without obvious clinical symptoms. In Figure 13.31 an advanced stage of the disease is demonstrated and in Figure 13.32, the earlier stages before complete fusion of the syndesmophytes. The diagnostic radiographic criteria include the presence of focal spinal ankylosis, intact vertebral end-plates, normal intervertebral disc height and, most importantly, flowing ossification of the anterior longitudinal ligament, especially along the right side of the thoracolumbar region. Absence of facet joint and sacroiliac joint sclerosis and fusion differentiates the disorder from ankylosing spondylitis. Approximately one-third of the older adult population has ankylosing hyperostosis at necropsy, more than half showing end-stage disease. The thoracic spine is involved twice as often as the lumbar spine, which in turn is involved twice as often as the cervical spine (Fig. 13.33). Both fluoride intoxication as well as 'excess' vitamin A intake are believed to favor the development of DISH. Calcaneal spurs are found radiographically in about 90% of individuals with DISH and occasionally ossification at other tendinous insertion may be present.

A peculiar variant of cervical ankylosing hyperostosis has been described, particularly in the Japanese literature, in which ossification of the posterior longitudinal ligament (OPL) occurs, sometimes leading to cord compression (Figs 13.34 and 13.35).

In patients who have undergone total hip replacement, a higher incidence of heterotopic bone formation after surgery has been found in patients with pre-existing ankylosing hyperostosis (Fig. 13.36).

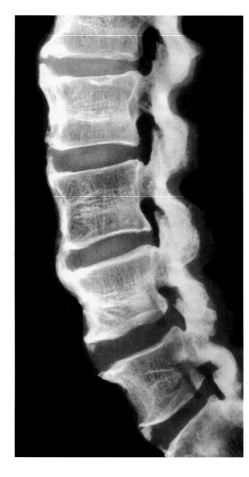

Figure 13.32 Radiograph of the lumbar spine to demonstrate various stages of syndesmophyte formation in a patient with DISH.

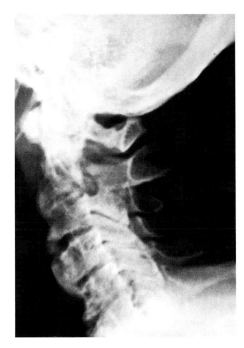

Figure 13.33 Lateral radiograph of the cervical spine of an elderly male who complained of difficulty in swallowing. There is an irregular severe anterior hyperostosis, which is largely the result of ossification of the anterior longitudinal ligament, typical of DISH. Neither the disc spaces nor the facet joints appear to be fused and the bone is not osteopenic, thus ruling out a diagnosis of ankylosing spondylitis.

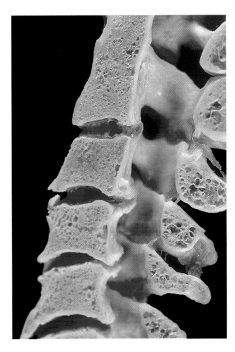

Figure 13.34 Photograph of a sagittal section through the cervical spine, which demonstrates ossification of the anterior longitudinal ligament (DISH) and severe ossification of the posterior longitudinal ligament (OPL).

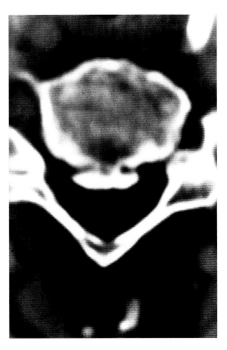

Figure 13.35 CT scan of the upper cervical spine of a patient with OPL and encroachment on the cervical canal. After minor trauma, this patient presented with myelopathy.

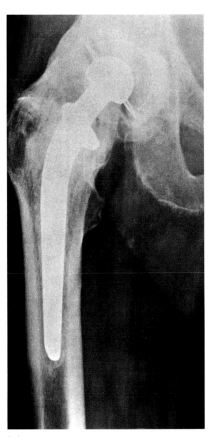

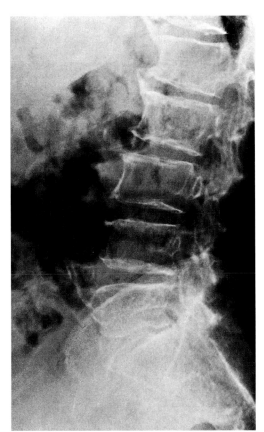

Figure 13.36 (a) Postoperative radiograph of a 65-year-old male with total hip replacement 3 years previously. Total bony ankylosis of the joint from ectopic ossification is seen. (b) A lateral radiograph of the lumbar spine shows the anterior cortical hyperostosis and nonmarginal syndesmophyte formation typical of ankylosing hyperostosis (DISH).

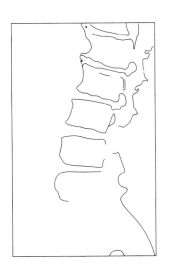

nonmarginal syndesmophytes

(a)

(b)

TISSUE RESPONSE TO IMPLANTED PROSTHESES

Foreign materials, introduced into the human body by accidental trauma, have long been known to cause damage and inflammation in the tissues. However surgeons, as a part of their therapy, also introduce foreign bodies, in the shape of drains and sutures (Figs 14.1–14.3).

The need to design artificial replacements for lost or diseased anatomic parts, especially in the form of joint prostheses, has resulted in a search for materials that can be implanted into the body to restore the lost function while not causing a deleterious reaction. The search for such biologically compatible materials has a long history and many materials have been used, including gold, animal bone, ivory, and in the early attempts at joint replacement, lucite (Fig. 14.4).

Until the middle of the last century the use of inorganic materials was restricted mostly to dentistry, although some metal was used for the internal fixation of fractures (Fig. 14.5). With the advances in artificial replacement of the hip joint by Charnley in the late 1950s, the use of metals and plastics by orthopaedic surgeons vastly increased. Since that time millions of arthroplasties have been performed worldwide, and in the USA alone it is estimated that over 500,000 such procedures including hips, knees and other joints are performed each year. Despite the success of the procedure, complications are eventually seen in about 10% of patients, in the form either of loosening of the implanted part,

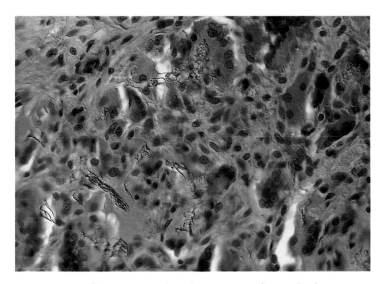

Figure 14.1   Photomicrograph to demonstrate a foreign body reaction to Gortex used in a blood vessel implant (H&E, × 10 obj.).

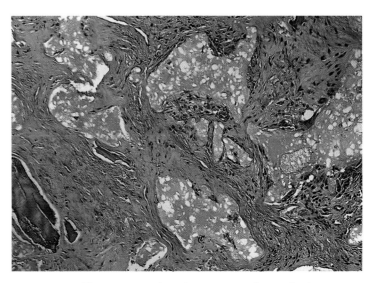

Figure 14.2   Photomicrograph to demonstrate a foreign body reaction to Collagraft used for ligamentous reconstruction (H&E, × 4 obj.).

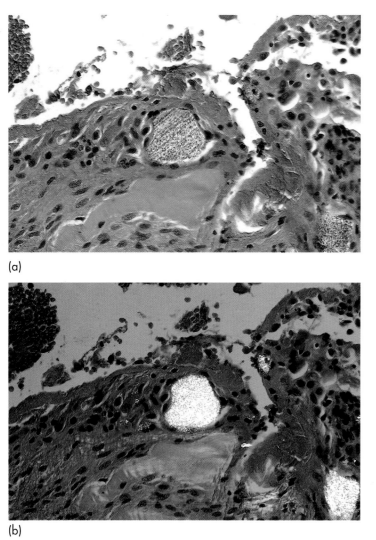

(a)

(b)

Figure 14.3   (a) Photomicrograph to demonstrate two large fragments of bone wax in tissue. (b) Polarized light (H&E, × 10 obj.).

Figure 14.4   A Judet-type prosthesis manufactured of lucite, which had been in place for many years before removal was necessary.

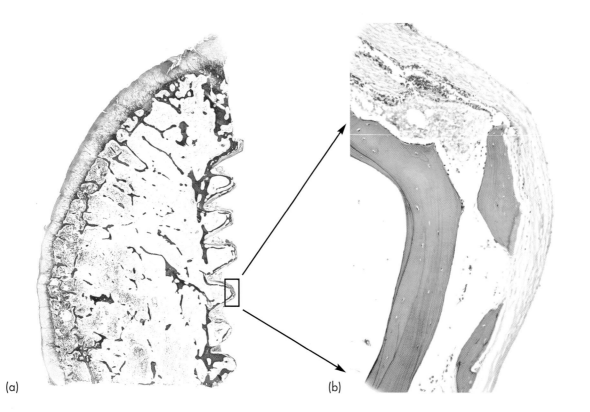

(a)

(b)

Figure 14.5   (a) Photomicrograph to show a screw track in a femoral head. The thread is outlined by a thin layer of bone and fibrous tissue (H&E, × 1 obj.). (b) A higher magnification of the boxed area shows the delicate fibrous cushion which has formed between the screw and its bony support (H&E, × 4 obj.).

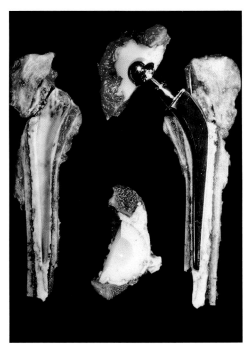

Figure 14.6 In this photograph the components of a total-hip replacement are seen to be attached to the bone. A layer of cement is interposed between the prosthesis (the plastic acetabular component and the metal stem of the femoral component) and the bone to obtain a close, optimally immobile fit of the prosthesis. Looseness of the prosthetic parts is a significant cause of failure in such operations.

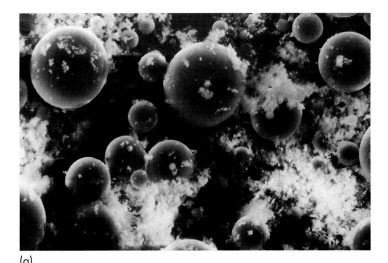

(a)

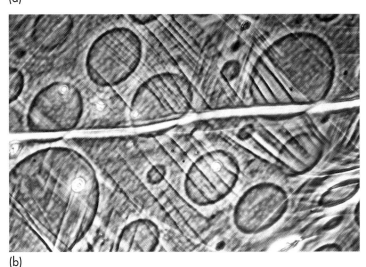

(b)

Figure 14.7 (a) Scanning electron micrograph of the polymer beads and admixed barium sulfate powder. A liquid monomer is added to this mixture to make bone cement ($\times$ 350 magnification). (b) Histologic section of a piece of cement reveals the 'two-phase' character of this material. The spherical objects are the microscopic equivalent of the bead-like polymer and the material between is the polymerized monomer (unstained, $\times$ 40 obj.).

which accounts for the majority of complications or less commonly, infection. A good deal of recent orthopaedic research and development has been directed toward reducing this morbidity.

Prostheses for replacement of large joints, such as the hip and knee, usually employ metal for the convex side of the joint (ceramic has also been used for this purpose) and high-density polyethylene, with or without a metal backing, for the concave side of the joint. Polymethylmethacrylate (PMMA) is usually used as a grouting material to secure fixation (Fig. 14.6). This is prepared from a mixture of its monomer, together with beads of fully polymerized PMMA, and a small amount of a radiodense barium sulfate, for imaging purposes during postoperative follow-up (Fig. 14.7). For use with metallic implants, various porous surfaces to promote the ingrowth of bone and fibrous tissues into the prosthesis have been developed and these are sometimes coated with a layer of hydroxyapatite to stimulate bone ingrowth (Fig. 14.8). Implants of silicone rubber have been usually reserved for the small joints of the hand, wrist, and feet, and are not cemented in place.

Despite extensive searches for materials that are biologically inert, it has become clear that no material implanted in living tissues is truly inert. On the contrary, experience indicates that there are essentially four types of response to implanted material:

1. If the material is toxic, the surrounding tissues are damaged or destroyed
2. If the material is nontoxic but can dissolve, the surrounding tissues remove and replace it
3. If the material is nontoxic and biologically relatively inactive, as is the case with most materials used in prostheses, a capsule of fibrous tissue is formed around it (Fig. 14.9)
4. If the material is nontoxic but biologically active, a bond can form between it and the surrounding tissue.

The metals and other inorganic materials that have been used in orthopaedic surgery abrade, corrode, or dissolve to variable degrees after implantation, producing both particulate debris and ionized constituents. With the use of moving parts, as in total joint replacement, the generation of particulate wear debris has been the cause of the greatest concern with respect to loosening of the prosthesis as well as possible cytotoxic effects (Fig. 14.10).

The cytotoxic effects of the different metals used in orthopaedic implants are varied. In cell culture using murine peritoneal macrophages, Rae studied the effects of particulate cobalt, chromium, molybdenum, nickel, titanium, and cobalt–chromium alloy on the release of lactate dehydrogenase (LDH) and the activity of glucose-6-phosphate dehydrogenase (G6PD). These investigations showed that cultures exposed to particulate molybdenum, chromium, or titanium did not produce elevations in extracellular LDH or reductions in intracellular G6PD. However, cultures exposed to particulate cobalt, nickel, or cobalt–chromium alloy produced elevations in LDH and reductions in G6PD. It has been suggested that the alterations in G6PD activity indicate decreased

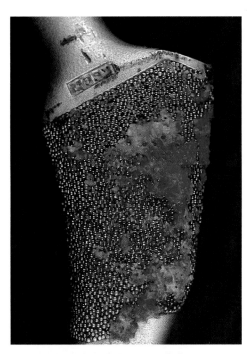

Figure 14.8   Portion of a femoral prosthesis covered with a layer of metal beads to provide for porous ingrowth. Fragments of attached bone and fibrous tissue are seen to be adherent to the beads.

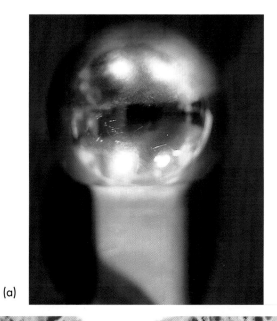

(a)

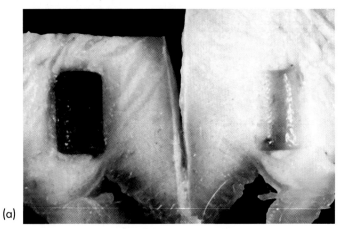

(a)

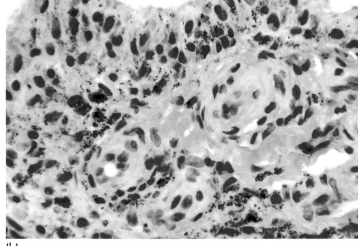

(b)

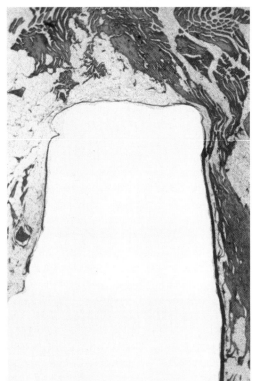

(b)

Figure 14.9   (a) Photograph demonstrating the appearance after a cylinder of inert metal had been implanted in skeletal muscle for 6 weeks. (b) Photomicrograph of a histologic section prepared from the specimen in (a) shows a very thin fibrous membrane around the space that was occupied by the metal implant (H&E, × 4 obj.).

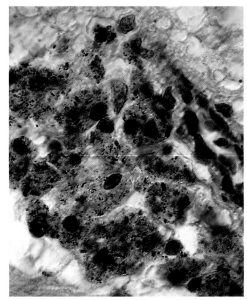

(c)

Figure 14.10   (a) Photograph of the articular surface of the femoral component of a total-hip replacement. This component, manufactured from titanium, shows severe burnishing of the articular surface, especially superiorly. (b) Photomicrograph of the synovial tissue surrounding the joint reveals extensive deposits of black metallic debris within the synovial and histiocytic cells (H&E, × 10 obj.). (c) High-power view of the metal-filled histiocytes (H&E, × 50 obj.).

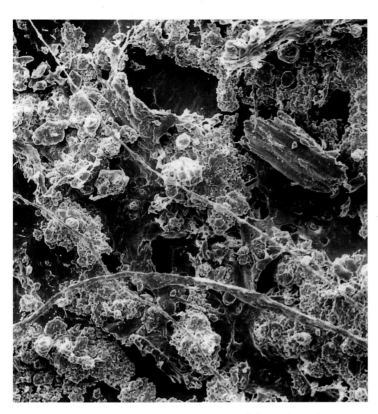

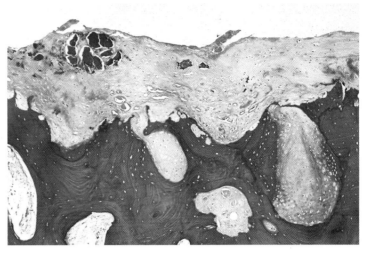

Figure 14.12 Photomicrograph showing the fibrocartilaginous membrane at the bone–cement interface of the acetabular component of a total-hip replacement. Fragments of bone are present in the fibrous membrane (H&E, × 4 obj.).

Figure 14.11 Scanning electron micrograph of the surface of a removed Silastic prosthesis showing gross irregularities and fragmentation (× 100 magnification).

phagocytic capacity. This may possibly contribute to increased incidence of delayed infections. In addition, the cells that ingested particles of chromium or molybdenum showed no morphologic alterations, whereas those that ingested particles of cobalt or cobalt–chromium alloy showed morphologic features of toxicity, characterized by shrunken cytoplasm and nuclear pyknosis.

Although there is little evidence that the fully polymerized PMMA is toxic to host tissues, the monomeric form has been shown to have local and systemic toxic effects, which will be discussed later. It has been hypothesized that biomedical polymers as a group, and polyethylene in particular, are capable of significantly affecting macrophage activation and production of interleukin-1.

In addition to their composition, the size, shape, and surface characteristics of implanted materials may have important effects on the surrounding tissue response (Fig. 14.11).

USUAL TISSUE RESPONSE TO CLINICALLY NONFAILED ARTICULAR IMPLANTS

CEMENTED IMPLANTS

At the time of initial fixation with PMMA, a rim of necrosis a few millimeters in thickness develops in the adjacent bone. It is likely that this rim of necrosis results from a combination of the effects of surgery with direct physical damage to the bone, disruption of the local blood supply, heat generated during polymerization, and

possibly a toxic effect of any residual monomer. The repair process begins with the ingrowth of granulation tissue and localized osteoclastic removal of damaged bone, and may occur as early as 1 week after implantation. This process is usually reckoned to be complete within 2 years.

Implants recovered at autopsy show that securely fixed prostheses have a cement–bone interface of variable composition. Most of the interface consists of a thin fibrous membrane, which is usually thicker at surfaces that are subjected to compressive forces, such as those on the acetabular side of the hip and the tibial side of the knee (Fig. 14.12). Histologically, this membrane is composed of densely packed collagenized tissue, which in some areas may show fibrocartilaginous metaplasia. Small amounts of fragmented cement, with macrophages and chronic inflammation, may be present in the membrane. Occasionally the membrane undergoes complete osseous replacement, so that bone comes into direct contact with the cement. This is most likely to occur at the more vertically oriented surfaces.

The surface appearance of the cement mantle varies according to the type of bone tissue with which it comes into contact. For example, proximally in the femoral neck, where cancellous bone predominates in the medullary canal, the cement mantle presents a nodular and papillary roughened surface, corresponding to the distribution of the bony trabeculae (Fig. 14.13). More distally in the femoral shaft, the cement comes into contact with the endosteal surface of the cortex, which is relatively smoother, and therefore the mantle has much less surface irregularity than the region of the neck.

NONCEMENTED IMPLANTS

In a similar way to the interface of a cemented implant, that of a noncemented implant has variable morphology, depending on whether the contact surface is vertically or horizontally oriented.

Along the more vertically oriented smooth surfaces of, for example, a Thompson–Moore prosthesis, the interface is composed of a dense, fibrous membrane which is usually a few millimeters thick. The collagen fibers in this membrane are oriented parallel to the implant surface (Fig. 14.14). Cellularity is sparse, and consists mostly of fibroblast and occasional aggregates of chronic inflammatory cells. An ill-defined layer of cells resembling synoviocytes may be present at the surface of the membrane in contact with the implant. Cells other than fibroblasts are not present in significant numbers in the membranes except in association with bone detritus, which is usually present in small amounts. When blood vessels are present, they are usually concentrated on the bone side and do not penetrate to the implant side of the membrane. Evidence of osteoclastic activity is not usually present on the bony surface of the membrane.

The interface membranes at implant surfaces that are more horizontally oriented, such as in the fenestration of interlocking femoral prostheses differ from those at the vertically oriented surfaces. A thick layer of fibrocartilage develops along the weight-bearing surfaces of the implant and is supported by a well-developed bony end-plate which overlies cancellous bone. The fibrocartilage may be so well developed as to mimic the features of articular cartilage. A small amount of metallic debris may be seen in these membranes.

The appearance of the tissue reaction at the coated porous surfaces of an implant also depends on the vertical or horizontal orientation of the bone–implant interface. In the vertically oriented regions, osseous tissue normally grows into the roughened surface of the implant without a well-defined intervening fibrous membrane (Fig. 14.15). On horizontal surfaces a visible fibrous membrane is more likely to develop despite the roughened surface (Fig. 14.16).

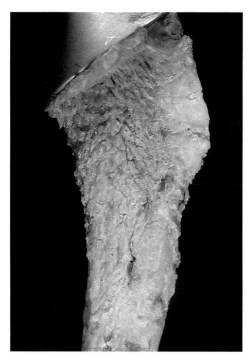

Figure 14.13
Photograph showing the cement mantle in a well-fixed femoral component. Note the irregularity of the surface of the cement where it interdigitates with the exposed cancellous bone.

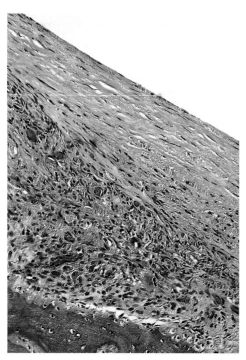

Figure 14.14
Photomicrograph of the fibrous membrane between the metal stem of a femoral prosthesis and the bone. Note at the surface the parallel arrangement of collagen fibers. Adjacent to the bone there is histiocytic and mild chronic inflammatory response (H&E, × 10 obj.).

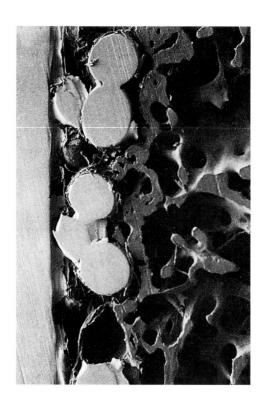

Figure 14.15
Scanning electron micrograph showing bone ingrowth on a porous metal surface. The cut surface of the metallic stem is seen at the left of the picture with the overlying cut metal beads. The bone trabeculae can be seen interdigitating between the metal beads.

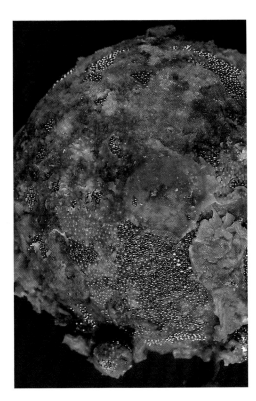

Figure 14.16 A photograph of the undersurface of the tibial component shows a fibrous membrane attached to the porous metal surface.

MORBIDITY ASSOCIATED WITH TOTAL JOINT REPLACEMENTS

The overall long-term failure rate for hip and knee replacements in recent experience is around 5–10%. The most commonly reported types of morbidity following joint replacement are listed in Table 14.1.

Some of the acute complications of total joint replacements represent familiar surgery-associated morbidity, e.g. pulmonary

embolism, and will not be discussed here. The complications that can be attributed to the joint replacement itself can be grouped into those that occur locally and those that are systemic.

LOCAL COMPLICATIONS

Infection

Today, the risk for orthopaedic device-related infection (ODRI) is < 1–2%. However, the absolute number of patients with infection continuously increases as the number of patients requiring such implants grows. Treatment of infected prostheses includes long-term antimicrobial treatment and removal of the implant.

All implants undergo physiological changes after implantation. Body fluids immediately coat all surfaces of the implant with a layer of host material, primarily serum proteins and platelets. Albumin, as the major serum component, is rapidly deposited on foreign material. The earliest and probably clinically the most important is the 'race for the surface', a contest between tissue cell integration and bacterial adhesion to that same surface. Adherence of *Staphylococcus aureus* to bioprosthetic materials is mediated by adhesion proteins such as fibronectin, fibrinogen, etc.

These communities of bacterial cells enclosed in a self-produced polymeric matrix and adherent to an inert or living surface are known as biofilms. Bacteria in a biofilm do not grow exponentially. They exist in a slow-growing or starved state (i.e. stationary phase) and, consequently, are not easily killed by antibiotics.

Acute or early infections of prosthetic implants (about 25% of infected cases) occur within 4 weeks of surgery. Subacute infections (about 25% of infected cases) occur within 1 year. Late infection (about 50% of infected cases) develops after 2 years of pain-free use (Table 14.2). The most common pathogens in the acute infections are shown in Table 14.3. Since infection around an implant cannot usually be cured by antibiotic therapy alone, removal of the prosthesis and extensive local debridement may be required.

Table 14.1 Morbidity of total joint replacements.

Time	Morbidity	Localization
Early	Intraoperative hypotension	Systemic
	Infection	Local
	Nerve disorders	Local
	Pulmonary embolism	Systemic
Late	Infection	Local
	Aseptic loosening	Local
	Hypersensitivity	Systemic
	Breakage of implant	Local
	Lymphadenopathy	Systemic
	Tumors	Local
	Pseudotumors	Local

Table 14.2 Infection as a complication of total-joint replacements.

Infection	Time of onset after surgery	Signs and symptoms	Representative microorganism
Early post operative	≤ 2–4 weeks	Persistent pain, fever, redness, swelling after surgery	*S. aureus*, coagulase-negative staphylococci
Subacute	≤ 1 year	Insidious onset	Coagulase-negative staphylococci, *Propionibacterium* species, anaerobes, *S. aureus*
Late infection	> 2 years	Fever, pain, redness, swelling after a long period of wellness	Streptococci, *S. aureus*, Gram-negative bacilli

Table 14.3 Microorganisms isolated from ODRI.

Microorganism	%
Coagulase-negative staphylococci	20–25
S. aureus	20–25
Polymicrobial	14–19
Gram-negative bacilli	8–11
Streptococci	8–10
Anaerobes*	6–10
Enterococci	3
Other	10

*Positive anaerobic culture depends on transport media used in operating room and microbiological technique

No preoperative tests are consistently sensitive and specific for infection in patients who need a revision arthroplasty. The only consistent clinical finding is pain at the site of the implant. The erythrocyte sedimentation rate (ESR), C-reactive protein (CRP) levels, and X-rays and bone scan results are highly variable.

Microbiological cultures

The reference standard for diagnosing infection is the isolation of the responsible pathogen. However, standard microbiological cultures are only moderately sensitive and specific for diagnosing an infected prosthesis. A very low inoculum, adherent bacteria, and the formation of small-colony variants of S. aureus may limit detection. Technical issues that can affect culture results include poor positioning of the aspiration needle or the addition of local anesthetic to the inflamed joint fluid.

Intraoperative cultures provide the most accurate specimens for microbiological cultures and are frequently used as the reference standard for diagnosing ODRI. Simple technical problems, such as routine antimicrobial prophylaxis before sampling, delay in sending the specimens to the laboratory, failure to ask for anaerobe cultures, and sending in swabs instead of biopsy material, may limit the ability of the laboratory to isolate the microorganism. A minimum of three specimens should be sent to the laboratory. The implant, if available, should be cultured as well. Sonication may increase the sensitivity of the culture technique by dispersing adherent bacteria.

Histopathology

Any single high-power field in the periarticular tissue that contains at least five stromal neutrophil granulocytes strongly

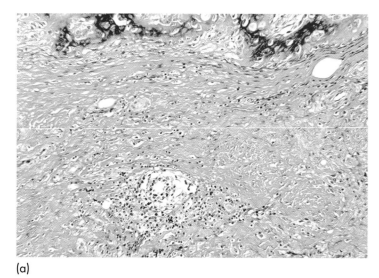

(a)

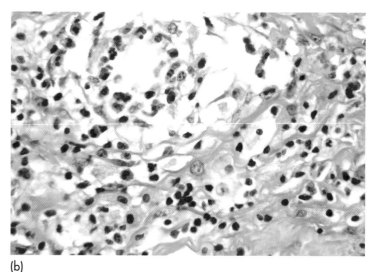

(b)

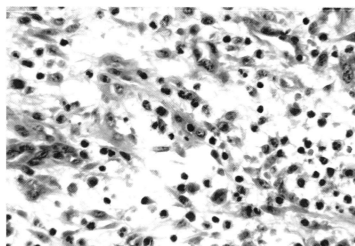

(c)

Figure 14.17 (a) Tissue removed from around an infected joint implant. There is reactive bone and scar tissue with some inflammatory cells which are focally prominent in the lower part of the photomicrograph (H&E, × 4 obj.). (b) At a higher magnification in addition to lymphocytes there are admixed eosinophils (H&E, × 25 obj.). (c) Some tissue breakdown with histiocytes and rare polymorphonuclear leukocytes are also present (H&E, × 25 obj.).

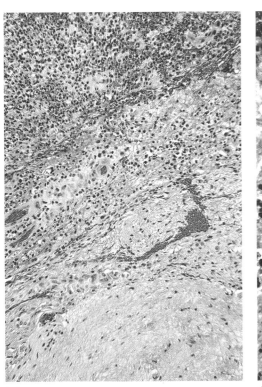 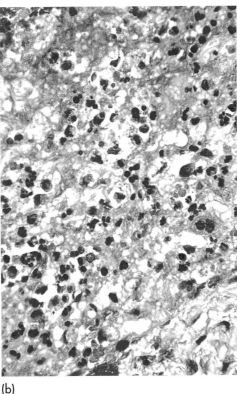

(a)   (b)

Figure 14.18   (a) At the time of revision a frozen section of the inflamed synovium will usually confirm the presence of infection and in the case shown there is a heavy infiltrate of inflammatory cells (H&E, × 4 obj.). (b) At a higher magnification both acute and chronic inflammatory cells are present (H&E, × 25 obj.).

suggests infection (Fig. 14.17). Frozen intraoperative sections correlate well with the permanent section of the capsular or granulation tissue. Permanent sections improve sensitivity by ~ 10% compared with frozen sections, but the specificity is > 95% with both methods. Frozen sections facilitate or allow the diagnosis of ODRI and help to distinguish true infection from contamination (Fig. 14.18). The accuracy of the technique depends on the experience and training of the histopathologist and the proper sampling of specimens from clinically inflamed tissue. Interobserver variability appears to be substantial, even in specialized institutions. Moreover, sampling errors will lead to false-negative results. The combination of two independent tests – histopathologic and microbiologic – allows an accurate diagnosis and should be used as the current reference standard for diagnosing ODRI.

Technical failure

Failure associated with alignment of the implant and the placement of the methylmethacrylate cement depends on surgical technique (Fig. 14.19). Improper cementing technique has been reported as the cause of such diverse complications as penetration of the medial wall of the acetabulum, obstruction of the small bowel caused by adhesions around a bolus of PMMA cement, unilateral ureteral obstruction, and postoperative hematuria. Other reported complications following total hip replace-

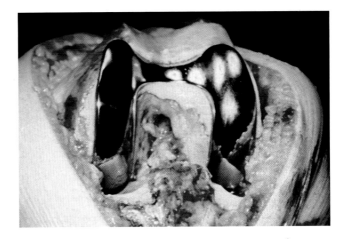

Figure 14.19   Total-knee replacement seen at necropsy. A large amount of cement has extruded around the prosthetic parts. Such excess cement is likely to break up and be ground between the articular surfaces, and will cause wear of the articulating surfaces of the artificial joint. The wear debris together with the powdered cement will enter the synovial cavity and eventually be incorporated into the synovial membrane, or depending on the rate at which the debris is generated by removal via the lymphatics. In joint-replacement procedures, the use of cement should be kept to a minimum, and any extruded cement, particularly around the prosthesis, should be carefully cleared from the joint before closure.

ment include delayed irritation of the sciatic nerve, false aneurysm of the external iliac artery, formation of various fistulas, and progressive dyspareunia.

Incorrect surgical alignment of the implant is a significant cause of fracture of the various components of the implant.

TUMORS AND PSEUDOTUMORS

Malignant tumors

A small number of malignant tumors have been reported in association with orthopaedic implants. The largest number have occurred in dogs treated for fracture of long bones using metallic plates for internal fixation. Osteosarcoma, fibrosarcoma, and undifferentiated sarcoma are the most common types of tumor seen in the dog.

As of 2002, at least 48 cases of malignant tumor have been reported in patients who have undergone total hip or total knee arthroplasty. However, since several million implants are in place, the incidence of malignancies developing in these patients may not be above that normally expected in an aging population (Fig. 14.20).

Pseudotumors

In the context of implant reactions, a pseudotumor is a space-occupying lesion resulting from the tissue reaction to accumulated particulate debris at or near the site of the implant.

The problem of pseudotumor formation plagued the early experience of Charnley when he used teflon for the acetabular component of his total-hip replacements. The problem largely disappeared after the introduction of high-molecular-weight polyethylene. However, reports of extensive reactions to large amounts of polyethylene debris in both total-hip and total-knee arthroplasties, with subsequent loosening resulting from endosteal bone resorption caused by the mass effect of the accumulating debris and its accompanying cellular infiltration, still continue to appear in the literature (Figs 14.21 and 14.22).

Pseudotumors in the bones of the wrist after replacement of carpal bones or joints by silicone rubber implants have also been reported (Fig. 14.23).

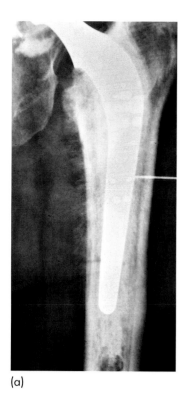
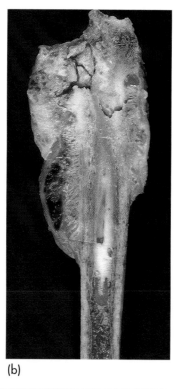

(a)   (b)

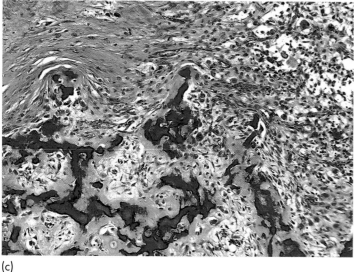

(c)

Figure 14.20   (**a**) Radiograph of a 53-year-old female who underwent total-joint replacement 8 years previously for secondary osteoarthritis (OA) following congenital dislocation of the hip. Recent pain in the hip prompted radiographic examination, which revealed the periosteal reaction seen here. (**b**) The resected specimen from the case illustrated in (**a**) shows a large tumor around the upper end of the femur. (The prosthesis has been removed.) (**c**) Photomicrograph of tissue obtained from the tumor shows an osteosarcoma (H&E, × 10 obj.).

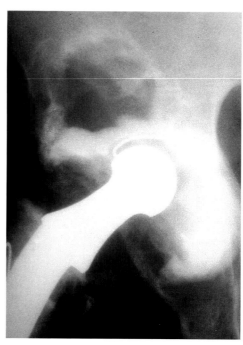

Figure 14.21
Radiograph of the pelvis in a patient with total-joint replacement of some years' duration. Recent pain prompted radiographic examination, which shows superior migration of the head into the acetabulum and a lytic defect in the ilium. Histological examination revealed an accumulation of polyethylene and cement, with an associated histiocytic response.

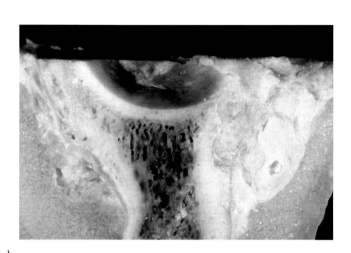

(a)

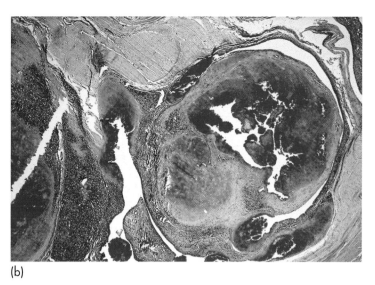

(b)

Figure 14.22 (a) Section through the acetabulum of a dog several months after total-hip replacement shows a juxta-articular tumor mass of yellowish-gray tissue. (b) Photomicrograph of a section through the specimen reveals large pink collections of fibrin, in which there was admixed cement and polyethylene debris, surrounded by histiocytes and chronic inflammatory cells (H&E, × 1.25 obj.).

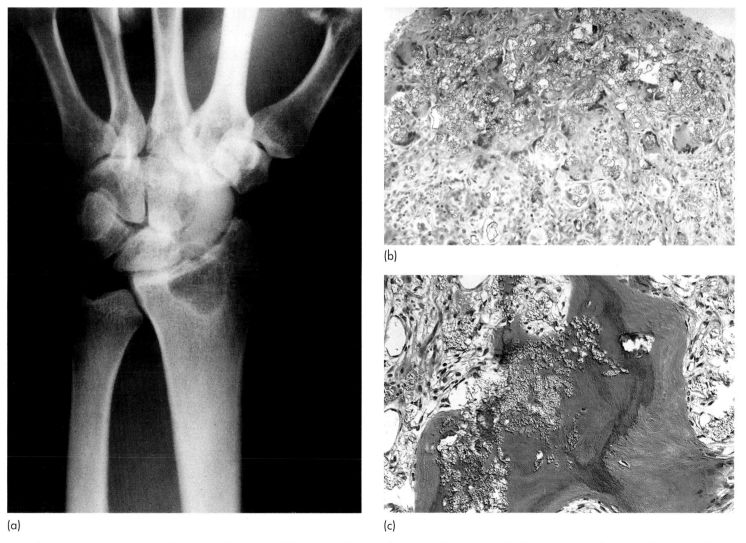

(a)

(b)

(c)

Figure 14.23 (a) Radiograph of the wrist of a patient following a Silastic replacement of the scaphoid. The large lytic defect in the lower end of the radius was found on microscopic examination to be secondary to a histiocytic and giant-cell reaction to particulate Silastic. (b) A lower-power photomicrograph of the synovium surrounding a failed silicone polymer prosthesis. A markedly cellular histiocytic and giant-cell reaction can be observed (H&E, × 10 obj.). (c) A higher power view from the tissue shown in (b). Within both the soft tissue and bone can be seen a bosselated inclusion of yellowish-gray material. This microscopic appearance is typical of silicone breakdown, and similar inclusions may be found around silicone injections used in plastic surgery procedures (H&E, × 25 obj.).

SYSTEMIC COMPLICATIONS

Hypotension and intraoperative death

Hypotension developing as a reaction to monomeric methyl-methacrylate seems to be fairly common during the instillation of methylmethacrylate; however, intraoperative death resulting from this complication is fortunately extremely rare.

Allergy/hypersensitivity

Tissue reactions due to hypersensitivity are difficult to evaluate in implant sites because of surgical scarring and the small amount of inflammation usually present in the tissues surrounding most types of implants during the early to intermediate postoperative time period. Hypersensitivity reactions may also be difficult to distinguish from low-grade infections, especially when the organism cannot be isolated.

Since the mid-1970s, attention has been drawn to the possibility that metals used in orthopaedic implants may induce a hypersensitivity reaction. However, the importance of sensitivity to metals in patients who receive metallic joint implants is not clear. In reports that suggest hypersensitivity has a causative role in loosening, the implants had already failed clinically and the timing of development of the sensitivity was not known. Even when metal sensitivity can be proved, it may be dose dependent and therefore may result from the loosening rather than being its cause. Inflammation and necrosis, as will be discussed later, often accompany failure of an implant, and in these cases the effects of hypersensitivity on the tissues may not be distinguishable from other causes of inflammation.

Lymph node and pulmonary spread

Autopsy studies have shown that careful dissection of the lymph nodal draining sites of replaced joints, and adequate sampling of lung tissue usually reveals the presence of particulate debris originating from the joint components, whether metal, plastic, or ceramic (Figs 14.24 and 14.25). The significance of these findings is not known; however, the presence of the implant material in lymph nodes may provide chronic stimulation to the lymphoreticular system, leading to various disturbances, possibly including lymphoreticular neoplasms.

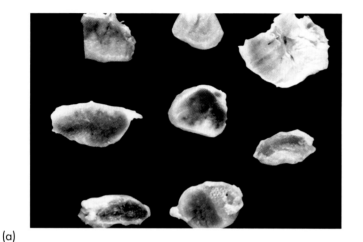

(a)

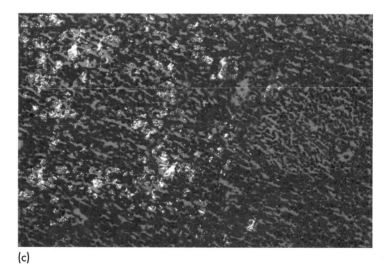

(b)

(c)

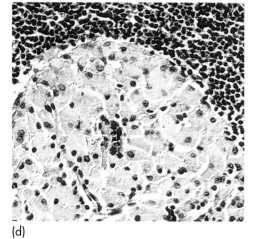

(d)

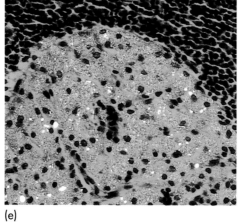

(e)

Figure 14.24 (a) Sections taken through enlarged para-aortic lymph nodes from a dog which had had a total-hip replacement some months previously. (b) Microscopy of a section of a lymph node showing an increase in histiocytes, which when examined by polarized light (c) can be seen to contain refractive material (H&E, × 4 obj.). (d) Photomicrograph of one of the lymph nodes illustrated taken at a higher power shows a nodular collection of pale histiocytes (H&E, × 25 obj.). (e) The same field, photographed with polarized light, shows refractive inclusions of polyethylene within the histiocytes.

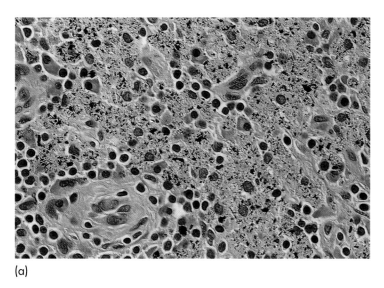

(a)

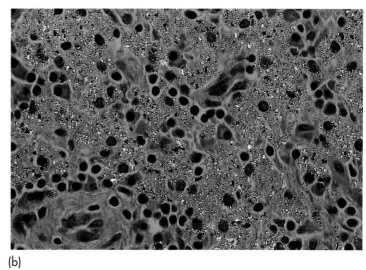

(b)

Figure 14.25   (**a**) Photomicrograph to demonstrate fine particulate debris in histiocytes within lymph nodes of a patient who had had a titanium implant (H&E, × 50 obj.). (**b**) Examination with polarized light shows a bright reflective edge to the particles.

TISSUES AROUND NONINFECTED, CLINICALLY FAILED ARTICULAR IMPLANTS

Fatigue fractures at the implant–bone interface or in the metallic or plastic components, as well as wear and tear on the articulating surfaces, are clear causes of failure of an articular prosthesis (Fig. 14.26). In this regard the quality of the bone is clearly of importance. Osteoporosis or other metabolic disturbances of the bone tissue will significantly affect the strength of the bone–prosthesis interface. Alterations in geometry and mechanics which result from fatigue and wear in the components can, in turn, potentiate and accelerate the process of failure of the prosthesis.

All failed implants that have been cemented in place have particulate cement in the surrounding bone and soft tissues. In addition it is usually possible to find particulate polyethylene in the tissues surrounding failed implants that have polyethylene components. Likewise, metallic debris can be found in many cases.

CEMENTED IMPLANTS

The surfaces of the cement mantle in failed loosened implants are generally smooth, polished, and devoid of the surface irregularities that characterize the tight interlock with bone in stable implants. This smooth appearance is due to fragmentation at the interface and results in pulverization of both cement and bone, which then accumulate in the surrounding tissues (Fig. 14.27).

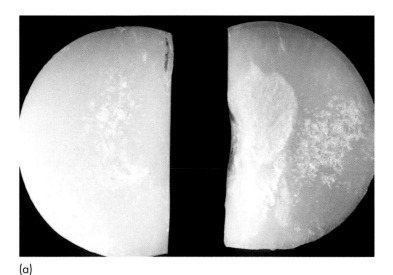

(a)

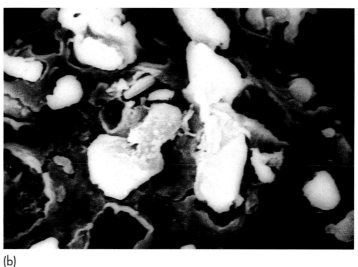

(b)

Figure 14.26   (**a**) The tibial components of total-knee prosthesis show extensive wear and scuffing on the articular surfaces of the polyethylene components. The material generated by this wear process is taken up by the synovium and may cause a considerable synovial reaction. Significant wear results from fragments of cement that are caught between the articular surfaces and ground into the polyethylene. (**b**) Scanning electron photomicrograph shows cement particles buried in the polyethylene surface of the tibial component (x 50 magnification).

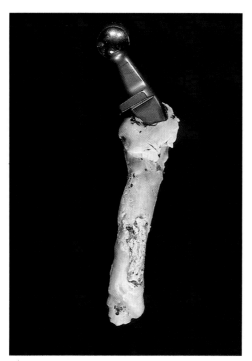

Figure 14.27
Photograph showing the surface of the cement mantle in a loose, failed prosthesis. Note the smooth, polished appearance which should be compared with the rough surface of a well-fixed prosthesis shown in Figure 14.13.

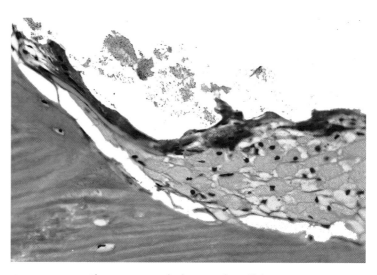

Figure 14.29   Photomicrograph showing the cellular response adjacent to cement. The upper part of the picture shows granules of barium sulfate in the space formerly occupied by cement. Immediately adjacent to that is a giant-cell reaction, and between the cement and the bone is a layer of foamy histiocytes with abundant granular eosinophilic cytoplasm (H&E, x 10 obj.).

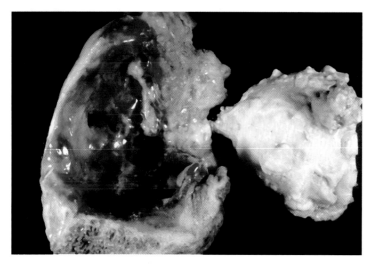

Figure 14.28   Photograph of the membrane lining the acetabulum in a patient with a failed prosthesis. The detached cement is shown on the right-hand side of the photograph. Note the edematous and hyperemic appearance of the membrane.

The most obvious feature observed after failure of a cemented implant is the presence of a thickened membrane around the cement. This membrane may measure up to several millimeters in thickness; it usually has a granular surface and a grumous, friable consistency (Fig. 14.28).

The microscopic features of the membrane include fibrosis, necrosis, and infiltrates of macrophages (Fig. 14.29). Macrophages are usually concentrated at the surface adjacent to the cement and may form a layer which has been said to resemble a synovial lining. Fibrosis is usually concentrated on the bone side of the membrane. Necrosis may be distributed throughout the membrane but is frequently seen nearer to the cement side.

NONCEMENTED IMPLANTS

Aseptically loosened noncemented implants also develop a thickened membrane, which usually has a granular, roughened surface, is friable and generally tan in color. There may also be regions of gray or black discoloration owing to metal debris. In our experience, failed implants made of titanium usually have the blackest appearance. Microscopic examination shows the presence of variable amounts of necrosis, fibrosis, and cellular infiltrates consisting mostly of macrophages.

METAL IN TISSUES

Metals are subject to chemical corrosion in the body, which results in coarsely granular brown–black debris. However, much more common are metallic particles produced as a result of wear at exposed surfaces and fractures of the metallic component (Fig. 14.30).

Microscopic examination of tissue sections from around metal implants, whether cemented or not, usually show sparse small, irregular black fragments measuring from 1–3 μm in greatest dimension. These fragments are opaque, but because of diffraction at their edges they can be more clearly seen in polarized light. Many of the fragments are present within macrophages. However, when there is heavy deposition, as in cases where a metal component has fractured, where metal components articulate with each other, or where the prosthesis is manufactured of Ti-Al-V alloy, the metallic debris can also be seen free in the necrotic or fibrous tissue (Fig. 14.31).

Ultrastructural studies demonstrate that many of the metal particles are in phagolysosomes and have a diameter of less than 0.5 μm, which is below the resolution of light microscopy (Fig. 14.32). The affected macrophages demonstrate a decrease in the endoplasmic reticulum and other distortions of cytologic ultrastructure.

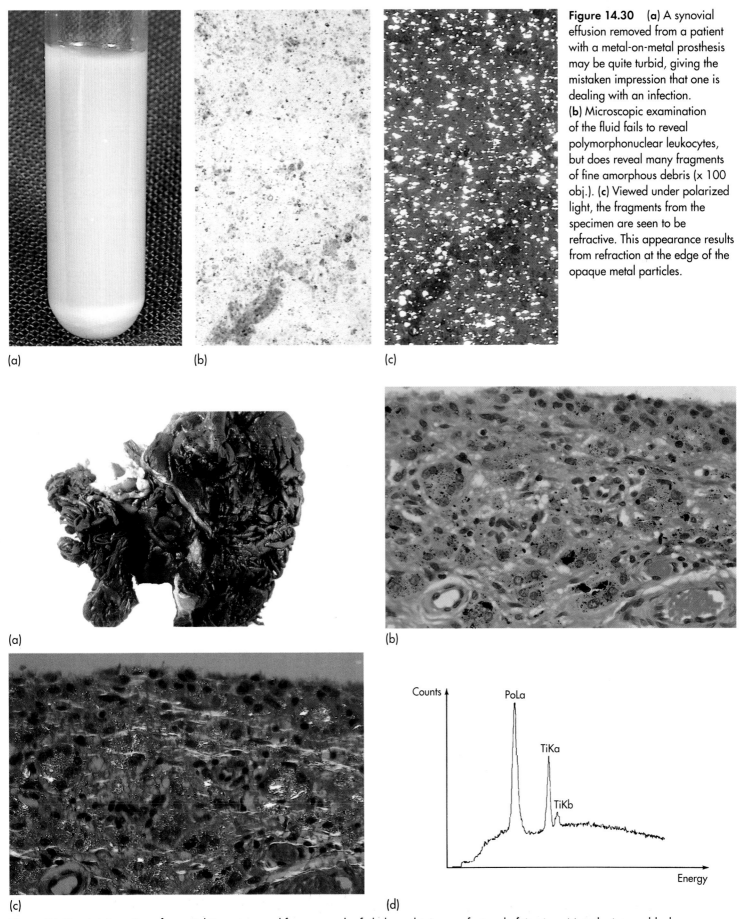

Figure 14.30   (a) A synovial effusion removed from a patient with a metal-on-metal prosthesis may be quite turbid, giving the mistaken impression that one is dealing with an infection. (b) Microscopic examination of the fluid fails to reveal polymorphonuclear leukocytes, but does reveal many fragments of fine amorphous debris (x 100 obj.). (c) Viewed under polarized light, the fragments from the specimen are seen to be refractive. This appearance results from refraction at the edge of the opaque metal particles.

Figure 14.31   (a) A portion of synovial tissue removed from around a failed prosthesis manufactured of titanium. Note the intense black discoloration of the synovial membrane. (b) Photomicrograph of a section taken through the synovium. Particulate black debris is seen both intracellularly and extracellularly in a chronically inflamed fibrous tissue stroma (H&E, × 25 obj.). (c) The same field as (b) photographed with polarized light, which shows many refractive particles of polyethylene as well as small points of reflected light over the metal particles. (d) Energy dispersive analysis shows a significant peak for titanium (TiKa and TiKb).

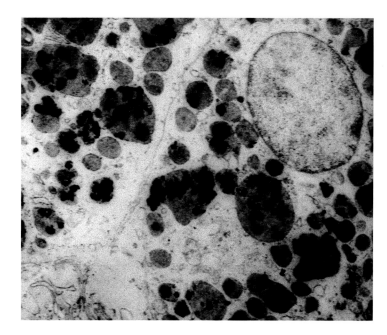

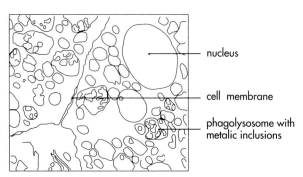

Figure 14.32 Electron photomicrograph of synovial cells from a patient with a total-hip replacement shows an accumulation of electron-dense material in phagolysosomes in the cytoplasm. These dense particles are metallic.

nucleus

cell membrane

phagolysosome with metalic inclusions

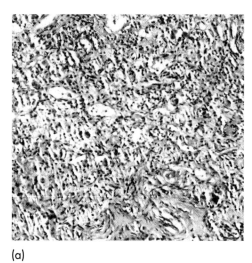

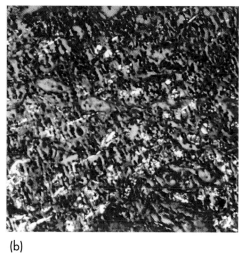

(a)   (b)

Figure 14.33 (a) Photomicrograph of a histologic section taken from the synovium of a patient with a hip prosthesis in which the acetabular component was made of polyethylene. In the transmission light photograph shown here, the subsynovium is infiltrated by large numbers of histiocytes and some chronic inflammatory cells (H&E, × 10 obj.). (b) On polarized light microscopy the cells are seen to be filled with thread-like particles of refractive material, which are derived from wear of the polyethylene surface.

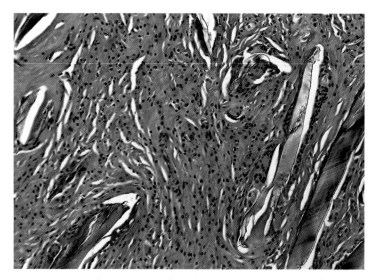

Figure 14.34 Photomicrograph to demonstrate large pieces of polyethylene within the capsular tissue of a rapidly failing joint (H&E, partially polarized × 4 obj.).

POLYETHYLENE IN TISSUES

Polyethylene debris is generated at the articulating surfaces by a number of mechanisms, including direct abrasion, three-body wear (often from entrapped particles of cement as has been illustrated in Fig. 14.26), and fatigue surface damage which increases with time.

Microscopic examination shows a cellular infiltrate of macrophages and giant cells, which may have a granulomatous pattern, or be confluent and appear as dense sheets of cells. The polyethylene, in the form of variably sized shards of glassy, refractile material, can easily be overlooked in transmitted light. However, examination under polarized light will readily and sometimes dramatically demonstrate their presence (Fig. 14.33). The largest pieces are surrounded by a layer of fibrous tissue (Fig. 14.34); the smaller pieces are surrounded or engulfed by giant cells and large mononuclear macrophages (Fig. 14.35). On occasion, many of the giant cells are seen to contain 'asteroid bodies' (Fig. 14.36).

Debris from a polyethylene component is usually concentrated

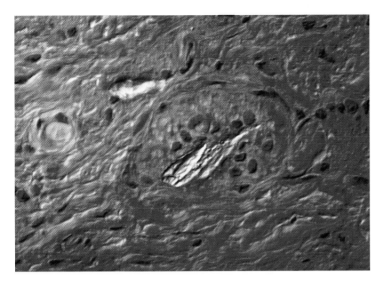

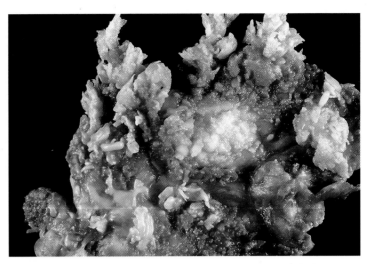

Figure 14.37 Photograph of synovium removed from a failed prosthesis showing marked papillary proliferation of the synovium with focal hemosiderin staining. Microscopic examination of this tissue revealed a foreign body reaction to polyethylene and cement debris.

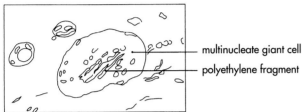

multinucleate giant cell

polyethylene fragment

Figure 14.35 Photomicrograph of a giant cell reveals fine thread-like particles of polyethylene within the cytoplasm (H&E, Nomarski, × 25 obj.).

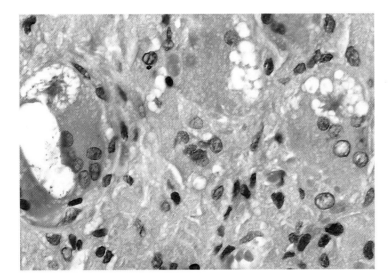

Figure 14.36 Photomicrograph of a histiocytic and giant-cell reaction to cement and polyethylene, showing the presence of asteroid bodies in two of the giant cells (H&E, × 40 obj.).

in the immediate vicinity of the component, in the synovial, pseudocapsular structures, and the joint margin (Figs 14.37 and 14.38). However, it may also be seen in small amounts deep within the bone and bone marrow (Fig. 14.39).

On occasion, the polyethylene component may have been a composite of carbon filaments. In this case it is possible to find fragmented carbon filaments in this tissue. Inflammation is usu-

ally not apparent, and in the absence of polyethylene debris there is no discernible foreign body giant-cell reaction to the carbon particles (Fig. 14.40).

METHYLMETHACRYLATE IN TISSUES

In histologic sections, methylmethacrylate is not seen because it dissolves in the solvents used to process tissues for paraffin embedding. In unstained frozen-tissue sections however, the particles are glassy and granular but are not birefringent in polarized light (Fig. 14.41). In paraffin sections the particles of PMMA instead appear as cleared-out spaces of widely variable size. The largest spaces are lined with giant cells and are partially filled with granular material, which can be shown by energy dispersive analysis (EDAX) to contain barium sulfate that was mixed with the PMMA to provide radiodensity (Fig. 14.42). Finely particulate PMMA is probably responsible for the extensive collection of histiocytes, without refractile material which are frequently present around failed cemented prosthesis (Fig. 14.43).

SILICONE RUBBER IN TISSUES

The tissue response to silicone debris is moderate to intense, and consists of an inflammatory infiltrate which includes lymphocytes, plasma cells, eosinophils, macrophages, and foreign body giant cells. The debris is bosselated, pale yellow and faintly refractile but not birefringent in polarized light. The particles range in size from 6–100 μm. The particles are usually intracellular but may also be free in the extracellular connective tissues (Fig. 14.44).

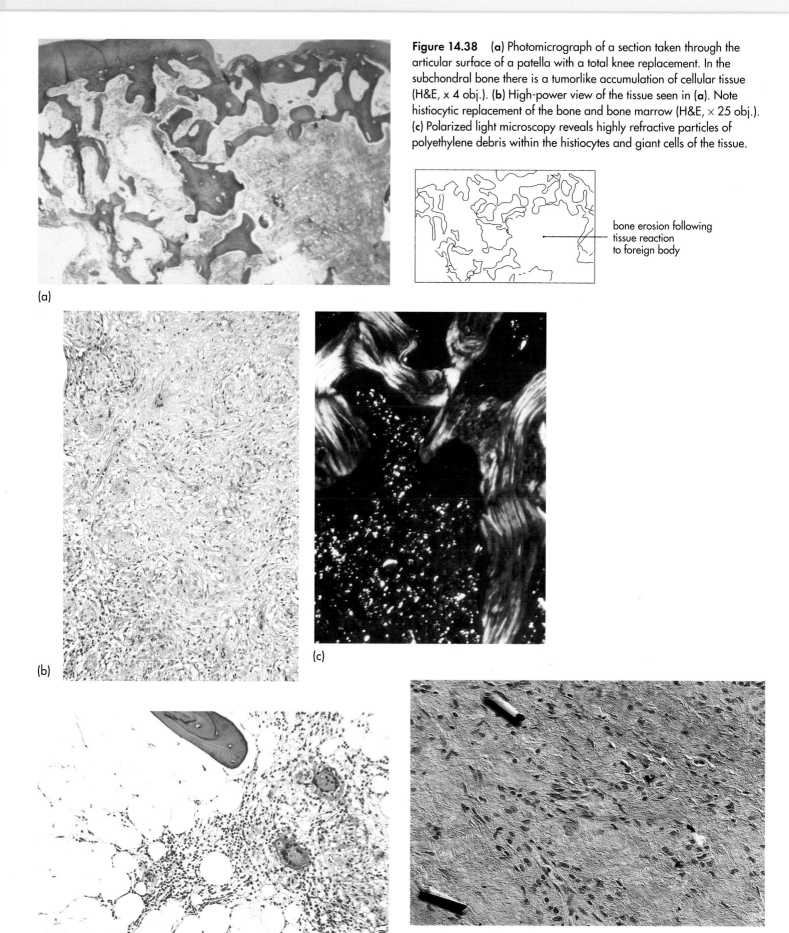

Figure 14.38 (a) Photomicrograph of a section taken through the articular surface of a patella with a total knee replacement. In the subchondral bone there is a tumorlike accumulation of cellular tissue (H&E, × 4 obj.). (b) High-power view of the tissue seen in (a). Note histiocytic replacement of the bone and bone marrow (H&E, × 25 obj.). (c) Polarized light microscopy reveals highly refractive particles of polyethylene debris within the histiocytes and giant cells of the tissue.

bone erosion following tissue reaction to foreign body

(a)

(b)

(c)

Figure 14.39 Photomicrograph of a small granulomatous mass in the marrow space at some distance from the site of a prosthetic implant (H&E, × 25 obj.).

Figure 14.40 Photomicrograph demonstrating cylindrical fragments of carbon fiber in the tissue from a patient who had a carbon fiber-reinforced implant. The section also shows a fibroblastic and histiocytic response, which with polarized light reveals extensive polyethylene debris (H&E, × 25 obj.).

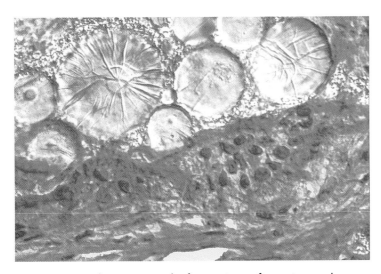

Figure 14.41 Photomicrograph of a specimen of synovium cut by frozen section without the use of solvents demonstrates cement in situ. Polymer balls are evident, and between these spheres a finely granular yellow material is seen. This appearance results from the barium sulfate that is mixed with the cement to render it radiopaque (H&E, Nomarski, × 25 obj.).

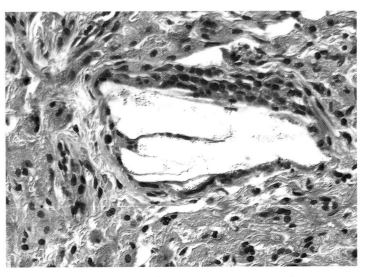

Figure 14.42 Photomicrograph demonstrating a giant-cell reaction around a large piece of cement, which appears as an irregular space in the center of the photograph because the cement itself has been dissolved by routine processing methods. The small collection of granular material seen within the space is barium sulfate, which is mixed into the cement to render it radio-opaque (H&E, × 40 obj.).

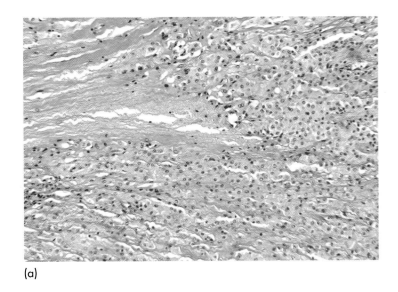

(a)

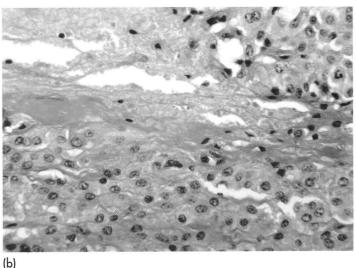

(b)

Figure 14.43 (a) Photomicrograph of tissue obtained from around a lucent cemented prosthesis shows abundant foamy histiocytes (H&E, × 10 obj.). (b) At a higher magnification there is no obvious foreign-body giant cell reaction (H&E, × 40 obj.).

CERAMIC IN TISSUES

The major feature of the reaction around a failed ceramic implant is the generation of a thickened membrane with necrosis, fibrosis, and macrophages similar to that seen in failure of the other types of implant (Fig. 14.45). Small particles of debris, < 5 μm in size, are numerous within the membrane and have a gray–black appearance. These particles are generally found within macrophages and foreign body giant cells are not usually seen (Fig. 14.46). By EDAX analysis the particles can be shown to contain both aluminum and silicon (Fig. 14.47).

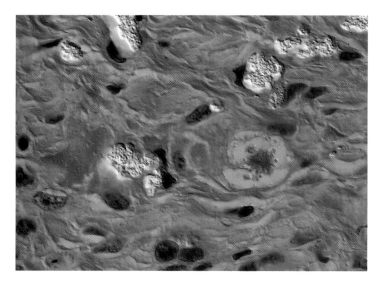

Figure 14.44 Photomicrograph to demonstrate breakdown products from a Silastic prosthesis. There is a histiocytic and giant-cell response in fibrous scar tissue. An asteroid body is present within a giant cell present in the middle of the field (Nomarski optics, H&E, × 25 obj.).

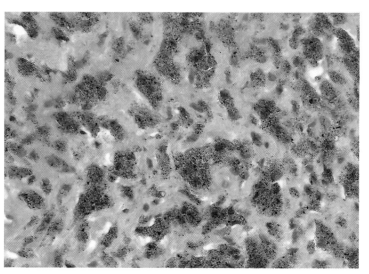

Figure 14.46 Photomicrograph of histiocytic response to ceramic. The ceramic particles are jagged in appearance and only faintly refractive (H&E, × 25 obj.).

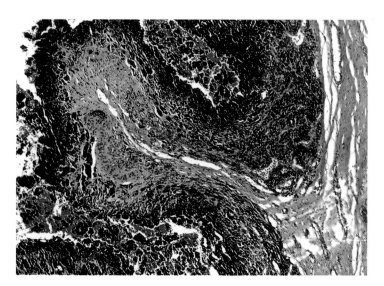

Figure 14.45 Photomicrograph of membrane adjacent to a failed ceramic prosthesis shows a gray to black discoloration of the tissue with secondary chronic inflammation and scarring (H&E, × 4 obj.).

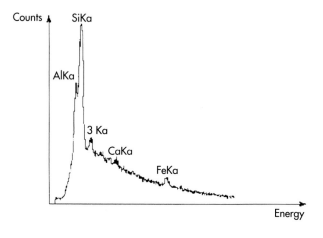

Figure 14.47 Energy dispersive analysis of the tissue shows peaks for aluminum and silica, consistent with ceramic (AlKa and SiKa).

CONCLUSION

There are at least three consequences of the shedding of wear particles from articulating implants. First, the total surface area of contact between implant material and the biologic environment is enormously increased by fragmentation, thus facilitating the exchange of potentially toxic elements at the interface for greater systemic dissemination. Second, wear particles of suitable sizes may be phagocytosed, resulting in a space-occupying lesion. Furthermore the particles become exposed to intracellular processes, which they might then alter. Third, particles that have been ingested may be transported to sites remote from the implant, such as regional lymph nodes, lungs, and spleen, and may interfere with the functions of these systems.

OSTEONECROSIS AND BONE INFARCTION

Tissue death (necrosis) results from one of five primary types of injury: (1) circulatory, (2) thermal, (3) toxic, (4) mechanical, or (5) radiation. When necrosis occurs secondary to a primary circulatory disturbance whether because of arterial disease, embolism, or obstruction of the venous return, the resultant region of necrosis is referred to as an infarct.

Bone death, in the form of a sequestrum, was first recognized as a complication of osteomyelitis. Later it came to be recognized that necrosis was also a feature of fracture and that in certain locations such as the hip, patella, and carpal scaphoid, the associated necrosis could be so extensive as to give rise to significant clinical complaints of non-union and/or secondary arthritis.

The occurrence of bone infarcts in caisson workers and other divers who have had decompression sickness as well as in patients with sickle-cell anemia, Gaucher's disease, and other hematologic disease, is now well recognized. Many cases involve the femoral head or other convex articular surfaces. However, infarction may also affect other bone sites, usually the metaphysis of a long bone or even, on occasion, a flat bone. The lesions may be multiple and occasionally symmetrical. Most of the patients are middle-aged or older, and some may complain of pain; in other cases the lesion is discovered as an incidental radiologic finding.

The early stage of a bone infarct can be observed only on MRI or at autopsy, where it appears grossly as an elongated pale area with a hyperemic border which is rather sharply demarcated from the surrounding bones (Fig. 15.1). At this stage, not enough time may have elapsed for changes in the architecture of the bone trabeculae to develop, and therefore little if any change is seen on the radiograph. Microscopically, large irregular spaces are seen in ischemic marrow fat, which result from breakdown of the walls of fat cells together with local hemorrhage (Fig. 15.2). The bone trabeculae are nonviable, as evidenced by lacunae that do not contain stainable osteocytes. However, the most obvious evidence of early infarction is seen in bone that contains hematopoietic tissue, since this tissue is extremely vulnerable to ischemia, and the necrotic hematopoietic tissue is readily recognized (Fig. 15.3).

With the passage of time, ingrowth of granulation tissue takes place at the periphery of the infarcted area, and a 'creeping substitution' of the nonviable cancellous bone by layering of new viable bone on the dead trabecular surfaces at the periphery is also seen. In most cases the healing process is aborted and a rim of highly collagenized connective tissue forms about the periphery of the lesion. This connective tissue wall generally becomes infiltrated with calcium salts (Fig. 15.4).

Radiographs of the lesion in the later stages of development have a typical appearance (Fig. 15.5). A moderately thick, radiopaque serpentine border can be observed, often outlining an elongated area of central radiolucency. This appearance may be likened to a coil of smoke. In some cases, particularly in solitary lesions, radiographs may suggest a calcified enchondroma. Usually, however, the foci of calcified matrix in enchondroma or chondrosarcoma are discrete and scattered diffusely throughout the lesion, and the margin of the lesion is not so clearly outlined as with an infarct. Some lesions which have been interpreted radiographically as bone infarcts may in fact represent calcified and cystified lipomas of bone (see Fig. 19.56).

The occasional development in a bone infarct of a malignant tumor, usually a malignant fibrous histiocytoma, is a well-recognized complication and will be referred to again in Chapter 18, p. 440.

SKELETAL MANIFESTATION OF DECOMPRESSION SICKNESS

Decompression sickness is the consequence of the liberation of gas bubbles (notably nitrogen) in the tissues and blood of subjects who have undergone rapid decompression after a period of exposure to a hyperbaric environment. In a subject who is exposed to a hyperbaric environment, greater amounts of the various gases, which go to make up the air we breathe, enter

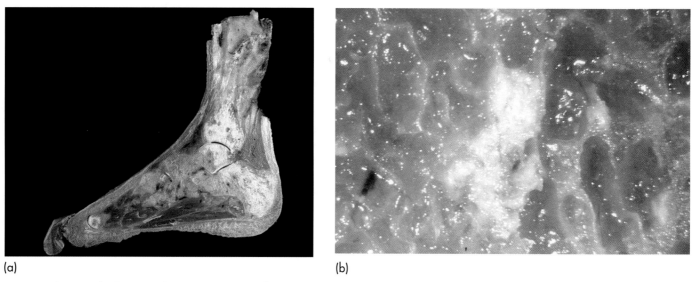

(a)   (b)

Figure 15.1   (a) Photograph of a sagittal section through the lower leg and foot of a 68-year-old male with multiple sclerotic lesions radiographically and a non-union of a fracture of the tibia. The multiple areas of sharply demarcated chalky white, opaque tissue in the tibia and in the bones of the foot are the result of infarction. (b) Close-up photograph of cancellous bone to demonstrate a small focus of marrow and bone necrosis recognized by its opacity, yellowish-white color, and failure to retract like the surrounding viable fatty marrow.

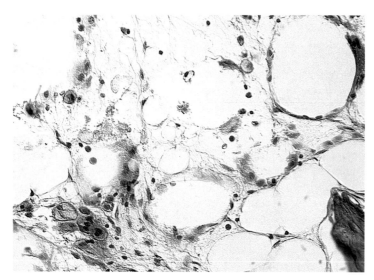

Figure 15.2   Photomicrograph to demonstrate early fat necrosis resulting from ischemia. There is breakdown of the walls of the fat cells, resulting in large irregular cystic spaces which are surrounded by foamy histiocytes and giant cells (H&E, × 10 obj.).

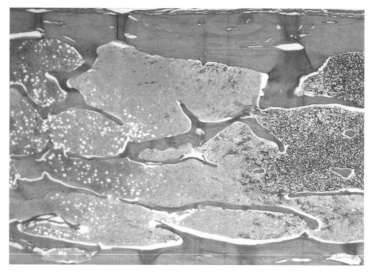

Figure 15.3   Photomicrograph to demonstrate necrosis of the hematopoietic marrow (viable blue-staining marrow, for comparison, is seen in the right-hand side of the photograph). Necrosis of the marrow is the most obvious microscopic finding associated with bone necrosis (H&E, × 4 obj.).

into solution until a state of saturation of the blood and tissues has been reached. The time required for saturation is not the same for all tissues, for example fat may require a much longer time before the saturation point for nitrogen is reached, since nitrogen is about five times more soluble in fat than in water. If a person who has been in a high-pressure environment, and whose blood and tissues are consequently saturated with the gases of the atmosphere, passes too quickly from the hyperbaric environment to one of normal atmospheric pressure, the various gases come out of solution.

By ventilation, the body readily disposes of the excess of oxy-gen and carbon dioxide. On the other hand the excess of nitro-gen, which has come out of solution and which is not ventilated by the lungs, forms bubbles. Nitrogen bubbles present in the cir-culating blood may act as air emboli, partially or completely blocking terminal vascular channels at a distant site or sites, giv-ing rise to neurologic impairment. Since the accumulation of nitrogen is greatest in tissues rich in fat such as bone marrow, the extravascular pressure upon the regional blood vessels may obstruct the blood supply to the bone.

The acute manifestations of decompression sickness are: firstly the bends, consisting of pain (most often at the knees) and secondly injury to vital organs (central nervous system, heart, lungs, etc.) due to bubbles of nitrogen arising or lodging in these organs. Organ damage sometimes leads to permanent disability or even death.

The late (or chronic) skeletal aspects of decompression sick-

ness are the result of ischemic necrosis, and are observed particularly in bone sites rich in fatty marrow. Months or even years may elapse between the occurrence of the underlying bone infarction and the appearance of clinical and/or radiographic evidence of the bone necrosis (Fig. 15.6).

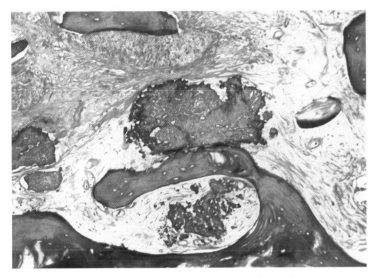

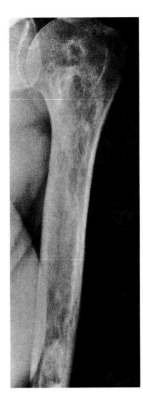

Figure 15.5 In a medullary bone infarction, seen here in the proximal humerus of a 36-year-old man with sickle-cell disease, there is no endosteal scalloping of the cortex, such as might be seen with a chondrosarcoma; this is the most important radiologic differential diagnosis. The calcified area is surrounded by a thin, dense sclerotic margin – the hallmark of a bone infarct.

Figure 15.4 Photomicrograph to demonstrate calcium deposition in necrotic marrow (H&E, × 10 obj.). (If there is heavy calcium deposition, it may lead to an obvious increase in radiodensity on clinical radiographs.)

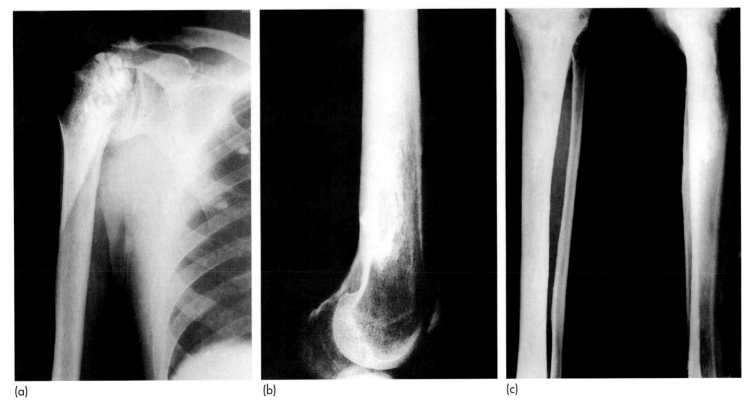

(a) (b) (c)

Figure 15.6 (a) A man who had worked as a caisson worker many years before presented with pain in the shoulder. The radiograph shows extensive areas of calcification within the medullary bone. (b) Within his distal femur there is a similar area of linear calcification. (c) Similar lesions are present in both the anteroposterior and lateral views of the proximal tibia.

OSTEONECROSIS OF THE FEMORAL HEAD

In 1915 Phemister described the microscopic findings in necrotic bone, comparing the changes in bone dying as a result of infection ('septic necrosis') with those resulting from a circulatory interference ('aseptic necrosis') following fracture. Later, he reported the histologic and radiologic changes seen in a dead bone, and the reparative processes occurring around dead bone coining the term 'creeping substitution' for the process whereby the dead bone is replaced by granulation tissue and a layer of living bone which is deposited onto the pre-existing dead bone.

Since the hip joint is a major focus of clinical orthopedic interest, the bulk of the pertinent literature is centered on osteonecrosis of the femoral head.

Early writers on necrosis of the femoral head frequently used the term 'aseptic necrosis' to stress the absence of infection. Later the term 'avascular necrosis of the hip' was applied since most of the recognized cases were associated with subcapital femoral neck fracture, which would be expected to interrupt the blood supply to the femoral head. Subchondral osteonecrosis without a history of femoral neck fracture was considered unusual.

The relationship between the occurrence of idiopathic sub-

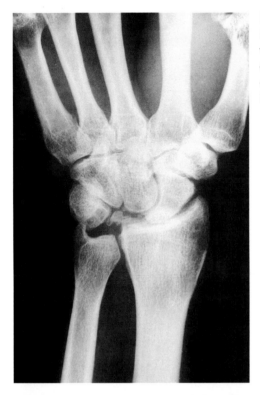

Figure 15.7
Radiograph of the wrist reveals collapse of the lunate bone characteristic of Kienböck's disease.

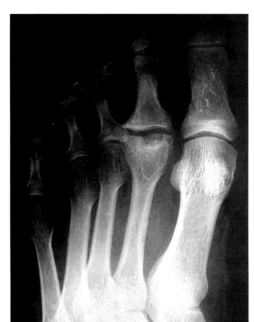

Figure 15.9
Radiograph of the forefoot of an adult showing collapse of the articular surface of the 2nd metatarsal: Freiberg's disease.

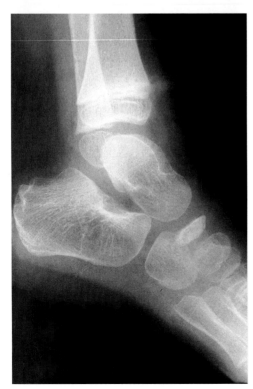

Figure 15.8
Radiograph of the hind foot of a child with collapse of the tarsal–navicular bone: Köhler's disease.

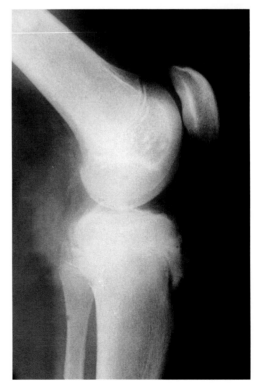

Figure 15.10
Lateral radiograph of a boy, showing disruption and fragmentation of the tibial tubercle; Osgood–Schlatter disease.

chondral avascular necrosis and steroid therapy or alcoholism was slowly recognized during the 1950s to 1960s. Although a circulatory disturbance is assumed to be the principle primary mechanism of idiopathic necrosis in the bones, unlike myocardial infarction the location of the occlusion cannot usually be shown by anatomical dissection.

Recently, as discussed in Chapter 11, p. 273, it has become clear that some instances of acute onset arthritic disease of the hip joint, particularly in elderly individuals, which until recently would have been regarded on the basis of history and magnetic resonance imaging (MRI) to be cases of primary osteonecrosis of the femoral head, are due to subchondral fractures, often without any clear history of trauma.

At one time it was also thought that most of that eponymous group of affections known as the osteochondritises, or osteochondroses, namely Kienböck's disease, Köhler's disease, Freiberg's disease, Osgood–Schlatter's disease (Figs 15.7–15.10), osteochondritis dissecans etc. were due to bone necrosis, but it has become increasingly clear that many of these lesions are consequent upon trauma, often repetitive and with a resulting fracture, and that where there is necrosis it is most probably the result of the fracture, i.e. a secondary phenomenon. In some cases necrosis and fractures are difficult to untangle and such a case is shown in Figure 15.11.

At the present time in our laboratory, of the 1700 femoral heads removed each year in total-hip replacement procedures for nontraumatic causes, about 10% show evidence of subchondral avascular necrosis as the primary etiology. Approximately 60% of the cases diagnosed as idiopathic osteonecrosis have bilateral disease and most of these patients have a history of either corticosteroid use or increased alcohol consumption.

Osteonecrosis as a secondary complication of osteoarthritis (OA) has been recognized grossly and confirmed microscopically in 38.2% of the femoral heads diagnosed in our laboratory as having primary OA. The foci of secondary osteonecrosis were categorized into two types based on shape, size and depth: a 'shallow' flat lesion (median axis 3–10 mm, depth 2–3 mm) with or without cysts (368 cases, 36.5%), and a 'deep, wedge-shaped'

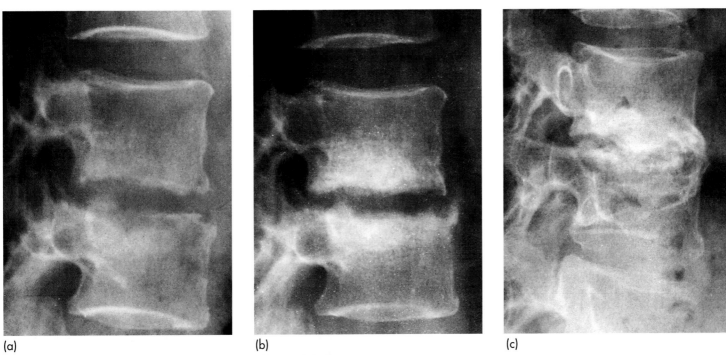

(a)   (b)   (c)

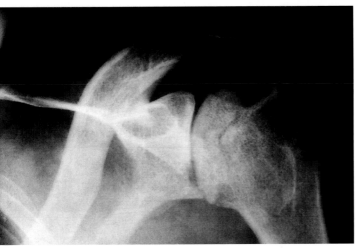

(d)

Figure 15.11   (a) Sequential radiographs of a man aged 50+, receiving cortisone therapy for a chronic skin condition. The time interval between the first and second films (b) is 8 months and the time between the second and third films (c) is 2 years. At the time of (b), the patient began to complain of pain in the shoulder (shown in d). The changes at the joint surfaces resulted from osteonecrosis secondary to cortisone therapy, although at first the radiologic changes were considered to be caused by tuberculosis. (d) Radiograph of the shoulder shows collapse of the humeral head secondary to SAVN.

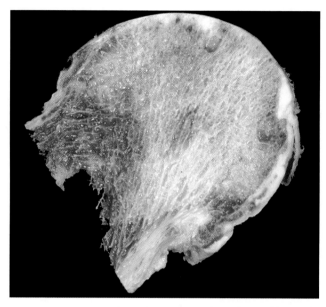

Figure 15.12 A section through an osteoarthritic femoral head shows an irregular linear area of osteonecrosis in the superior eburnated articular surface.

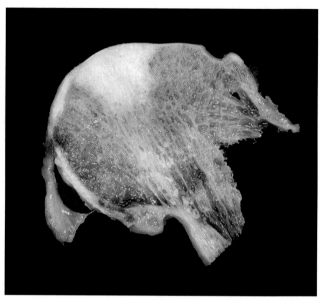

Figure 15.13 A section through an osteoarthritic femoral head shows a large wedge-shaped area of necrosis at the superior portion of the head.

large lesion (> 20 mm across and depth 10 mm) with or without cysts (17 cases, 1.7%). In the 'shallow' flat lesion, the age ranged from 25–88 (average 66), the female/male ratio was 0.8 and the location of osteonecrosis correlated best with the direction of migration in OA (Fig. 15.12). In the 'deep, wedge-shaped' lesion, the age ranged from 56–92 (average 70), the female/male ratio was 1.8 and the location of osteonecrosis was similar to that found in primary osteonecrosis (Fig. 15.13).

NECROSIS FOLLOWING FRACTURE

Fractures of the femoral neck are occasionally encountered in children and young adults, however, they occur predominantly in elderly persons. In young subjects a complete fracture of the femoral neck may follow a stress fracture and is likely to occur in young men undergoing basic military training or in other youthful subjects who are subjecting themselves to exceptional physical exertion, e.g. shin splints in young ballet dancers.

In elderly persons, especially women, a subcapital fracture frequently follows upon a trivial injury, often occurring during walking and resulting merely from a slip or misstep. In older individuals underlying bone disease (osteoporosis or osteomalacia) together with neuromuscular deterioration are very important contributing factors.

A fracture of the femoral neck is regularly followed by more or less complete ischemic necrosis of the femoral head, due to an interruption of its blood supply. However even though the femoral head becomes necrotic, a majority of fractures treated by internal fixation unite with a sound bony union, sometimes within a few months. During this period the necrotic head is in most cases undergoing revascularization and repair.

Since the repair of the necrotic femoral head usually lags behind the healing of the fracture of the neck, perhaps it is not surprising that collapse of the upper weight-bearing segment of the femoral head constitutes a fairly common late complication, occurring in upward of 20% of the patients with intracapsular fractures. This complication usually does not develop until about a year and a half after the occurrence of the fracture, and sometimes is delayed for 2 years or more after the fracture. The patient may have been ambulatory and free of pain for many months before the segmental collapse of the femoral head. However, the collapse results not only in pathologic incongruity of the articulating surfaces and therefore a dysfunctional joint, but also pain which is often severe.

In 1965, Catto published two classic papers describing in detail the destructive and reparative changes in subchondral avascular necrosis of the femoral head after subcapital fractures of the neck of the femur.

Four stages in the development of subchondral avascular necrosis were defined morphologically and these may be shown to correlate with the observed radiographic appearances:

1. Characterized predominantly by the presence of necrosis of both bone and bone marrow without evidence of repair.
2. Reparative processes are evident at the periphery of the necrotic region.
3. The major feature is segmental collapse of the articular surface.
4. Features of secondary OA have developed.

It is important to recognize that the morphological features of subchondral avascular necrosis are a composite of both necrotizing and reparative processes, and that at least some of the apparently degenerative features – for example, segmental collapse in stage three – often may be the result of reparative processes.

STAGE I

In stage one external examination of the joint shows no abnormalities, though an ill defined focal yellow discoloration may be seen through the articular cartilage. On cut section of the femoral head, a necrotic wedge-shaped region in which the marrow is dull, yellow, chalky and opaque, will be seen. This is generally in an immediately subarticular location extending for some distance into the underlying epiphyseal bone. The region is usually well demarcated and separated from the surrounding bone marrow by a thin, red, hyperemic border (Fig. 15.14). The marrow beyond this border shows no specific abnormality referable to the necrotizing process, but may have an abnormal appearance depending on an associated or predisposing condition – for example, sickle-cell disease with its dark red bone marrow, or Gaucher's disease with its pale and waxy marrow. At this stage changes in the trabecular architecture are not appreciable on specimen radiographs (Fig. 15.15).

On microscopic examination the overlying articular cartilage is viable. The subchondral bone, corresponding to the opaque yellow region seen grossly, is characterized by necrotic bone marrow, which is granular, eosinophilic, and lacking in cellular elements except for the occasional ghosts of disrupted fat cells (Fig. 15.16). There may also be focally calcified lipid cysts (Fig. 15.17). In the bone the osteocytic lacunae may be either empty, contain cellular debris, or have a ghost nucleus.

At the margin of the infarct there is increased osteoclastic activity with removal of necrotic bone as well as an infiltration of proliferating fibroblasts and capillaries (granulation tissue) into the necrotic marrow. This zone corresponds to the thin red rim seen in the gross specimen. Beyond the infarct and the hypervascular zone the bone and bone marrow are unchanged and reflect the state of the tissue before the necrotizing event.

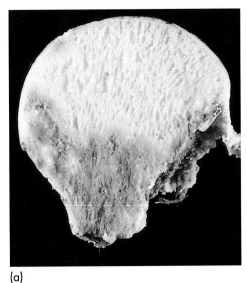

(a)

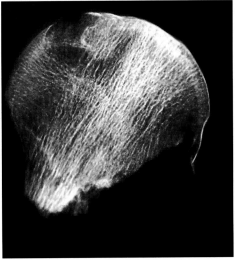

(b)

Figure 15.15 (a) Femoral head excised from a patient approximately 1 week after a subcapital fracture exhibits extensive bone necrosis. (b) Specimen radiograph of (a).

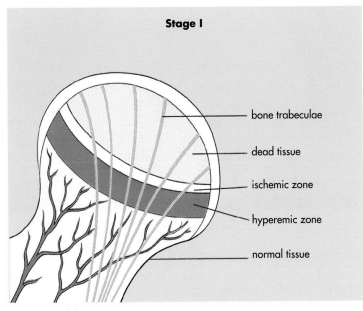

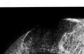

Figure 15.14 Diagrammatic representation of changes occurring in stage I SAVN.

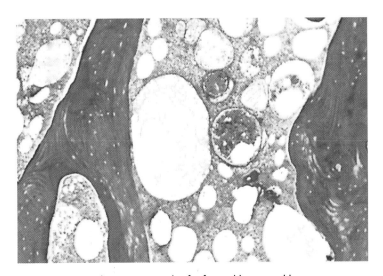

Figure 15.16 Photomicrograph of infarcted bone and bone marrow reveals the acellular nature of the tissue and large, fat cysts characteristic of infarcted bone marrow (phloxine & tartrazine, × 4 obj.).

STAGE II

As in stage I the articular surface appears intact (Fig. 15.18). However, on sectioning the femoral head a rim of bony sclerosis, best seen on specimen radiographs, can be identified at the boundary between the necrotic zone and the unaffected marrow (Fig. 15.19).

On microscopic examination an advancing front of granulation tissue, composed of lipid-laden macrophages, proliferating fibroblasts, and capillaries, is seen extending into the necrotic zone (Fig. 15.20). Following closely behind this 'clean up' front is a second front where osteoblasts can be seen, depositing a layer of new bone on the pre-existing dead trabecular bone – 'creeping substitution' (Fig. 15.21).

The overall effect of these processes is to remove the necrotic marrow and bone while maintaining the structural integrity of the bone. The increased vascularity with osteoblastic activity and new bone formation give rise both to the clinical radiographic appearances of bony sclerosis at the margin of the infarct, and to the increased uptake of radioactive technetium diphosphonate isotope on a bone scan (Fig. 15.22).

STAGE III

An obvious alteration in the shape of the articular bone is first encountered in this stage (Fig. 15.23). This disturbance in shape is the result of fracture either within the necrotic region or at the junction of the necrotic bone and reparative tissue. It may be apparent on external examination of the bone as a buckling of the articular surface (Fig. 15.24). On sectioning the femoral head fracture can be seen to occur most often either just below the articular bone end-plate (i.e. superficial) (Fig. 15.25) or on the

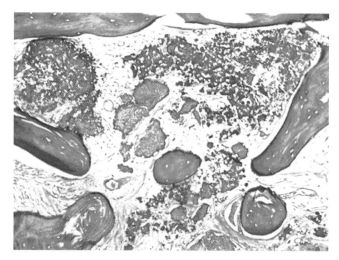

Figure 15.17   Calcification is sometimes a prominent feature in infarcted bone marrow and may on occasion give rise to increased density on radiographs (H&E, × 4 obj.).

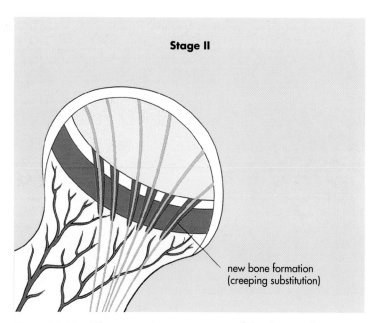

Figure 15.18   Diagrammatic representation of the changes that occur in stage II SAVN.

new bone formation (creeping substitution)

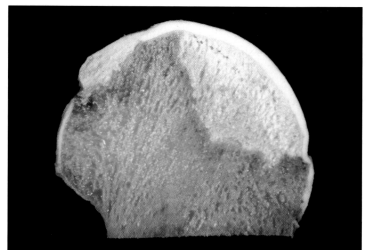

(a)

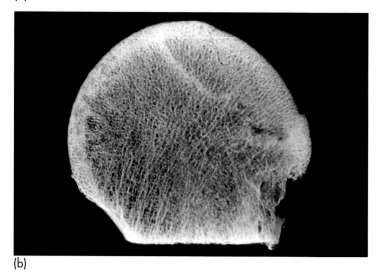

(b)

Figure 15.19   (a) Photograph from a patient with stage II SAVN shows a well-demarcated hyperemic border. A fine fracture line can be seen running through the necrotic bone close to the articular surface.
(b) Specimen radiograph showing a line of bone sclerosis which corresponds to the zone of hyperemia seen in the gross photograph. At the inferior edge of the infarcted area there is a small fracture involving the subarticular bone, resulting in a step deformity.

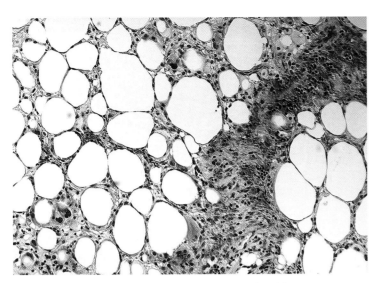

Figure 15.20 Photomicrograph to demonstrate focal fat necrosis as well as fibroblastic and vascular proliferation at the margin of the infarcted area (H&E, × 10 obj.).

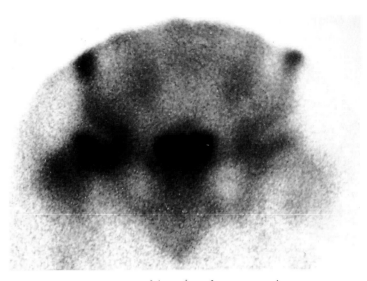

Figure 15.22 Scintigram of the pelvis of a patient with symptoms suggestive of SAVN, but without radiographic changes, shows increased uptake of isotope in the affected femoral head.

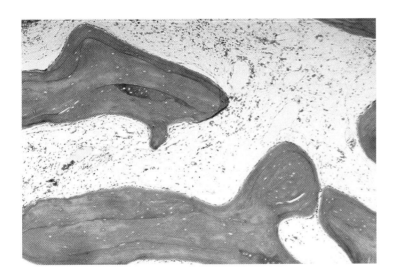

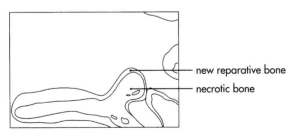

Figure 15.21 In the process of healing an infarcted area of bone, a layer of living bone is deposited on the surface of the necrotic bone. This process, referred to as 'creeping substitution', gives rise to increased radiodensity at the healing margin of the infarct. Note also the vascularized fibrous tissue in the marrow spaces (H&E, × 10 obj.).

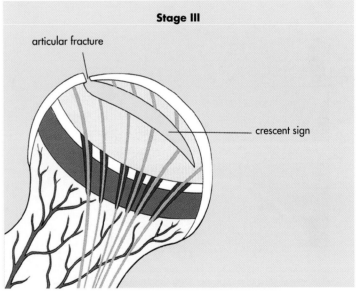

Figure 15.23 Diagram illustrating the associated tissue changes with the crescent sign in stage III SAVN.

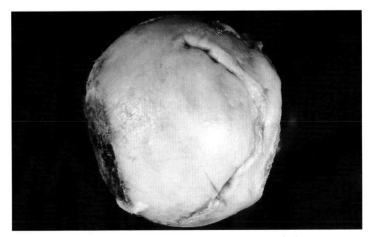

Figure 15.24 Gross photograph of a femoral head removed surgically after clinical signs and symptoms of avascular necrosis were detected. On the articular surface of the femoral head there is a linear dimpling of the articular cartilage, marking the site of an underlying fracture.

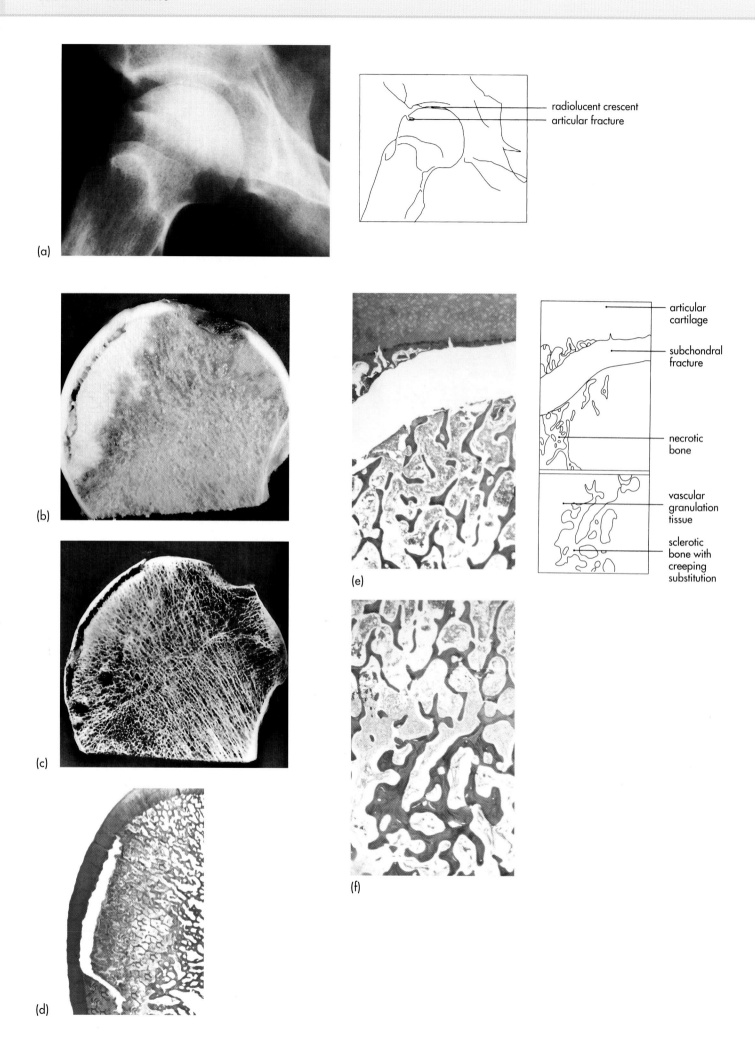

(a)

radiolucent crescent
articular fracture

(b)

(c)

(d)

(e)

articular
cartilage

subchondral
fracture

necrotic
bone

vascular
granulation
tissue

sclerotic
bone with
creeping
substitution

(f)

necrotic side of the advancing sclerosis in the reparative front (i.e. deep) (Fig. 15.26).

Fracture may be the result of the cumulative effect of microfractures induced by fatigue within the necrotic zone. On the other hand it may be because of weakness of trabeculae in the reparative front because of increased osteoclastic resorption with interruption of trabecular continuity and associated inadequacy of repair bone. A focal concentration of stress at the junctions between the thickened sclerotic trabeculae of the reparative zone and necrotic trabecula resulting from the bioengineering concept of 'stress risers' may be yet another cause (15.27).

STAGE IV

The major feature of this stage is articular deformity. Depending on the degree of bone loss and the severity of the deformity, it

may be no longer possible on clinical radiographs to recognize the initial events as those of subchondral avascular necrosis. In many cases, however, there is sufficient evidence on gross and microscopic examination to allow for proper diagnosis (Fig. 15.28).

A frontal section of the femoral head at this stage of subchondral avascular necrosis may show residual fragments of articular cartilage and dense fibrous connective tissue in the area of infarction. The articular surface at the margin of the infarct will usually demonstrate a densely sclerotic eburnated articular surface (Fig. 15.29).

Two useful clues to the diagnosis of subchondral avascular necrosis may be the absence of clearly eburnated bone at the articular surface overlying the area of infarction, and the presence of bony and cartilaginous debris in the accompanying synovial and capsular tissue. When the changes of secondary OA are

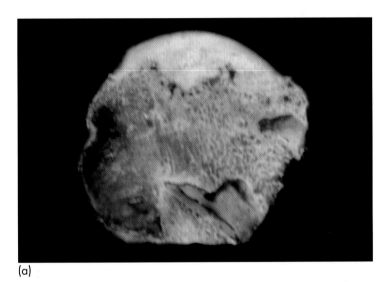

(a)

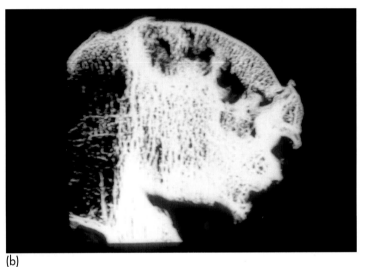

(b)

Figure 15.26   (a) Photograph of a slice through a femoral head showing an area of infarction seen as a triangular, opaque yellow area lying immediately beneath the articular surface. Also seen in this photograph is the track of the nail that was used for fixation of the subcapital fracture that preceded the necrosis. (b) Radiograph of the specimen shown in (a). Note the unaltered trabecular pattern of the infarcted bone. [In contrast, the viable bone at the base of the infarct is dense, resulting from the formation of new bone in this area by the process of creeping substitution (see text).] The lucent area at the base of the infarction results from fibrous granulation tissue eroding the necrotic bone. The collapse of the necrotic segment is well demonstrated by the fracture through the subchondral plate, which is seen at both edges of the infarct.

Figure 15.25   (a) Radiograph of a young patient who complained of sudden onset of pain in the hip. Although the joint space is normal in this frog-lateral view, a crescentic lucent zone outlining the articular surface can be seen on the superior aspect of the femoral head. This crescent sign is often an early radiologic manifestation of avascular necrosis and may be best appreciated in the frog-lateral view. (b) Photograph of a slice taken through the femoral head removed from a patient who has stage III osteonecrosis. The subchondral infarct is demarcated from the viable bone by a zone of hyperemia. The lucent crescent seen on the radiograph in (a) represents a space between the articular cartilage and the underlying infarcted bone. This results from collapse of the subchondral bone following fracture in the zone between the infarct and the underlying viable bone; the more elastic articular cartilage maintains its contour. (c) Specimen radiograph of the slice shown in (b). Again the crescent sign is clearly seen. The dense lucent line evident on the superior surface of the femoral head is an image of the subchondral bone end-plate and the calcified cartilage, which remain adherent to the articular cartilage after the collapse of the infarcted area. After collapse the articular surface probably springs back like a ping-pong ball, giving rise to this radiologic phenomenon. (d) Photomicrograph of a histologic preparation of the femoral head shown in (b) and (c). The thickened trabeculae in the viable bone at the base of the infarct can be clearly appreciated (H&E, × 1 obj.). (e) Photomicrograph through an area of stage III osteonecrosis. At the top can be seen viable articular cartilage as well as the necrotic bone and bone marrow of the infarcted area; between them is the subchondral crescent. The lower frame (f) shows the junction between the necrotic and viable bone. At the bottom of the picture the thickened trabeculae of viable bone are evident. This thickening is the result of new bone deposition on the trabecular surfaces, which occurs as part of the healing of the infarct (H&E, × 4 obj.).

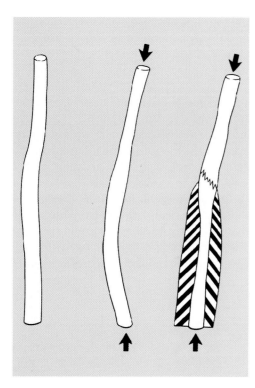

Figure 15.27 Diagram demonstrating the effect of creeping substitution. Increased stiffening of the bone causes focal stress concentration at the junction between the existing bone and the sclerotic bone. When a bending force is applied to the bone, fracture is likely to occur at this point.

Table 15.1 Staging osteonecrosis (University of Pennsylvania Classification and Staging).

Stage	Criteria
0	Normal or nondiagnostic radiograph, bone scan, and MRI
I	Normal radiograph; Abnormal bone scan and/or MRI A – Mild (< 15% of head affected) B – Moderate (15–30%) C – Severe (> 30%)
II	Lucent and sclerotic changes in femoral head A – Mild (< 15%) B – Moderate (15–30%) C – Severe (> 30%)
III	Subchondral collapse (crescent sign) without flattening A – Mild (< 15% of articular surface) B – Moderate (15–30%) C – Severe (> 30%)
IV	Flattening of femoral head A – Mild (< 15% of surface and < 2 mm depression) B – Moderate (15–30% of surface or 2–4 mm depression) C – Severe (> 30% of surface or > 4 mm depression)
V	Joint narrowing and/or acetabular changes A – Mild (Average of femoral head involvement B – Moderate as determined in stage IV, and estimated C – Severe acetabular involvement)
VI	Advanced degenerative changes

(with permission from: Steinberg ME, Hayken GD, Steinberg DR. **Classification and staging of osteonecrosis.** In: Urbaniak JR, Jones, JP Jr, eds. *Osteonecrosis, etiology, diagnosis and treatment.* American Academy of Orthopaedic Surgeons; 1997:279.)

advanced, the only clue that the initial event might have been subchondral avascular necrosis is that the femoral head may have a deep, saddle-shaped deformity.

Most of the recent imaging criteria for staging have developed from Catto's classic description (Tables 15.1 and 15.2).

Table 15.2 Unified system (Proposed by Enneking).

Stage	Event	Criteria*	Quantitation		Location
I	Infarction/repair	(+) MRI, CT, radiograph	Size of infarct A – < 15% B – 15–30% C – > 30%		A – Medial B – Central C – Lateral
II	Stalled repair/fracture	(+) CT, radiograph	Length of fracture A – < 15% B – 15–30% C – > 30%		A – Medial B – Central C – Lateral
III	Deformation	Radiograph	Amount of deformation A – < 2 mm B – 2–4 mm C – > 4 mm		
IV	Arthritis	Radiograph	Degree of arthritis A – Narrowed cartilage B – Subchondral sclerosis C – Osteophytes		

* MRI = magnetic resonance imaging; CT = computed tomography

(with permission from: Enneking WF. **Classification of nontraumatic osteonecrosis of the femoral head.** In: Urbaniak JR, Jones, JP Jr, eds. *Osteonecrosis, etiology, diagnosis and treatment.* American Academy of Orthopaedic Surgeons; 1997:274.)

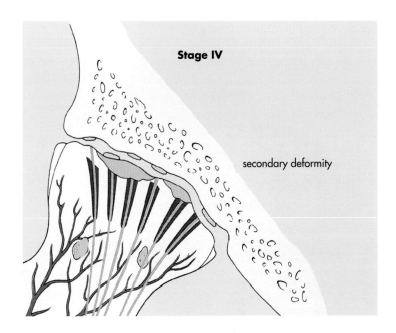

Figure 15.28 Diagrammatic representation of stage IV SAVN.

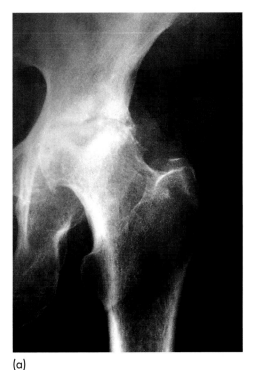

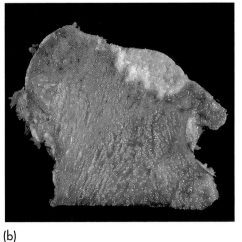

(b)

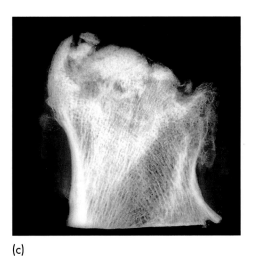

(c)

Figure 15.29 (a) Radiograph of a patient with severe hip disease secondary to SAVN shows marked deformity of the superior margin of the femoral head secondary to collapse. (b) A frontal section through the femoral head resected from the patient illustrated in (a). (c) Specimen radiograph of the case illustrated in (a) and (b).

(a)

LEGG–CALVÉ–PERTHES DISEASE

Osteonecrosis of the femoral head also occurs in children, usually between the ages of 5–9 years. The disease is more likely to affect boys, and in about 13% of patients, the condition is bilateral. In some instances, a familial predisposition has been noted.

Injection studies have demonstrated that the most important vessels supplying the epiphysis are the lateral epiphyseal vessels. Because the growth plate of the femoral head lies above the insertion of the capsule of the hip joint in children, and the vessels track along the surface of the neck of the femur to enter the epiphysis above the growth plate. These vessels are therefore vulnerable to interruption of blood flow by trauma or by increases in

intra-articular pressure (Fig. 15.30). In Perthes disease, the ischemic events may be episodic in nature and result from intermittent increased intra-articular pressure.

One of the earliest radiologic signs of Legg–Calvé–Perthes disease is widening of the joint space. This is probably caused by the cessation of endochondral ossification and resultant failure of cartilage to be converted to bone. Therefore, on the radiologic film the continuous growth of the cartilage will be appreciated as an increase in the width of the joint space (Fig. 15.31). Although the necrotic bony epiphysis may undergo collapse and subsequent deformation, deformity may also result from the irregular growth of new bone as a result of revascularization on the surface of the necrotic secondary center of ossification

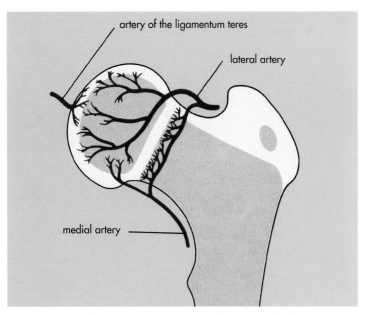

Figure 15.30 Blood supply to the femoral head in a child.

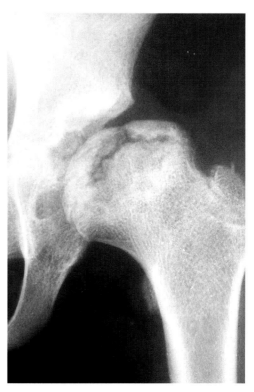

Figure 15.32 Radiograph of a patient with Legg–Calvé–Perthes disease. There is marked irregularity of the acetabulum and fragmentation of the femoral epiphysis, as well as irregularity of the metaphyseal bone.

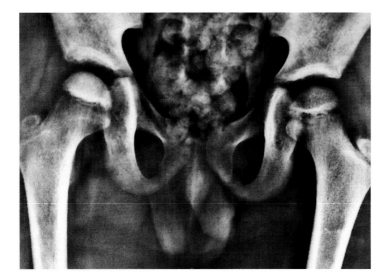

Figure 15.31 In the early stage of Legg–Calvé–Perthes disease, there is cessation of growth in the bony epiphysis with continued growth of the cartilage. Therefore, radiographic studies reveal widening of the joint space. Interference with the vascular supply to the growth plate results in defects in the metaphysis, seen here as a lytic area on the lateral side of the left femoral head.

(Fig. 15.32) Characteristic radiologic findings in patients with Legg–Calvé–Perthes disease include enlargement of the femoral head and sometimes alterations in the femoral neck. Since the growth plate is dependent upon the epiphyseal vasculature for growth and nutrition, it can be expected that secondary changes will occur in the growth plate after necrosis of the epiphysis. In the early stages of the disease, lytic lesions are often present in the metaphysis, and as a late consequence of cessation of growth, there is a widening and shortening of the neck of the femur.

IDIOPATHIC, NONTRAUMATIC OR PRIMARY OSTEONECROSIS OF THE FEMORAL HEAD

As already noted, before 1960 aseptic necrosis without a history of fracture was considered unusual. In 1962, Mankin and Brower could collect only 27 cases of idiopathic femoral head necrosis from the world literature. Nowadays, it is recognized to be an important cause of arthritis, a high proportion of the cases being attributable to either treatment with corticosteroids or chronic alcoholism, less commonly to sickle-cell disease and Gaucher's disease.

The most frequent site of subarticular osteonecrosis is the proximal femur. It is most commonly seen in men in the fifth decade of life and in women in the sixth and seventh decades. In our own cases of idiopathic osteonecrosis of the femoral head, about half of the patients showed radiographic evidence of another site of involvement, either at the time of initial presentation or shortly afterwards. The other sites included the opposite hip, proximal humerus, knee and spine. However the most common site of involvement was the opposite femoral head.

NATURAL HISTORY AND DIAGNOSIS

In approximately half of the patients, the onset of symptoms relating to the affected joint is likely to be sudden and acute, though in the rest the onset may be insidious with only vague pain and dysfunction. (The history of acute onset of symptoms is in marked contrast to OA or rheumatoid arthritis, though it is typical in spontaneous subchondral insufficiency fracture, where the pain is generally very severe and unremitting.) However, even in cases of osteonecrosis of the hip where the onset is insidious, eventually the patient will usually experience a sudden increase in the level and frequency of pain as well as of joint dysfunction. Radiographs taken at this stage will often show the 'crescent sign', which is characterized by a radiolucent line paralleling the subchondral bone end-plate, and overlying the area of bone necrosis. Visualization of this radiolucent line requires correct positioning of the joint when taking the X-ray. For example, in osteonecrosis of the hip, although an AP view may appear to be normal, a frog lateral view will usually show the radiolucent line if it is present. Prior to the appearance of the 'crescent sign', technetium diphosphonate imaging will generally show a markedly increased uptake of the isotope. MRI will help visualize the bone marrow changes. In general, from the time of the initial radiographic diagnosis of osteonecrosis, the radiographic changes of secondary OA take about 5 years to develop, though they may be delayed for up to 15 years.

In osteonecrosis stages I and II, plain radiographs are generally insufficient for diagnosis and staging, and are diagnostic only in some cases of stage III, in which a characteristic pattern is clearly visible when the hip is correctly positioned. The main advantage of CT compared to the other imaging modalities is the accurate detection of a subchondral fracture in stage III (Fig. 15.33). The disadvantage of CT is that small lesions might be overlooked.

On bone scintigraphy, a cold spot is an unspecific pattern and can be found in several other bone marrow processes. The repair process with revascularization, detected as a hot spot, is the most common finding in osteonecrosis but is also nonspecific. Only the combination of a cold and a hot spot represents a diagnostic pattern for osteonecrosis (if osteonecrosis involves both hip joints, bone scans could be misinterpreted as negative in some cases).

It is believed that MRI is the most accurate imaging modality used for the diagnosis of osteonecrosis of the femoral head, especially in the early stages. Characteristic MRI signal alterations in the antero-superior portion of the femoral head surrounded by a band of low-signal intensity on T_1- and T_2-weighted images are thought to be diagnostic of osteonecrosis. The occurrence of a double line on the T_2-weighted image is thought to be a pathognomonic sign of osteonecrosis, however its absence does not eliminate the diagnosis of osteonecrosis. Because the morphologic changes in the necrotic area are mainly the result of the repair process, the MR image may show a wide range of more or less inhomogeneous signal alterations.

Diffusely distributed MRI abnormalities, with a hypointense signal on T_1-weighted and an iso- or hyperintense signal on T_2-weighted images indicate bone marrow edema, and represent a nonspecific pattern seen with several bone pathologies (tumor, infection, insufficiency or stress fracture, and bone marrow edema syndrome or transient osteoporosis).

The limitation of MRI in osteonecrosis is indicated by the lack of clear criteria for the signal alterations and the limited understanding of the histopathologic correlates of the imaging findings with regard to the repair processes. MRI is less sensitive than radiography and especially CT in detecting subchondral fractures or early femoral flattening.

The pathological findings both gross and microscopic in idiopathic AVN are for the most part similar to those already described for postfracture osteonecrosis of the femoral head.

ETIOLOGY OF IDIOPATHIC NECROSIS

Perhaps the most important factors rendering the bone liable to infarction at its articular end are:

- Small diameter of the terminal vessels in the subchondral region
- Lack of a collateral circulation, particularly at the convex surfaces
- Reduced blood flow in the bone which has fatty marrow as compared with that associated with hematopoietic marrow
- Inexpandable nature of the bone tissue.

Necrosis may result from decreased blood flow in the arterial system, due to either narrowing of the lumen, or increased viscosity of the blood such as occurs with sickling, or embolism. Necrosis may also be caused by increased intraosseous pressure obstructing venous outflow.

Increased intraosseous pressure occurs in caisson disease, and in replacement of the marrow tissue by an infiltrative process. In the case of patients undergoing cortisone therapy, it has been suggested that there is an increase in the size of the fat cells, which in turn will result in an increase in intraosseous pressure. The importance of increased intraosseous pressure has been particularly stressed by Zizic *et al*. They found that in patients treated with corticosteroids, in which intraosseous pressures were measured, a raised level was predictive of osteonecrosis in 50% of cases. Only rarely did patients with normal pressures develop osteonecrosis.

Hyperlipidemia with associated embolism, hypercoagulability and hypofibrinolysis has been postulated to be a potent cause of osteonecrosis. Cortisone and alcohol have been implicated as causative factors in fat embolism. It has been proposed that fat embolism may appear from one or more of three sources: (1) a fatty liver; (2) destabilization and coalescence of plasma lipoproteins to form fat droplets; and (3) by disruption of the marrow fat.

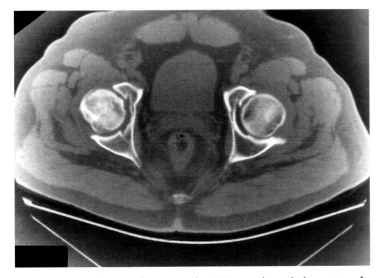

Figure 15.33 Computed tomography (CT) scan through the region of the femoral heads shows increased density in the right femoral head associated with stage II SAVN.

In the case of the fatty liver, for example in an alcoholic, fat may be released by blunt trauma. Focal liver necrosis may also contribute to embolization and it may follow use of certain types of anesthesia, as in halothane, and certain drug treatments such as isoniazid and Imuran.

A number of investigators have reported that in experimental studies in rabbits, cortisone use results in hyperlipemia, fatty livers and fat embolism of the femoral head. (In this regard there is a need for much more careful autopsy studies of the bones in patients who have been on long-term cortisone therapy.) It has also been suggested that fat embolism in the bone results in local vascular damage with a subsequent inflammatory response, further that free fats may favor platelet adhesiveness and aggregation, thereby increasing the local coagulability of the blood.

We have measured the serum levels of cholesterol and triglycerides in a series of patients with osteonecrosis of the hip and like others, we have not found significantly different levels from control subjects. However, we have also studied the tissue lipids in 18 resected osteonecrotic femoral heads. We found that the lipids associated with osteonecrotic bone have higher cholesterol content than those associated with normal bone and the total lipids in the affected supero-lateral regions of the osteonecrotic bone were found to be elevated as compared with both the unaffected infero-medial regions and the supero-lateral regions of the nondiseased femoral heads. Cholesterol content was elevated in both the affected and unaffected regions of the osteonecrotic bones when contrasted with the cholesterol content of control bones. The greatest elevations were noted for those patients with histories of combined steroid use and alcohol abuse.

Episodic infarction in patients receiving cortisone therapy has been proposed by Inoue and Ono, who reported that 83% of femoral heads they examined showed histological evidence of recurring necrosis, that is, evidence of death in previously healing areas. However, our own studies have failed to confirm this finding.

Attempts to produce infarcts experimentally have not been too successful. Kahlstrom *et al.* were unsuccessful in producing experimental bone infarcts in dogs by air emboli. Foster *et al.* produced both cortical and medullary bone infarcts in young rabbits by cutting the nutrient artery and stripping the periosteum. However, these lesions healed within 2 months and late changes, such as the advanced sclerosis and fat necrosis seen in our patients, were not observed.

BONE INFARCTIONS NOT ASSOCIATED WITH CAISSON DISEASE

Single or multiple bone infarcts not associated with caisson or sickle-cell disease are uncommon.

Men and women are equally affected and the average age is around 50. Many of the patients will have an associated diffuse connective-tissue disease which has usually been treated with cortisone. In about two-thirds of the cases, only a single bone is involved, whereas in the remainder multiple bones, often bilateral, are affected. The lesions have a predilection for the upper end of the tibial shaft and the lower end of the femoral shaft.

In approximately one-half of cases, it appears reasonable to attribute the patient's symptoms directly to the lesion.

BONE TUMORS

Chapter 16

BONE-FORMING TUMORS AND TUMOR-LIKE CONDITIONS

REACTIVE OR POST-TRAUMATIC LESIONS WHICH MAY BE MISTAKEN FOR MALIGNANT TUMORS

In bone, the tissue response to mechanical injury may be mistaken for a malignant neoplasm. Some of the problems in differential diagnosis of stress fractures as well as traction injuries at various ligamentous insertions have already been alluded to in Chapter 4 (p. 107). Most pseudosarcomas present on the surface of the bone and are likely to be mistaken for osteosarcomas or chondrosarcoma.

Although various names have been given to the pseudosarcomatous conditions described below, depending on their location and clinical presentation, they are certainly all very closely related entities.

FLORID REACTIVE PERIOSTITIS

Florid reactive periostitis is a rare calcifying and ossifying soft-tissue lesion which occurs most commonly in the hands and less commonly in the feet. Most of the affected patients are between 20 and 40 years of age; there is no sex predilection. It is likely to originate along the margin of one of the short tubular bones, most commonly the proximal and middle phalanges. A history of trauma may not be given, but it is generally believed that, as in the case myositis ossificans circumscripta and subungual exostosis (lesions to which reactive periostitis is closely related), the lesion is post-traumatic. Although in the early stages no mineralization may be seen radiographically at the time of clinical presentation, calcification is usually present. Radiographically the lesion appears to arise from the underlying cortical surface but without any alteration of the surface architecture.

Microscopically, especially in the early phases, the disordered loose myxomatous fibroblastic proliferation, mitotic activity, and immature bone formation may suggest osteosarcoma (Fig. 16.1). However, as with myositis ossificans, there is zonal arrangement with the bone elements being centrally located and the cartilage peripheral.

SUBUNGUAL EXOSTOSIS

Subungual exostosis is a rare osteocartilaginous lesion arising from a distal phalanx, most commonly that of the big toe. Clinically, the lesion must be differentiated from other subungual lesions that may cause ulceration of the nail bed, includ-

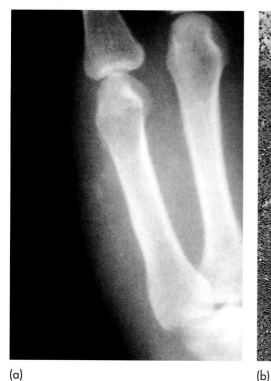

(a)

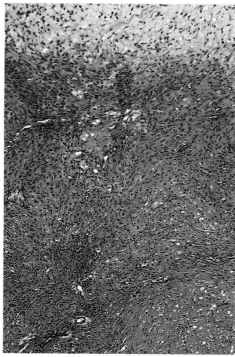

(b)

Figure 16.1 (a) Radiograph of a 31-year-old drummer who had had a 5-month history of pain in the little finger. In addition to soft-tissue swelling along the ulnar side of the proximal phalanx there is poorly defined extraosseous calcification. In this case, the differential diagnosis would include myositis ossificans or another reactive lesion, synovioma, as well as a benign or malignant cartilage lesion. (b) Photomicrograph of the tissue obtained from this case of reactive periostitis showing the zoning phenomenon seen at the edge of such lesions. A loose myxoid tissue gives way to more dense proliferative fibrous tissue. In the lower part of the picture extracellular matrix is being formed, giving rise to tissue resembling primitive bone or cartilage (H&E, × 10 obj.). (Courtesy of Dr Leonard Kahn.)

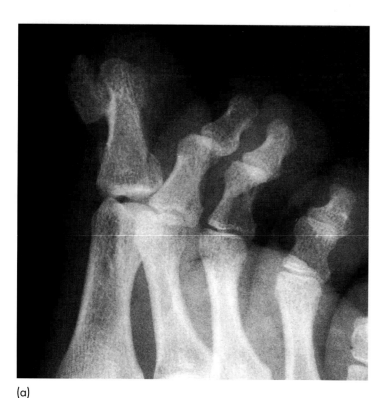

(a)

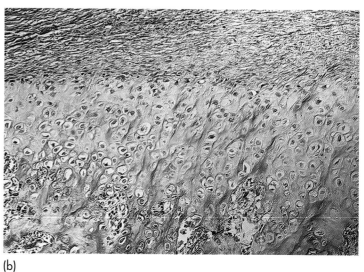

(b)

Figure 16.2 (a) Radiograph of the forefoot to demonstrate a subungual exostosis of the big toe. (From Pavlov H, Torg JS, Hirsh A, Freiberger RH. **The Roentgen Examination of Runners' Injuries.** *Radiographics* 1981, 1: 17–34.) (b) Photomicrograph of a portion of the periphery of a subungual exostosis showing the merging of the cartilaginous portion with overlying proliferative fibrous tissue and underlying bone formation (H&E, × 25 obj.).

ing verrucae, glomus tumor, epidermal inclusion cyst, subungual melanoma, carcinoma of the nail bed, and pyogenic granuloma.

Most patients are adolescents or in their early 20s, but occasionally older individuals are affected. The symptoms are likely to have been present for a few months and growth of the lesion may be rapid, although it is limited. A history of trauma is rarely elicited, although it seems most likely that the lesion is post-traumatic rather than representing a true osteochondral or osteocartilaginous exostosis.

On radiographic examination, the exostosis arises from the dorsal aspect of the tip of the distal phalanx and grows distally. Early in the clinical course of the lesion it appears as a soft-tissue density without attachment to the underlying bone. Later, however, as it calcifies it begins to show a trabecular pattern and eventually connects to the underlying bone.

The microscopic appearance depends on the stage of maturation. In the early stages the lesion appears as a foci of proliferating cellular fibrous tissue with areas of cartilaginous metaplasia. Later in its development it shows focal calcification and ossification. However, even in a mature lesion there is no distinct layer of periosteum covering the cartilage cap, as is seen with a true osteocartilaginous exostosis (Fig. 16.2); rather, the fibrocartilaginous tissue at the periphery of the lesion blends with the overlying fibrous connective tissue.

The microscopic findings are quite similar to those of florid reactive periostitis and, like that lesion, may be mistaken for a malignant lesion, especially if biopsy tissue has been obtained only from the periphery of the lesion or early in the course of its development.

The lesion is likely to recur unless it is completely excised, especially if it is removed in the early stages of the disease. Similar lesions when present in other parts of the phalanges are often referred to as turret exostoses.

BIZARRE PAROSTEAL OSTEOCHONDROMATOUS PROLIFERATION (NORA'S LESION)

Bizarre parosteal osteochondromatous proliferations (BPOPs) are rare lesions closely related to reactive periostitis and subungual exostoses. More common in the hands than the feet, they occur most commonly on the proximal and middle phalanges, metacarpals, or metatarsals; they are rare in the long tubular bones. Usually, there is no history of trauma (Figs 16.3 and 16.4).

Complaints are most commonly related to the local mass or limitation of movement of the nearby joints. Patients are usually young or early middle aged, and the sexes are equally affected. Following excision, about 50% recur. Metastasis does not occur.

Radiographically, the lesions may resemble ordinary osteochondromas. However, in contrast to the osteochondroma, in which the cortex and the spongiosa of the lesion is continuous with that of the underlying bone, BPOPs arise directly from the cortical surface of the bone and do not show the seamless continuity of lesional and cortical bone characteristic of an osteochondroma.

Microscopically, there usually is a transition from bizarre fibroblastic proliferation at the periphery to cellular cartilage, to disorganized bone adjacent to the cortex. The fibrous and cartilage cap is usually very cellular, and may in the presence of cytologic atypia be mistaken for an osteosarcoma or chondrosarcoma. However, like florid reactive periostitis on low-power examination, the lesion shows a zonal pattern.

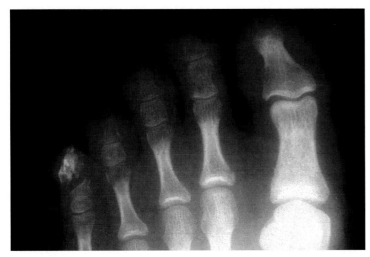

(a)

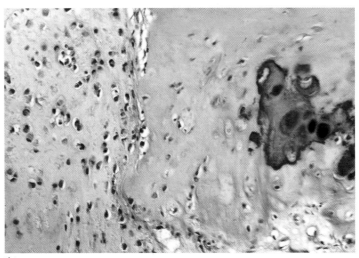

(b)

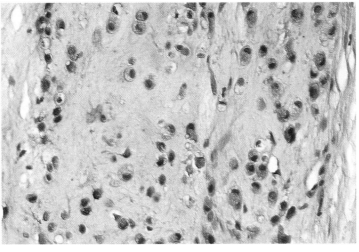

(c)

Figure 16.3 (a) Radiograph of the forefoot of a 28-year-old male complaining of pain in the 5th toe. There is a well-defined lobulated and ossified mass in the soft tissue distal to the distal phalanx. This mass does not seem to be attached to the bone of the phalanx. (b) A low-power photomicrograph of the resected lesion to demonstrate the lobulated cellular cartilaginous tissue and fibrocartilagenous tissue found at the periphery of the lesion. The focal basophilic calcification seen in the middle right hand part of the lesion is a characteristic finding (H&E, × 4 obj.). (c) A higher power photomicrograph of the cartilaginous component of the lesion to demonstrate the hypercellularity of the cartilage and the large chondrocytes which are typically seen in bizarre parosteal osteochondromatous proliferation (BPOP) of bone or Nora's lesion (H&E, × 25 obj.).

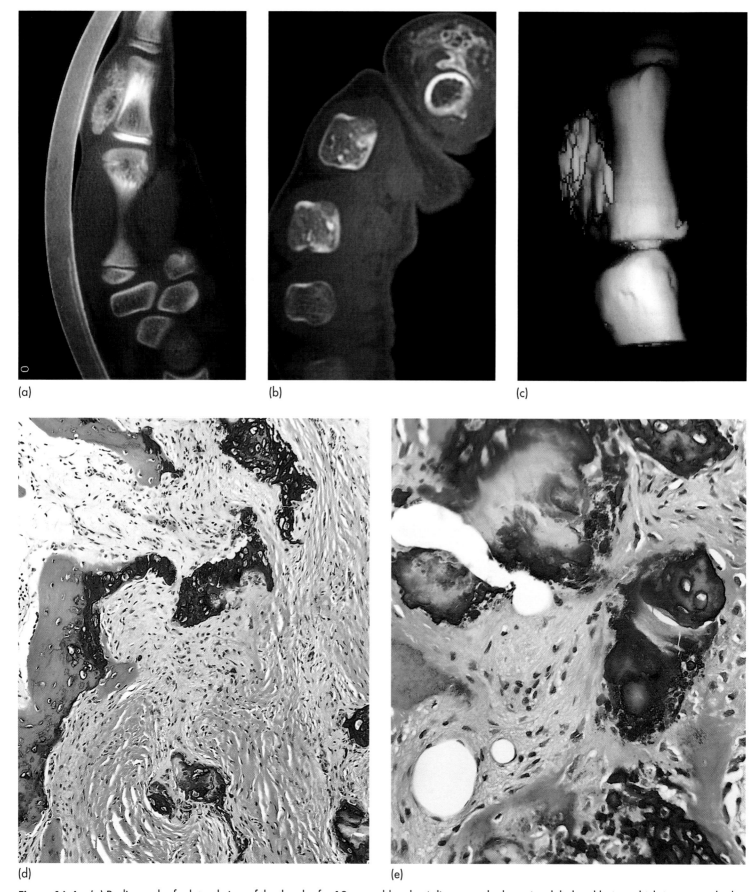

(a) (b) (c)

(d) (e)

Figure 16.4 (a) Radiograph of a lateral view of the thumb of a 13-year-old male. Adjacent to the bone is a lobulated lesion which is not attached to the phalanx and which is forming bone. (b) A CT scan of the lesion shows the lesional bone to have varying degrees of maturation. (c) A three-dimensional CT reconstruction of the lesion. (d) Photomicrograph taken at the periphery of the lesion demonstrates a mixture of bone, fibrous tissue and calcified cartilage arranged in a bizarre pattern (H&E, × 4 obj.). (e) Photomicrograph at a higher power to demonstrate the transition of bone and cartilage in this lesion. The bone appears to be quite benign. The tissue seen here is typical of BPOP (H&E, × 25 obj.). (Courtesy of Dr Sharon Wallace, Victoria, Australia.)

DEVELOPMENTAL OR HAMARTOMATOUS TUMORS

BONE ISLAND (SOLITARY ENOSTOSIS)

A solitary fleck of increased density in cancellous bone is not an uncommon incidental finding on radiographs. On gross examination, these foci are found in the intramedullary spongy bone and are composed of compact bone which merges with the surrounding trabecular bone to give a spoke-like pattern at the periphery (Fig. 16.5). Microscopic examination of this tissue reveals mature lamellar bone with well-developed haversian and interstitial lamellar systems (Fig. 16.6). No endochondral ossification or calcified cartilage is observed.

Usually these lesions are only 1 or 2 mm in diameter, but occasionally they may be as large as 1 cm or even larger. Occasionally scintigraphy may reveal increased uptake of isotope in these lesions, suggesting active growth (Fig. 16.7).

The lesions are probably developmental in origin and significant only in differential diagnosis (e.g. of osteoid osteoma when they are small or of sclerosing osteosarcoma if they are large).

OSTEOPOIKILOSIS

Osteopoikilosis (multiple bone islands) is a rare, symptomless, and clinically benign condition. It is inherited as an autosomal dominant trait. On radiographs, the bones show multiple discrete or clustered foci of radiopacity with uniform density, giving the bone a spotted appearance. The disorder is usually symmetrical and affects both the epiphyseal and metaphyseal zones. It most commonly involves the small bones of the hands and feet, and the ends of the long bones of the extremities. The microscopic features of the lesions are similar to those of solitary bone islands (Fig. 16.8).

Some cases of osteopoikilosis have been reported in association with cutaneous nodules which usually prove on microscopic examination to be fibrous tissue (resembling scleroderma-like lesions, or keloids). This suggests a general mesenchymal defect in these patients.

MELORHEOSTOSIS

Melorheostosis is a rare, nonfamilial condition in which the affected bones display a peculiar irregular cortical hyperostosis,

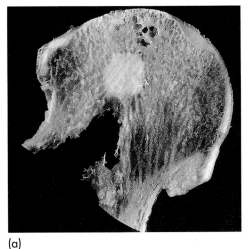
(a)

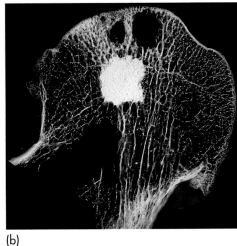
(b)

Figure 16.5 (a) Coronal section through an osteoarthritic femoral head reveals a whitish, circumscribed piece of bone, clearly demarcated from the surrounding cancellous bone. (b) Radiograph of the specimen illustrated in (a) demonstrates the marked density of the solitary bone island and its connectedness with the surrounding cancellous bone.

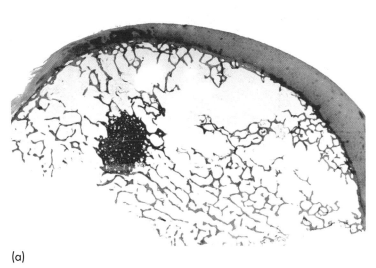
(a)

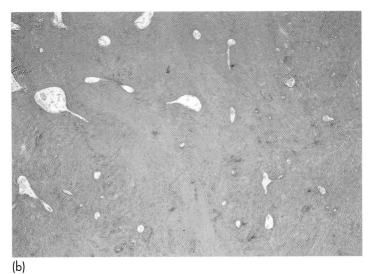
(b)

Figure 16.6 (a) The bone island consists of dense but normal bone distinctly separated from the surrounding cancellous bone spicules. Note that the spicules merge with the nodule in a radial fashion. The bone is found to be lamellar when viewed under polarized light (H&E, × 1 obj.). (b) High-power view of the bone island illustrated in (a) shows the mature appearance of the bone (H&E, × 4 obj.).

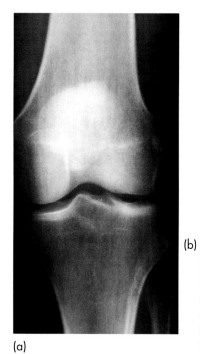

(a)

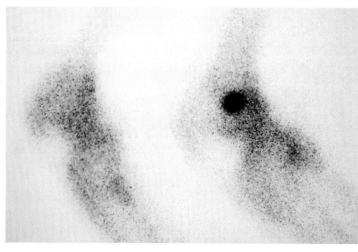

(b)

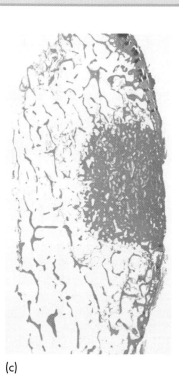

(c)

Figure 16.7 (a) Antero-posterior radiograph of a knee, showing in the lateral femoral condyle, a peripheral island of dense bone delineated by a fine osteolytic rim. (b) Scintigram showing increased uptake of ⁹⁹Tc diphosphonate in the lesion. (c) Photomicrograph of a section through the lesion demonstrated in (a) reveals dense cortical bone which merges imperceptibly with the surrounding cancellous bone (H&E, × 1 obj.). (Courtesy of Dr Leon Sokoloff.)

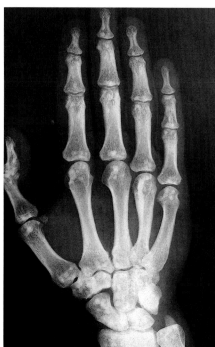

(a)

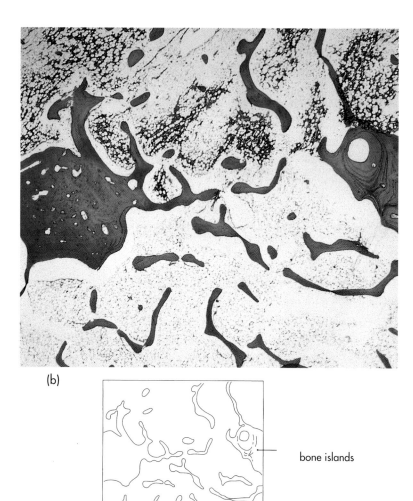

(b)

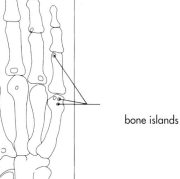

bone islands

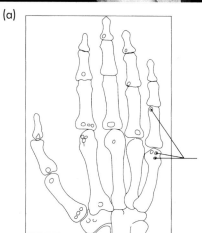

bone islands

Figure 16.8 (a) Radiograph reveals circumscribed dense foci of bone distributed throughout the hand of a patient with osteopoikilosis. (b) Nodules of bone with connected spicules of cancellous bone are evident in this photomicrograph of a specimen from a patient with osteopoikilosis (H&E, × 4 obj.).

similar in appearance to melting wax dripping down the sides of a candle (Fig. 16.9). The lesions occur on both the periosteal and endosteal surfaces. The lesions may be monostotic, monomelic or polymelic. Radioisotope bone scans usually show increased uptake in the lesional tissue. Associated cutaneous lesions, including vascular malformations and focal subcutaneous and para-articular fibrosis, are common and in children, prominent soft-tissue fibrosis may predate osseous abnormalities.

In affected children, the skeleton is characterized by hyperostoses of the bones of the extremities and pelvic girdle, by inequality in the length of the extremities, and by contractures resulting in joint deformity. On radiographs, the lesions may be found to involve the epiphysis, and osseous tissue may be seen to cross the growth plate. Attempts at surgical management of the contractures have been unrewarding.

In adult melorheostosis, the patients present with pain, deformity, or limitation of joint motion. The lesion may involve one or many bones. Ectopic bone may be present in para-articular locations. The involvement of one side of a bone (or row of bones, in some cases) has suggested a sclerotome distribution.

On gross examination of the affected bones, the periosteal and endosteal surfaces are irregular, and the bones display thickened cortices. The marrow cavity is narrowed. Histologic examination reveals that the new bone is either woven or lamellar (Fig. 16.10). Even when the new bone tissue is lamellar, its cancellous architecture is irregular, and there is a distinct differentiation between the normal and melorheostotic bone.

OSTEOPATHIA STRIATA (VOORHOEVE'S DISEASE)

Osteopathia striata is a benign, asymptomatic disorder characterized radiographically by usually symmetrical, axially oriented, dense striations. Its presence in association with sclerosis of the base of the skull has been determined to be genetically transmit-

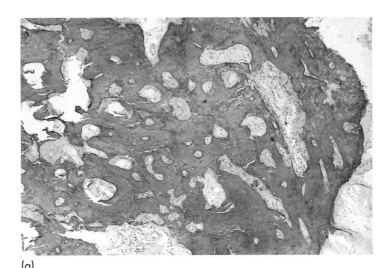

(a)

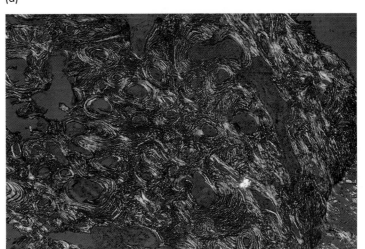

(b)

Figure 16.10 (a) Biopsy specimen of cortical bone from a patient with melorheostosis reveals markedly irregular bone with relatively little cellular activity on the endosteal surfaces. The marrow may show mild fibrosis (H&E, × 4 obj.). (b) The same histologic field shown in (a), photographed with polarized light. Note the irregular mixture of lamellar and woven bone.

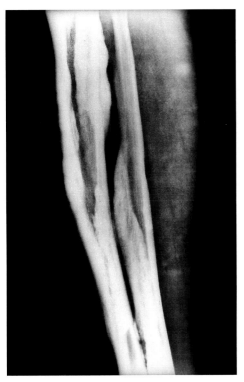

Figure 16.9
Radiograph of forearm in a 35-year-old man with generalized bone pain and melorheostosis shows the thickened endosteal and periosteal bone which has the characteristic appearance of 'candle wax dripping'.

ted as an autosomal dominant condition (Fig. 16.11). Osteopathia striata may be seen in association with osteopoikilosis and/or melorheostosis, in which case the condition is usually referred to as mixed sclerosing bone dystrophy (Fig. 16.12).

BENIGN TUMORS

SURFACE OSTEOMAS OF THE CRANIUM, FACIAL BONES AND OTHER BONES

These lesions are relatively uncommon, asymptomatic, benign slow-growing bony tumors on the calvaria and facial bones, and although it is very rare, they may be seen in other skeletal sites. Osteomas appear on the outer surface of the calvaria as circumscribed, ivory-like excrescences composed of mature lamellar bone (Fig. 16.13). Surface osteomas similar to those seen on the calvaria are extremely rare in the long or flat bones. The initial

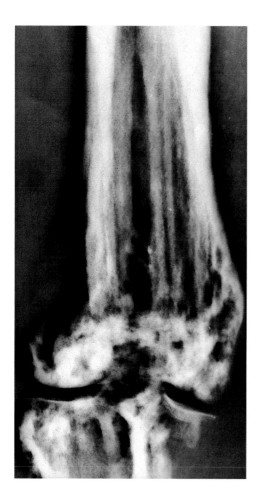

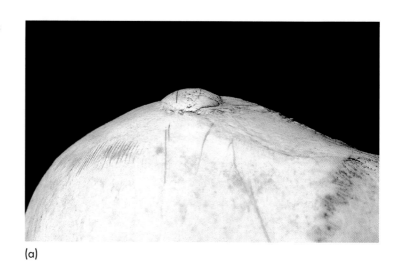

Figure 16.11 In this radiograph of the lower femur, the striated pattern of Voorhoeve's disease can be clearly seen.

(a)

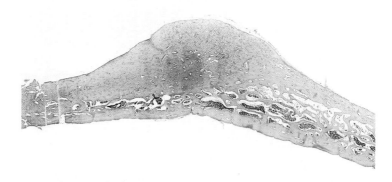

(b)

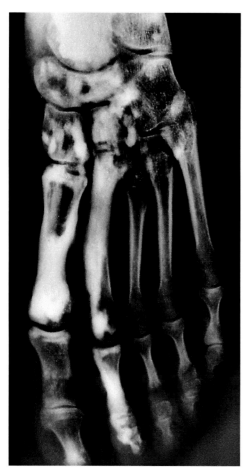

Figure 16.12 Many bone islands as well as evidence of melorheostosis can be seen in this radiograph of a foot. This rare pattern of mixed sclerosing bone dystrophy was generalized throughout the skeleton in this particular specimen.

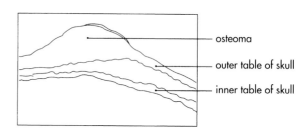

— osteoma

— outer table of skull

— inner table of skull

Figure 16.13 (a) Gross photograph of an osteoma (or ivory exostosis) of the calvaria shows a well-circumscribed nodular growth distorting the smooth contour of the skull. (b) Photomicrograph of the lesion shown in (a) demonstrates that the lesion is composed of mature lamellar bone (H&E, × 1 obj.).

radiographic diagnosis in such a case is most likely to be surface osteogenic sarcoma. However, microscopic examination will reveal only mature bone without an associated low-grade fibrous component and usually only nondescript adipose tissue in the marrow spaces (Fig. 16.14).

Osteomas on the facial bones are generally associated with the sinuses, and are formed of dense immature bone, often with a central area characterized by fibrosis with active osteoblasts and osteoclasts (Fig. 16.15). The etiology of this facial osteoma is obscure, however, microscopically the lesion has a close kinship with osteoblastoma. The lesion does not recur after surgical excision and it is not associated with malignant change.

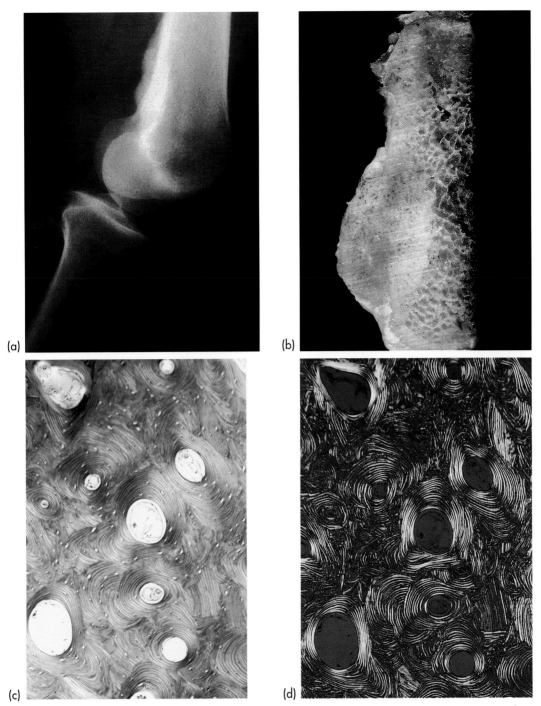

Figure 16.14   (a) Lateral radiograph of the left knee in a 28-year-old obese female complaining of pain in the knee for 2–3 months. There is an irregular heavily mineralized mass just above the condyles, very suggestive of parosteal osteosarcoma. (b) A section through the resected specimen shows that the lesion has a dense appearance and is well demarcated from the adjacent cancellous bone. (c) Photomicrograph of a typical area of the mass shows compact cortical bone typical of a benign osteoma (H&E, × 4 obj.). (d) Polarized light image of the same field shows the mature lamellar bone which makes up the lesion.

Very rarely osteomas of the facial bones may be associated with colonic polyps (Gardner's syndrome). Other disorders characteristically grouped with this syndrome are odontomas, supernumerary and unerupted teeth, and soft-tissue tumors, including fibromas and epidermal inclusion cysts. Gardner's syndrome is an autosomal dominant genetic disorder, and is of particular importance because of the malignant change that frequently occurs in the adenomatous intestinal polyps.

OSTEOID OSTEOMA

Osteoid osteomas are relatively common, small (less than 1 cm in diameter), usually solitary, benign but generally painful lesions of bone. They are characteristically seen in children and adolescents, with males affected more than twice as frequently as females (Fig. 16.16). Most commonly presenting in a lower extremity, the lesions tend to occur near the end of the diaphysis,

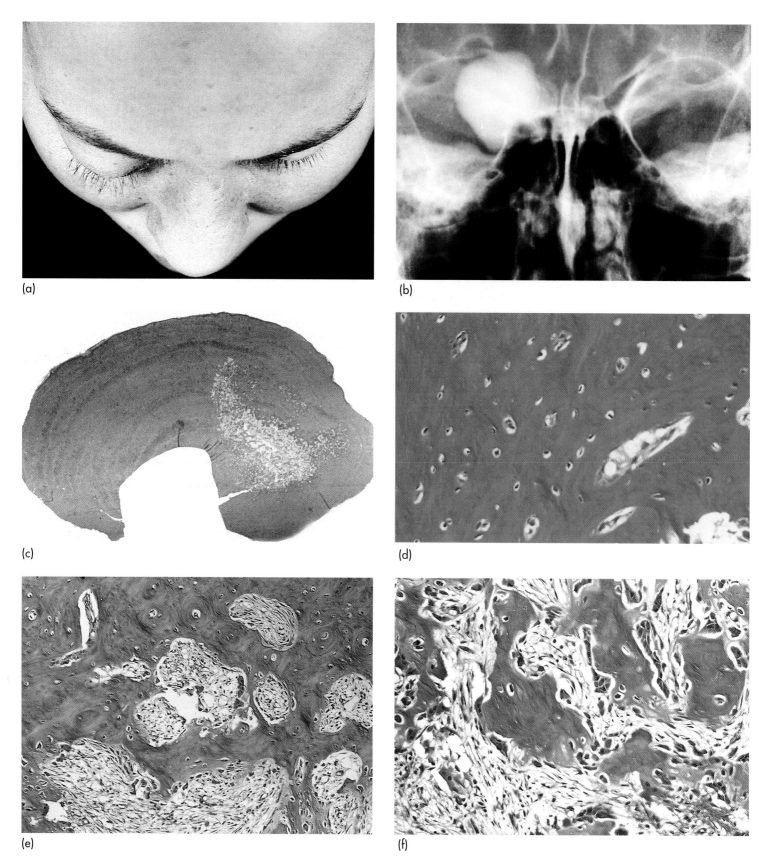

Figure 16.15 (a) The protrusion of the orbit seen in this patient is caused by tumor arising from the bone of the frontal sinus. (b) Radiograph demonstrates a well-circumscribed dense lesion which is distorting the frontal sinus (the cause of the orbital protrusion in the clinical photograph). (c) Histologic section through the lesion excised from the frontal sinus of the patient shown in (a) and (b). The lesion consists of dense immature bone with a focal area of active bone modeling. Although this lesion is usually referred to as an osteoma, the immature bone and osteoblastoma-like features clearly distinguish it from a routine osteoma (H&E, × 1 obj.). (d) Photomicrograph of the more solid area of the lesion to demonstrate the cellular woven character of the bone (H&E, × 10 obj.). (e) Photomicrograph to include part of the more active area to demonstrate the fibrous nature of the lesion and the active bone modeling (H&E, × 10 obj.). (f) Photomicrograph of a higher power demonstrates active osteoblastic and osteoclastic components (H&E, × 25 obj.).

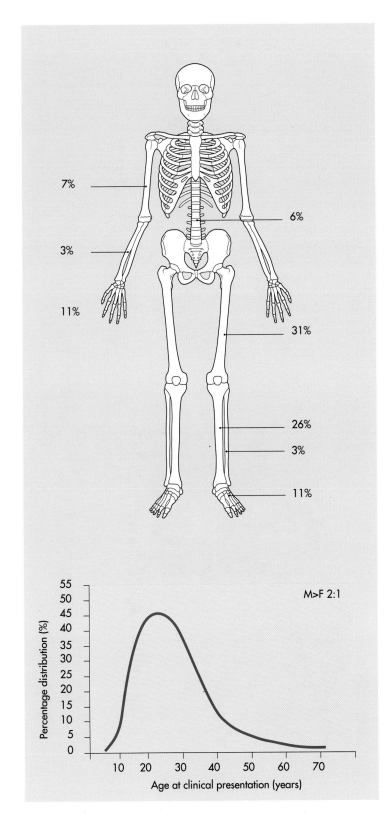

The typical lesion is located within the cortex of a long bone, and exhibits on radiographs a central lucent zone (or nidus) with increased sclerosis of the surrounding bone which may also show marked periosteal new bone formation (Figs 16.19 and 16.20). (Osteoid osteomas located subperiosteally or in the cancellous portion of the bone may have much less surrounding sclerosis.) On bone scans the lesions show up with increased uptake of radioactive isotope. The differential diagnosis includes a small focus of osteomyelitis or a stress fracture (Fig. 16.21).

When the lesion is close to or within a joint, often the hip, the patient may present with a joint effusion and symptoms of synovitis. Indeed in such a case synovial biopsy will often reveal a marked lymphoproliferative synovitis. This type of clinical presentation, which is not likely to be immediately diagnosed as osteoid osteoma, is seen in approximately 20% of the cases that are juxta-articular.

Another group of patients in which the diagnosis may be obscured are individuals with lesions in the vertebral column, who may present with scoliosis (Fig. 16.22).

At surgery, the area of involvement is sometimes difficult to ascertain, although there may be a mild pinkish cast to the overlying cortical bone due to the periosteal reaction and increased vascularity. The lesion itself may appear as a well-demarcated nodule, often cherry red (Fig. 16.23), but occasionally very dense and white.

Osteoid osteomas are characterized microscopically by a maze of small spicules of immature bone, most often lined with prominent osteoblasts and osteoclasts. In more mature lesions the intervening stroma is sparsely cellular, with readily apparent vascular spaces (Figs 16.24 and 16.25). Cartilage matrix formation does not occur. Very rare cases have been observed in which multiple nidi were present.

The minute size of the lesion often makes it difficult to locate both for the surgeon and the pathologist. A fine-grain radiograph may be helpful in determining the location of the nidus of an osteoid osteoma in the curetted tissue submitted at the time of operation for microscopic examination (Fig. 16.26). However, even with this technique, the lesion may be difficult to localize. Preoperative technetium (^{99}Tc) isotope injections with intraoperative localization of radioactivity and postoperative localization by specimen autoimaging on undeveloped film can also help.

The etiology of this bizarre condition remains obscure.

OSTEOBLASTOMA

An osteoblastoma is a very rare solitary, benign, osteoid- and bone-forming neoplasm which contains many well-differentiated osteoblasts and osteoclasts and usually has a vascular stroma. Osteoblastomas predominantly affect young adults and are often painful. Swelling and tenderness are usually the symptoms that prompt the patient to seek medical attention. In most cases, the long bones or vertebrae are the sites of involvement. In long bones, the lesion may arise in either the metaphysis or the diaphysis (Fig. 16.27). However, approximately 40% of osteoblastomas originate in the spine.

Osteoblastomas arise with about equal frequency in the cervical and lumbar regions, with the thoracic region being less frequently involved (Fig. 16.28). Occasionally they may involve the pelvis or sacrum. Mainly they affect the vertebral arch, involving the spinous and transverse processes as well as the laminae and pedicles. In only a few cases does the lesion appear to originate

Figure 16.16 Location and age distribution of osteoid osteoma.

however almost any bone may be involved (Figs 16.17 and 16.18).

The characteristic clinical presentation is nocturnal pain, which is usually relieved by aspirin. On physical examination, local swelling may be apparent and the lesion may be exquisitely tender; mild leukocytosis may be present.

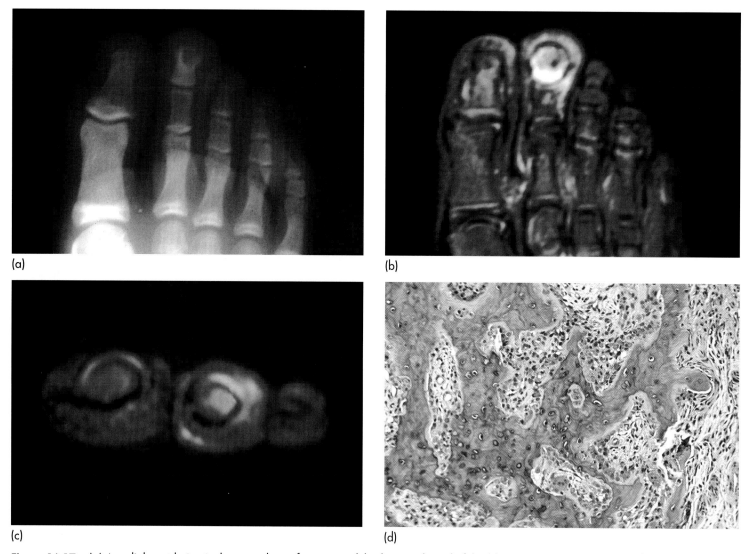

(a)   (b)

(c)   (d)

Figure 16.17   (**a**) A radiolucent lesion in the second toe of a young adult who complained of throbbing pain. (**b**) An MR image shows increased bloodflow or edema, both of the bone and surrounding tissues. (**c**) Same MRI in cross-section. (**d**) Photomicrograph of the curetted tissue reveals woven immature bone with prominent osteoblasts and osteoclasts consistent with an osteoid osteoma (H&E, × 10 obj.).

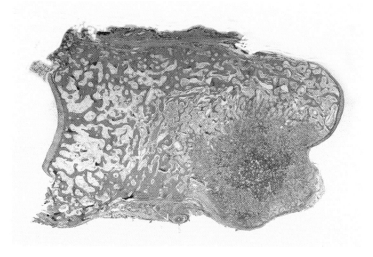

Figure 16.18   Low-power photomicrograph of the middle phalanx of a finger. A subperiosteal osteoid osteoma is seen adjacent to the joint margin (H&E, × 1 obj.).

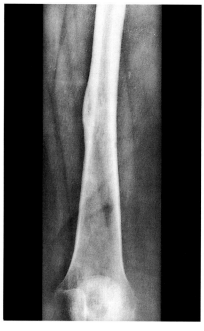

Figure 16.19   A 20-year-old man complained of pain in the midshaft of the right femur. Radiograph shows an area of cortical thickening, in the center of which is a lucent defect which proved on microscopic examination to be the result of an osteoid osteoma. An osteoid osteoma in cortical bone usually produces a considerable amount of reactive bone tissue, as seen in this case. (However, in the cancellous area of the bone it may be difficult to see the lesion because of a lack of reactive bone sclerosis.)

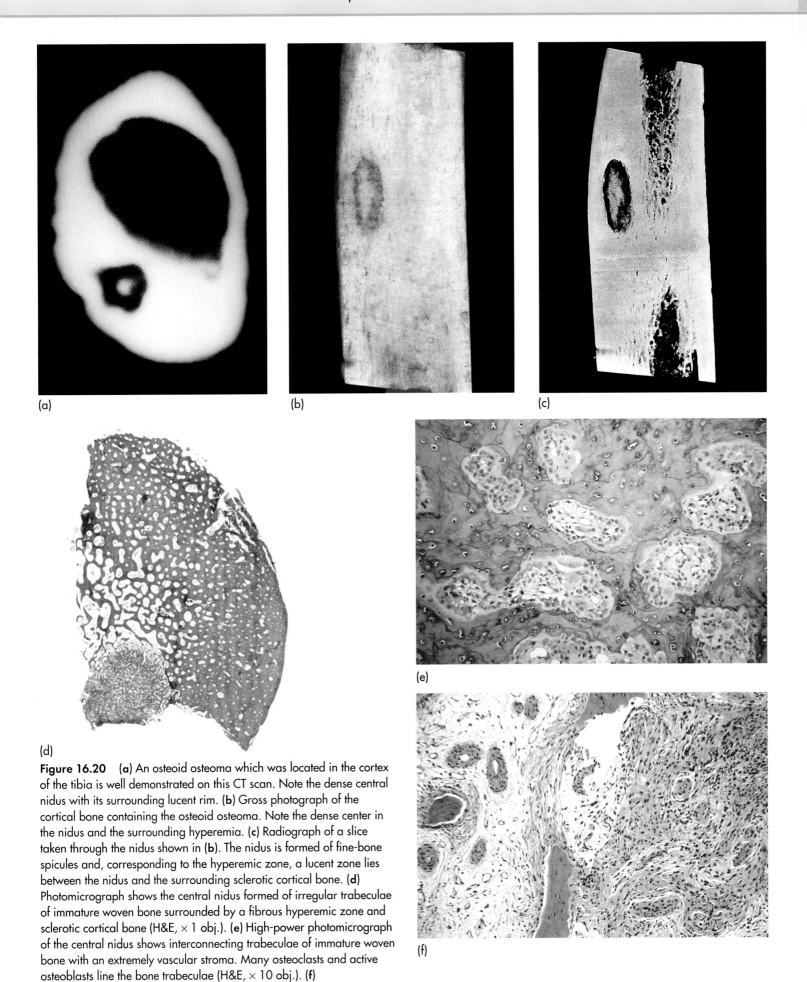

(a)

(b)

(c)

(d)

(e)

(f)

Figure 16.20 (a) An osteoid osteoma which was located in the cortex of the tibia is well demonstrated on this CT scan. Note the dense central nidus with its surrounding lucent rim. (b) Gross photograph of the cortical bone containing the osteoid osteoma. Note the dense center in the nidus and the surrounding hyperemia. (c) Radiograph of a slice taken through the nidus shown in (b). The nidus is formed of fine-bone spicules and, corresponding to the hyperemic zone, a lucent zone lies between the nidus and the surrounding sclerotic cortical bone. (d) Photomicrograph shows the central nidus formed of irregular trabeculae of immature woven bone surrounded by a fibrous hyperemic zone and sclerotic cortical bone (H&E, × 1 obj.). (e) High-power photomicrograph of the central nidus shows interconnecting trabeculae of immature woven bone with an extremely vascular stroma. Many osteoclasts and active osteoblasts line the bone trabeculae (H&E, × 10 obj.). (f) Photomicrograph at the margin of the lesion shows loose fibrous connective tissue with increased vascularity (H&E, × 4 obj.).

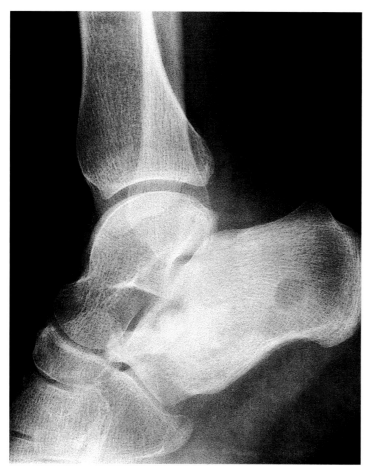

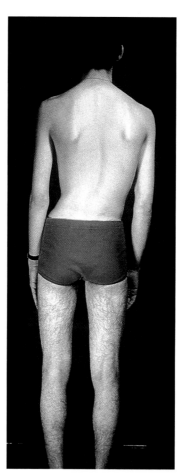

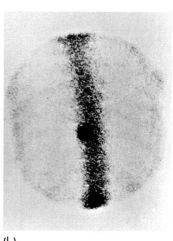

(b)

Figure 16.22 (a) Clinical photograph demonstrating mild scoliosis in a teenaged boy with an osteoid osteoma in the spine. (Courtesy of Dr David Levine.) (b) Technetium scan of the spine shows a localized area of high uptake.

Figure 16.21 Radiograph of a lateral view of the hind foot. The lytic lesion in the posterior third of the body of the os calcis was shown at an excisional biopsy to be an osteoid osteoma. There is only minimal reactive osteosclerosis and the nidus is not very obvious. (Courtesy of Dr Robert Freiberger.)

(a)

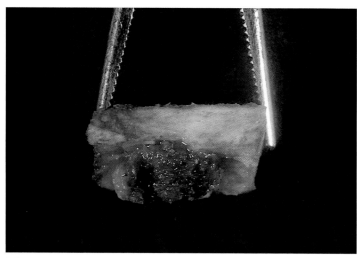

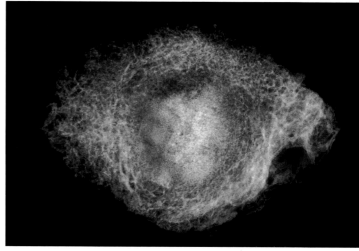

(a)

(b)

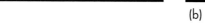

Figure 16.23 (a) Gross photograph of an excised osteoid osteoma which appeared on radiographs as a completely lucent lesion. Note the hyperemic appearance of the tissue. (b) Radiograph of the specimen demonstrating the relative lucency of the nidus. However, there are fine-bone trabeculae coursing through the lesion.

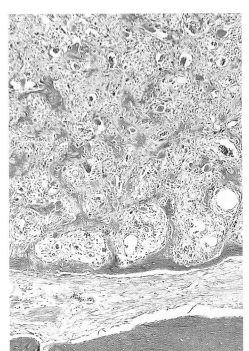

Figure 16.24
Photomicrograph showing a portion of an osteoid osteoma nidus and a part of the normal bone at the edge of the lesion. The nidus is composed of vascular fibrous tissue in which there are small, irregular but connected trabeculae of woven bone, demonstrating both prominent osteoblasts and prominent osteoclasts (H&E, × 10 obj.).

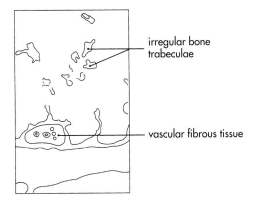

irregular bone trabeculae

vascular fibrous tissue

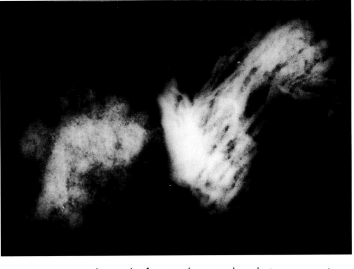

Figure 16.26   Radiograph of curetted tissue taken during surgery in a patient with a suspected osteoid osteoma. Radiographs of the specimen were taken immediately (see Chapter 2, p. 42 for methodology). In the portion of the specimen illustrated, it is possible to discern a piece of bone with a very fine trabecular pattern typical of an osteoid osteoma (left), and a fragment of more normal cancellous bone (right). When many specimens are received from a patient with an osteoid osteoma, radiographs of the specimens not only help the pathologist to inform the surgeon whether he or she has removed the lesional tissue or not, but also enable the pathologist to select the proper pieces for histologic examination.

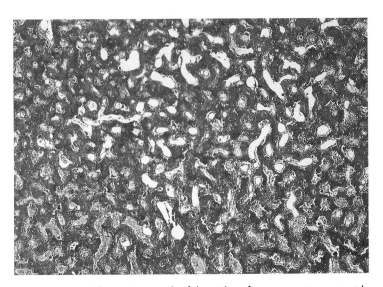

Figure 16.25   Photomicrograph of the nidus of a more mature osteoid osteoma, with more dense interconnecting trabeculae of bone and less cellular activity than is seen in Figure 16.24 (H&E, × 4 obj.).

within the vertebral bodies. The clinical presentation of osteoblastoma in the spine may include myelopathic and/or radicular symptoms, and suggest a herniated disc. Progressive scoliosis may also appear. If the cervical spine is affected, reversal of the lordotic curve may occur and torticollis may be prominent.

On radiographic examination, the lesion characteristically appears as a lucent defect with various degrees of central density. They are usually well circumscribed, without extensive surrounding bone sclerosis. They are therefore very similar in appearance to osteoid osteoma, with the difference that the nidus generally exceeds 1.5 cm. CT scanning may be particularly helpful in delineating these lesions (Fig. 16.29) and isotope scanning will show increased uptake (Fig. 16.30). Treatment consists of curettage or en-bloc excision.

At surgery, an osteoblastoma is found to be composed of hemorrhagic, granular, friable, and calcified tissue (Fig. 16.31). On microscopic examination, the lesion consists of a vascular spindle-cell stroma with abundant irregular spicules of mineralized bone and osteoid (Fig. 16.32). Osteoblasts and multinucleated osteoclasts are readily evident on the bone surfaces, but generally no cartilage can be seen in the lesion.

Microscopically, it is difficult to differentiate an osteoblastoma from an osteoid osteoma. However, the tissue pattern usually appears less regular in an osteoblastoma than in an osteoid osteoma. Furthermore, osteoid osteomas do not exceed 1 cm in

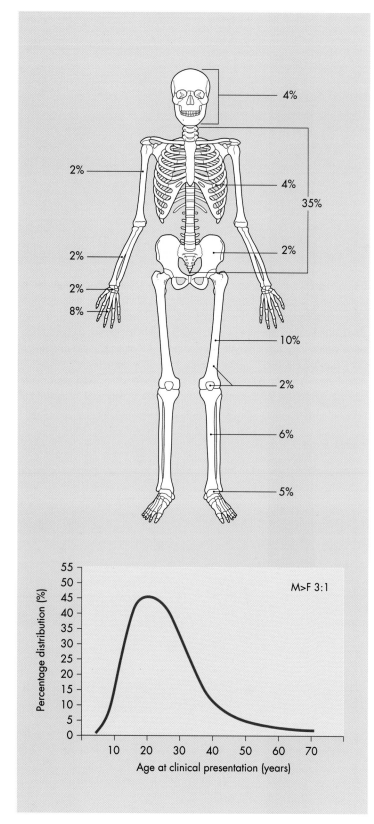

Figure 16.27   Location and age distribution of osteoblastoma.

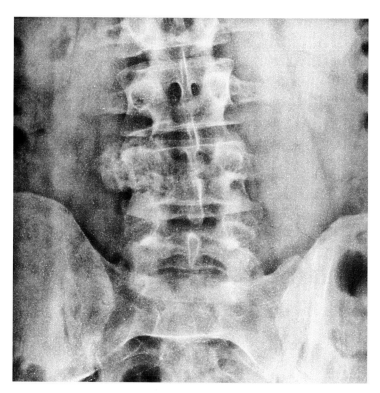

Figure 16.28   A 20-year-old man complained of low back pain and was admitted to the hospital with an expanding, destructive lesion affecting the pedicle and transverse process on the right side of L4. On radiographic examination, the margin of the lesion is well defined and there is a patchy increase in density. An excisional biopsy of the lesion proved it to be a benign osteoblastoma.

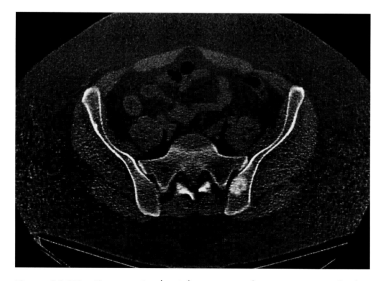

Figure 16.29   Computerized axial tomogram shows a circumscribed sclerotic lesion in the ilium adjacent to the sacroiliac joint, which proved to be an osteoblastoma.

diameter and are self-limiting lesions, whereas osteoblastomas may be several centimeters in diameter and have a tendency to enlarge. Nevertheless, the lesions are similar enough that osteoblastomas have in the past been referred to in the literature as giant osteoid osteomas.

On rare occasions, osteoblastomas have been noted to act aggressively, with significant bone destruction and extension into adjacent soft tissues. In these cases microscopic analysis has revealed large, plump osteoblasts which have epithelioid features and may form sheets of cells in the intertrabecular spaces

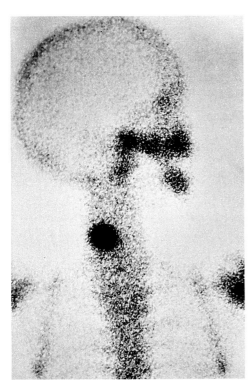

Figure 16.30
Radioisotope scan of an osteoblastoma in the transverse process and pedicle of C5. The intense focal uptake is typical of that seen in association with both osteoblastomas and osteoid osteomas. In this case, the size of the lesion indicates that this is an osteoblastoma.

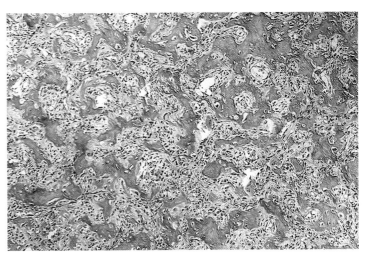

(a)

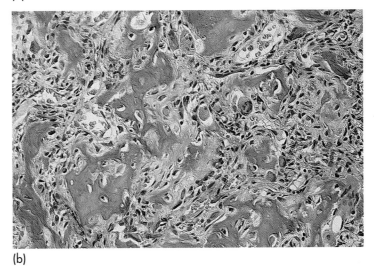

(b)

Figure 16.32   (a) Photomicrograph of an osteoblastoma shows the usual pattern of disorganized trabeculae of immature bone set in a cellular vascular stroma (H&E, × 4 obj.). (b) Photomicrograph of an osteoblastoma at a higher magnification shows marked osteoblastic and osteoclastic activity at the bone surfaces (H&E, × 25 obj.).

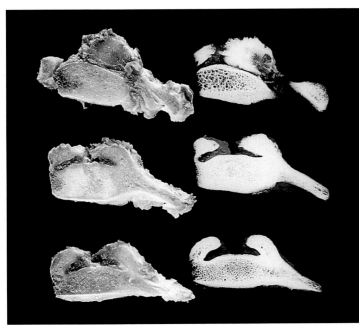

Figure 16.31   A series of slices through an osteoblastoma are matched with fine-grain radiographs, to demonstrate the mixed lytic and sclerotic areas which may be seen in osteoblastoma. (Courtesy of Dr Alberto G. Ayala.)

(Fig. 16.33). The nucleoli of these cells may be prominent. Mitoses may be present. In some cases it may be very difficult to differentiate an aggressive osteoblastoma from a low-grade osteosarcoma.

Changes characteristic of an aneurysmal bone cyst may be present within some osteoblastomas, adding to the problem of differential diagnosis.

MALIGNANT TUMORS

OSTEOSARCOMA (OSTEOGENIC SARCOMA)

Osteosarcoma is the second most common primary skeletal neoplasm (myeloma being the commonest) accounting for approximately 20% of all primary malignant bone tumors. Osteosarcoma is defined as a malignant neoplasm in which bone matrix is formed by the malignant cells (Fig. 16.34). However, the pluripotential nature of the malignant cells is evident in the abundant fibrous or cartilaginous matrix present in many of these tumors. Roughly 50% of all osteosarcomas are principally osteoblastic; the rest may have a predominantly chondroblastic, fibroblastic, small-cell- or a giant-cell-rich pattern. Occasionally large areas of the tumor may not be making a discernible extracellular matrix so that histologic diagnosis depends on adequate sampling (Box 16.1).

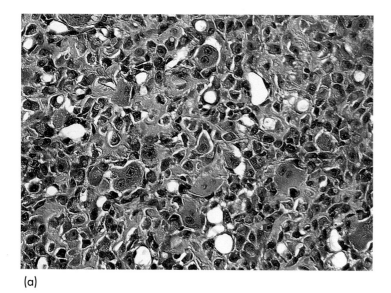

(a)

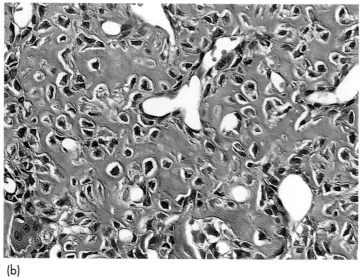

(b)

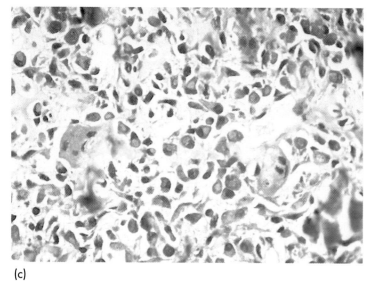

(c)

Figure 16.33 (a–c) Photomicrographs of three separate fields of an atypical osteoblastoma with crowded, large epithelioid stromal cells; small irregular foci of woven bone are present. It is important for the pathologist to recognize that an osteoblastoma may be cellular, and to distinguish this pattern from osteosarcoma, a histologic differentiation that can at times be very difficult [(**a**) and (**b**) H&E, × 25 obj.; (**c**) H&E, × 40 obj.).]

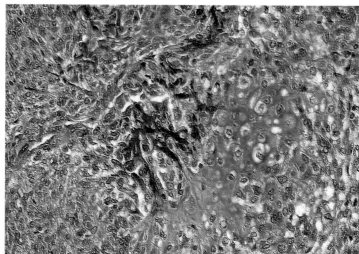

Figure 16.34 Photomicrograph of a cellular osteosarcoma showing foci of both bone and cartilage matrix differentiation (H&E, × 25 obj.).

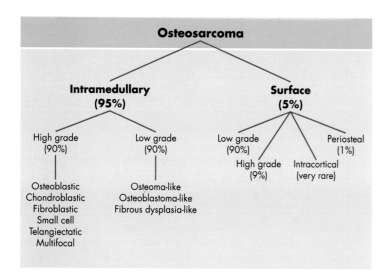

Box 16.1 Osteosarcoma

Heterogeneity may lead to confusion of this lesion with a number of other entities, including fracture callus (especially following a stress fracture without a clinical history of injury), aneurysmal bone cyst, chondrosarcoma, Ewing's tumor and even giant-cell tumor. The diagnostic difficulties may be aggravated if a pathologic fracture has complicated the underlying lesion (Table 16.1).

In very rare cases, an osteosarcoma may present with more than one focus of tumor. In such a case it may be difficult to

Table 16.1 Differential diagnosis of osteosarcoma

Post-traumatic lesion – fracture callus
Pathologic fracture through a pre-existing benign lesion, e.g. fibrous
    dysplasia
Nonossifying fibroma
Osteoblastoma – aggressive osteoblastoma
Giant bone island
Surface osteoma
Ewing's sarcoma with reactive bone formation
Giant-cell tumor with reactive bone formation

determine whether it is a tumor of multifocal origin or whether the other lesions are metastatic. However there are some points that characteristically suggest a multifocal origin, including symmetrical and simultaneous involvement with metaphyseal lesions in long bones, and sparing of the visceral organs.

Multicentric osteosarcoma may also on occasion be associated with genetic disturbances as with Rothmund–Thompson syndrome or Bloom's syndrome (see Fig. 16.46).

From the genetic standpoint, there is an interesting association with the inherited form of retinoblastoma. Children with this condition are at high risk for developing a second primary non-ocular tumor, notably osteosarcoma. Two genes have been implicated: R_b (on chromosome 13) and p53 (on chromosome 17p). The potential importance of these observations is firstly the use of techniques to study gene expression in the differential diagnosis of osteosarcoma and secondly the potential for gene therapy.

Most osteosarcomas are high-grade lesions, although less commonly low-grade osteosarcomas may also be encountered, usually as a surface lesion. The discussion that follows will consider high-grade central lesions (the most common), low-grade central lesions, low-grade surface lesions (so-called parosteal or juxtacortical osteosarcomas), high-grade surface lesions, periosteal osteosarcomas and intracortical osteosarcomas. Finally, osteosarcomas that complicate Paget's disease, radiation therapy and other conditions will be considered (Table 16.2).

Central osteosarcoma, high grade
Central high-grade osteosarcoma, the most common variant, usually affects children (before the closure of the growth plates) and occurs more often in boys than in girls. About 80% of the lesions occur at the ends of long bones, especially around the knee joint (Fig. 16.35). Localized swelling, often accompanied by pain (and sometimes by a pathologic fracture), develops in children who are otherwise in good health. Alkaline phosphatase

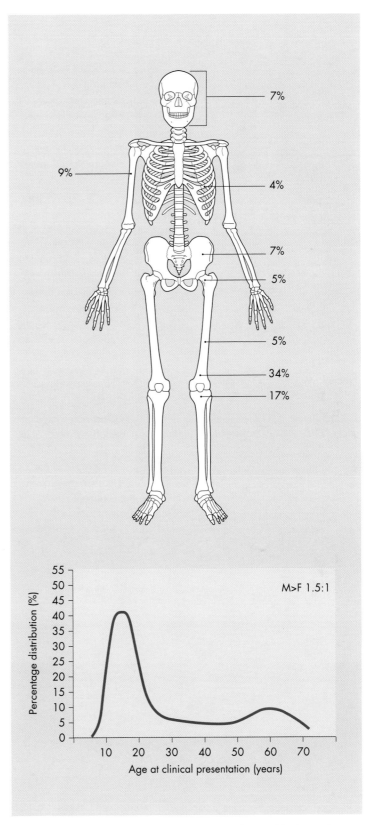

Figure 16.35 Location and age distribution of central high-grade osteosarcoma.

Table 16.2 Conditions occasionally associated with osteosarcoma

Paget's disease
Bone infarction
Chronic osteomyelitis
Post-irradiation (especially giant-cell tumor or fibrous dysplasia)
Metallic prosthetic implants
Retinoblastoma
Rothmund–Thompson syndrome

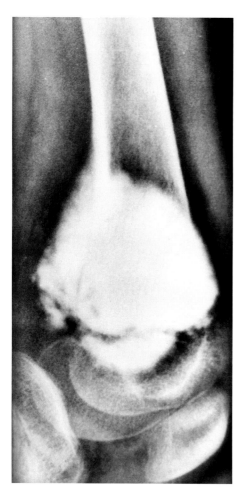

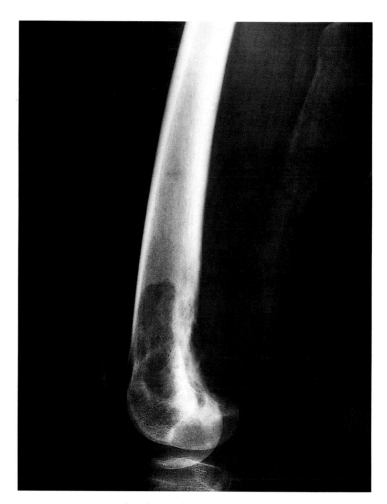

Figure 16.36 A 10-year-old boy presented with complaints of pain around the knee joint. On physical examination, some fullness was felt in the lower femur, which was noted to be warmer than the surrounding tissue. Radiograph shows a radiodense tumor involving the metaphyseal end of the femur, with extension of the tumor both anteriorly and posteriorly into the soft tissue. It is difficult to determine whether or not the epiphyseal end of the bone is involved because of the two-dimensional radiologic image of the three-dimensional bone. (This radiograph should be compared with that in Figure 16.41, photographs of the specimen resected from this patient.)

Figure 16.37 Lateral radiograph to show a lytic osteosarcoma of the lower femur. Posterior extension of the tumor into the soft tissue is evident.

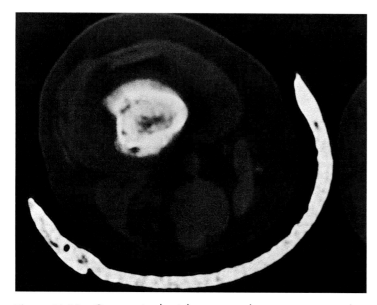

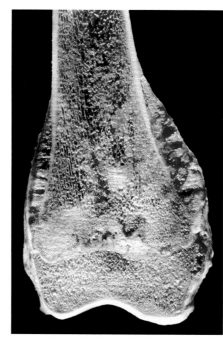

Figure 16.39 In this photograph of a frontal section through the distal femur of a young patient with osteosarcoma, the tumor has extended through the cortex elevating the periosteum. The new bone formed beneath the periosteum is perpendicular to the underlying cortex resulting in a 'sunburst' appearance.

Figure 16.38 Computerized axial tomogram demonstrates expansile subperiosteal bone matrix formation in a case of central osteosarcoma.

levels in these patients are two to three times those found in normal individuals.

Radiographic examination may reveal a sclerotic (in about 35%) (Fig. 16.36), lytic (in about 25%) (Fig. 16.37), or mixed destructive lesion generally in the metaphysis, although rarely the diaphysis or even the epiphysis is the primary site of involvement. The tumor has often invaded the cortex and extended into the soft tissues at the time of presentation (Fig. 16.38), and in many cases there is abundant periosteal new bone formation (which sometimes shows a 'sunburst' pattern) (Fig. 16.39). As with other malignant tumors in the bone, at the edge of the tumor, elevation of the periosteum may result in a triangle of reactive bone, which is visible on radiologic films; this is referred to as Codman's triangle (Fig. 16.40). The sides of the triangle are formed by the periosteum, the underlying cortex, and the

narrow margin of the tumor mass. However, the triangle itself is made up of benign reactive bone and this tissue may cause diagnostic problems if biopsy specimens are obtained only from this area.

The gross and microscopic appearance of osteosarcoma varies according to the type of matrix (bony, fibrous, or cartilaginous) produced by the lesion (Figs 16.41 and 16.42). Penetration of the cortex is common and of the epiphysis less so, however the joint space is rarely involved.

Most osteosarcomas have in common a pleomorphic and anaplastic cell population that produces an immature and disorganized bone matrix and, as previously stated, may also form cartilage matrix or may be mainly fibroblastic. However, the histologic diagnosis rests on the finding of malignant bone matrix formation; in small cell tumors this may not be very obvious (Fig. 16.43).

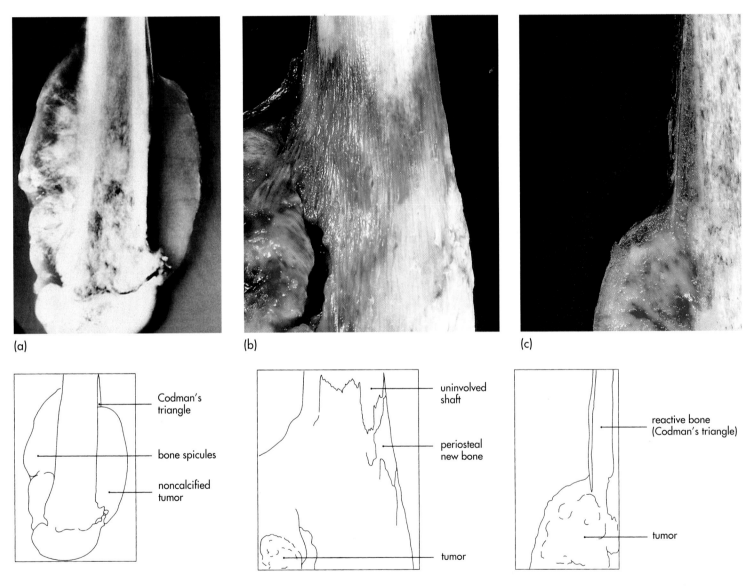

(a)   (b)   (c)

Codman's triangle

bone spicules

noncalcified tumor

uninvolved shaft

periosteal new bone

tumor

reactive bone (Codman's triangle)

tumor

Figure 16.40 (a) Specimen radiograph of an osteosarcoma demonstrates that in the anterior part of the tumor the lesion is purely lytic, that is without calcified bone formation. Posteriorly, bone formation has occurred, and the newly formed bone spicules are oriented at right angles to the surface of the bone, producing a sunburst pattern. A well-defined Codman's triangle is apparent at the upper end of the lesion anteriorly. (b) At the upper end of the photograph a portion of the uninvolved femoral shaft can be seen, while at the lower end the tumor is seen to break through the cortex of the bone. Between the tumor and the normal cortex is a hyperemic zone which has an irregular margin with the cortical bone. This hyperemic zone is composed of reactive bone formed by the periosteum, and would appear on a radiograph as a Codman's triangle. (c) A close-up of a slice through the superior anterior aspect of the specimen demonstrates the reactive periosteal bone above and the tumor below. If this reactive periosteal bone is the site of biopsy, it will fail to produce any histological evidence of malignant tumor.

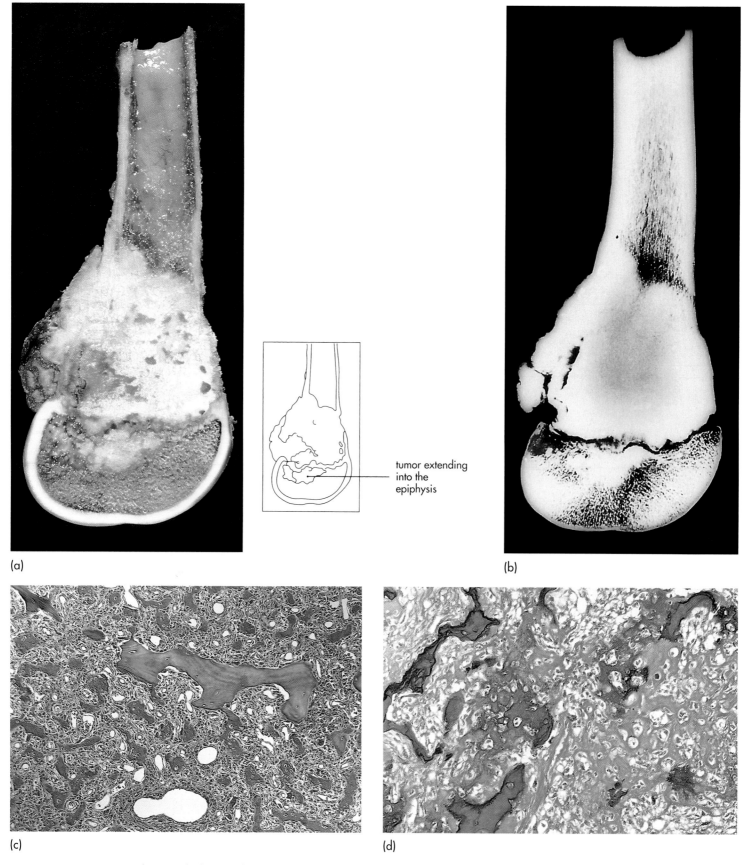

(a)

(b)

tumor extending
into the
epiphysis

(c)

(d)

Figure 16.41   (a) Gross photograph shows a dense osteoblastic osteosarcoma in the lower end of the femur. It has extended through the cortex into the soft tissue and is also present in the epiphysis. Although epiphyseal extension is rarely seen on clinical radiographs, it is commonly present when the resected specimen is examined (compare with Figure 16.36). (b) Specimen radiograph of the lesion shown in (a) reveals extensive bone formation (i.e. an osteoblastic osteosarcoma). (c) A characteristic feature of osteosarcoma is the abundant mineralized matrix which infiltrates through the marrow spaces between the existing trabeculae of the bone. The malignant tumor tissue may become firmly attached to the surface of the existing bone (H&E, × 4 obj.). (d) Photomicrograph shows an area of extensive primitive bone matrix formation which is focally calcified. Sometimes, as seen here, it is difficult to distinguish bone matrix formation from cartilage matrix formation (H&E, × 25 obj.).

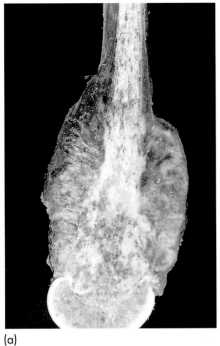

Figure 16.42 (a) Gross photograph of the lesion shown in Figure 16.40 (a) shows a bulky and more vascular osteosarcoma. Extensive soft-tissue extension and involvement of the epiphysis may be observed. (b) Low-power photomicrograph of tissue from this tumor shows a cellular pleomorphic tumor which is producing a noncalcified collagenous matrix; focally, this matrix has the appearance of primitive bone (H&E, × 10 obj.).

(a)

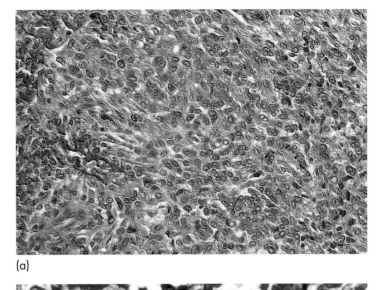

(a)

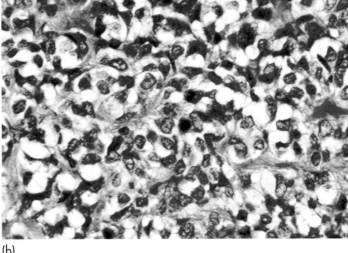

(b)

Figure 16.43 (a) Photomicrograph of an intraosseous tumor principally characterized by packed small, round spindled cells, a small cell osteosarcoma. As can be appreciated in this photograph, fine spicules of bone matrix are being formed by the tumor cells in one focus at the left-hand edge of the photograph (H&E, × 25 obj.).
(b) Photomicrograph of a small-cell osteosarcoma. Note the regular Ewing's-like cells with only small wisps and islands of matrix production (H&E, × 25 obj.).

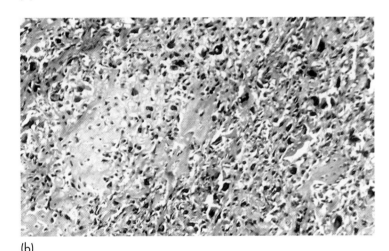

(b)

Telangiectatic osteosarcoma is a rare variant of central high-grade osteosarcoma which is characterized radiographically by a large lytic defect which is usually expansile and is accompanied by an extensive soft tissue component. Magnetic resonance imaging will usually show fluid levels similar to those seen in an aneurysmal bone cyst (Fig. 16.44).

Gross examination will reveal blood-filled cavity, and microscopically there are dilated vascular channels lined with multinucleated giant cells and an anaplastic sarcomatous stroma with evident bone formation (Fig. 16.45). Occasionally this lesion may be very difficult to distinguish from an aneurysmal bone cyst.

Osteosarcomas metastasize, primarily hematogenously and most commonly to the lungs. Favorable prognostic factors include small and/or distal lesions.

As mentioned earlier, osteosarcomas may be seen in association with chromosomal abnormalities. An example of Rothmund–Thompson syndrome is shown in Figure 16.46.

Central osteosarcoma, low grade

Rarely, an intramedullary bone-forming tumor of low-grade malignancy may be encountered. This tumor is usually seen in somewhat older individuals than the conventional high-grade lesion, although individuals in a wide age range may be affected. Males and females are affected with equal frequency.

Radiographically, these lesions are usually either sclerotic, mimicking large bone islands (Fig. 16.47), or resemble foci of solitary fibrous dysplasia (Figs 16.48 and 16.49). On microscopic examination, they most commonly have a fibrous stroma with

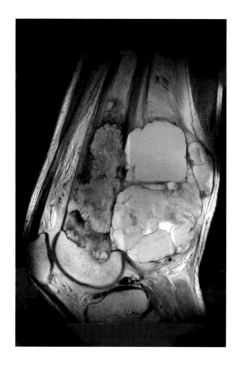

(a)

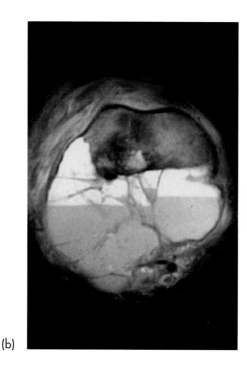

(b)

Figure 16.44 (a) In this MRI, there is an aggressive mass in the distal femur extending from the epiphysis proximally for 14 cm. There is a large posterior soft tissue mass which is mostly cystic with areas of lower signal which may be related to calcification or clot formation. (b) In cross section images multiple fluid-fluid levels were present.

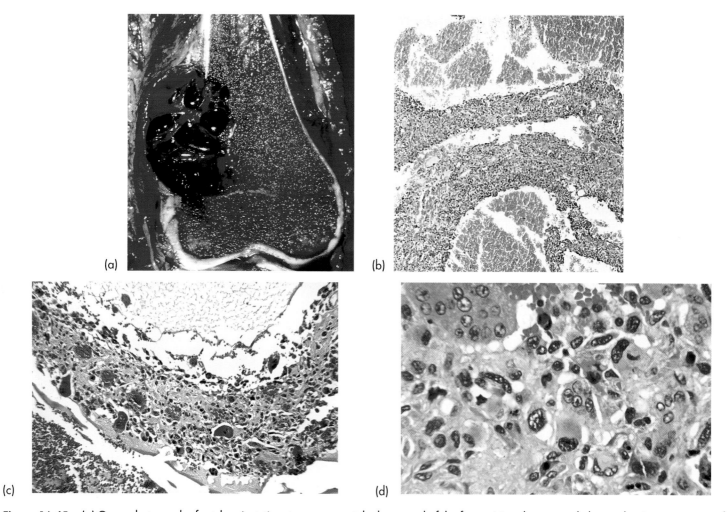

(a)

(b)

(c)

(d)

Figure 16.45 (a) Gross photograph of a telangiectatic osteosarcoma at the lower end of the femur. Note the extremely hemorrhagic appearance of this tumor, which on radiographic examination appeared to be completely lytic. (b) Low-power photomicrograph of this telangiectatic osteosarcoma. Septae of cellular tissue are separated by large blood-filled spaces. At this magnification the lesion can easily be confused with an aneurysmal bone cyst (H&E, × 4 obj.). (c) Higher power view of one portion of the tumor illustrated in (b) demonstrates the anaplastic malignant quality of the tumor tissue with tumor bone formation. Such tissue may be difficult to find in a telangiectatic osteosarcoma and must be carefully looked for in this type of hemorrhagic tumor (H&E, × 10 obj.). (d) Higher power view shows anaplastic cells (H&E, × 25 obj.).

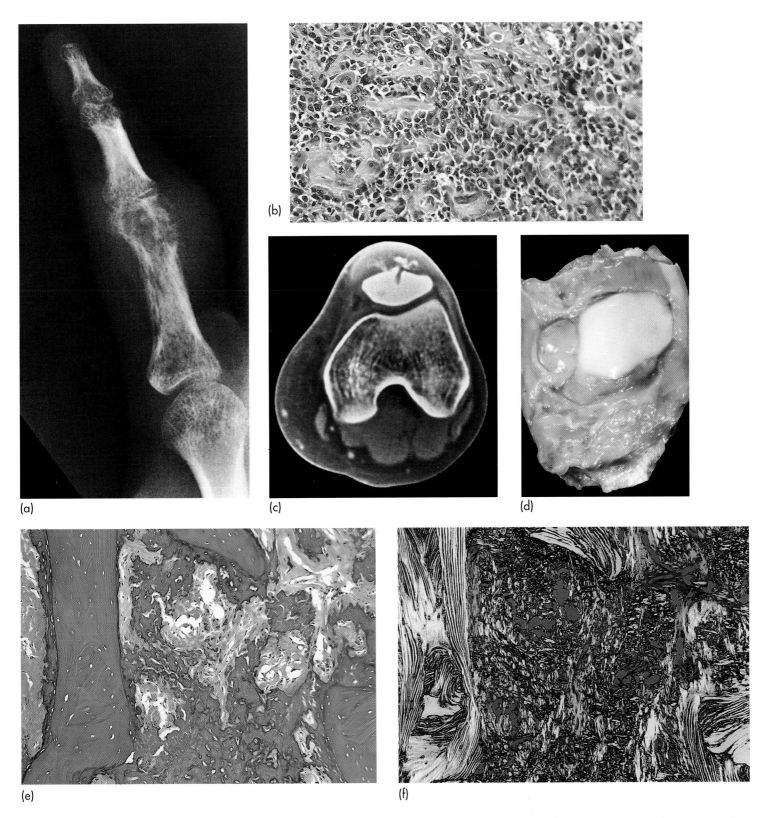

Figure 16.46 (a) A radiograph shows a destructive lesion of the distal end of the proximal phalanx, with soft-tissue invasion. (b) Photomicrograph of the lesional tissue obtained from the lesion demonstrated in (a). There are foci of immature bone formation and the cellular components show pleomorphic nuclei. This was interpreted as osteosarcoma, though there were considerable differences in the expert opinions which were obtained (H&E, × 25 obj.). (c) Computerized axial tomogram through the right knee of the same patient. The patella is extremely dense and an osseous mass is seen in the prepatellar region. The linear defects in the anterior part of the patella represent the area of the biopsy. (d) Gross photograph of the articular surface of the patella resected at a later date with surrounding soft tissue. Adjacent to the patella is a pink/gray nodule which represents part of the soft-tissue extension of the patellar tumor. Resection of the tumor was delayed because of differences of opinion in the interpretation of the original biopsy. Resection was performed only after obvious soft-tissue extension. (e) Photomicrograph of the patellar lesion showing sclerosing osteosarcoma of poor cellularity, which is invading the marrow space and is plastered onto the surface of residual trabecular bone within the medullary cavity (H&E, × 10 obj.). (f) Photomicrograph of the same field shown in (e), photographed in polarized light, demonstrates the 'irregular' woven appearance of the collagen matrix produced by the tumor bone. The lamellar pattern of the residual bone is clearly seen.

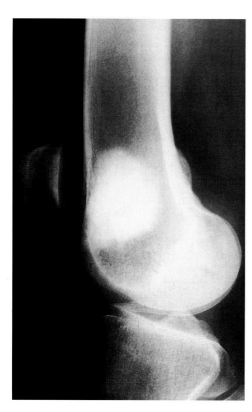

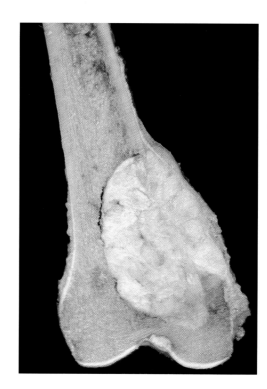

Figure 16.47
Lateral radiograph of a knee shows a large intramedullary sclerotic lesion which has a spiculated periphery suggestive of a large bone island. On biopsy, this lesion proved to be a low-grade osteosarcoma. (Courtesy of Dr Lauren Ackerman.)

Figure 16.49
Photograph of a low-grade fibrous osteosarcoma in the distal femur. Note the cortex has been eroded and the overlying periosteum is being elevated.

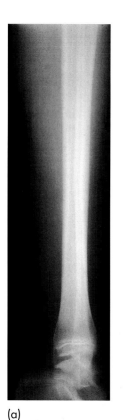

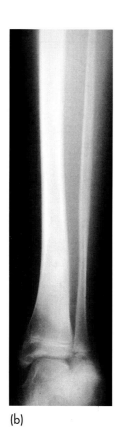

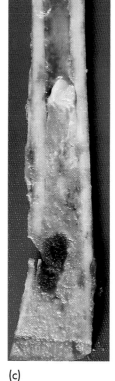

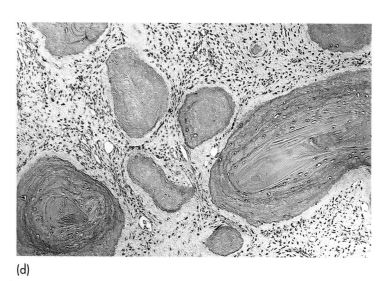

(a)   (b)   (c)   (d)

Figure 16.48   Antero-posterior **(a)** and lateral **(b)** views of the leg in a young patient complaining of vague pain around the ankle. The radiograph shows an ill-defined sclerotic lesion involving the distal diaphysis and metaphysis of the tibia. The initial impression was that this represented fibrous dysplasia. However, a biopsy proved it to be a low-grade osteosarcoma. **(c)** Gross photograph of a longitudinal section of the tibia in the case illustrated in **(a)** and **(b)**. There is an intramedullary mass characterized by firm pink/gray tissue, the upper margin of which is well-delineated from the bone marrow. **(d)** Photomicrograph of the lesion illustrated in **(c)**. The fibrous stroma, although somewhat cellular, has a relatively bland appearance. However, islands of bone are being formed by the tumor and, significantly, this bone is seen to surround residual trabecular bone. This was a feature of the case and is not seen with fibrous dysplasia. The diagnosis was a low-grade osteosarcoma (H&E, × 25 obj.).

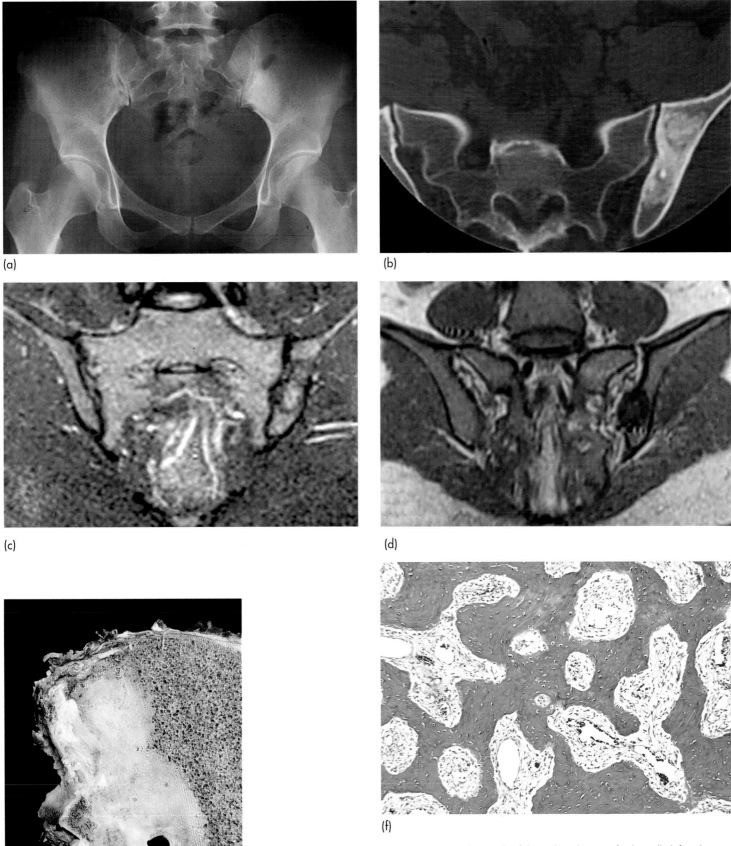

Figure 16.50   (a) An antero-posterior radiograph of the pelvis shows a fairly well-defined radiodense lesion abutting the sacroiliac joint on the left side. (b) A CT scan reveals a bone-forming tumor which appears in this cut to be confined to the bone, and this is confirmed by an MRI (c). (d) In another MRI the tumor is seen pushing the sacroiliac joint, but there is no evidence of extension into the sacrum. (e) A photograph of the resected ilium shows the bony nature of the tumor. At the margins there is slight irregularity as the tumor invades the marrow space (the hole in the tumor is the site of biopsy). (f) Photomicrograph at low magnification shows a bone-forming tumor with a vascularized cellular fibrous stroma (H&E, × 4 obj.).

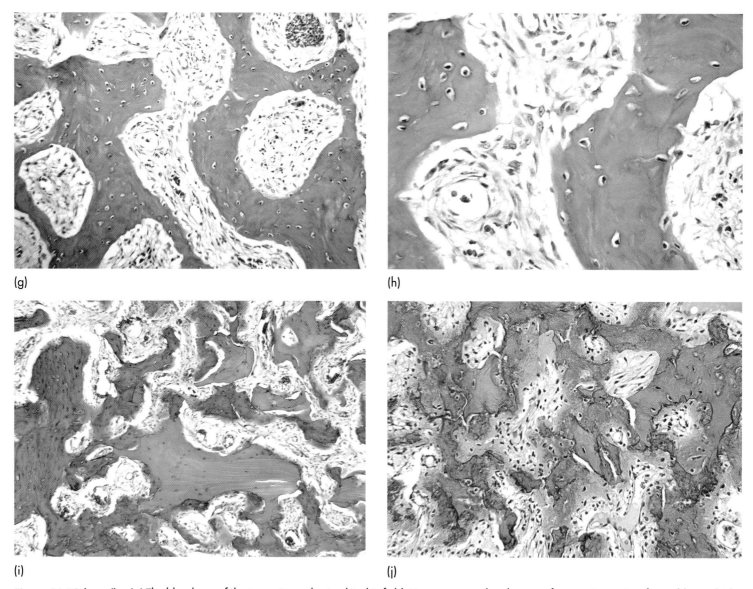

(g)

(h)

(i)

(j)

Figure 16.50 (contd)   (g) The blandness of the tumor is emphasized in this field. However, note the absence of a prominent rim of osteoblasts which is generally seen in an osteoblastoma, which would be the differential diagnosis in this case. Furthermore there is some atypia and loss of an organized pattern in the fibrous stroma (H&E, × 10 obj.). This is better seen at the somewhat higher magnification (H&E, × 10 obj.) **(h)**. **(i)** The best evidence of malignancy is the stuccoing of tumor bone on fragments of the normal lamellar bone (H&E, × 4 obj.) **(j)**, seen here at higher magnification (H&E, × 10 obj.).

rather bland-looking foci of bone formation similar to the appearance of a conventional surface or parosteal lesion and mimicking fibrous dysplasia. In other cases, a pattern suggesting osteoblastoma may be seen (Fig. 16.50). However, in these latter cases the osteoblastic rimming of the bone trabeculae characteristic of osteoblastoma is missing.

The key to the recognition of these lesions is the identification of the invasive character of the lesion, which is typified by the presence of islands of residual lamellar bone within the lesion and evidence of malignant tumor bone plastered on and surrounding these islands of residual as shown in Figure 16.48d.

In cases of low-grade central osteosarcomas, the prognosis is much better than that of the classic high-grade intramedullary

osteosarcoma. However as with other low-grade sarcomas, dedifferentiation may occur.

Parosteal osteosarcoma, low grade (juxtacortical osteogenic sarcoma)

A surface osteosarcoma is most commonly a histologically low-grade, slow-growing neoplasm that occurs on the external surface of a bone, most commonly on the back of the lower end of the femur (the popliteal region) in patients over 20 years of age (Fig. 16.51). In general, this lesion has a much better prognosis than the classic high-grade intramedullary osteosarcoma. (However, it is important to recognize that some fully malignant osteosarcomas may present as juxtacortical lesions.)

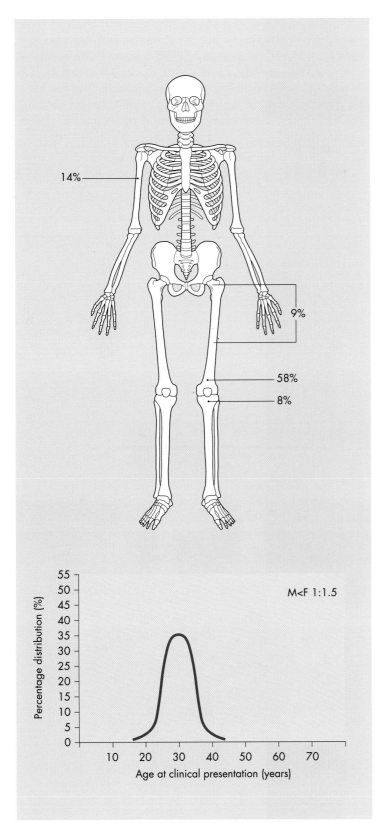

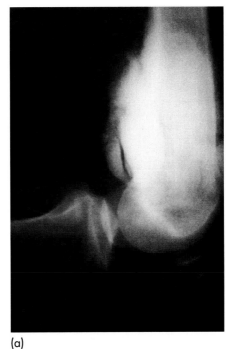

(a)

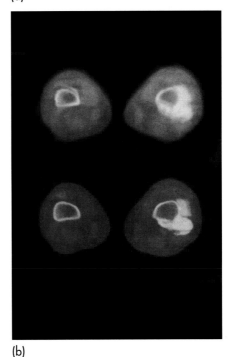

(b)

Figure 16.52 (a) Lateral radiograph of the knee demonstrates a sclerotic bone-forming tumor involving the lower end of the femur. In this view it is not possible to determine the involvement of the bone itself. (b) Computerized axial tomograms of the lesion shown in (a) demonstrate that the tumor is entirely confined to the periphery of the bone, with no involvement of the intramedullary bone. (Courtesy of Dr Leonard Kahn.)

Figure 16.51 Location and age distribution of juxtacortical osteosarcoma.

On radiographic examination, the lesion appears as a large, well-circumscribed, generally dense juxtacortical mass, although lytic areas may be present (Fig. 16.52). The mass may be separated from the cortical bone by a fine, relatively lucent line (Fig. 16.53). It is not usually possible to distinguish between high-grade and low-grade tumors on the radiographic images.

Grossly the tumor is firmly adherent to the bone and on cut section may exhibit bony, cartilaginous, and fibrous areas (Fig. 16.54). Microscopically, the lesion consists of a well-defined lob-

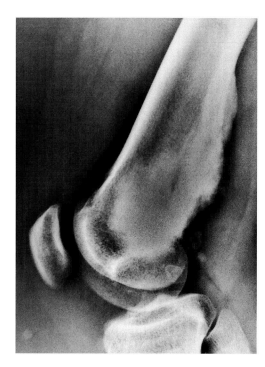

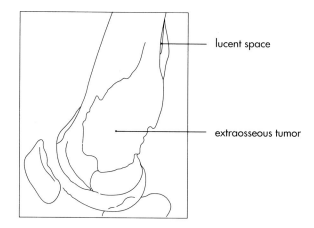

Figure 16.53   Radiograph of a 35-year-old woman who complained of pain above the knee. An irregular radiodense tumor can be seen on the surface of the bone, particularly posteriorly but also to some extent laterally at the lower end of the femur. The margins of the tumor are well defined, and between the tumor and the underlying cortex a fine radiolucent line is focally apparent. In a case of a juxtacortical osteosarcoma/parosteal osteosarcoma such as this, it is difficult to determine radiographically whether or not the medullary cavity is involved. For this reason, a CT scan can be extremely useful in determining the extent of the tumor.

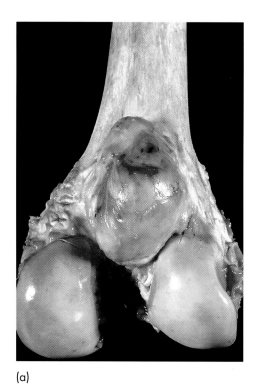

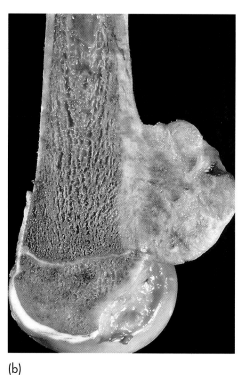

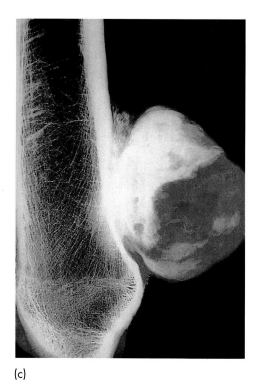

(a)   (b)   (c)

Figure 16.54   (a) Gross photograph of the lower end of the femur resected from a patient with a juxtacortical osteosarcoma. A large mass is present on the cortex of the bone just above and between the two femoral condyles. This location is typical for juxtacortical osteosarcoma. (b) Gross photograph of a sagittal section through the lesion shown in (a) demonstrates that the lesion is well encapsulated and formed of bone-producing tissue. As in the case shown here, the lesion frequently extends for a short distance through the cortex into the medullary cavity. For this reason, when surgical treatment of a juxtacortical osteosarcoma is planned, medullary extension should be carefully sought and taken into account if local recurrence is to be prevented. (c) Radiograph of the specimen in (b). A low-grade juxtacortical osteosarcoma, as shown here, may contain a large area of tumor which is either purely fibrous or cartilaginous, and therefore radiolucent.

ulated mass, with extensive bone and (occasionally) cartilage formation. Most tumors contain a bland, well-differentiated fibrosarcomatous stroma (Fig. 16.55).

The treatment of choice is surgical removal of the mass. However, in some cases intramedullary extension of the lesion may have occurred, so that excision of the lesion and the attached cortex may not be adequate treatment. Computerized axial tomography should be performed on all these lesions to gauge the extent of intramedullary extension. Rarely these lesions may undergo de-differentiation (Fig. 16.56).

The differential diagnosis should include that of surface osteoma as well as a high-grade surface lesion.

Surface osteosarcoma, high grade

It should not be assumed that because a bone-forming lesion has a juxtacortical location it necessarily has a better prognosis. Fully malignant parosteal lesions may account for as much as 25% of all parosteal lesions. On microscopic examination, the features of a malignant parosteal osteosarcoma are those of a high-grade central lesion. There are no radiographic features which distinguish low-grade from high-grade surface lesions. In a high-grade lesion with an intramedullary component, it can sometimes be difficult to decide whether a particular case is a surface lesion or a central lesion with a large soft-tissue component. However, in either case the prognosis is similar (poor).

Periosteal osteosarcoma

Periosteal (peripheral) osteosarcoma is a rare, predominantly cartilage-forming osteosarcoma characterized on radiographs by ill-defined swelling and formation of periosteal new bone, which often has a 'sunburst' appearance. The lesion usually occurs at the midshaft of the femur or tibia in children. It is usually small at the time of presentation (Fig. 16.57), although larger lesions may be encountered (Fig. 16.58). The microscopic appearance is

typical, with abundant cartilage formation and a cellular stroma (Fig. 16.59). However, malignant bone matrix formation is present and distinguishes the lesion from a juxtacortical chondroma or chondrosarcoma.

Intracortical osteosarcoma

Cases of osteosarcoma that have an intracortical origin have been only rarely described. One such case of intracortical osteosarcoma is illustrated in Figure 16.60. Intracortical osteosarcoma may be and has been mistaken for an osteoid osteoma.

PAGET'S SARCOMA

Rarely patients with symptomatic Paget's disease develop sarcoma. These patients usually have advanced polyostotic Paget's disease. However, on rare occasions sarcoma may occur in patients with nonsymptomatic monostotic disease (for example, in a single vertebral body) (see also Fig. 7.34).

The presenting symptom is likely to be localized pain which is sometimes associated with a pathologic fracture. Typically the patients are over 50 years of age. The commonest sites are the humerus, femur and pelvis.

The tumor most frequently associated with Paget's disease is osteosarcoma (Fig. 16.61), although occasionally other patterns of sarcoma (e.g. chondrosarcoma, malignant fibrous histiocytoma) may be encountered. The prognosis for sarcomas arising in patients with Paget's disease is very poor. Rarely, a benign giant-cell tumor, often in the facial bones, occurs in a patient with Paget's disease and even metastatic disease may appear in Pagetoid bone. For these reasons it should not be assumed that because a patient with Paget's disease has evidence of a tumor associated with the disease, that the tumor is necessarily a sarcoma (see also Figs 7.36 and 7.37).

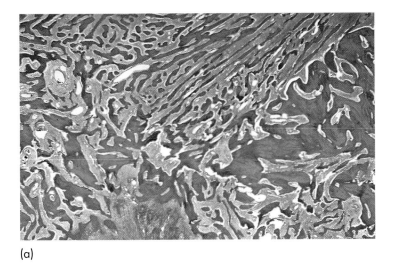

(a)

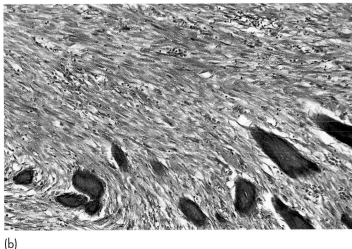

(b)

Figure 16.55 (a) Low-power photomicrograph of a juxtacortical osteosarcoma shows the typical appearance of a heavily collagenized fibrous matrix with irregular trabeculae of bone (H&E, × 4 obj.). (b) Higher power photomicrograph shows the cellular, though unremarkable, fibrous stroma of a juxtacortical osteosarcoma with islands of bone tissue (H&E, × 25 obj.).

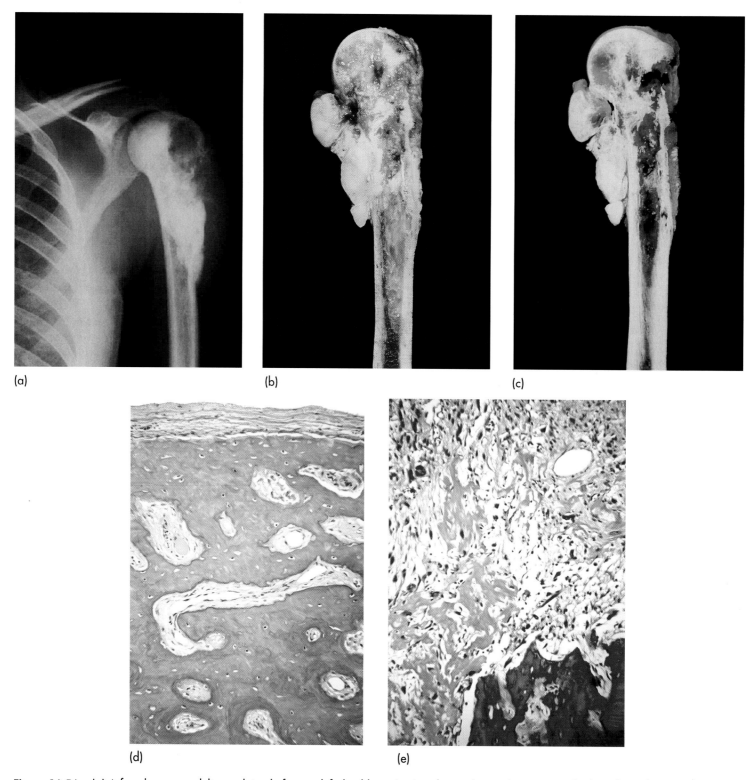

(a)   (b)   (c)

(d)   (e)

Figure 16.56   (a) A female young adult complained of recent left shoulder pain. A radiograph reveals an extremely dense bone-forming tumor which, although not obvious from this single view, is probably a surface lesion. Additionally there is a destructive lesion affecting the humeral head. (b) A section through the resected humerus shows a dense surface lesion and in addition an intramedullary lesion which is destroying the lateral cortex. (c) A specimen radiograph clearly distinguishes the dense surface lesion, which has a radiolucent line between much of the tumor and the cortex, and the destructive intramedullary component. (d) A photomicrograph of the dense osteoblastic surface tumor shows the classic pattern of a low-grade parosteal osteosarcoma (H&E, × 10 obj.). (e) A photomicrograph of the intramedullary portion of the tumor reveals the anaplastic de-differentiated tumor tissue in the intramedullary cavity. Although uncommon, low-grade osteosarcoma, either on the surface or as a central lesion, may de-differentiate into a high-grade sarcoma (H&E, × 10 obj.).

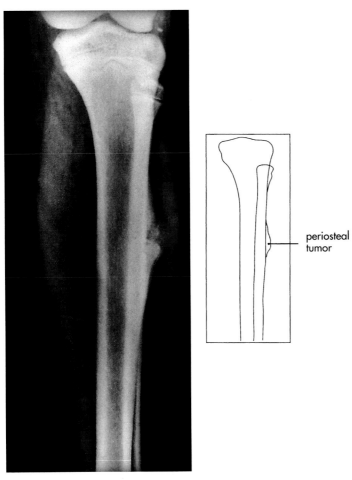

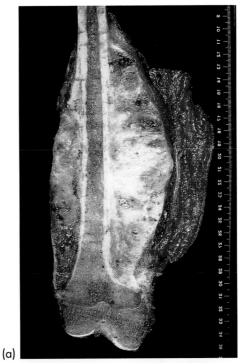

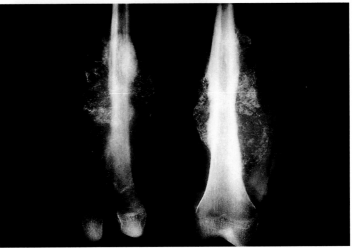

Figure 16.58
(a) Gross photograph of a longitudinal section through the lower end of the femur demonstrates a large surface tumor composed of gray/white glistening tissues and admixed bone. (b) Radiograph of the dissected specimen shown in (a) demonstrates the extent of bone formation in the tumor. (Courtesy of Dr Leonard Kahn.)

(a)

(b)

Figure 16.57   Radiograph of a 14-year-old boy who complained of pain in the upper part of the leg. In the proximal tibial diaphysis is a peripheral lesion apparently confined to the surface of the bone. It is composed of an irregular bone-forming lesion, and there is reactive periosteal new bone both superiorly and inferiorly. Histologic examination proved this to be a cartilage-rich periosteal osteosarcoma.

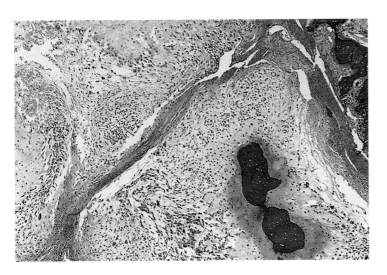

Figure 16.59   Photomicrograph demonstrating the features of a periosteal osteosarcoma. These lesions tend to be more cellular than juxtacortical osteosarcoma and for the most part to form, as here, a cartilaginous extracellular matrix; however, foci of bone formation can be found if searched for (H&E, × 10 obj.).

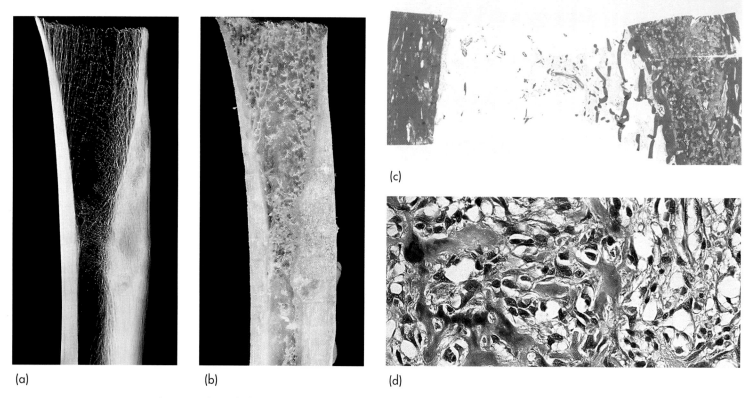

(a)   (b)   (d)

Figure 16.60   (a) A teenage boy complained of pain in the shin. Radiograph shows marked cortical thickening with a dense intracortical lesion, which was interpreted as an osteoid osteoma. A biopsy showed an osteosarcoma. (b) The resected specimen from the patient in (a) demonstrates tumor confined to the cortical area of the bone. (c) Histologic section through the shaft of the tibia shown in (b) shows an osteosarcoma confined to the cortex of the bone (H&E, × 1 obj.). (d) Close-up view of the tumor (H&E, × 25 obj.).

RADIATION SARCOMA

Osteosarcoma and fibrosarcoma were the most commonly diagnosed radiation-induced sarcomas, although at the present time malignant fibrous histiocytomas, are perhaps more commonly seen. The time interval between radiation and the diagnosis of postirradiation sarcoma may be as long as 40 years, but the average is around 10–12 years. If the interval between radiation and tumor diagnosis is less than 2 years, a causal relationship should be seriously doubted. The vast majority of cases have received a radiation dose of more than 3000 rad and usually much more than that. The incidence of sarcomatous degeneration appears to be related to the dose given. In general radiation sarcomas behave in a highly malignant way.

The tumors present in the radiation field and the most commonly treated lesions that give rise to postirradiation sarcomas are gynecologic cancer and breast cancer (Fig. 16.62). Among primary bone lesions which have been treated by radiation therapy, giant-cell tumors seem to be particularly associated with postirradiation sarcoma.

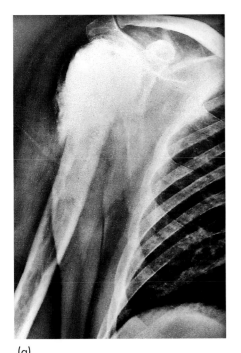

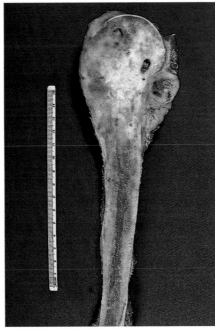

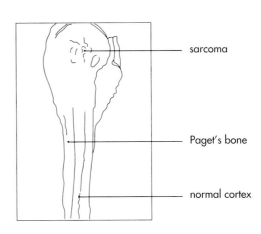

(a)   (b)

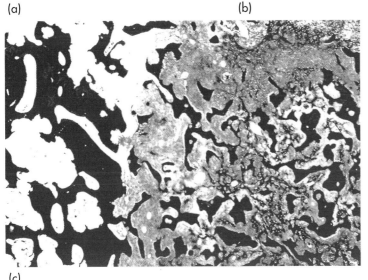

(c)

Figure 16.61 (a) Radiograph of a 65-year-old man who presented with severe pain in the upper end of the right humerus shows a large destructive and sclerotic tumor in the upper end of the humerus extending into the soft tissue. Note that the cortex of the bone below the tumor is thickened and indistinct, characteristic of Paget's disease. (b) Sagittal section through the humerus of the patient shown in (a) shows a large destructive tumor at the upper end. The tumor has extended through the cortex into the soft tissue. (Often, sarcoma in Paget's disease occurs in the midshaft of the bone, and this finding contrasts with that of primary osteosarcoma, which is more often seen in the rnetaphysis.) Note the thickened hyperemic cortical bone involved by Paget's disease. (c) Photomicrograph of tissue removed from the patient in (b). On the left, is pagetoid bone; on the right, a cellular bone-forming tumor (H&E, × 4 obj.).

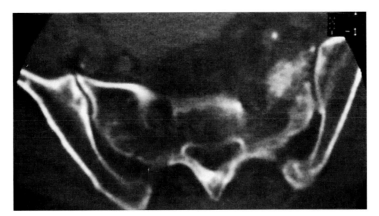

Figure 16.62 Computerized axial tomogram through the sacroiliac joint of a 52-year-old woman shows an expanding and destructive bone-forming tumor involving the left ala of the sacrum. Biopsy confirmed the diagnosis of sarcoma secondary to previous irradiation of a cervical carcinoma.

Chapter 17

CARTILAGE-FORMING TUMORS AND TUMOR-LIKE CONDITIONS

This chapter deals with those benign and malignant tumors where a cartilaginous extracellular matrix is formed by the neoplastic cells. Occasionally foci of bone matrix are seen in tumors which are essentially cartilaginous but in these cases the bone will be found to be reactive rather than having been formed by the neoplastic cells.

REACTIVE OR POST-TRAUMATIC TUMORS

In post-traumatic reactive lesions on bone surfaces, cartilage may be a prominent feature. For a discussion of these lesions see Chapter 16 (reactive periostitis, subungual exostosis and BPOP, pp. 363–365).

DEVELOPMENTAL OR HAMARTOMATOUS TUMORS

OSTEOCHONDROMA (OSTEOCARTILAGINOUS EXOSTOSIS)

Osteochondroma is a common nonfamilial developmental aberration, with the majority of cases presenting clinically in the first 2 decades of life. It is approximately 1.5 times more common in boys than in girls (Fig. 17.1).

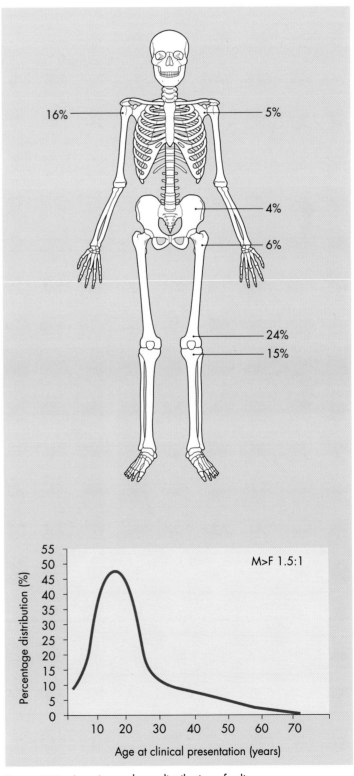

Figure 17.1 Location and age distribution of solitary osteocartilaginous exostosis.

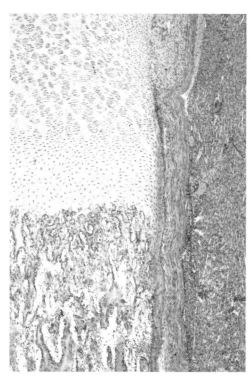

Figure 17.2
Histologic section taken from a normal 12-week-old fetus. The cartilage on the left and the underlying bone metaphysis can be seen. To the right of the epiphysis is a thin layer of periosteal bone which forms a cuff around the cartilaginous epiphysis. The perichondral bone cuff is important to the mechanical integrity of the epiphyseal growth plate cartilage (H&E, × 40 obj.).

The lesion is thought to result from the herniation and separation of a fragment of epiphyseal growth plate cartilage through the periosteal bone cuff that normally surrounds the growth plate (Fig. 17.2). Persistent growth of the herniated cartilage fragment and its subsequent endochondral ossification result in a cartilage-capped subperiosteal bony projection from the bone surface. Rarely, osteochondromas may arise after radiation therapy in children.

The most common sites of occurrence are the long bones, usually the lower end of the femur and upper end of the tibia. However, involvement of the flat bones, ilium, and scapulae occurs in about 5% of cases. Osteochondromas of the spine are rare.

The lesion generally manifests clinically before the third decade of life, often with the patient complaining of juxta-articular pain or a mass. On radiographs, the lesions appear as either a flattened (sessile) or a stalk-like (exostosis) protuberance on the bone shaft in a juxta-epiphyseal location. This bony protuberance is contiguous with the adjacent cortical bone and generally points away from the adjacent joint (Figs 17.3–17.5). Radiographically the stalk merges imperceptibly with the adjacent bone cortex.

Following surgical excision the pathologist usually receives an irregular bony mass with a bluish-gray cartilaginous cap resembling a cauliflower; the base of the lesion consists of a rim of cortical bone and central cancellous bone which is contiguous with

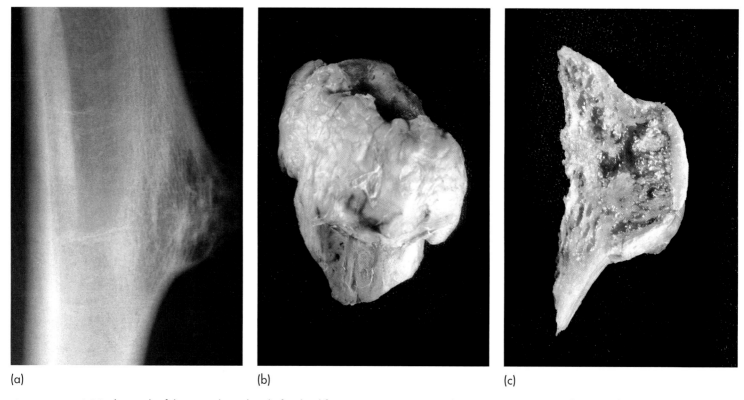

(a)   (b)   (c)

Figure 17.3   (a) Radiograph of the metaphyseal end of a distal femur in a young patient shows an eccentric irregularity on the cortex, with a lucent cap. The margins of the lesion are contiguous with the surrounding cortex. (b) Photograph of the specimen removed from the femur seen in (a). An irregular, cauliflower-like, bluish-gray cartilage mass overlies the cortical bone. (c) Cross-section of the specimen shown in (b) demonstrates that the lesion seen radiologically is contiguous with the surrounding cortex, but is capped by a thin layer of bluish-gray cartilage.

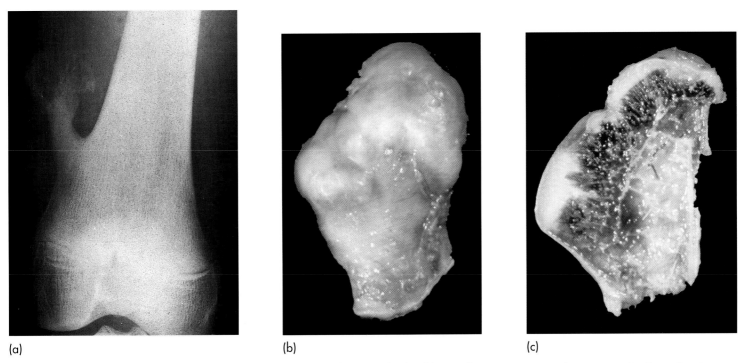

(a) (b) (c)

Figure 17.4 (a) Clinical radiograph of a pedunculated osteochondroma in the distal femur of a young patient. Characteristically, the stalk points away from the adjacent joint surface and the cortex of the osteochondroma is contiguous with the femoral cortex. Surface (b) and cross-section (c) of the osteochondroma removed from the patient seen in (a). The cartilage cap varies considerably in thickness.

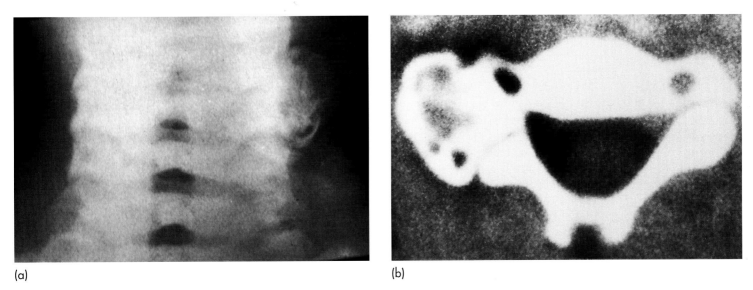

(a) (b)

Figure 17.5 Antero-posterior radiograph (a) of the lower cervical spine shows a well-corticated bubbly expansile lesion lateral to the lateral masses of C4 and C5. A CT section (b) through C4 shows an expansile lesion extending from the left lateral mass. The cortex is thick and is contiguous with that of the pedicle. The neural foramina and spinal canal are uninvolved. The matrix is similar to that of a medullary cavity with coarse trabeculations. There is no evidence of calcified cartilage within the matrix and no associated surrounding soft-tissue component. (From Novick GS, Pavlov H, Bullough PG. **Osteochondroma of the cervical spine: Report of two cases in preadolescent males.** *Skeletal Radiol* 1982, **8**:13–15.)

the underlying normal shaft. On cut section the cartilage cap may vary considerably in thickness and often shows areas with an opaque yellow appearance due to calcification within the cartilage matrix. Microscopic examination reveals the cartilaginous cap to be somewhat disorganized in its structure and cellular organization, and covered with a thin layer of fibrous periosteum (Fig. 17.6). The older the patient, the thinner the cartilaginous

component becomes. After adolescence and closure of the growth plates there is usually no further growth of the osteochondroma. The lesion may recur if it is inadequately excised, and this is particularly a problem with sessile lesions where a part of the cartilage cap may be left behind. In very rare cases, a malignant tumor (usually a chondrosarcoma) may be engrafted onto the lesion.

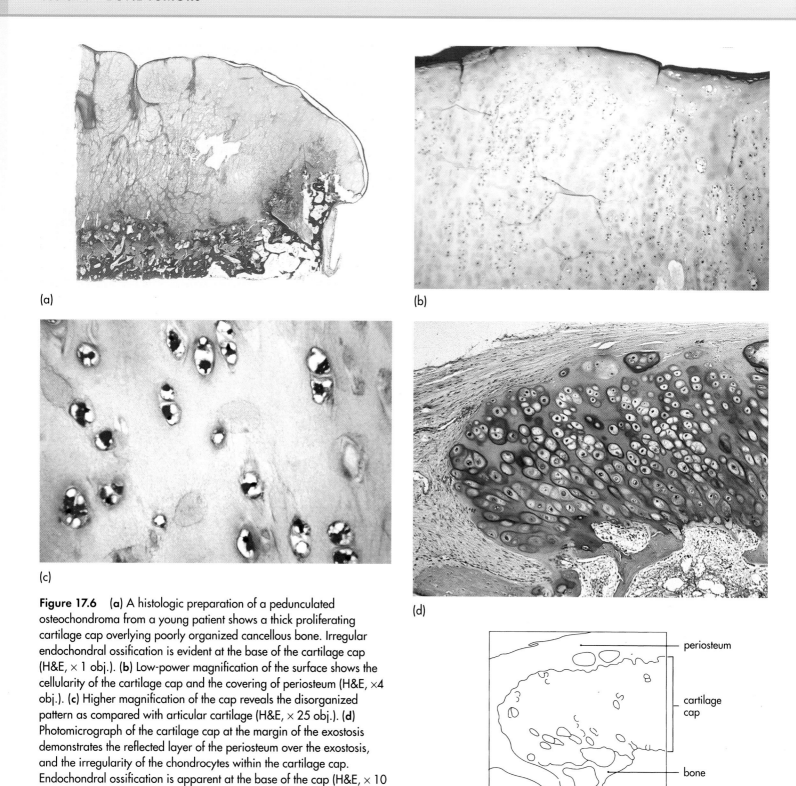

(a)

(b)

(c)

(d)

Figure 17.6   **(a)** A histologic preparation of a pedunculated osteochondroma from a young patient shows a thick proliferating cartilage cap overlying poorly organized cancellous bone. Irregular endochondral ossification is evident at the base of the cartilage cap (H&E, × 1 obj.). **(b)** Low-power magnification of the surface shows the cellularity of the cartilage cap and the covering of periosteum (H&E, ×4 obj.). **(c)** Higher magnification of the cap reveals the disorganized pattern as compared with articular cartilage (H&E, × 25 obj.). **(d)** Photomicrograph of the cartilage cap at the margin of the exostosis demonstrates the reflected layer of the periosteum over the exostosis, and the irregularity of the chondrocytes within the cartilage cap. Endochondral ossification is apparent at the base of the cap (H&E, × 10 obj.).

periosteum

cartilage cap

bone

MULTIPLE OSTEOCHONDROMAS (HEREDITARY MULTIPLE OSTEOCARTILAGINOUS EXOSTOSES)

The occurrence of multiple osteocartilaginous exostoses is rare. Inherited as an autosomal dominant trait, this condition is usually associated with short stature and other bony deformities (Fig. 17.7). The patients present with disfigurement or with pain induced by pressure on surrounding soft-tissue structures. Individual lesions are radiographically, grossly, and microscopi-

cally similar to solitary osteochondromas, although frequently the multiple lesions are more disorganized in structure and tend to have bosselated cartilage caps.

The significance of this disorder for the surgeon lies in the management of the multiple lesions; however, the pathologist must consider that the incidence of malignant transformation, compared with that in solitary osteochondromas, is much higher (about 10%). A lesion with suspected malignant transformation is shown in Figure 17.8.

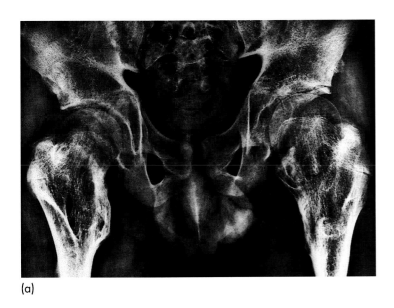

(a)

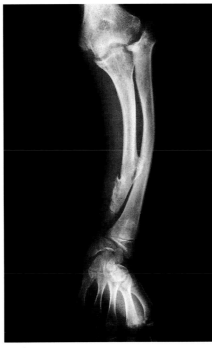

(b)

Figure 17.7
(a) Radiograph of an adolescent boy with hereditary multiple exostoses. Note the short, wide, deformed femoral necks, on which can be seen several exostoses. (b) Radiograph of the forearm of the patient shown in (a). Note multiple exostoses, with shortening and deformity of the forearm associated with malformation of the distal ulna.

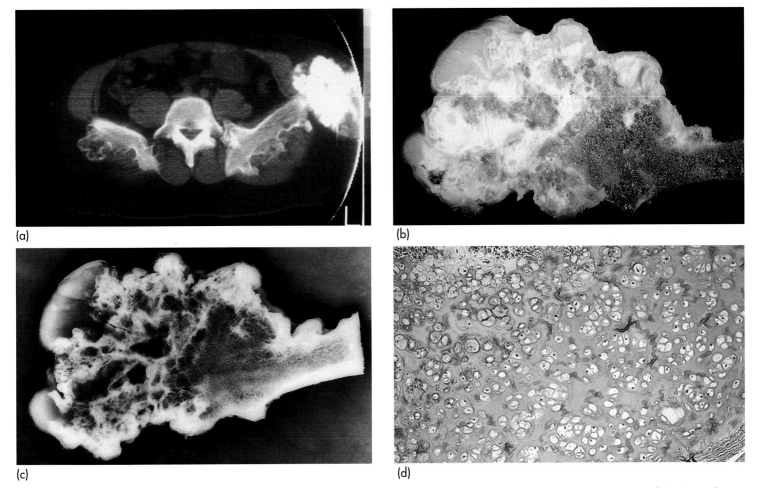

(a)

(b)

(c)

(d)

Figure 17.8   (a) This CT scan of the pelvis in a 36-year-old man with known multiple exostoses reveals a large mass on the wing of the ilium. The patient's history revealed that this mass had been increasing in size. (b) Transected specimen removed from the patient shown in (a). Note the thick cartilage cap on the surface and the extensive calcification (calcified cartilage) within the irregular bosselated lesion. (c) Radiograph of the specimen shown in (b) again reveals the thick cartilage cap and extensive calcification of the cartilage matrix. (d) Photomicrograph of the cartilage cap in the specimen shown in the previous three figures. The cartilage cap is covered with a dense fibrous capsule, seen in the lower right-hand corner and the cartilage matrix is filled with crowded viable chondrocytes. The finding of a thick, active cartilage cap on an exostosis in a skeletally mature individual (especially if the lesion has a history of recent growth) must alert the clinician and pathologist to the possibility of malignant transformation (H&E, × 10 obj.).

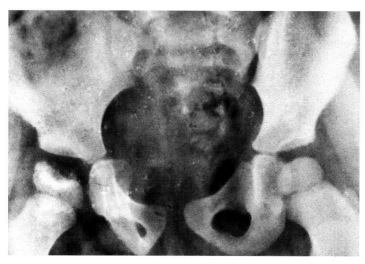

Figure 17.9   Radiograph of a child with an eccentrically enlarged, irregular, capital femoral epiphysis due to an epiphyseal osteochondroma (Trevor's disease). It is important not to confuse this condition with Legg–Calvé–Perthes disease.

DYSPLASIA EPIPHYSEALIS HEMIMELICA (OSTEOCHONDROMA OF THE EPIPHYSIS; TREVOR'S DISEASE)

Dysplasia epiphysealis hemimelica is a nonfamilial developmental disorder of the skeleton, usually manifested in young children who present with unilateral irregular enlargement of an epiphysis (Fig. 17.9). The disorder most commonly involves the lower femur, the upper tibia, or the talus. Although it is a benign condition, varus or valgus deformities of the limb may ensue. Surgical excision is the treatment of choice.

When excised and examined microscopically, the lesion somewhat resembles an osteochondroma, with a cartilage cap of disorganized cartilage, as compared with the surrounding articular cartilage. Underlying the cartilage cap there is endochondral ossification, and normal progression of cancellous bone formation (Fig. 17.10).

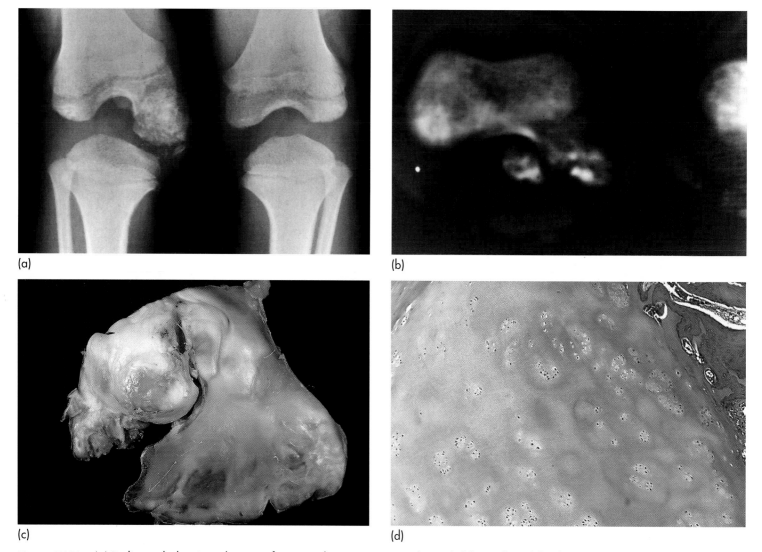

(a)

(b)

(c)

(d)

Figure 17.10   (a) Radiograph showing a large ossifying protuberance arising in the medial femoral condyle of a patient with Trevor's disease. (b) A computerized axial tomogram through the left medial femoral condyle shown in (a) demonstrates the origin of the lesion from the underlying bone. (c) A gross photograph of the resected specimen of the lesion shown in (b). Note the cartilaginous appearance of the lesion, which has focal ossification at its periphery and is partially covered by a fibrous membrane. (d) Photomicrograph of a portion of the cartilage cap on the articular surface demonstrated in (c), showing the increased irregular cellularity of the lesional cartilage (H&E, × 10 obj.).

ENCHONDROMATOSIS (OLLIER'S DISEASE)

Ollier's disease is a rare developmental abnormality which appears to have no familial association and usually presents in early childhood. The disease is characterized by scattered clones of immature chondrocytes within those parts of the skeleton which develop through the process of endochondral ossification (Fig. 17.11). Characteristically, multiple cartilaginous tumors, ranging from microscopic foci to bulky masses, appear throughout the epiphyses, metaphyses, and diaphyses of the skeleton (Fig. 17.12). The lesions may be either central or subperiosteal in location. Their distribution is most often unilateral and confined to one limb.

Radiographic examination reveals multiple lucent lesions, often within deformed or shortened bone. A short ulna, as is also seen in association with multiple exostoses, is not uncommon. Stippled calcification within the tumors is common, and occasionally the affected bone may have a striated appearance (Fig. 17.13).

The histologic features of these lesions somewhat resemble those of solitary enchondromas (see later), but in enchondromatosis the tumors are more cellular, frequently myxoid and, in general, have a more ominous appearance (Fig. 17.14). Malignant transformation (rare in solitary enchondromas) is reported to occur in approximately one-third of cases and seems to be particularly common in Maffucci's syndrome, a condition

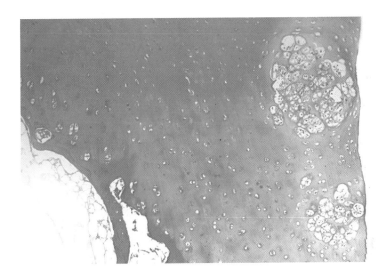

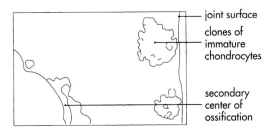

Figure 17.11 Histologic section of the cartilaginous end of a bone in a young child with enchondromatosis. Proliferating clones of markedly atypical chondrocytes are seen within the cartilaginous epiphysis, thus demonstrating that this condition arises from abnormal clones of chondrocytes within the cartilage anlage of the affected limb (H&E, × 2.5 obj.).

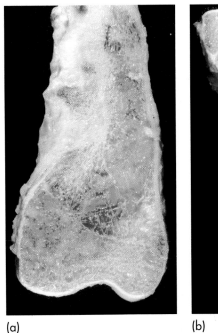

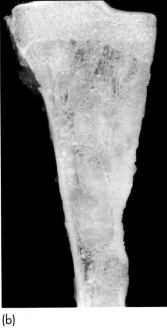

(a)   (b)

Figure 17.12 In the coronal section of a femur (**a**) and tibia (**b**) involved by enchondromatosis, note replacement of the cancellous portion of the bone with circumscribed grayish-blue nodules. In addition to the metaphysis and diaphysis, the epiphysis and periosteal surface are also affected by the disease.

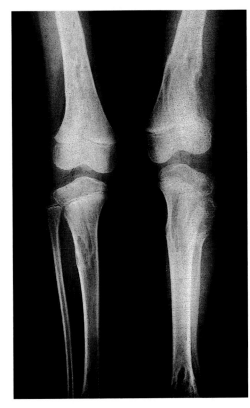

Figure 17.13 Radiograph of the lower limbs in a patient with multiple enchondromas. Typically, the lytic lesions are most prominent in the metaphysis and have a striated appearance. However, the lesions also affect the epiphysis and the periosteal surfaces, and may result in bone shortening as well as deformity of the articular ends.

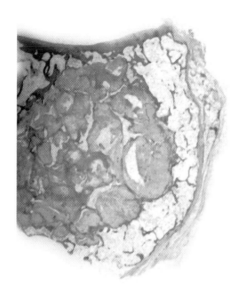

(a)

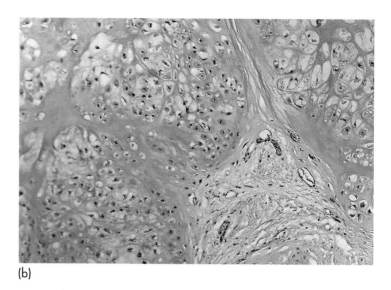

(b)

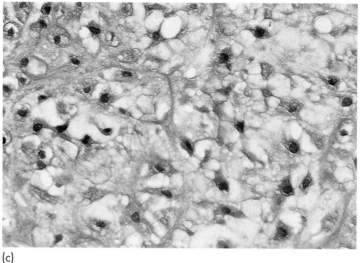

(c)

Figure 17.14 (a) Low-power photomicrograph of the articular end of a bone from a patient with multiple enchondromatosis demonstrates a cartilaginous nodule extending up to the articular surface. Note the lobular arrangement of the cartilage and the lesion's bony rim (H&E, × 1 obj.). (b) Photomicrograph of a portion of the lesion shown in (a) demonstrates the lobular and cellular appearance of the cartilaginous nodules in enchondromatosis. These lesions usually exhibit more cellularity than is seen in solitary enchondromas (H&E, × 10 obj.). (c) Higher power view to show a myxoid appearance of the tumor with crowded stellate cells (H&E, × 25 obj.).

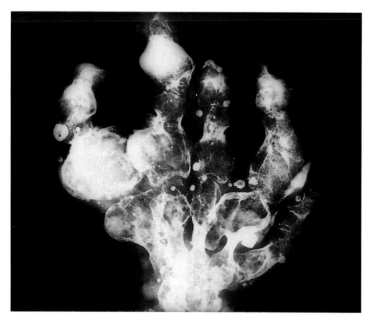

Figure 17.15 Radiograph of a hand in a patient with multiple enchondromas reveals many calcified phleboliths in association with soft-tissue hemangiomas. This combination of soft-tissue hemangiomatosis and enchondromatosis is known as Maffucci's syndrome.

characterized by the occurrence of multiple enchondromatosis in association with soft-tissue hemangiomas, including visceral hemangiomas (Fig. 17.15). (See also Fig. 21.44).

BENIGN TUMORS

ENCHONDROMA

Enchondroma is a relatively common, often asymptomatic, benign intramedullary cartilaginous neoplasm. Enchondromas most often present clinically in the short tubular bones of the hands and feet of adults, but may also occur as an incidental finding in the long bones (Fig. 17.16). When they are in long bones or in the axial skeleton, they may be very difficult to distinguish radiographically or microscopically from low-grade chondrosarcoma. Indeed such differentiation may be amongst the most difficult problems in bone tumor pathology. However, although it may be difficult on histologic examination to differentiate an enchondroma from a low-grade chondrosarcoma, small peripheral cartilage tumors are usually benign, whereas large axial tumors are more likely to be malignant.

In the short tubular bones an enlarging lesion may fracture, and this complication is the usual reason for clinical presentation. In rare cases, an eccentric chondroma may cause bulging of the cortex. (This appearance has been referred to as enchondroma protuberans.)

Radiographically enchondroma usually appears as a well-delineated solitary lucent defect in the metaphyseal region of the bone and in the small tubular bones, most of the shaft is usually involved. The cortex is generally intact unless a fracture through the weakened bone has occurred (Fig. 17.17). Calcification is usually present in the lesion, appearing as fine, punctate stippling or small broken rings of radiodensity (Fig. 17.18). In long bones, when calcification is pronounced, the lesion may be suggestive of a bone infarct. However a bone infarct generally shows peripheral calcification and on the radiograph the lesion more resembles a coil of smoke.

Gross inspection of an enchondroma reveals bluish-gray lobules of firm, translucent tissue. On microscopic examination these lobules are found to be proliferating nests of cartilage cells without obvious atypia. Foci of calcification are usually present, and a thin layer of lamellar bone rimming the cartilage nodules is sometimes observed. Occasionally, evidence of endochondral ossification is seen. However, invasive infiltration of the bone marrow spaces is not a characteristic of benign enchondromas, and this finding is probably the most helpful microscopic feature in trying to distinguish an enchondroma from a low-grade chondrosarcoma. Rarely, a chondrosarcoma develops in a pre-existing enchondroma, more often in long tubular bones (Fig. 17.19).

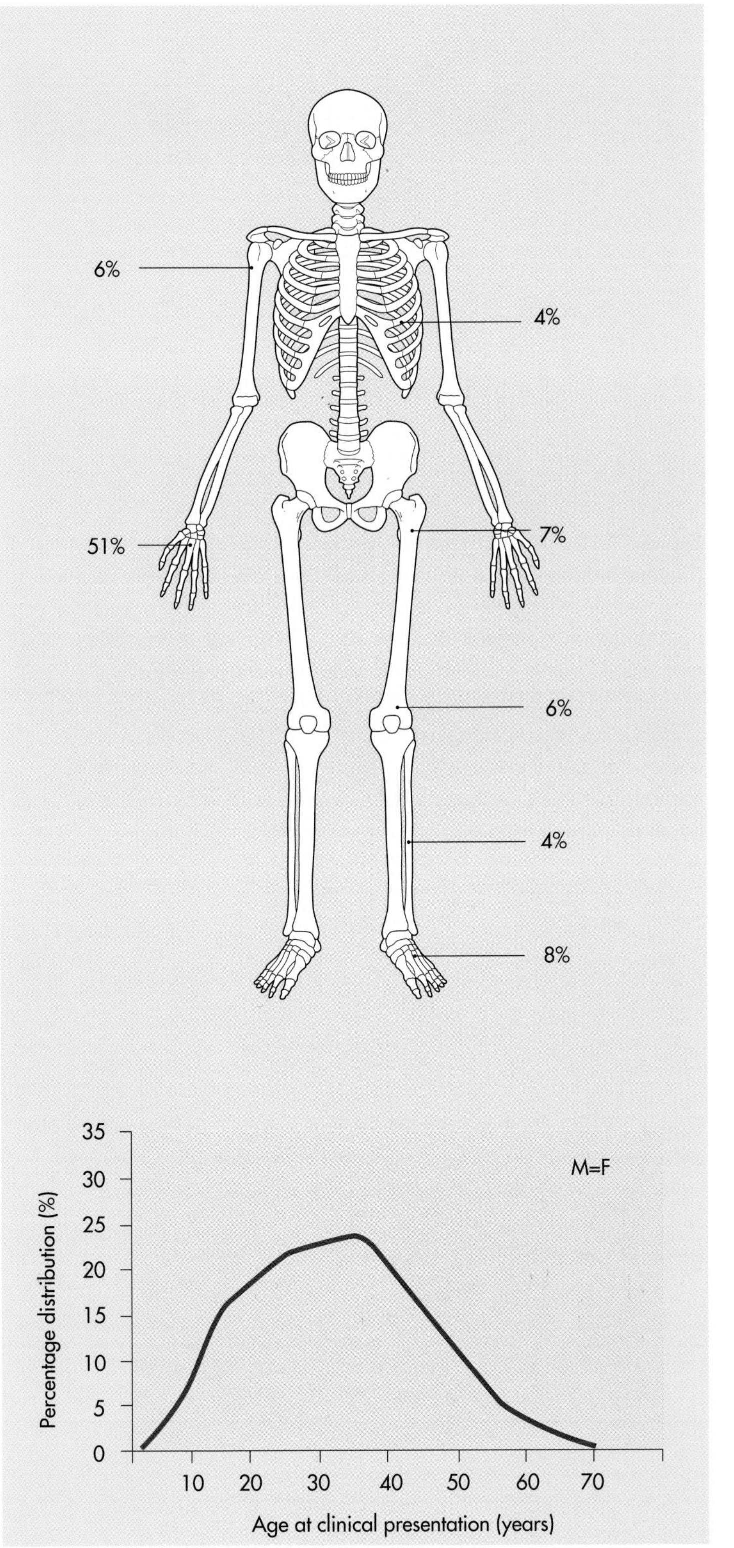

6%

4%

51%

7%

6%

4%

8%

35
30
25
20
15
10
5
0

M=F

Percentage distribution (%)

10 20 30 40 50 60 70

Age at clinical presentation (years)

Figure 17.16 Location and age distribution of solitary enchondroma.

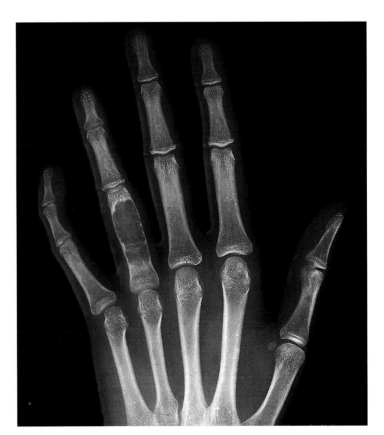

Figure 17.17 Radiograph of a hand shows a well-defined lytic lesion with small punctate calcifications in the proximal phalanx of the ring finger. This appearance is characteristic of enchondroma. At the proximal end of the lesion is a line of density, suggesting a fracture through the tumor.

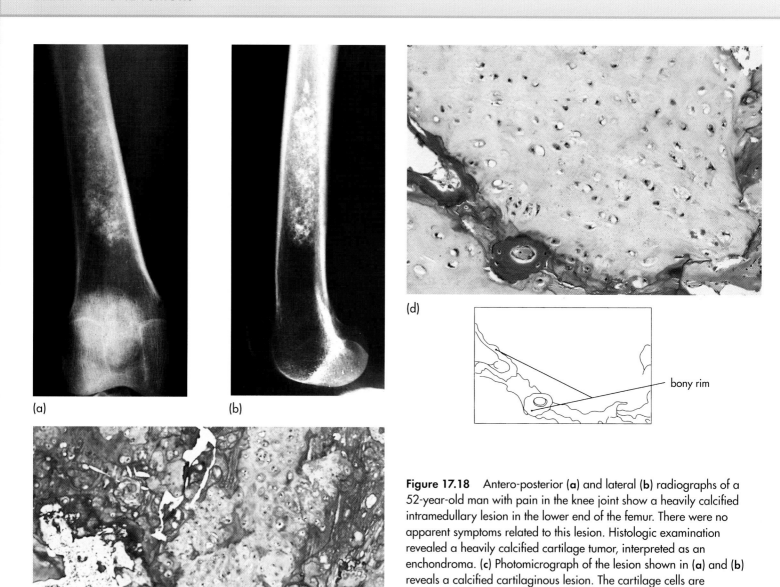

(a)   (b)

(d)

(c)

Figure 17.18   Antero-posterior (**a**) and lateral (**b**) radiographs of a 52-year-old man with pain in the knee joint show a heavily calcified intramedullary lesion in the lower end of the femur. There were no apparent symptoms related to this lesion. Histologic examination revealed a heavily calcified cartilage tumor, interpreted as an enchondroma. (**c**) Photomicrograph of the lesion shown in (**a**) and (**b**) reveals a calcified cartilaginous lesion. The cartilage cells are uncrowded and unremarkable (H&E, × 10 obj.). (**d**) Frequently in enchondroma, the cartilage lobules are surrounded by a narrow rim of bone, as shown in this photomicrograph (H&E, × 25 obj.).

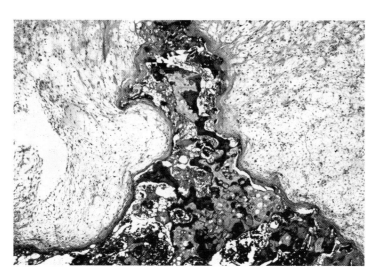

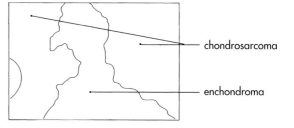

Figure 17.19   Photomicrograph to demonstrate the development of a chondrosarcoma in a patient with pre-existing enchondroma. In the lower center part of the photomicrograph, a heavily calcified enchondroma is apparent. In the upper left and right parts a cellular myxoid chondrosarcoma is present (H&E, × 4 obj.).

The examination of cross-sections of a large number of surgically removed femoral heads occasionally reveals small nodules of cartilage within the bone, which are usually less than 1 cm in diameter. Such nodules are perhaps best regarded as benign cartilage rests (Figs 17.20 and 17.21).

JUXTACORTICAL CHONDROMA (PERIOSTEAL CHONDROMA)

Juxtacortical chondroma is a benign cartilaginous lesion characterized by its location on the metaphyseal cortex of both long and short tubular bones. On radiographic examination a cup-shaped or scalloped cortical defect with a sclerotic margin is usually evident, and the lesion, which is rarely more than 3–4 cm in diameter, typically has overhanging edges (Fig. 17.22). On gross inspection, juxtacortical chondroma is a well-circumscribed lesion which is partially embedded in cortical bone and covered by the periosteum. Its cut surface is grayish-white or bluish and lobulated. When examined microscopically, proliferating chondrocytes show minimal pleomorphism and nuclear abnormalities. Focal calcification and ossification may occur within the cartilage (Fig. 17.23).

The treatment of a juxtacortical chondroma is en-bloc resection.

CHONDROBLASTOMA

Chondroblastoma is an uncommon, benign cellular neoplasm most often located in the epiphysis of long bones, and usually diagnosed in the patient's second decade of life. On rare occasions these lesions may occur in older individuals and in odd locations, such as the spine or a flat bone (Fig. 17.24).

The characteristic radiographic signs of chondroblastoma include a well-demarcated lucent defect with mottled calcifica-

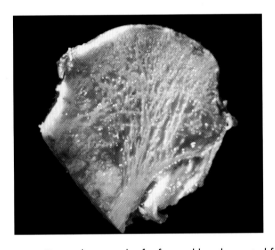

Figure 17.20 Gross photograph of a femoral head resected for osteoarthritis. A small cartilage rest is present in the neck of the femur. Note the glistening, lobulated, bluish-white appearance of the cartilaginous tissue.

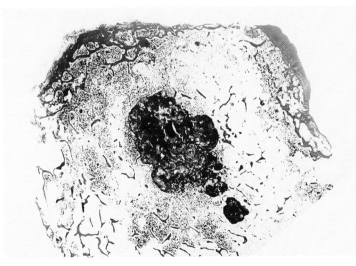

Figure 17.21 Photomicrograph of a section through a femoral head that contains a large multilobular cartilage rest (H&E, × 1 obj.).

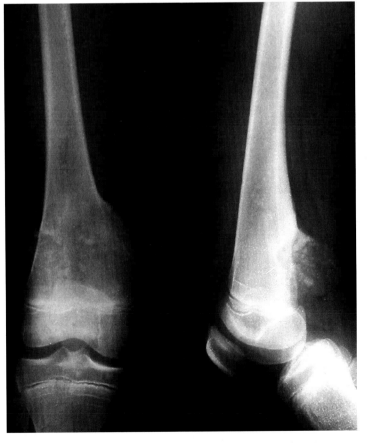

Figure 17.22 Antero-posterior and lateral radiographs of the lower femur of a young girl with a palpable mass behind the knee. This proved after resection to be a large juxtacortical chondroma.

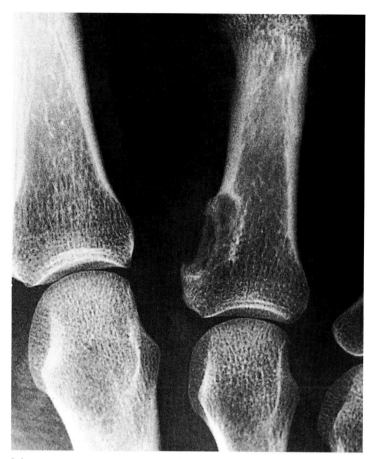

(a)

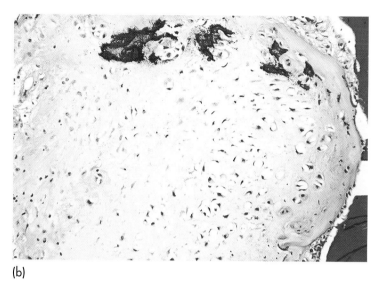

(b)

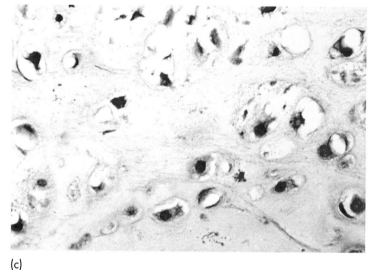

(c)

Figure 17.23   (a) Radiograph of a hand shows a well-defined saucer-like depression of the cortex at the proximal end of one phalanx. This radiographic picture is typical of a juxtacortical chondroma.
(b) Photomicrograph of the lesion illustrated in (a) shows a cellular and focally calcified benign cartilaginous lesion (H&E, × 4 obj.). (c) Higher magnification of (b) shows mild to moderate atypia (H&E, × 25 obj.).

tion, located in the epiphysis and sometimes extending into the metaphysis of long bones (Figs 17.25 and 17.26). The cortical bone may be intact or expanded. The lesion has a predilection for the upper end of the humerus, the upper and lower ends of the femur, and the upper end of the tibia, and in most cases the diagnosis can be made with some confidence from the radiographs because of the characteristic location and the patient's age.

Curettage generally produces a gritty, grayish-pink tissue (Fig. 17.27) which is characterized microscopically by round and ovoid cells, mixed with varying numbers of scattered giant cells. Focally, an intercellular chondroid matrix is produced in which a lace-like deposit of calcium granules is typically observed (so-called 'chicken-wire' calcification) (Figs 17.28–17.30).

In about 20% of cases, the lesions are cystic and hemorrhagic (cystic chondroblastoma). Since the majority of lesions may be cystic, inadequate sampling may give rise to a diagnosis of aneurysmal bone cyst. The presence of cartilage and giant cells in chondroblastomas may on occasion lead to diagnostic confu-

sion of the lesion with either chondrosarcoma or giant-cell tumors of bone. In typical cases of chondroblastoma the S-100 protein is strongly positive in the mononuclear cells though negative in the giant cells. In the presence of cystic changes however the S-100 protein is only focally positive in the mononuclear cells.

Curettage or local excision is the treatment of choice. In very rare cases, soft-tissue implants and/or lung metastases may occur; when present, they are usually rimmed with bone (Fig. 17.31). These implants or metastases should be surgically removed.

CHONDROMYXOID FIBROMA

Chondromyxoid fibroma is a very rare, benign bone neoplasm most often discovered during the patient's second or third decade of life. The lesion usually occurs eccentrically in the metaphysis of the lower femur or upper tibia, or in the short tubular bones of

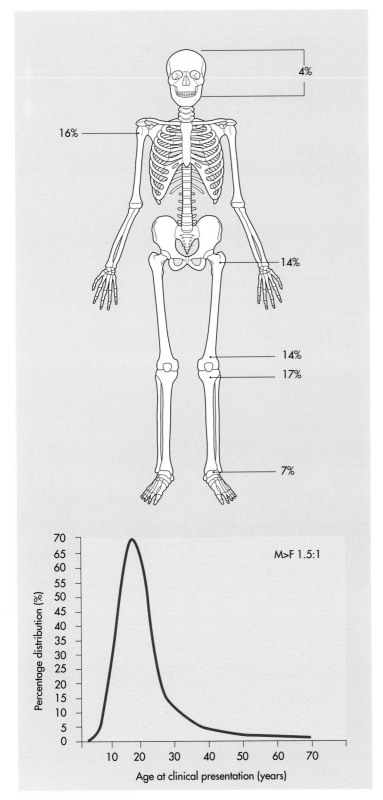

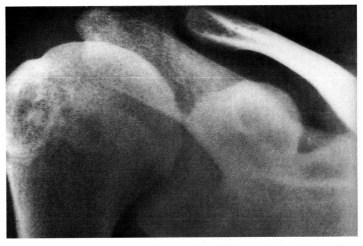

Figure 17.25 Radiograph of an 11-year-old boy with complaints of pain and limitation of motion in the right shoulder. An eccentric lytic lesion with patchy calcification involves the apophysis of the humerus laterally. Curettage of this lesion proved it to be a chondroblastoma. The radiographic appearance and location shown here are typical.

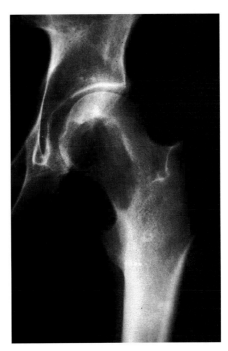

Figure 17.26 An antero-posterior radiograph of the left hip of a young woman with pain. An eccentric lytic lesion extends to the articular surface and into the neck of the femur.

Figure 17.24 Location and age distribution of chondroblastoma.

M>F 1.5:1

Percentage distribution (%)

Age at clinical presentation (years)

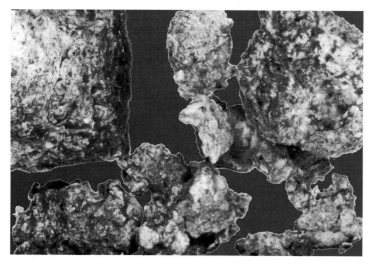

Figure 17.27   Photograph of a curetted chondroblastoma. Note the granular appearance and the clearly yellow calcified areas. (Courtesy of Dr Miguel Calvo.)

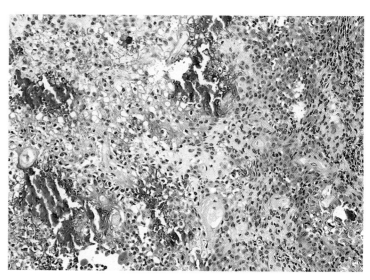

Figure 17.28   Photomicrograph of a chondroblastoma demonstrates the variegated appearance of this lesion. Cellular areas mixed with areas of cartilage matrix formation and calcification can be seen (H&E, × 10 obj.).

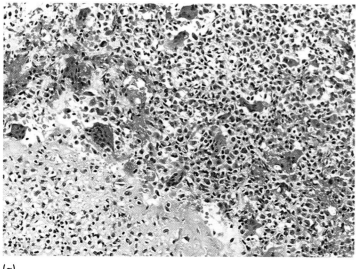

(a)

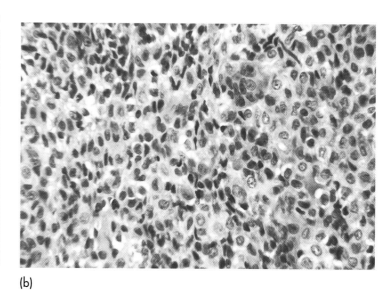

(b)

Figure 17.29   (a) Photomicrograph reveals the juxtaposition of an area of chondroid matrix on the lower left, with a more cellular area of polyhedral cells and admixed giant cells on the upper right (H&E, × 4 obj.). (b) Photomicrograph shows a higher magnification of the cellular area (H&E, × 25 obj.) and (c) of the matrix-producing area (H&E, × 25 obj.).

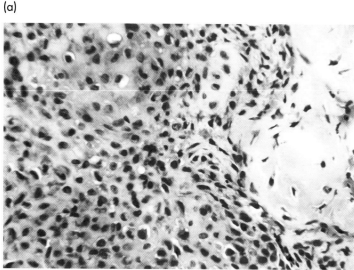

(c)

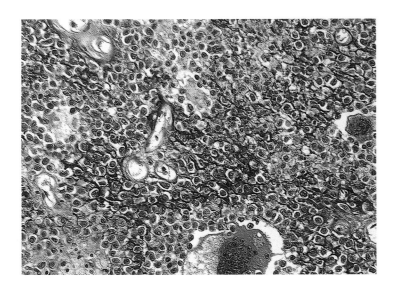

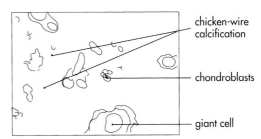

Figure 17.30   Fine stippled calcification is characteristic of chondroblastoma and frequently extends around the individual chondroblasts, producing a 'chicken-wire' appearance (H&E, × 25 obj.).

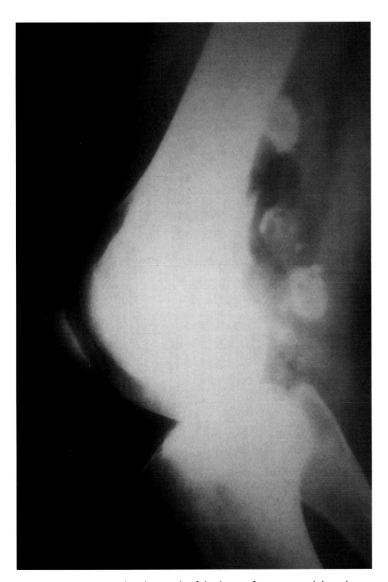

Figure 17.31   Lateral radiograph of the knee of a young adult male who, 18 months before, had had a curettage of a chondroblastoma of the lower femur. There are now three implanted nodules, which proved to be chondroblastoma in the popliteal space; each is surrounded by a rim of bone.

the foot, but it may occasionally develop in other bones (Fig. 17.32). Patients usually present with pain and/or local swelling.

On radiographs, the lesion is characterized by an eccentric well-demarcated lucent defect with a thin, well-defined scalloped border of sclerotic bone (Figs 17.33 and 17.34). [When imaging any cartilage-containing lesion, the bright signal which characterizes the T_2 image on magnetic resonance imaging (MRI) helps to differentiate these lesions from fibrous or cellular lesions.]

Inspection of intact gross specimens shows that the lesion is usually sharply demarcated and covered on its outer surface with a thin rim of bone or periosteum. Examination of the cut surface demonstrates a firm, lobulated, grayish-white mass, sometimes with small cystic foci and areas of hemorrhage.

On microscopic examination, chondromyxoid fibroma has a lobulated pattern, with sparsely cellular lobules alternating with more cellular zones. The sparsely cellular lobules show spindle and stellate cells without distinct cytoplasmic borders in a myxoid or chondroid matrix. Running between the lobules are fibroblastic septae of increased cellularity, with scattered multinucleated giant cells. Some nuclear pleomorphism may be evident but mitotic figures are rare (Fig. 17.35).

Because recurrence of the lesion after curettage is frequent, en-bloc excision is the preferred treatment.

The cells in the myxoid areas generally are weakly positive for the S-100 protein.

FIBROMYXOMA

Fibromyxoma is microscopically superficially similar to a chondromyxoid fibroma, but it is even more rare and occurs in older individuals. In addition, fibromyxoma lacks both the lobular pattern and the chondroid matrix that typify a chondromyxoid fibroma.

This lesion is so rare that no radiographic characteristics have been substantiated. The radiograph shown was thought to be of a giant-cell tumor (Fig. 17.36). However, histologic examination showed it to be of a fibromyxoma. Follow-up of the few cases described in the literature has revealed no instances of local recurrence or metastases.

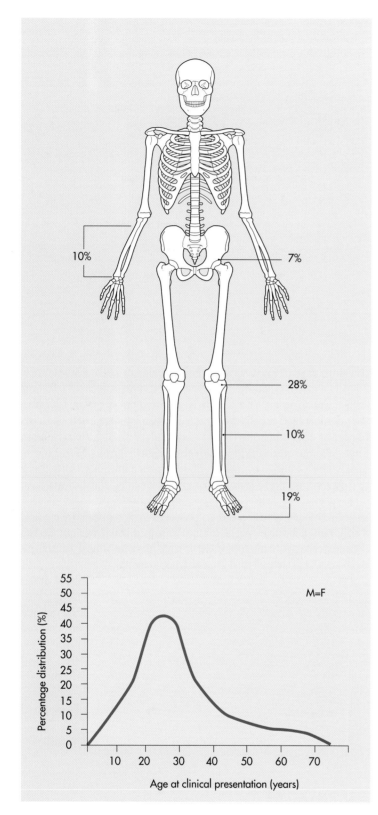

10%

7%

28%

10%

19%

M=F

Percentage distribution (%)

55
50
45
40
35
30
25
20
15
10
5
0

10   20   30   40   50   60   70

Age at clinical presentation (years)

Figure 17.32   Location and age distribution of chondromyxoid fibroma.

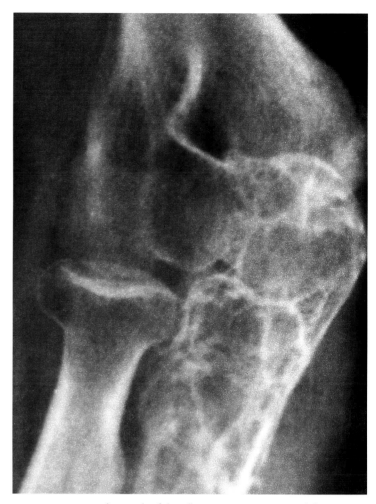

Figure 17.33   Radiograph of the elbow joint in a young adult man who complained of pain shows a well-defined, trabeculated lytic lesion with cortical thinning but no obvious soft-tissue extension. This soap-bubble appearance is typical of chondromyxoid fibromas, although these lesions are so rare that the diagnosis is usually not made until after histologic examination.

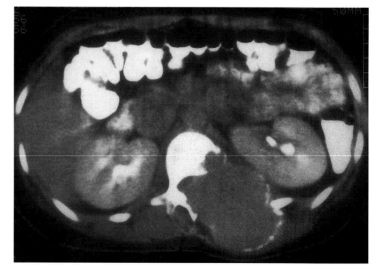

Figure 17.34   Computed axial tomogram through the lumbar region of a young woman who presented clinically with weakness in the right leg. It shows an expanded lesion involving both the posterior elements and the vertebral body. On biopsy, this lesion proved to be a chondromyxoid fibroma. (Courtesy of Dr Julius Smith.)

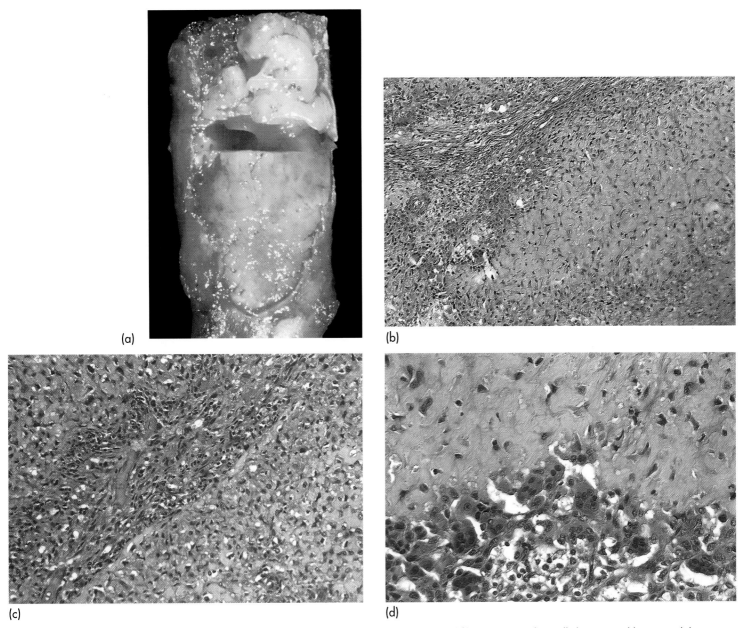

(a)

(b)

(c)

(d)

Figure 17.35   (a) Gross photograph of a segment of resected fibula with a chondromyxoid fibroma. Note the well-demarcated lesion and the glistening fleshy appearance. (b) Photomicrograph of a chondromyxoid fibroma shows the typical lobulated and variegated appearance of this lesion. Lobules of chondromyxoid tissue and septa of cellular fibrous tissue are evident, with occasional multinucleated giant cells running between the lobules (H&E, × 10 obj.). (c) Higher power view of another field of the same tumor (H&E, × 20 obj.). (d) Another view to demonstrate a layer of osteoclasts eroding the chondroid area of the tumor (H&E, × 25 obj.).

MALIGNANT TUMORS

INTRAMEDULLARY CHONDROSARCOMA

Chondrosarcoma is a malignant neoplasm with cells that produce cartilage matrix. Bone matrix made by the malignant cells is not present in chondrosarcoma, although on occasion there may be foci of benign reactive bone. Chondrosarcoma is characteristically seen in adults in their fifth and sixth decades of life (Fig. 17.37). Clinically, it occurs most frequently in the pelvis and in the medullary cavity of the femur, humerus, and ribs (Figs 17.38 and 17.39). Patients initially complain of persistent mild pain and often of local swelling.

On radiography, chondrosarcomas in the long bones are located in the metaphysis and often extend into the diaphysis to produce a fusiform, lucent defect with a scalloped inner cortex. Thickening and inequality of the cortex are common radiographic findings and, when associated with pain, help to distinguish a chondrosarcoma from an enchondroma. Extension into the soft tissue should be looked for. Frequent punctate or stippled

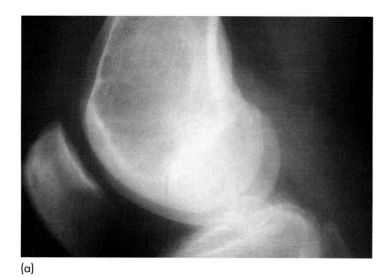

(a)

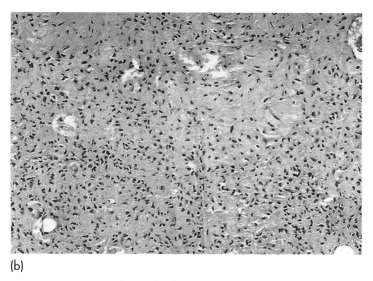

(b)

Figure 17.36   (a) Radiograph of the lower end of the femur in a 38-year-old man who complained of pain in the knee joint. A lytic destructive lesion involves both the epiphysis and the metaphysis of the femur; radiographically, this lesion is most consistent with a giant-cell tumor. (b) Photomicrograph of the lesion shown in (a) shows loose fibromyxomatous tissue without lobulation and without obvious chondroid areas. A few such cases have been reported, usually in older people, and these lesions have been designated as fibromyxomas (H&E, × 10 obj.).

Figure 17.37   Location and age distribution of chondrosarcoma.

calcifications are characteristic (Fig. 17.40). Occasionally, extensive calcification may give rise to the radiologic confusion of chondrosarcoma with a bone infarct. MRI will show a characteristic bright signal on T_2 images and is most helpful in showing the extent of the tumor.

Grossly, chondrosarcomas are lobulated, grayish-white or blue, focally calcified masses, often with areas of mucoid degeneration or necrosis.

Microscopically chondrosarcomas are graded into three groups:

1. Grade I: low-grade chondrosarcomas are cytologically so similar to enchondromas that the diagnosis is mostly dependent on the clinical and radiologic presentation, and on the location. Pain, cortical thickening and possible soft-tissue extension are important findings. Lesions located in the pelvis, scapula or

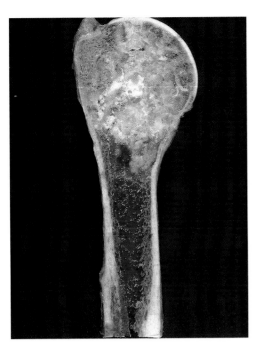

Figure 17.38
Gross photograph
of a central
chondrosarcoma
arising from the
medullary cavity of a
humerus. Although
much of the lesion
appears like calcified
cartilage at the distal
margin, it is much
more fleshy.

3. Grade III: high-grade chondrosarcomas are comparatively rare. They are characterized by marked cellular atypia, hypercellularity and high mitotic activity. They are generally rapidly growing, aggressive and frequently metastasize. They have an aneuploid pattern on flow cytometry and show complex aberrations on chromosomal analysis (Figure 17.41–17.44).

It is generally true that lesions in the axial skeleton and proximal portions of the appendicular skeleton are more likely to pursue a malignant course than tumors in the distal skeleton. [However, it is important to recognize that on rare occasions chondrosarcomas may arise in the digits (Fig. 17.45).] Furthermore, infiltration of the marrow spaces occurs in chondrosarcomas, so that trabeculae of normal bone may be found embedded in the tumor. In assessment of low-grade chondrosarcomas, this microscopic finding is most helpful in distinguishing the lesion from an enchondroma (Fig. 17.46).

The clinical course of chondrosarcoma depends on several factors. In general, well-differentiated tumors rarely metastasize, but they recur locally after incomplete excision. Anaplastic, fully malignant tumors metastasize early, primarily to the lung. Grade II chondrosarcoma may metastasize in about 10–15% of cases. Complete surgical excision of the tumor is the treatment of choice. (Cartilage lesions do not usually respond to chemotherapy or radiation therapy.)

About 10% of all chondrosarcomas undergo dedifferentiation in one area or another and become highly malignant sarcomas with spindle cells and bizarre giant cells [features of fibrosarcoma or malignant fibrous histiocytoma (Fig. 17.47)]. These dedifferentiated tumors carry a poor prognosis and often metastasize widely, the metastases frequently showing only the spindle-cell component of the tumor. Radiographs in such a case may reveal

ribs in general behave aggressively. Microscopic evidence of invasion of the haversian canals or of the medullary space with embedded fragments of trabecular bone is the most helpful finding in making the distinction from a benign enchondroma.

2. Grade II chondrosarcomas show a definite increased cellularity with increased nuclear size and distinct nucleoli in many of the cells. Binucleate cells are common. Focal myxoid change is a frequent occurrence.

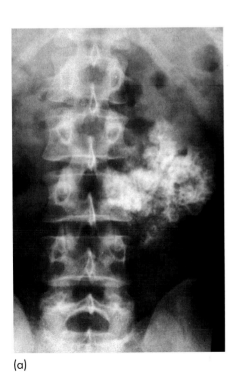

(a)

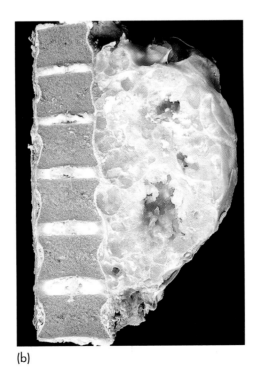

(b)

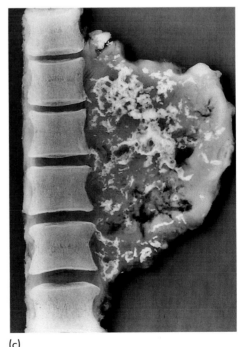

(c)

Figure 17.39   (a) In this radiograph a large calcified mass is present adjacent to the lumbar spine. This lesion proved to be a low-grade chondrosarcoma. (b) Gross photograph of the lesion. (c) Radiograph of the specimen shown in (b) demonstrates irregular areas of calcification.

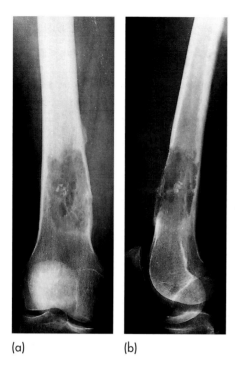

(a)   (b)

Figure 17.40   Antero-posterior (**a**) and lateral (**b**) radiographs of the lower femur in a 50-year-old man complaining of acute onset of pain. The margin of the lesion is fairly well defined and thinning of the cortex gives rise to a trabeculated appearance. Soft-tissue extension of the tumor is evident anteriorly and medially, showing that this is a malignant tumor. In the center of the lesion, small foci of punctate calcifications are apparent, consistent with a diagnosis of a cartilage tumor.

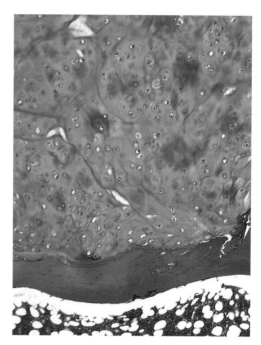

Figure 17.41 Photomicrograph of a low-grade chondrosarcoma. The chondrocytes though somewhat crowded, are not particularly atypical. (H&E, × 4 obj.).

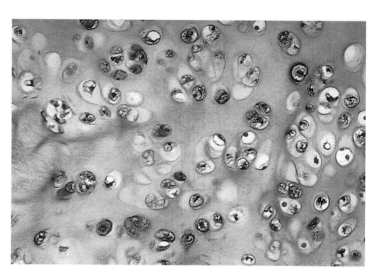

Figure 17.43   Photomicrograph of a malignant, grade II chondrosarcoma shows cellular atypia and crowding (H&E, × 40 obj.).

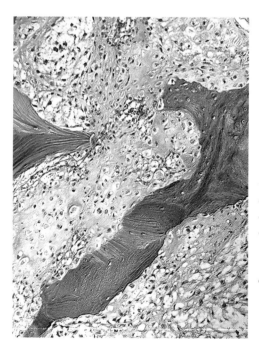

Figure 17.42   In a chondrosarcoma, the hallmark of the lesion is that the tumor invades between the bone spicules, as illustrated here. In addition, when compared with the low-grade lesion, there is much more crowding and atypicality of the chondrocytes indicating a grade II lesion. (H&E, × 10 obj.).

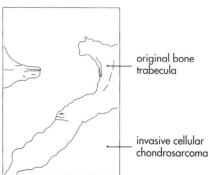

original bone trabecula

invasive cellular chondrosarcoma

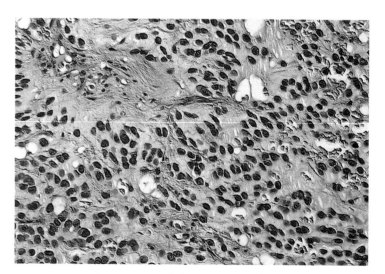

Figure 17.44   Photomicrograph from an area within a grade III chondrosarcoma that exhibits crowded round cells in a myxoid matrix (H&E, × 10 obj.).

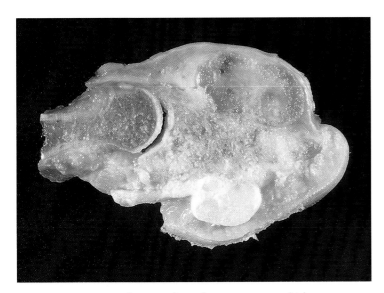

Figure 17.45 Sagittal section through a great toe in which a chondrosarcoma of the distal phalanx has extensively grown out into the surrounding soft tissues. Microscopically, this proved to be a high-grade tumor.

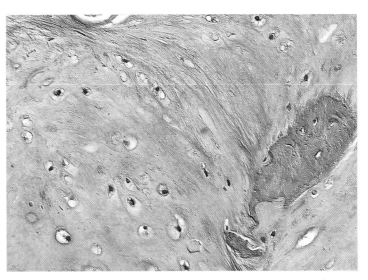

Figure 17.46 Photomicrograph taken from a low-grade chondrosarcoma illustrating the invasive quality of the lesion, with islands of mature lamellar bone embedded within the cartilaginous tumor tissue. From its cellularity, the cartilage gives no obvious evidence of malignancy in this field (H&E, × 40 obj.).

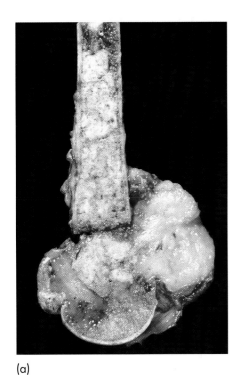

(a)

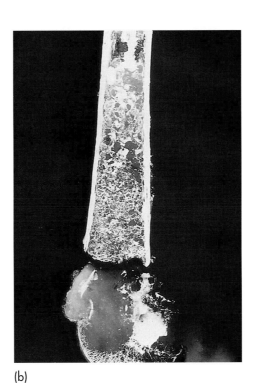

(b)

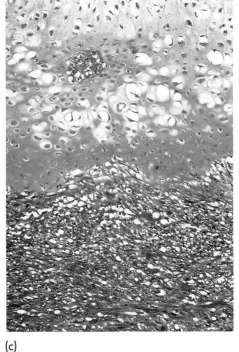

(c)

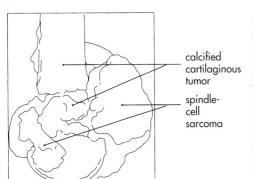

calcified cartilaginous tumor

spindle-cell sarcoma

Figure 17.47 (a) Gross photograph of the lower end of a femur removed from a patient with a longstanding cartilaginous tumor that had recently begun to grow rapidly. The transected specimen exhibits a lobulated bluish-gray tissue filling the medullary cavity of the bone. However, at the lower end of the femur, filling the medulla and extending to the soft tissue, a fleshy yellow–tan tumor can be seen. This area proved to be a malignant spindle-cell tumor. (b) Specimen radiograph of the dedifferentiated chondrosarcoma shown in (a). Although the cartilaginous portion of the tumor is heavily calcified, the dedifferentiated spindle-cell component is entirely radiolucent. (c) Photomicrograph of the dedifferentiated spindle-cell tumor that developed in the chondrosarcoma illustrated in (a) and (b). The spindle-cell tumor has the pattern of a malignant fibrous histiocytoma and is seen here abutting the chondrosarcoma (H&E, × 10 obj.).

a poorly defined and destructive lucent zone in an otherwise typical chondrosarcoma with stippled calcification.

MESENCHYMAL CHONDROSARCOMA

Mesenchymal chondrosarcoma is a very rare, malignant bone tumor which has been seen most commonly in individuals in the second and third decades of life. Almost any bone may be affected, although there is a reported predilection for the maxilla, mandible and ribs. Approximately one-third of the lesions have been found in soft tissue. Patients may experience pain and/or swelling.

An ill-defined osteolytic lesion with irregular calcification may be noted on radiographs, and this radiologic appearance corresponds to the grayish-white or yellow tumor mass with evident foci of cartilage and calcification found on gross examination. On microscopic examination, the characteristic feature of these lesions is a biphasic pattern. The majority of the tumor is composed of small, uniform, round- to spindle-shaped cells that resemble those of Ewing's tumor with a perivascular arrangement of cells which results in a hemangiopericytoma pattern of the cellular component. There are focal admixed areas of a cartilaginous or chondroid matrix arranged in a lobular pattern (Fig. 17.48). Reciprocal translocation (11:33)(q24:q12) has been

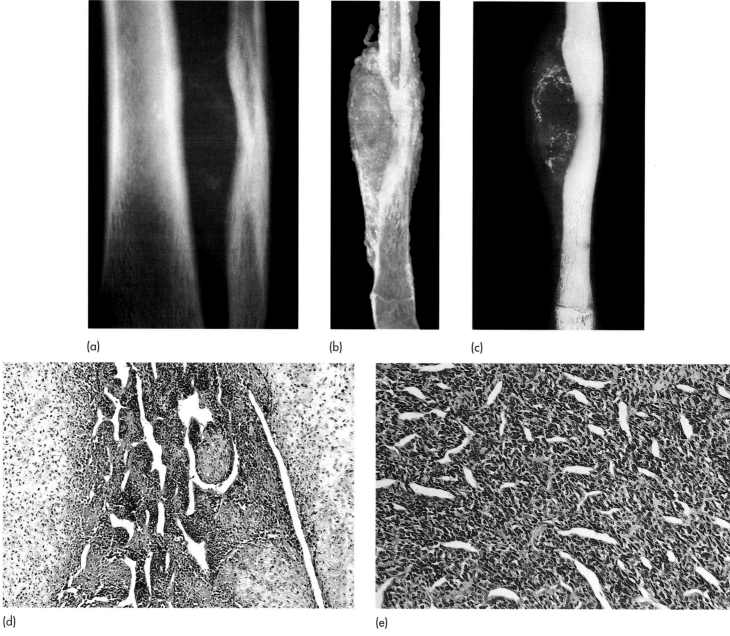

(a)   (b)   (c)

(d)   (e)

Figure 17.48   (a) Clinical radiograph of a young man who presented with leg pain and swelling. A soft-tissue mass is eroding the adjacent bone between the fibula and tibia. Focal calcification is evident within the tumor mass. In this case, the differential diagnosis would have to include synovial sarcoma. (b) Gross photograph of the resected specimen from the patient in (a) shows a soft-tissue tumor eroding the cortex of the adjacent fibula. (c) Specimen radiograph of the lesion shown in (b). Focal calcification is seen, particularly at the periphery of the lesion. (d) Photomicrograph of a portion of a mesenchymal chondrosarcoma showing nodules of cellular chondroid tissue on either side and between a vascular cellular tumor (H&E, × 4 obj.). (e) Higher power photomicrograph of the cellular vascular component shown in (d). Note the small closely packed spindle cells surrounding the vascular spaces and resembling the pattern of a hemangiopericytoma (H&E, × 40 obj.).

reported in the small cell component. The S-100 protein is found only in the cartilaginous components of the tumor.

Mesenchymal chondrosarcoma metastasizes primarily to the lungs, but osseous and soft-tissue metastases have been documented.

CLEAR-CELL CHONDROSARCOMA

Clear-cell chondrosarcoma (considered by some to represent an aggressive variant of chondroblastoma), is a destructive low-grade malignant tumor which presents most commonly in young adults, predominantly males. It was originally thought to only affect the epiphyseal ends of long bones, most often the upper femur. However, as these lesions have become more commonly recognized, it has become clear that by no means are all clear-cell chondrosarcomas located in the epiphysis or in the upper femur.

On radiographs, these tumors are well-circumscribed mixed lucent and sclerotic defects, often with a thin sclerotic border (Figs 17.49 and 17.50) and scattered calcification. When located in the epiphysis, they are most likely to be diagnosed radiologically as chondroblastomas or giant-cell tumors.

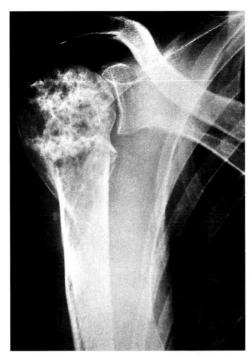

Figure 17.49 Radiograph of a 35-year-old man with a 7-year history of pain in the right shoulder. The patient was seen because of acute pain secondary to a pathologic fracture. There is extensive replacement of the cancellous bone by a calcified tumor which is extending to the articular surface and which proved to be a clear-cell chondrosarcoma. (Courtesy of Dr Takeo Matsuno.)

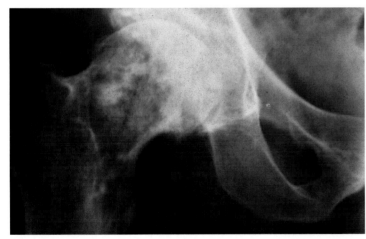

(a)

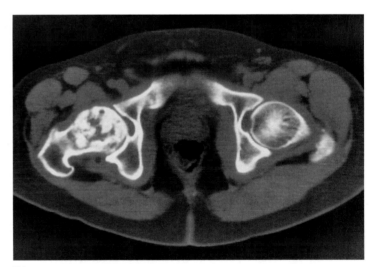

(b)

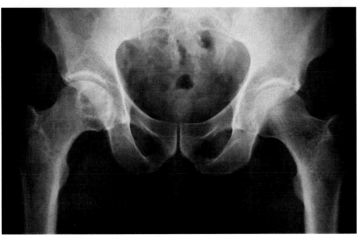

(c)

Figure 17.50 (a) Radiograph of the right hip in a middle-aged man with a long-term history of pain in the hip, who recently developed acute pain due to pathologic fracture. A heavily calcified tumor involves a good deal of the femoral head and neck. No soft-tissue extension is evident. (b) Computerized axial tomogram through the body of the lesion illustrated in (a) demonstrates the focal character of the calcification within the lesion. (c) Radiograph of the pelvis of the patient shown in (a) and (b), taken 13 years previously, shows a clearly defined lytic lesion which is mostly confined to the right capital femoral epiphysis. When this was eventually excised, it proved to be a clear-cell chondrosarcoma.

On histologic examination, a clear-cell chondrosarcoma contains many cells with abundant clear, vacuolated cytoplasm rich in periodic acid–Schiff (PAS)-positive glycogen, which often lie between heavily calcified trabeculae of cartilage matrix that may superficially resemble bone. Frequently, scattered giant cells are seen and, between the cells, a scant chondroid matrix (Fig. 17.51). The vacuolated clear cells may suggest a renal-cell carcinoma, but the scattered giant cells and the scant chondroid matrix should help to differentiate the two lesions. The cells of clear-cell chondrosarcoma are strongly positive for the S-100 protein.

Clear-cell chondrosarcomas are locally aggressive, and metastases have been reported.

CHORDOMA

Chordoma, though it may have a superficial similarity to a cartilage lesion, is a neoplasm that arises from remnants of the notochord, and therefore in almost all cases it occurs in the midline of the axial skeleton. About half the cases occur in the sacrococcygeal region, whereas one-third are present at the base of the skull. The remaining cases arise at different sites along the vertebral column, most commonly in the cervical region. Chordoma is a slow-growing neoplasm, causing clinical symptoms which depend on its location. (Cranial lesions usually are smaller than sacrococcygeal lesions at the time of initial presentation.) Males are more frequently affected than females; the average age at diagnosis for sacral lesions is approximately 55 years and for spheno-occipital lesions somewhat younger (Fig. 17.52).

Bone destruction is the radiographic hallmark of chordoma; about half of the patients exhibit focal calcifications within the lesion (Fig. 17.53). Localization of the lesion is greatly aided by the use of MRI, particularly in cases of intracranial chordoma (Fig. 17.54). When chordomas affect areas of the spine other than the two common sites (i.e. sacrococcygeal and cervical), the lesions are likely to be lytic, located centrally within the vertebral body, and slowly expansile (Fig. 17.55). When the cervical vertebrae are affected, extension anteriorly into the soft tissues may result in dysphagia (Fig. 17.56), whereas posterior extension may lead to neurologic complications. Systemic metastases to the regional lymph nodes, lung, liver, and bone have been reported in about half the cases.

On examination, chordomas are generally soft and appear to be well encapsulated. Lobulations are apparent on cut section, and the tumor usually has a bluish-gray color with extensive gelatinous translucent areas which are focally cystic and hemorrhagic (Fig. 17.57). Grossly, the tissue may suggest a chondrosarcoma or even a mucinous carcinoma.

Microscopic examination reveals a characteristic arrangement of tumor cells separated into lobules by fibrous septa of different thicknesses. The tumor cells are of various sizes and shapes, arranged in both cords and sheets, with an eosinophilic cytoplasm associated with both extracellular and intracellular mucin that may be minimal or abundant. The vacuoles may be very prominent and thus may displace the nucleus to one edge, producing the so-called physaliphorous cell (Fig. 17.58). The tumor cells express both the S-100 protein and epithelial markers.

Approximately one-third of spheno-occipital chordomas contain a significant chondroid component, and these lesions can easily be confused with chondrosarcomas, especially with chondrosarcomas having a predominantly myxoid structure (Fig. 17.59). Rarely, an associated malignant mesenchymal tumor has

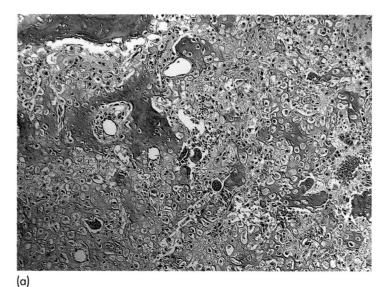

(a)

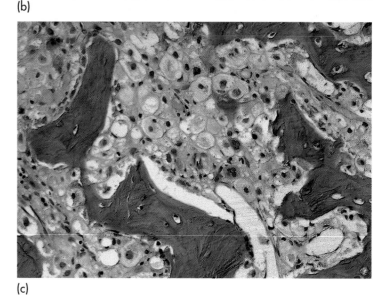

(b)

(c)

Figure 17.51   Photomicrographs at low (a) and intermediate (b) magnification demonstrating the typical histology of a clear-cell chondrosarcoma. Note the crowded vacuolated cells, with minimal cartilage matrix between them and scattered giant cells and foci of bone embedded within the lesional tissue (H&E, × 10 and × 25 obj.).
(c) Higher power photomicrograph from a clear-cell chondrosarcoma shows the clear vacuolated cytoplasm of the tumor cells typical of the lesion, together with occasional giant cells (H&E, × 25 obj.).

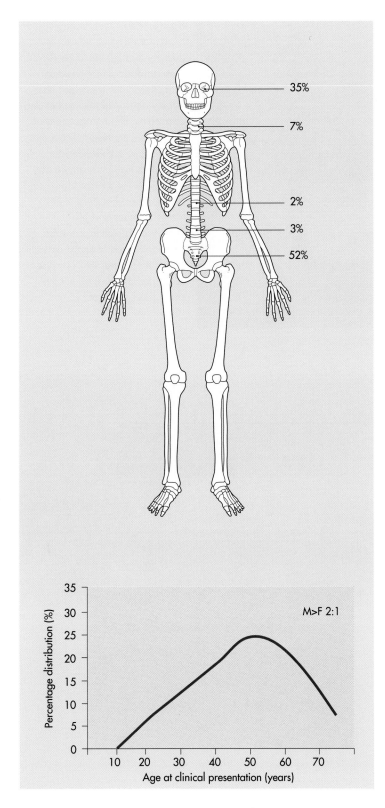

Figure 17.52   Location and age distribution of chordoma.

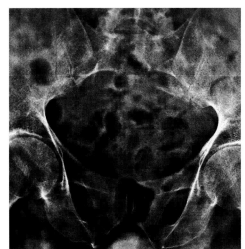

Figure 17.53
Radiograph of a 60-year-old man who complained of pain in the coccygeal region reveals destruction of the sacrum and the coccyx by a large, lytic, expansile lesion, which on biopsy proved to be a chordoma.

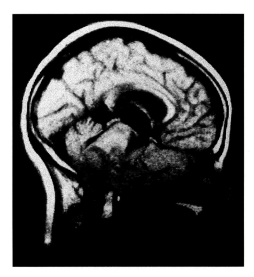

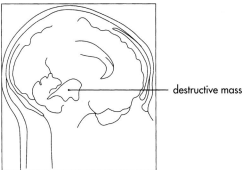

destructive mass

Figure 17.54   A sagittal spin–echo MRI shows a large mass filling the nasal cavity and ethmoid sinus anteriorly. It has obliterated the nasopharynx, extending inferiorly into the hypopharynx. Rostral to the odontoid process, it extends into the cranial cavity, completely destroying the clivus. It has invaded or displaced the brainstem, extending directly to the anterior aspect of the fourth ventricle.

been described in association with a chordoma, either a malignant fibrous histiocytoma or another poorly differentiated sarcoma; at least some of these cases have been associated with a history of radiation therapy.

On occasion a large notochordal rest in a vertebral body may be discovered as an incidental finding on MRI. In such a case the differentiation from a chordoma may be a problem, though in a chordoma there is generally a lytic lesion seen on radiographic imaging, whereas this is not the case with the notochordal rests which have been reported.

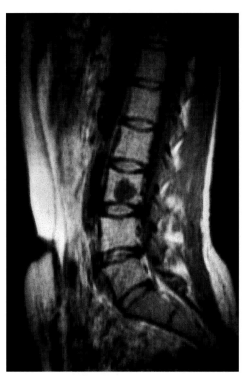

Figure 17.55 MR T$_1$-weighted image, demonstrating a large defect in the body of L3, which was not visible on the plain radiograph. Biopsy revealed tissue consistent with a chordoma (S-100 and cytokeratin positive) which would be regarded now by most as a large notochordal rest. (Courtesy of Dr German Steiner.)

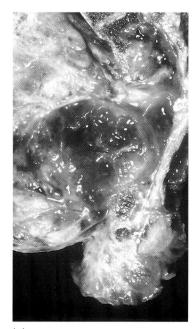

(a)

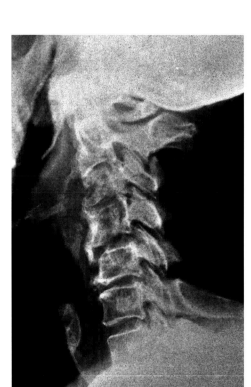

Figure 17.56 Lateral radiograph of a 40-year-old male who presented with dysphagia and myelopathy. There is a destructive lesion involving C3 and C4, with an anterior soft tissue extension which partially occludes the airway.

Figure 17.57 (a) Photograph of a sagittal section obtained at autopsy through the lower lumbar spine and sacrum of a patient with chordoma. The tumor has largely destroyed the sacrum and is involving L5. A large anterior component is present. The tumor tissue shows a characteristic lobulated, firm blue–gray tissue mass, with focal hemorrhage and cystification. (Courtesy of Dr Mario Campanacci.) (b) Photomicrograph to show the nests and cords of tumor cells with abundant eosinophilic cytoplasm separated by lakes of mucoid tissue (H&E, × 10 obj.).

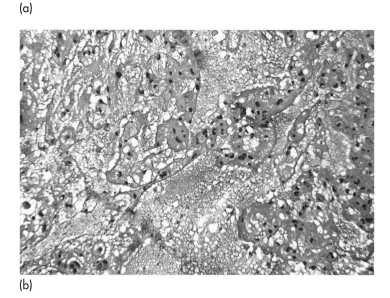

(b)

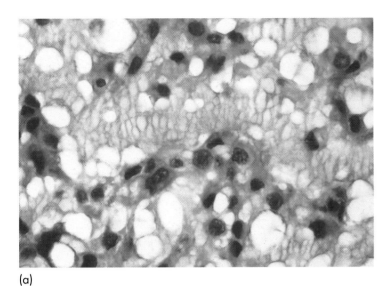

(a)

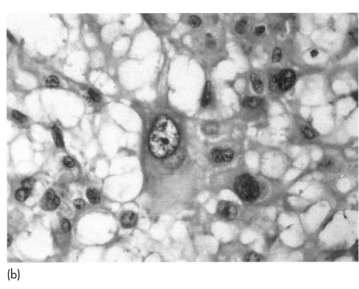

(b)

Figure 17.58   (a) In some areas of chordoma, large mucoid foci are present; in these mucoid areas, cords of eosinophilic cells may be present (as in this photomicrograph) (H&E, × 40 obj.).
(b) Photomicrograph shows the large variegated and vacuolated cells characteristic of chordoma (physaliphorous cells) (H&E, × 40 obj.).

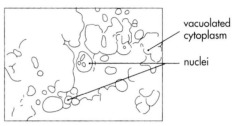

vacuolated
cytoplasm

nuclei

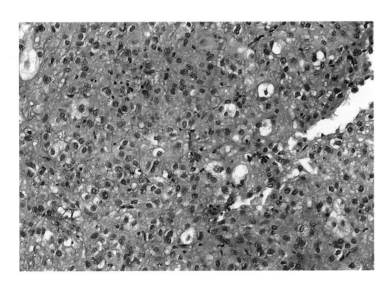

Figure 17.59   In some patients with chordomas arising in the area of the clivus, the tumor has a distinctly chondroid appearance (as in this photomicrograph). This chondroid pattern is important to recognize, since the prognosis for patients with chondroid chordomas in the base of the skull is believed to be better than for patients with a conventional pattern of chordoma in that area (H&E, × 10 obj.).

Chapter 18

FIBER-FORMING TUMORS AND TUMOR-LIKE CONDITIONS

In this chapter, both those tumor-like conditions and neoplasms in which there is a collagenous extracellular matrix of a simple fibrous character are considered.

REACTIVE OR POST-TRAUMATIC TUMORS

PERIOSTEAL 'DESMOID' TUMORS

Periosteal desmoid is a fairly common periosteal fibrous lesion that most commonly affects boys in the first 2 decades of life. It arises on the postero-medial aspect of the lower metaphysis of the femur. Radiographic examination reveals erosion of the cortex, with a sclerotic base. Periosteal desmoids are composed microscopically of dense collagenized tissue with uniform, unremarkable fibroblasts and reactive bone formation (Fig. 18.1).

The lesion almost certainly occurs as the result of previous trauma. It is characteristic in location and does not warrant a biopsy.

DEVELOPMENTAL OR HAMARTOMATOUS TUMORS

NONOSSIFYING FIBROMA (FIBROUS CORTICAL DEFECT; BENIGN FIBROUS HISTIOCYTOMA)

A nonossifying fibroma is a very common benign, well-circumscribed, eccentric, solitary (but occasionally, multiple) lesion in the metaphysis of a long bone of a child. Most commonly the femur or tibia is involved. These lesions usually regress spontaneously (Fig. 18.2).

Radiologic surveys have shown a 35% incidence of fibrous cortical defects in normal children. Most clinical cases are detected as incidental findings on radiographic examination, although occasionally a pathologic fracture through a large lesion causes the patient to seek medical attention (Fig. 18.3). The lesions range in size from a few millimeters to several centimeters and are characterized on radiographs by their cortical, eccentric location, as well as by their well-demarcated central lucent zones surrounded by scalloped sclerotic margins (Figs 18.4 and 18.5). Often a nonossifying fibroma is elongated in the longitudinal axis of the bone. Serial radiographs have demonstrated the migration of the defect away from the epiphyseal plate with time. As the lesions regress the affected area often shows residual sclerosis (Fig. 18.6).

Gross inspection of surgical curetting reveals the lesions to be formed of soft, somewhat friable yellow or brown tissue (Fig. 18.7). The microscopic findings include a cellular tissue of unremarkable spindle cells arranged in an interlacing, whorled pattern and interspersed with multinucleated giant cells and foamy, pale histiocytes. Hemosiderin deposits and scattered lymphocytes are characteristic features (Fig. 18.8). The microscopic features may on occasion cause diagnostic confusion of a nonossifying fibroma with other giant-cell-containing lesions. However, the clinical and radiographic presentation of nonossifying fibroma is so typical that it should rarely be confused with anything else.

Although the vast majority of cases of nonossifying fibroma occur in children, very rarely lesions that are histologically indistinguishable from them may be seen in adults. (In adults, such a lesion is often reported as a benign fibrous histiocytoma or a fibroxanthoma.) Radiographically, the lesions differ from those seen in children by having less distinct borders and being central rather than eccentric; they may either be lucent or more scle-

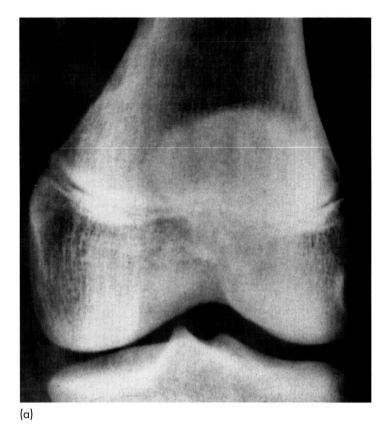

(a)

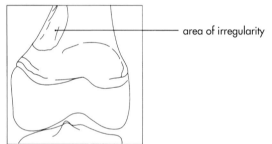

area of irregularity

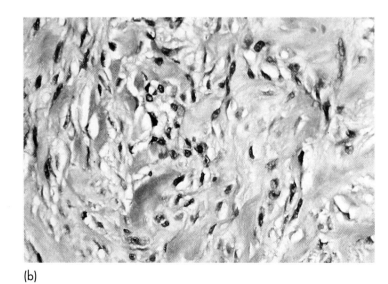

(b)

Figure 18.1 (a) A scalloped periosteal defect with a sclerotic base in the medial metaphysis of the femur is the characteristic radiographic appearance of a periosteal desmoid tumor, a benign lesion, possibly post-traumatic. (b) Photomicrograph of the dense fibrous tissue removed from the lesion illustrated in (a). Abundant collagen production by poorly organized but unremarkable fibroblasts has occurred (H&E, × 25 obj.).

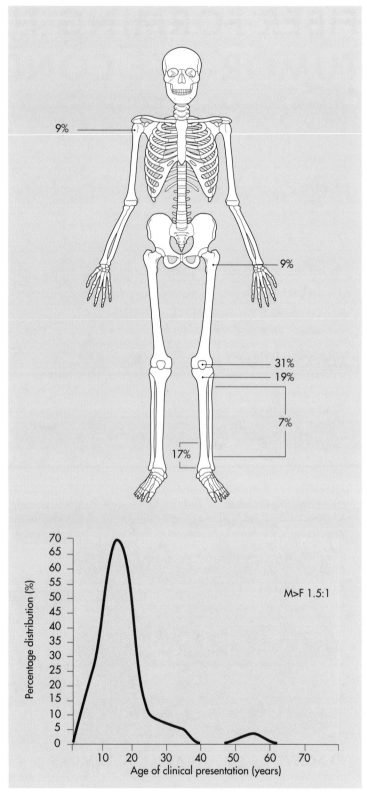

Figure 18.2 Location and age distribution of nonossifying fibroma.

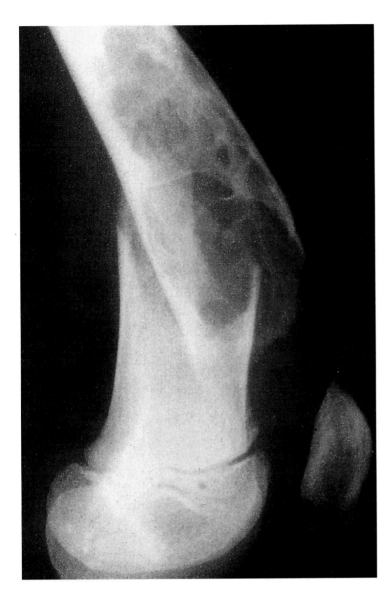

Figure 18.3   Radiograph showing a pathologic fracture through a large trabeculated lytic lesion of the lower femoral diaphysis, which proved on biopsy to be a nonossifying fibroma. Such a lesion may, because of subimposed fracture callus, be overdiagnosed as a malignancy.

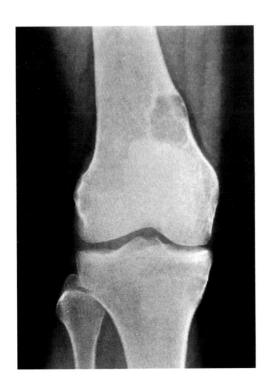

(a)

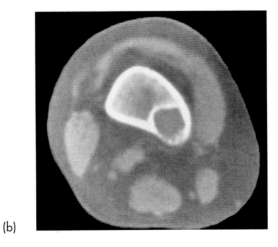

(b)

Figure 18.4   (a) Radiograph showing a typical nonossifying fibroma eccentrically located in the lower femoral metaphysis. (b) Computerized axial tomogram through the lesion demonstrated in (a) emphasizes the sclerotic margin.

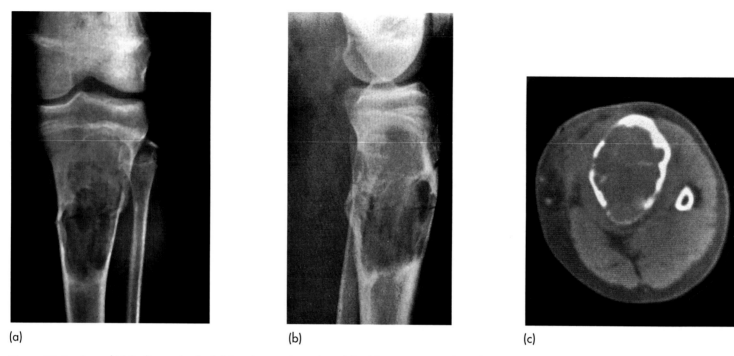

(a)   (b)   (c)

Figure 18.5   (a and b) Radiograph of a left leg shows a large lytic defect due to a nonossifying fibroma involving the upper end of the tibia. A pathological fracture through the lesion has occurred. (c) Computerized axial tomogram of the lesion shown in (a).

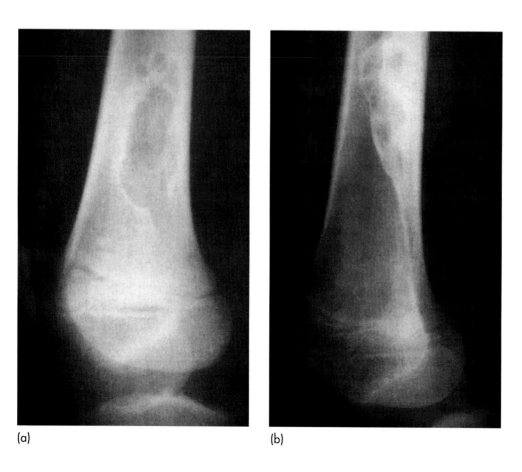

(a)   (b)

Figure 18.6   In this pair of radiographs, the healing of a nonossifying fibroma (a) has occurred 3 years later without any treatment (b).

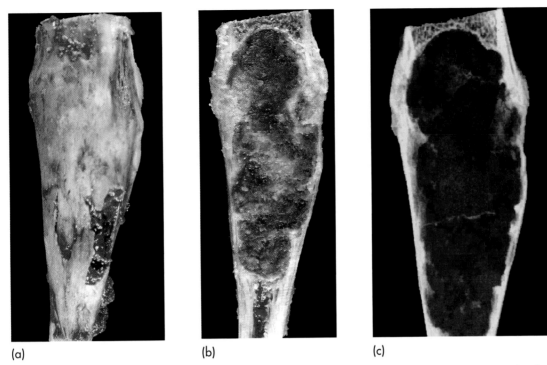

(a)   (b)   (c)

Figure 18.7   (a) Gross photograph of a resected segment of fibula which contains a nonossifying fibroma. Note the irregular thinning of the cortical bone, which focally reveals underlying mahogany brown lesional tissue. (b) Section through the specimen demonstrated in (a) shows the scalloped margin of the lesion and the cortical thinning. The reddish-brown color is typical. The focal areas of gray probably represent fibrous tissue, and the areas of yellow discoloration, lipid accumulation. (c) Specimen radiograph of the lesion illustrated in (b). The radiograph shows cortical erosion, with a thin layer of periosteal bone covering the expanded tumor.

rotic, and the bones involved are also likely to be different from those seen in children (Figs 18.9 and 18.10). Patients may experience mild pain or they may be asymptomatic. On microscopic examination, however, just as in childhood lesions the spindle-cell stroma has a whorled or 'storiform' pattern. The predominant underlying cell, a fibroblast, is mixed with polygonal histiocytic cells, which have a more vacuolated cytoplasm. Iron deposits, multinucleated giant cells, sparse chronic inflammatory cells, or lipid-laden cells may be evident.

FIBROUS DYSPLASIA (FIBRO-OSSEOUS DYSPLASIA; FIBRO-OSSEOUS LESION)

Fibrous dysplasia is a relatively common, usually solitary (monostotic), slow-growing hamartomatous lesion composed mainly of bone and fibrous tissue, but occasionally containing foci of cartilage. Rarely, an associated soft-tissue tumor may be present, usually an intramuscular myxoma (Fig. 18.11). This association is known as Mazabraud syndrome.

The condition is most often first seen in children and adolescents, and remains relatively unchanged throughout life, though the lesion may slowly increase in size. Deformity may occur because of repeated minor fractures through the affected bone. The clinical course of fibrous dysplasia is most consistent with that of a developmental abnormality, and no familial association is known.

Fibrous dysplasia is usually asymptomatic, and in most instances the lesion is discovered incidentally at radiographic examination. Occasionally a patient with fibrous dysplasia will exhibit symptoms, such as a mass, a pathologic fracture or impingement. The classic 'shepherd's crook' deformity of the upper end of the femur is the result of multiple sequential fractures, each of which is followed by some residual deformity (Fig. 18.12). The femur, tibia, skull, or ribs are most commonly affected, but almost any bone can be involved. Involvement of the cranio-facial bones may result in marked asymmetry and disfigurement (unilateral cranial hyperostosis) (Fig. 18.13).

On radiographic examination, the lesion is usually well defined, although the rim is not usually sclerotic and the tissue often has a 'ground-glass' appearance due to the finely scattered bone islands in the lesional tissue. Scintigraphy reveals increased isotope uptake in these lesions.

The classic gross appearance of fibrous dysplasia may be seen in Figure 18.14 in a rib, a commonly affected bone in which typically there is fusiform expansion, thinning of the cortex and replacement of bone tissue by a firm, whitish tissue of gritty consistency, which may often contain cysts. In a few cases the cysts can be quite large and associated with secondary changes (Fig. 18.15).

Microscopic examination reveals irregular foci of woven (nonlamellar) bone trabeculae in a cellular but otherwise unremarkable fibrous stroma (Fig. 18.16). The bony spicules in fibrous dysplasia are often described as resembling the letters C and Y, or Chinese characters. Microscopic evidence of osteoclastic resorption (Fig. 18.17) is frequently associated with these configurations. Osteoblastic rimming of bone, if present, is minimal.

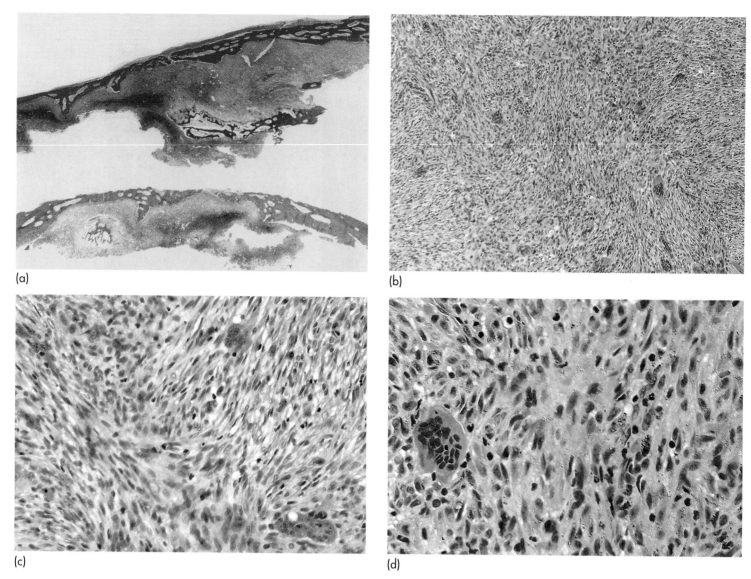

(a)

(b)

(c)

(d)

Figure 18.8   (**a**) Low-power photomicrograph of a histologic section demonstrates the variegated appearance of a nonossifying fibroma. In some areas the lesion is more cellular; in others it has a pink collagenous stroma (H&E, × 1 obj.). (**b**) Low-power photomicrograph of a nonossifying fibroma shows the spindle-cell stroma with occasional giant cells and mitoses. Note that the stromal cells are crowded, with little collagen formation (H&E, × 4 obj.). (**c**) Intermediate-power photomicrograph, demonstrating the matted storiform pattern (H&E, × 10 obj.). (**d**) High-power photomicrograph of the stromal cells shows foamy cytoplasm in some of the cells and one multinucleated giant cell (H&E, × 25 obj.).

In a few cases, we have observed areas which, instead of immature bone, contained dense blue nodules, or 'cementicle'-like structures, in the fibrous stroma (Fig. 18.18). Occasionally the fibrous stroma exhibits a storiform pattern similar to that seen in a benign fibrous histiocytoma (Fig. 18.19).

Cartilage in lesions of fibrous dysplasia may be either intrinsic to the lesion or secondary to fracture, or may result from disruption of an affected growth plate during childhood. In any event, the amount of cartilage present in the lesion may lead to confusion in diagnosis and the lesion may be mistaken for a chondrosarcoma (Fig. 18.20).

Patients with fibrous dysplasia in addition to islands of cartilage may also exhibit other secondary reactive changes caused by

a pathologic fracture. These changes include areas of multinucleated giant cells, foamy histiocytes, and fracture callus (Fig. 18.21). If these reactive areas are the only tissues biopsied, the lesion may be mistaken on histologic examination for a primary neoplasm or even a metastatic carcinoma.

Polyostotic involvement by fibrous dysplasia is decidedly rare. Usually but not always, the multiple lesions affect predominantly one side of the body or a single limb (Fig. 18.22). The histologic features of polyostotic lesions are identical to those of monostotic lesions. The polyostotic involved may result in severe deformities, and it is sometimes, mostly in females, associated with patchy skin pigmentation and various endocrinopathies usually with precocious puberty (Albright–McCune syndrome).

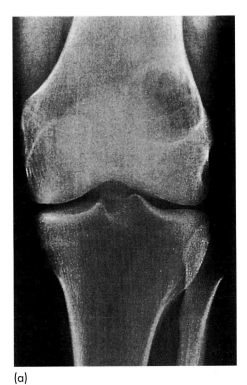

(a)

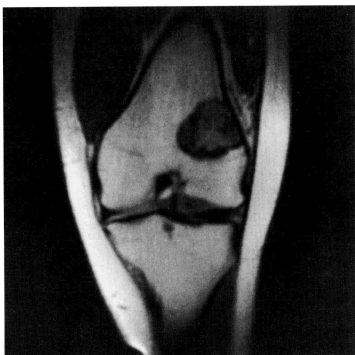

(b)

Figure 18.9 (a) Radiograph of the right knee of a 30-year-old female complaining of 'dull pain' around the knee joint. There is an eccentric, well-defined radiolucency in the metaphysis abutting the peripheral region, which proved on biopsy to be a benign fibrous histiocytoma. (b) Magnetic resonance image of the lesion shown in (a).

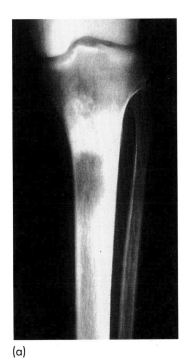

(a)

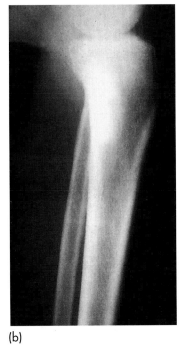

(b)

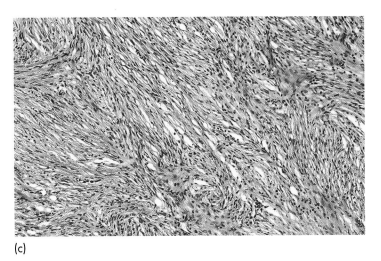

(c)

Figure 18.10 Antero-posterior (a) and lateral (b) radiographs of the tibia in a 64-year-old man who had had a bone scan for suspected metastatic disease. The lesion in the tibia was discovered incidentally, and the radiographs show a dense lesion in the metaphysis which is well defined and shows no periosteal reaction. (c) Photomicrograph of tissue removed from the patient shown in (a) and (b). The lesion twas composed of a benign but cellular spindle-cell stroma, with scattered chronic inflammatory cells, and giant cells and a matted storiform pattern. This histologic appearance is similar to that seen in the typical nonossifying fibroma in children; in an adult, this lesion is sometimes referred to as a fibroxanthoma or a benign fibrous histiocytoma (H&E, × 10 obj.).

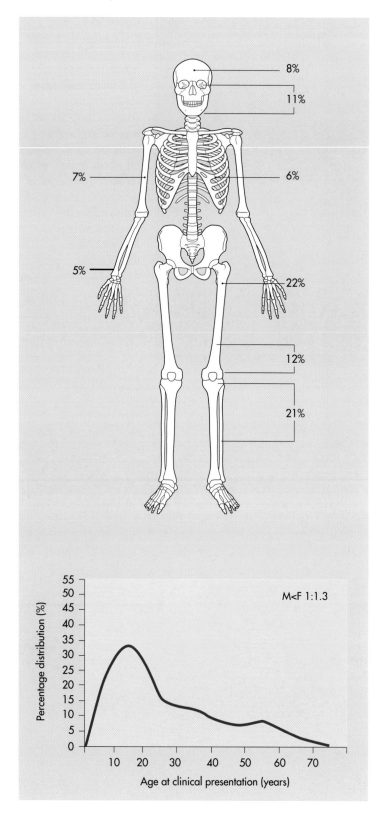

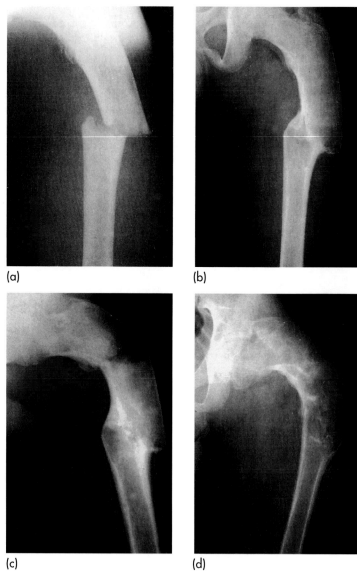

(a)

(b)

(c)

(d)

Figure 18.12 **(a–d)** Radiographs of the upper end of the femur in a patient with fibrous dysplasia shows the development of marked varus ('Shepherd's crook') deformity. This typical deformity in patients with polyostotic fibrous dysplasia results from repeated fractures through the involved section of the proximal femur, with residual deformity after each fracture.

Figure 18.11 Location and age distribution of fibrous dysplasia.

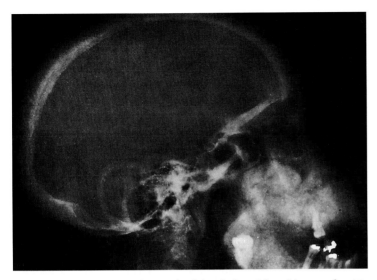

Figure 18.13 Lateral radiograph of the skull and facial bones of a 45-year-old woman who had suffered with progressive deformity of the face for a few years. Note the 'ground glass' texture of the mandible and facial bones, with loss of cortical differentiation and floating teeth. (Courtesy of Dr German Steiner.)

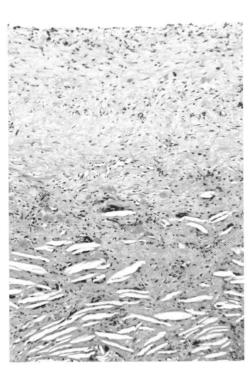

Figure 18.15
Photomicrograph of a portion of the lining of a cyst found in a case of fibrous dysplasia shows extensive cholesterol deposition with an associated histiocytic and giant-cell response (H&E, × 10 obj.).

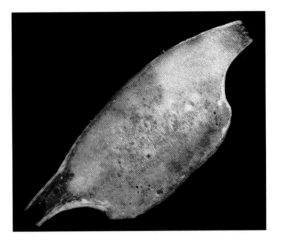

(b)

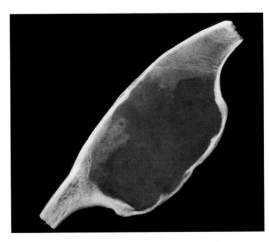

(c)

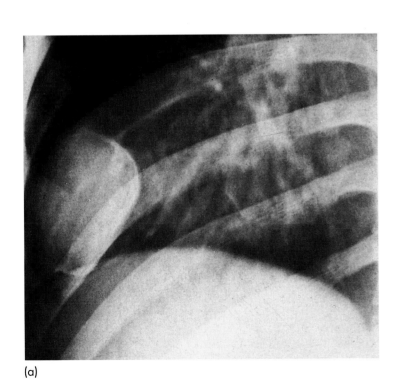

(a)

Figure 18.14 (a) Radiograph of the chest in a 20-year-old man who complained of a swollen area on the seventh right rib. Note the uniform density of the expanded tumor, which is often referred to as a 'ground-glass' appearance. (b) This gross photograph of fibrous dysplasia in the resected rib reveals a well-circumscribed expansile lesion with a solid white and tan appearance. Note the normal cancellous and cortical bone of the rib on both sides of the lesion. In such a lesion, the cut surface has a gritty consistency due to the presence of fine bone spicules, which are responsible for the ground-glass appearance on radiography. (c) Radiograph of the specimen shown in (b) reveals a relatively lucent expanded zone with marked thinning of the cortex. Throughout the lesion there is a ground-glass appearance due to diffusely distributed fine spicules of bone.

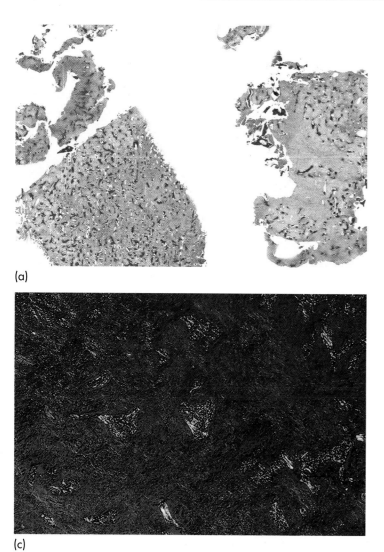

(a)

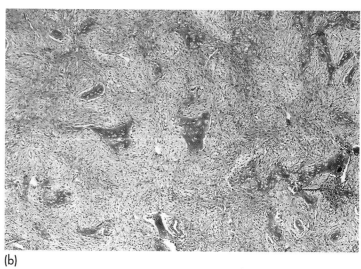

(b)

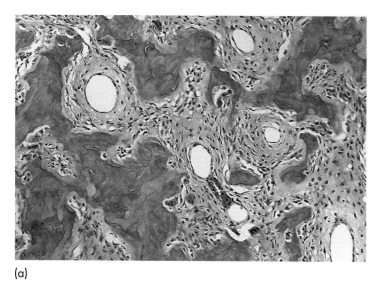

(c)

Figure 18.16   (a) Low-power view of curetted fragments from a patient with fibrous dysplasia shows a fibrous tissue stroma with islands of immature bony tissue-woven bone throughout (H&E, × 1 obj.). (b) Photomicrograph of fibrous dysplasia shows a background of collagenized fibrous tissue, within which are irregularly shaped spicules of immature bone. Although bone production is readily evident, there are relatively few osteoblasts rimming the bone spicules. This finding suggests a direct metaplasia of bone from the underlying fibrous tissue (H&E, × 10 obj.). (c) The same tissue seen in (b) viewed with polarized light demonstrates the woven appearance of the collagen within the bone matrix. [This photograph should be compared with the appearance of osteofibrous dysplasia in Figure 18.25(c).]

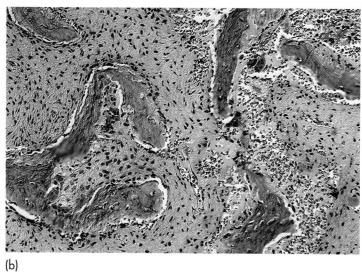

(a)   (b)

Figure 18.17   (a) Photomicrograph of tissue obtained from a case of fibrous dysplasia. Note the irregular trabeculae and the osteoclastic activity (H&E, × 4 obj.). (b) Photomicrograph demonstrating a feature of fibrous dysplasia not usually illustrated but nevertheless common, i.e. osteoclastic resorption of the bone spicules in the fibrous stroma (H&E, × 10 obj.).

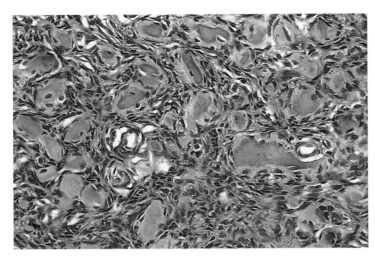

Figure 18.18 Photomicrograph showing small, discrete foci of calcified matrix within a case of fibrous dysplasia, which resemble the cementicles occasionally seen in fibromas of the jaw (H&E, × 10 obj.).

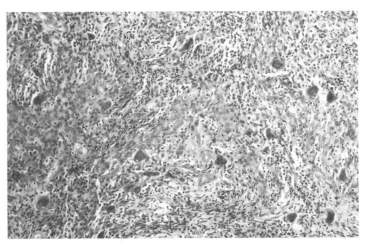

Figure 18.21 Photomicrograph taken through an area of fracture in a patient with fibrous dysplasia demonstrates a spindle-cell stroma with many giant cells and a sprinkling of chronic inflammatory cells. A biopsy taken through such an area may be confusing in differential diagnosis (H&E, × 10 obj.).

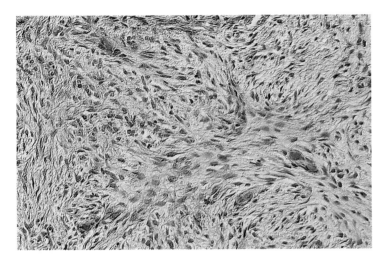

Figure 18.19 Photomicrograph of a purely fibrous area within a lesion of fibrous dysplasia demonstrates the 'whirling pinwheel' storiform pattern of benign fibrous histiocytoma (H&E, × 10 obj.).

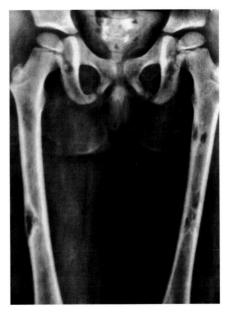

Figure 18.22
Radiograph of a 4-year-old girl with multiple bilateral cystic lesions in the femur and pelvis that proved, on histologic examination, to be fibrous dysplasia. With time, the lesions seen here undoubtedly would enlarge and result in deformity.

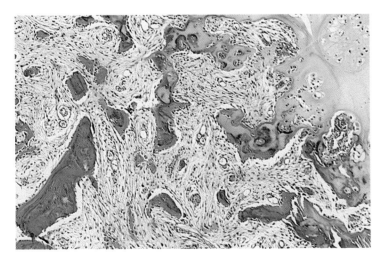

Figure 18.20 Photomicrograph demonstrating focus of cellular cartilage within fibrous dysplasia. Occasionally, the cartilaginous areas occupy a considerable portion of the lesion and therefore can be diagnostically confused with chondrosarcoma; this has been designated by some as fibrocartilaginous mesenchymoma (H&E, × 10 obj.).

BENIGN TUMORS

OSTEOFIBROUS DYSPLASIA (OSSIFYING FIBROMA)

Osteofibrous dysplasia occurs almost exclusively in the tibia and fibula, though rarely the forearm bones are involved. Although it has been considered by many to be a variant of fibrous dysplasia, it is most often seen in young children who present with tibial tumors that may be rapidly enlarging but are usually painless. The deformity of the involved leg may be quite dramatic and the lesion initially behaves in an aggressive fashion. The natural history of this lesion is the subject of much debate, but it appears that osteofibrous dysplasia behaves less aggressively as the affected child gets older.

Imaging studies show that the lesion is usually extensive, involving the anterior cortex either of the diaphysis or the metaphysis of the tibia; the epiphysis is usually not affected. Characteristic eccentric intracortical osteolysis, with distortion and thinning of the cortex, is normally evident (Figs 18.23 and

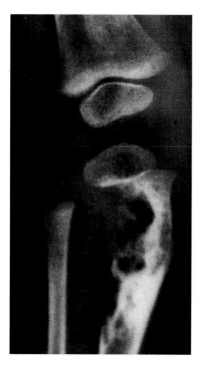

Figure 18.23   Radiograph of a 15-month-old boy with a large, lytic, eccentric defect in the upper end of the tibia, which proved on histologic examination to be an osteofibrous dysplasia.

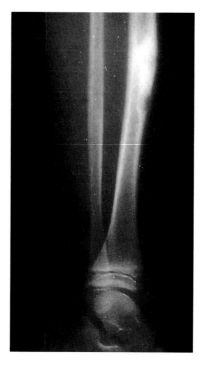

Figure 18.24   Lateral radiograph of the right leg of an 8-year-old boy with local pain and deformity. Cortical thickening with a stress fracture as well as a lytic defect is present in the midshaft. This proved, on biopsy, to be due to osteofibrous dysplasia.

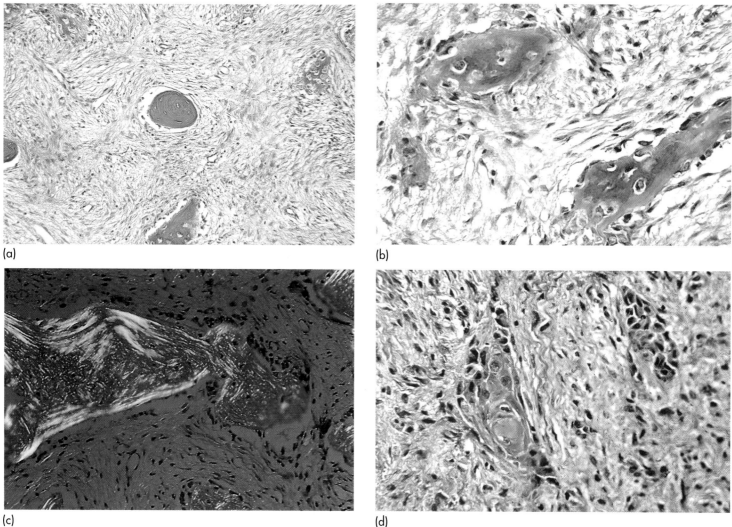

(a)

(b)

(c)

(d)

Figure 18.25   (a) Photomicrograph of tissue obtained from a patient with osteofibrous dysplasia reveals a cellular spindle-cell stroma, with spicules of bone, both mature lamellar and immature woven bone (H&E, × 4 obj.). (b) A higher magnification shows focally rimming of woven bone spicules by osteoblasts (H&E, × 25 obj.). (c) In some areas the surface is covered by lamellar bone with a core of woven bone. This finding of peripheral maturation is characteristic of osteofibrous dysplasia (Polarized light, × 10 obj.). (d) In most cases of osteofibrous dysplasia, immunoperoxidase staining will show single keratin-positive cells within the fibrous matrix. In a very few cases there are also rare clusters of keratin-positive cells, occasionally showing keratinization as shown here. In such a case the term 'differentiated adamantinoma' has been applied (H&E, × 25 obj.).

18.24). The cortical bone may actually be absent in places. Anterior bowing of the tibia is common, as is a multiloculated appearance. The periosteum is usually well preserved.

The histologic appearance of the affected tissue is similar to that seen in fibrous dysplasia, with irregular spicules of trabecular bone and unremarkable spindle cells that produce a collagenous stroma. However, in contrast to fibrous dysplasia, the bone spicules are characteristically lined with osteoblasts that produce a rim of lamellar bone, even though the center of these spicules of bone may have a woven appearance (Fig. 18.25). Foci of hemorrhage and foamy histiocytes, as well as an occasional area of cartilage (usually in the vicinity of a fracture), may be observed.

Using immunohistochemical stains for cytokeratin, it has been shown that in most cases of osteofibrous dysplasia it is possible to demonstrate isolated cells scattered in the matrix which are cytokeratin positive; very occasionally small nests of cytokeratin-positive cells are present. Electron microscopy has demonstrated occasional cells with tonofilaments, even in the absence of cytokeratin-positive stains. These findings suggest that this condition should be regarded as being related to adamantinoma and possibly to represent a differentiated adamantinoma. It is certainly a distinct entity to be differentiated from fibrous dysplasia.

DESMOPLASTIC FIBROMA

Desmoplastic fibroma is a rare, intraosseous, collagen-producing well-differentiated fibrous tumor characterized clinically by pain.

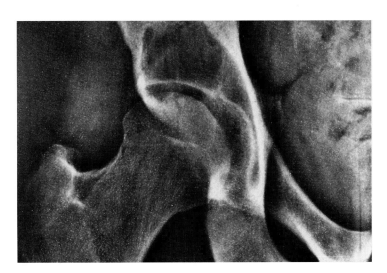

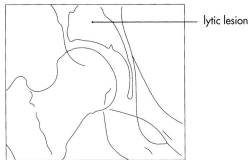

Figure 18.26 Radiograph of a young adult patient who complained of pain in the hip joint reveals a large lytic defect in the ilium, just above the acetabulum. The margins of the lesion are fairly well defined, without obvious sclerosis. On curettage, this lesion proved to be a densely collagenous fibrous tumor, characterized microscopically as a desmoplastic fibroma.

The tumor usually presents during the first 3 decades of life, and most commonly develops towards the end of a long bone, in the pelvis or mandible. In most cases radiographs reveal a lucent defect which may expand the cortex and on occasion has a trabeculated appearance due to irregular thinning of the cortex (Fig. 18.26). In some cases there may be cortical destruction, suggesting a malignant tumor. Microscopically, the most prominent features are interlacing bundles of dense collagen. The cells are usually sparse and exhibit no cytologic atypia (Fig. 18.27). The histologic similarity of desmoplastic fibroma to certain fibrous lesions elsewhere (such as palmar fibromatosis and desmoid tumors) suggests that it is an intraosseous counterpart of those lesions (Fig. 18.28). The tumor has a tendency to recur locally but does not metastasize. The lack of bone production in this lesion characteristically distinguishes it from fibro-osseous lesions of bone.

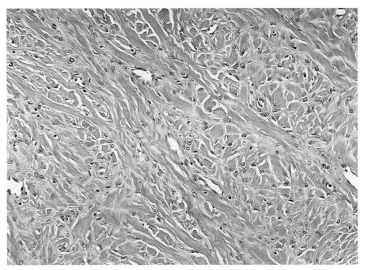

Figure 18.27 Low-power photomicrograph of a desmoplastic fibroma shows the dense, collagenized matrix of this lesion (H&E, × 10 obj.).

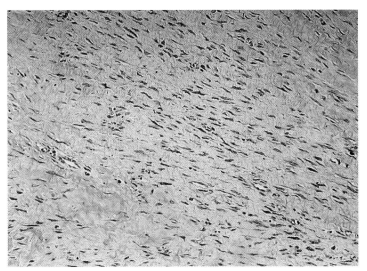

Figure 18.28 Photomicrograph of another area of desmoplastic fibroma which is somewhat more cellular than that seen in Figure 18.27. Note the innocuous appearance of the fibroblasts and the extensive collagen production (H&E, × 10 obj.).

MALIGNANT TUMORS

FIBROSARCOMA

Fibrosarcoma is a rare malignant spindle-cell neoplasm which produces a sparse to moderate amount of collagen matrix and has no other matrix differentiation. The lesion usually occurs in the metaphyseal ends of the long bones, especially around the knees of adults who are usually between 20 and 60 years of age (Fig. 18.29). Pain or swelling in the affected area is frequently exacerbated by a pathologic fracture. About one-quarter of the reported cases have been associated with a pre-existing condition such as Paget's disease, fibrous dysplasia, an irradiated giant-cell tumor, bone infarct or longstanding osteomyelitis.

On radiographic examination, fibrosarcomas appear as lucent lesions, often with cortical destruction and extension into soft tissue. The involved bone often has a mottled or moth-eaten pattern. The tumor margins are irregular (Fig. 18.30). On gross examination the tumor is usually tan to grayish-white, and rubbery in consistency (Fig. 18.31).

On microscopic examination, fibrosarcomas contain homogeneous spindle-shaped fibroblasts with ovoid nuclei which are arranged in a characteristic 'herringbone' pattern; there is relatively little pleomorphism and infrequent mitoses (Fig. 18.32). Poorly differentiated tumors with pleomorphic cells, abundant mitotic activity, and bizarre hyperchromatic nuclei are better classified as malignant fibrous histiocytomas (Fig. 18.33). The well-differentiated tumors grow slowly and the treatment of choice is radical surgical excision.

The differential diagnosis of primary fibrosarcoma should include leiomyosarcoma either primary or metastatic, metastatic carcinoma, which may demonstrate a spindle-cell pattern (e.g. carcinoma of the kidney), and metastatic melanoma, and in this regard immunohistochemical studies can be most helpful.

MALIGNANT FIBROUS HISTIOCYTOMA

Malignant fibrous histiocytoma is a sarcoma which was first described in soft tissue about 30 years ago and is characterized microscopically by a heterogeneous population of pleomorphic spindle cells organized in a characteristic storiform or 'starry-night' pattern. In the older literature, cases in the bone were usually classified as poorly differentiated fibrosarcoma, malignant giant-cell tumors, or osteosarcoma.

When these tumors occur in bone, they primarily affect adults, who may be of any age; they usually involve the lower femur or upper tibia.

On radiographic examination, malignant fibrous histiocytoma appears as a poorly delineated lucent defect, often with cortical destruction. Minimal periosteal new bone formation may be evident (Fig. 18.34). In some cases this tumor has been found in association with a pre-existing bone infarct (Fig. 18.35).

The characteristic microscopic features of malignant fibrous histiocytoma are bundles and whorls of pleomorphic spindle-shaped cells with patchy or extensive collagen fiber production. The cells and fibers often meet at right angles, and sometimes take on a pinwheel (storiform) pattern (Fig. 18.36). Foci of rounded cells with foamy or vacuolated cytoplasm may be observed, as well as giant cells and multiple, often atypical, mitotic figures. There is often evidence of phagocytosed intracytoplasmic material, including hemosiderin, hematin, and lipo-

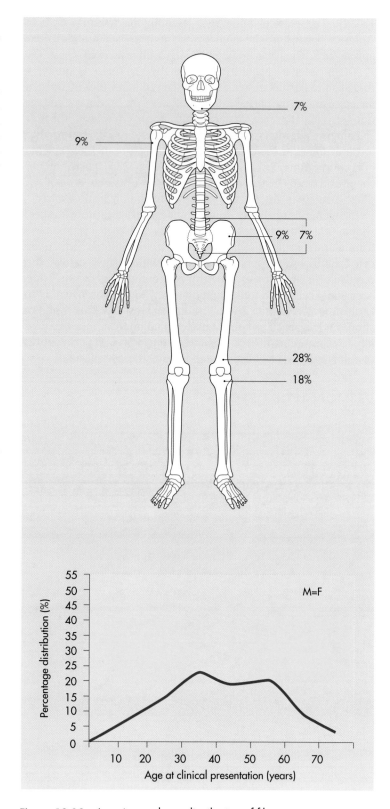

Figure 18.29 Location and age distribution of fibrosarcoma.

fuchsin pigments. An infiltration of chronic inflammatory cells is characteristically present. The complicated microscopic appearance of the tumor is best understood in light of evidence supporting a pluripotential cell that has features of both a macrophage (hence 'histiocyte') and a collagen-producing cell (hence 'fibroblast').

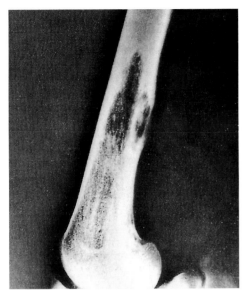

Figure 18.30
Radiograph of the lateral aspect of the femur in a 40-year-old man who complained of pain in the lower thigh shows an intramedullary lytic area extending into the posterior cortex. The margin is ill defined and the lesion has at its periphery a permeative appearance. On biopsy, this lesion proved to be a fibrosarcoma.

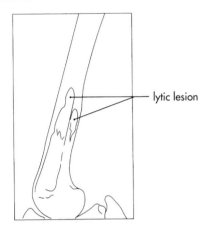

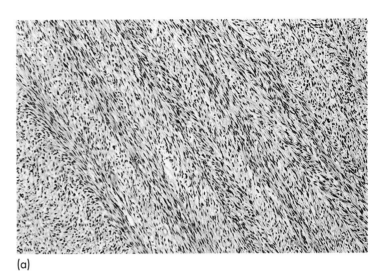

(a)

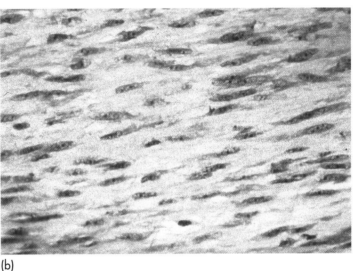

(b)

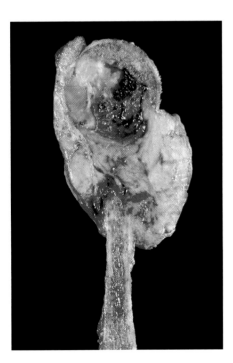

Figure 18.31
Photograph of a transected humerus shows a solid tumor at the upper end of the humerus, extending into the soft tissue. Focal hemorrhage is evident. When examined histologically, this tumor proved to be a fibrosarcoma. Multiple sections would be required in such a case to exclude the diagnosis of fibroblastic osteosarcoma.

Figure 18.32 (a) Photomicrograph of a fibrosarcoma clearly demonstrates the typical herringbone pattern of these lesions (H&E, × 4 obj.). (b) Most fibrosarcomas of bone are well differentiated, as seen in this high-power view (H&E, × 25 obj.).

Studies using various immunologic markers have shown that many lesions which had been classified as malignant fibrous histiocytoma are in fact poorly differentiated liposarcomas, or malignant muscle tumors. Therefore before making the diagnosis of malignant fibrous histiocytoma, it is imperative to obtain a suitable panel of immunohistochemical stains.

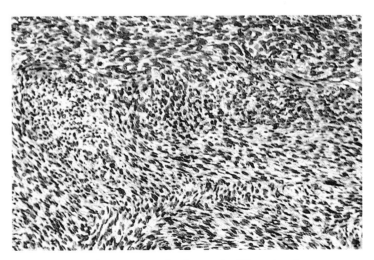

Figure 18.33 Photomicrograph of a poorly differentiated fibrosarcoma shows cell crowding and pleomorphism typical of a high-grade lesion (H&E, × 10 obj.).

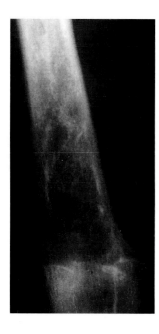

Figure 18.34 Radiograph of the lower femur in a man with a long history of pain, recently increasing in intensity. This extensive lytic and sclerotic lesion proved on biopsy to be a malignant fibrous histiocytoma.

Although malignant fibrous histiocytoma is not as aggressive as osteosarcoma, it is a fully malignant and metastasizing tumor, and radical treatment is recommended.

Rare instances of multicentricity have been reported.

ADAMANTINOMA OF LONG BONES

Adamantinoma is an extremely rare slow-growing neoplasm that sometimes occurs in long bones, over 90% in the diaphysis of the tibia and most of the rest in the fibula or forearm bones. It is somewhat similar to the much more common odontogenic adamantinoma of the jawbones. Patients with long-bone lesions are usually between 20 and 30 years of age. Males are somewhat more frequently affected than females. The principal clinical sign of adamantinoma is the insidious onset of pain, sometimes developing over many years. The characteristic radiographic finding is a multicystic ('soap-bubble') osteolytic lesion with surrounding sclerosis, cortical thinning, and expansion (Figs 18.37 and 18.38).

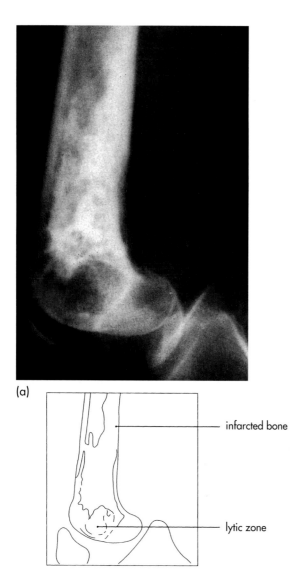

(a)

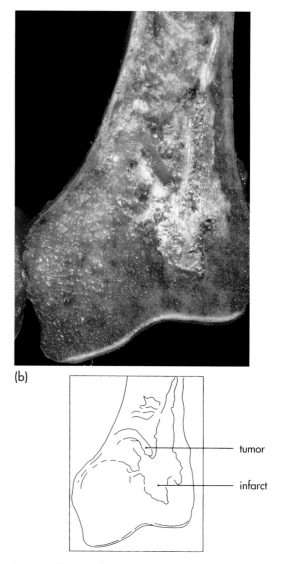

(b)

Figure 18.35 (a) Lateral radiograph of the femur in a patient with a longstanding history of bone infarction, resulting from his being a caisson worker. Recently, the patient had experienced severe pain in the lower end of the femur, and on the radiograph a lytic area can be discerned at the lower end of the infarcted zone. (b) Photograph of frontally sectioned specimen of the femur removed from the patient in (a). The infarcted bone, seen as an area of opaque yellow tissue, is clearly delineated from the surrounding normal bone. The center left portion of the lesion exhibits admixed, fleshy gray tissue which, on microscopic examination, proved to be a malignant tumor.

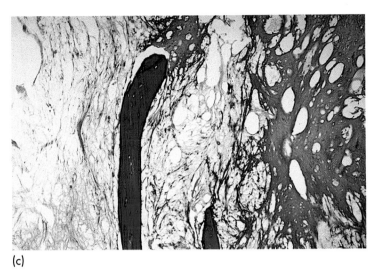

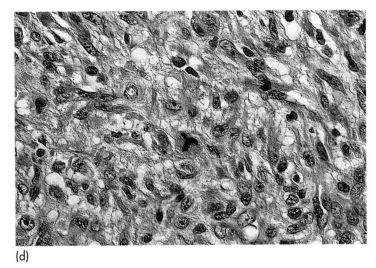

(c)   (d)

Figure 18.35 (contd)   (c) Photomicrograph of the infarcted area of the lesion illustrated in (a) and (b) (H&E, × 4 obj.). (d) Photomicrograph of a portion of the fleshy tumor shown in (b) demonstrates the pleomorphic cellular pattern of the tumor, with vacuolated cytoplasm and, in the center, a tripolar mitosis (H&E, × 40 obj.).

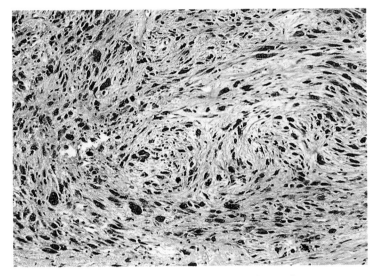

Figure 18.36   Photomicrograph of a malignant fibrous histiocytoma demonstrating the marked nuclear pleomorphism, with giant-cell forms and the typical storiform or 'starry-night' pattern (H&E, × 25 obj.).

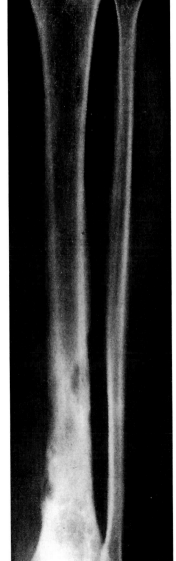

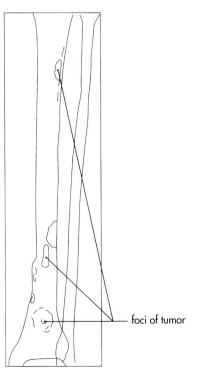

Figure 18.37   Radiograph of the left leg in a young adult patient who complained of aching leg pain shows multiple lytic lesions in the bone, particularly in the lower third of the diaphysis. The lytic, bubbly appearance of the tumor, together with the presence of satellite lesions, is characteristic of adamantinoma in the tibia. Occasionally, adamantinomas may also be seen in the fibula, and even more rarely in the long bones of the forearm.

foci of tumor

On gross inspection the tumor is generally well circumscribed and rubbery in texture; however, focal areas of hemorrhage or necrosis may be evident. The microscopic finding of a biphasic pattern of spindle-shaped, collagen-producing cells, alternating with sinewy cords or nests of epithelioid cells, is characteristic (Figs 18.39 and 18.40). The epithelioid cells are strongly positive for keratin.

Adamantinomas present complex chromosomal abnormalities with multiple translocations and some extra chromosomes.

The etiology and histogenesis of this tumor has been disputed, but on the basis of immunohistochemical studies an epithelial origin is now generally accepted (see also the discussion of osteofibrous dysplasia, p. 437).

Adamantinoma is a neoplasm of relatively low-grade malignancy. It is locally invasive and may metastasize late in its course in about 20% of cases.

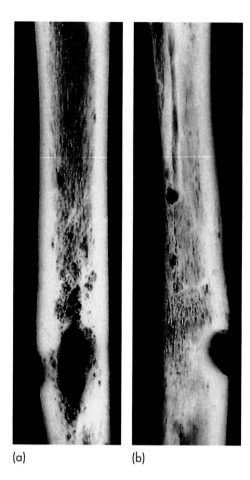

(a)   (b)

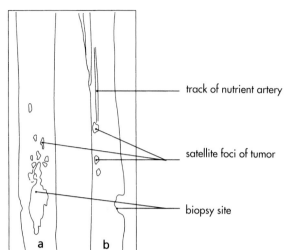

— track of nutrient artery

— satellite foci of tumor

— biopsy site

a   b

Figure 18.38   Antero-posterior (**a**) and lateral (**b**) radiographs of a portion of the tibial diaphysis removed from a 9-year-old boy with adamantinoma of the tibia. Small punch-out lesions not connected with the main tumor mass are clearly evident; on histologic examination, each of these lesions contained tumor. When such satellite lesions are found, radical resection is necessary if recurrence is to be avoided.

Treatment of adamantinoma consists of adequate surgical excision; the margins of resection should be carefully planned if recurrence is to be avoided, because satellite lesions may occur at some distance from the major tumor mass.

Limited biopsies may result in confusion with metastatic carcinoma or with fibrous dysplasia, however the characteristic clinical presentation should help to avoid this dilemma.

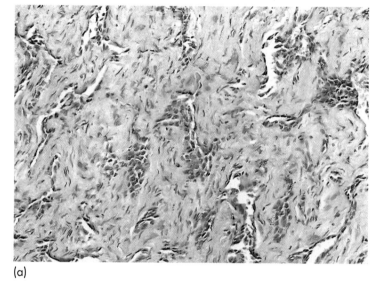

(a)

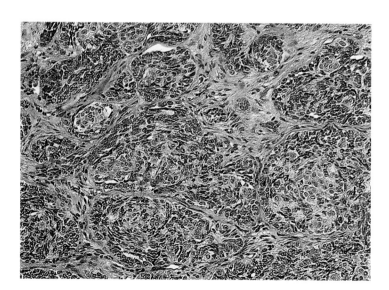

Figure 18.39   Photomicrograph of an adamantinoma of the tibia shows a fibrous stroma with islands of basophilic epithelioid cells which may be focally sparse and show cleft-like spaces (as shown in Figure 18.40) (H&E, × 10 obj.).

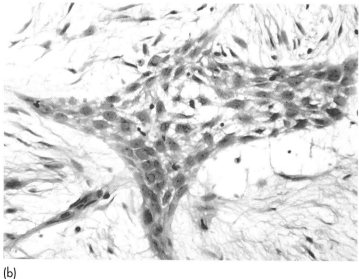

(b)

Figure 18.40   (**a**) Photomicrograph of an adamantinoma with a dense fibrous stroma and cleft-like spaces lined with epithelioid cells (H&E, × 4 obj.).   (**b**) Higher magnification of an island of epithelioid cells (H&E, × 25 obj.).

BENIGN NONMATRIX-PRODUCING BONE TUMORS

This chapter will consider those benign lesions either cystic, vascular or solid, where matrix production is not an essential part of the lesion.

REACTIVE OR POST-TRAUMATIC TUMORS

EPIDERMOID INCLUSION CYSTS

Epidermoid inclusion cysts are cysts bounded by a wall of stratified squamous epithelium and filled with keratin debris (Fig. 19.1). Although these lesions occur only rarely in bone, they may occur as a result of a puncture wound or from pressure erosion when the bone surface is close to the skin. They present radiologically as sharply outlined, intraosseous lytic areas with a sclerotic border. They are most commonly found in the distal terminal phalanx (Fig. 19.2) or the calvaria, but cases in larger bones such as the proximal tibia and pelvis have been reported.

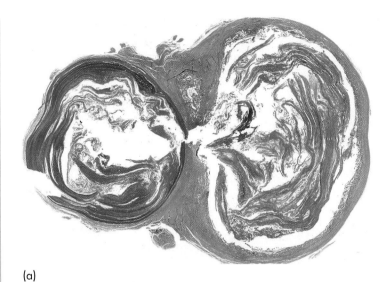
(a)

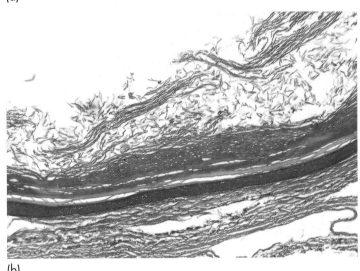
(b)

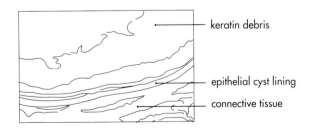

keratin debris

epithelial cyst lining

connective tissue

Figure 19.1   (a) Photomicrograph of an epidermoid inclusion cyst. The space on the left is lined with stratified squamous epithelium and is filled with keratin debris. In the right half of the photograph, the contents of the cyst have ruptured into the adjacent soft tissue, resulting in a foreign body histocytic and giant-cell reaction (H&E, × 1.25 obj.). (b) A higher power view of the cyst wall lined with squamous epithelium (H&E, × 4 obj.).

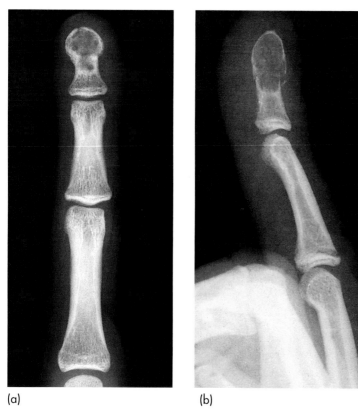

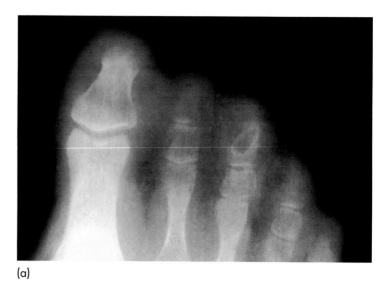

(a)

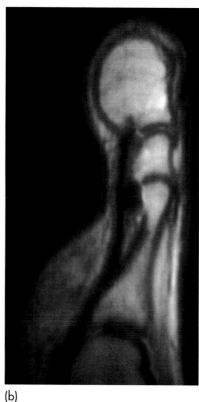

(b)

Figure 19.2   Antero-posterior (**a**) and lateral (**b**) radiographs showing an epidermoid inclusion cyst. A well-circumscribed lucent defect with a thinned cortical rim is present in the distal portion of the terminal phalanx. No calcification is evident, and this, together with the location, helps to differentiate this lesion from an enchondroma.

Figure 19.3   (**a**) A radiograph of the right foot. In the terminal phalanx of the third toe, there is a defect (**b**), which on a T₂-weighted image is consistent with cartilage. Curettage proved this to be a chondroma.

The radiologic differential diagnosis of an epidermoid inclusion cyst in the finger includes enchondroma [which does occasionally occur in the distal phalanx (Fig. 19.3)], giant-cell reparative granuloma, acral metastases and intraosseous extension of a glomus tumor (Fig. 19.4) or of a subungual melanoma.

GANGLION CYST OF BONE

Intraosseous ganglion cysts are rare. On radiographic examination they present as uniloculated or multiloculated well-demarcated lytic defects with a thin rim of sclerotic bone. Patients with this disorder are usually middle-aged and present with mild, localized pain that is increased by weight bearing. The lesion is most frequently seen at the epiphyseal end of long bones, commonly in the medial malleolus of the ankle, though the knee and shoulder are other common sites (Figs 19.5 and 19.6). Despite

proximity to a joint, a ganglion cyst rarely involves the joint. Occasionally an overlying soft-tissue ganglion is present on clinical examination, and it may communicate with the intraosseous ganglion.

At surgery, the lesion is a unilocular or multilocular cyst lined with a thick, fibrous membrane and filled with a whitish or yellowish gelatinous material. On microscopic examination, the wall of a ganglion cyst is composed of a dense, fibrous connective tissue layer with focal mucoid degeneration, flattened membrane-lining cells, and occasional mononuclear inflammatory cells (Fig. 19.7).

The lack of communication between the cystic bone defect and articular cavity, and the absence of arthritic change distinguish this disorder from those marginal cysts and subchondral bone cysts associated with degenerative joint disease.

Treatment by curettage or excision has been curative. Recurrences are rare.

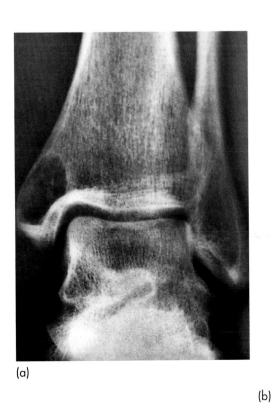

(a)

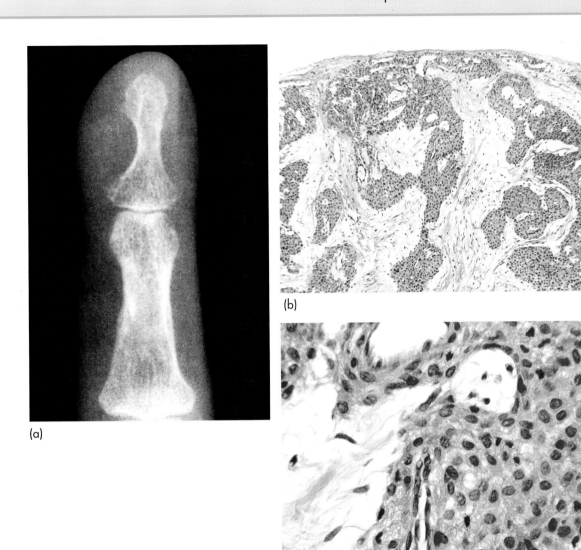

(b)

(c)

Figure 19.4 **(a)** Radiograph shows a lytic defect in the terminal phalanx of the little finger, caused by the intraosseous extension of a soft-tissue glomus tumor. (Courtesy of Dr Isao Sugiura.) **(b)** Photomicrograph of a glomus tumor shows fibrous connective tissue contains connecting cords of round to oval homogeneous cells with pinkish cytoplasm which surround branching vascular channels (H&E, × 4 obj.). **(c)** Higher power photomicrograph shows the bland appearance of the distinctive, rounded and regular glomus cells (H&E, × 10 obj.).

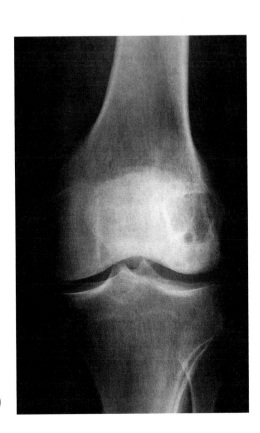

(a)

(b)

Figure 19.5 **(a)** Ganglionic cyst of bone. In this radiograph of the lower end of the tibia, a well-demarcated, roundish lucent area is evident. Although this lesion is close to the joint space, the joint space is not narrowed; this finding helps to differentiate a ganglionic cyst from an osteoarthritic cyst. **(b)** Antero-posterior radiograph of a knee, showing a well-defined peripheral trabeculated lytic lesion of the lateral femoral condyle, which proved to be an intraosseous ganglion.

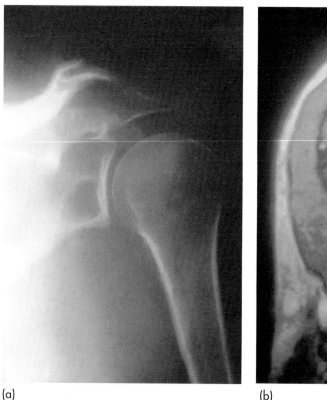
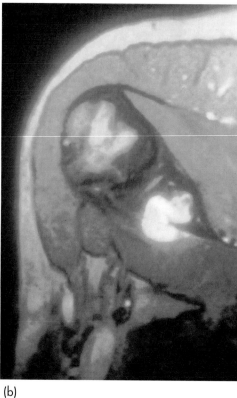

Figure 19.6 (a) A middle-aged female with a history of chronic shoulder pain has a lytic lesion in the glenoid, which on MR (b) shows a bright signal consistent with a fluid-filled cyst. Histology showed this to be a ganglion. The development of a soft-tissue ganglion following a labral tear is not uncommon and the lesion may, as in this case, erode into the bone.

(a)   (b)

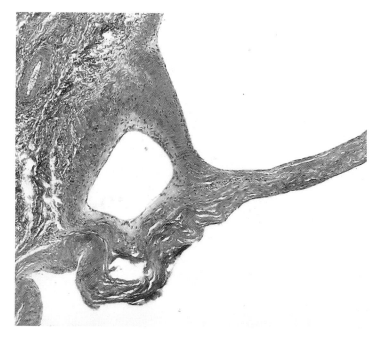

Figure 19.7 Microscopic examination of a ganglionic cyst of bone reveals the wall of the lesion to consist of fibrous connective tissue, with focal areas of mucoid degeneration and patchy dense collagen. The membrane may be lined with flattened lining cells resembling a synovial lining (H&E, × 10 obj.).

UNICAMERAL BONE CYST (SOLITARY CYST; SIMPLE BONE CYST)

A simple bone cyst is a benign, solitary cystic defect in the metaphyseal region of long bones, usually presenting clinically in children or young adolescents; males are more commonly affected (Fig. 19.8). The classic location for such a lesion is the proximal humerus but it is also commonly found in the proximal femur. The most common clinical presentation is a pathologic fracture through the area of weakened bone.

On radiographic studies, the lesion appears as a well-defined lucent area with a thin sclerotic margin (Figs 19.9 and 19.10). A pseudo-loculated appearance may result from irregular thinning of the cortex by the expanding cyst (Fig. 19.11). Apparent expansion of the bone results from cortical erosion by the cyst associated with periosteal new bone formation (Fig. 19.12). However, Codman's triangle is not a feature of a simple bone cyst, indicating that growth is not rapid. The lesion, when observed in serial radiographs, appears to migrate from the epiphyseal plate (although in reality the growth plate grows away from the cyst) (Fig. 19.13).

On both gross and microscopic inspection, an unaltered lesion appears as a clear, fluid-filled cyst lined with a thin fibrous membrane without obvious lining cells (Figs 19.14 and 19.15). However, because fractures are common complications, secondary changes, such as hemorrhage, hemosiderin deposits,

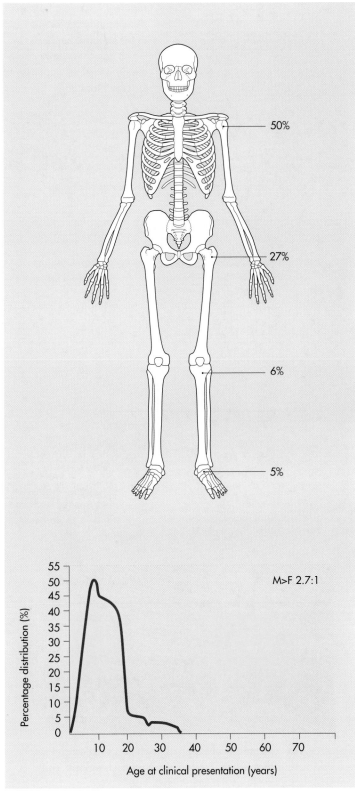

Figure 19.8   Location and age distribution of a simple bone cyst.

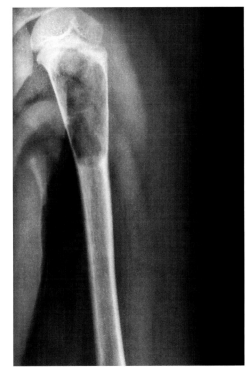

Figure 19.9
Radiograph of a simple bone cyst in the proximal humerus of an 8-year-old boy reveals a well-circumscribed lucent area in the metaphysis, extending to the diaphysis. Although the lesion extends up to the growth plate, the epiphysis is not involved. Thinning of the cortex is evident. (Because these lesions typically present after a fracture, the radiologic appearance may be complicated by callus formation.)

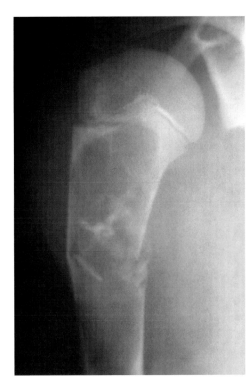

Figure 19.10
Antero-posterior radiograph of the right shoulder of a 12-year-old boy with sudden pain in the arm, demonstrating a fracture through a bone cyst. (Courtesy of Dr Alex Norman.)

granulation tissue, cholesterol clefts, fibrin, calcification, and reactive bone (Fig. 19.16), may be observed microscopically in focal areas of the tumor. In such instances, the lesion may mimic the histologic features of an aneurysmal bone cyst or even a giant-cell tumor. A rarely observed histologic feature is the accumulation of calcified amorphous material which superficially resembles the contents of a cementoma of the jaw (Fig. 19.17). This material probably represents calcified fibrin.

Because of the difficulty of complete surgical removal of the lesion, there is a high rate of recurrence after surgical curettage, particularly in children under 10 years of age in whom the lesion is characteristically juxta-epiphyseal. Nonsurgical treatment by aspiration and injection with corticosteroids is now widely used.

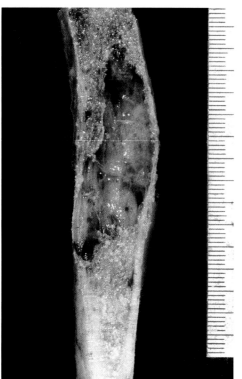

Figure 19.11 Longitudinal section of a segment of resected humerus reveals a well-demarcated cystic cavitation in the medullary portion of the bone, with cortical thinning and periosteal elevation leading to a bulging cortex. Note also the glistening cystic lining. (These lesions usually contain a clear, serous-like fluid.)

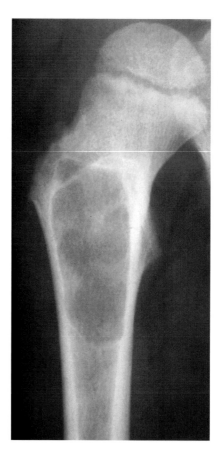

Figure 19.13 Radiograph showing a large, simple cyst in the femoral diaphysis which has grown away from the growth plate. (Courtesy of Dr Alex Norman.)

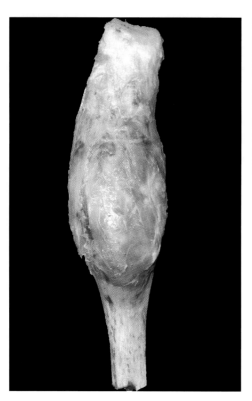

Figure 19.12 Gross photograph of a fibula with a central bulb-like expansion caused by a simple bone cyst. Note the pink color at the margin of the cyst, due to periosteal bone formation.

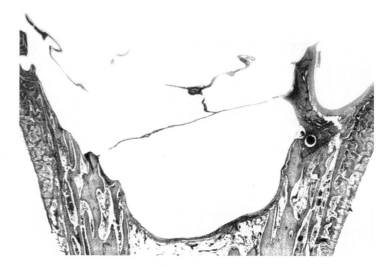

Figure 19.14 Low-power photomicrograph of a simple bone cyst reveals a fibrous membrane. Erosion of the cortex is evident, as is periosteal bone formation (H&E, × 1 obj.).

ANEURYSMAL BONE CYST

An aneurysmal bone cyst is a solitary, expansile lesion of unknown etiology which is generally eccentric in location. These lesions are most commonly seen in individuals under 20 years of age, where swelling, pain, and/or tenderness may be the presenting complaint (Fig. 19.18).

Although the lesion most often involves the long bones or the spine, any bone can be involved, including flat bones. Approximately 15% of all aneurysmal bone cysts arise in the spine, where they may occur at any level, with the exception of the coccyx. Occasionally multiple vertebrae are affected. Generally the tumor involves principally the vertebral arches, however they occasionally extend into the vertebral bodies (Fig.

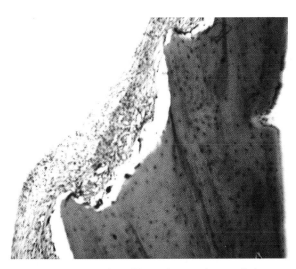

Figure 19.15 High-power view of the fibrous lining of a simple bone cyst (H&E, × 4 obj.). Note the osteoclastic resorption of the cortical bone.

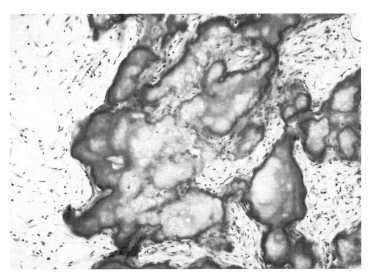

Figure 19.17 The membranous wall of this simple bone cyst reveals a peculiar, irregularly arranged calcific matrix which morphologically resembles the tissue present in a cementoma of the jaw. Such lesions are sometimes referred to as 'cementifying bone cysts', though the material is likely to be calcified fibrin (H&E, × 10 obj.).

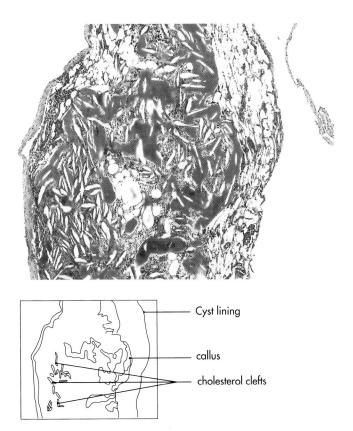

Cyst lining

callus

cholesterol clefts

Figure 19.16 Photomicrograph of tissue curetted from a simple bone cyst after fracture. Local hemosiderin deposits, chronic inflammation with many cholesterol clefts, and a rapidly forming callus are present (H&E, × 4 obj.).

19.19). Extradural cord compression is fairly common and may cause neurologic complications.

When a long bone is affected, serial radiographs generally demonstrate a rapidly expansile, eccentric, lucent lesion in the shaft of the bone. The periphery of the lesion is often indistinct, and the tumor itself often has a trabeculated appearance. Magnetic resonance imaging (MRI) studies will show the loculated pattern of the lesion and often demonstrate fluid levels.

On external gross examination, the wall of an aneurysmal bone cyst is usually soft and fibrous. When the cyst is opened, separated spaces containing friable, brownish blood clot usually become apparent (Fig. 19.20).

On histologic examination, the lesion is found to contain cystic spaces of different sizes which are filled with blood but are not lined with vascular endothelium. Between the blood-filled spaces are fibrous septa containing giant cells and foci of immature bone or unmineralized osteoid (Figs 19.21 and 19.22). Focal or diffuse collections of hemosiderin or reactive foam cells and chronic inflammatory cells may be seen in the septal zone. Characteristically, the cell morphology appears to be innocuous.

It is believed that in many cases aneurysmal bone cyst is a secondary reactive lesion and in some instances it is clear from microscopic examination that the lesion coexists with another, usually benign, tumor such as an osteoblastoma, chondroblastoma, nonossifying fibroma or fibrous dysplasia (Fig. 19.23). In about 50% of patients the lesion recurs once or several times after curettage.

It is important to differentiate this lesion both radiographically and microscopically from a telangiectatic osteosarcoma, a differential diagnosis that may on occasion be difficult.

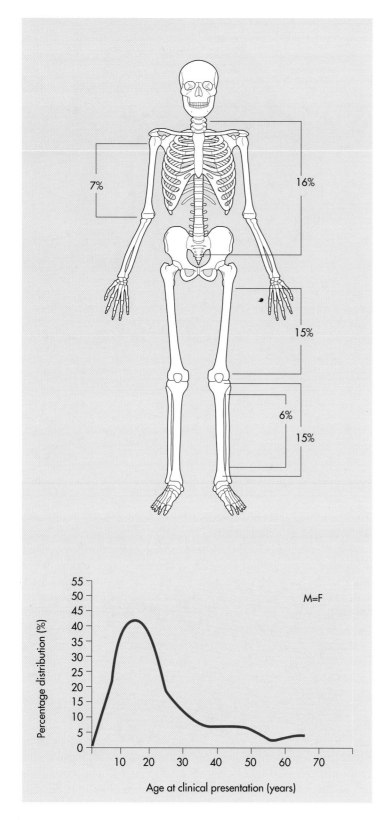

Figure 19.18 Location and age distribution of an aneurysmal bone cyst.

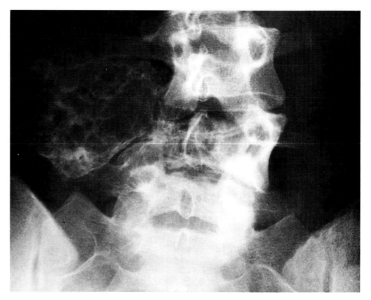

Figure 19.19 Antero-posterior radiograph of the lumbar spine of a woman in her mid-twenties with complaints of low back pain. Examination revealed a scoliotic deformity and slight local tenderness. This film shows collapse of the L4 body, with a huge expansion of the transverse process. The cortex is intact and the bone has a honeycombed trabeculated appearance; the pedicle is not seen on the affected side. The mild scoliotic deformity has developed as a result of the lesion.

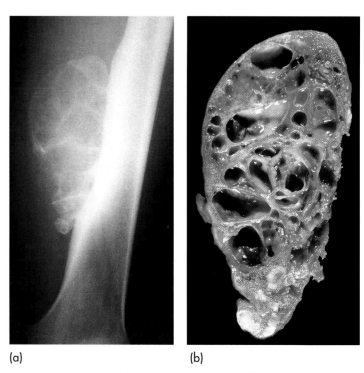

(a)   (b)

Figure 19.20 (a) Radiograph of an aneurysmal bone cyst shows a septated, subperiosteal blowout lesion. Note the irregular cortical margins at the lesion's interface with the shaft of the bone. (b) Viewed grossly, the lesion resected from the patient shown in (a) is a spongy, honeycombed, blood-filled mass with cystic spaces of various sizes, some containing osseous tissue within the septated walls.

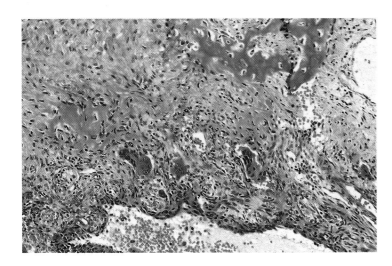

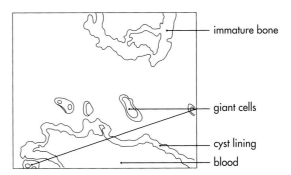

Figure 19.21 Low-power photomicrograph reveals that the tissue of an aneurysmal bone cyst contains a cellular stroma, often with many giant cells and bone formation (H&E, × 4 obj.). Note that the blood-filled spaces are not lined by vascular endothelium.

— immature bone
— giant cells
— cyst lining
— blood

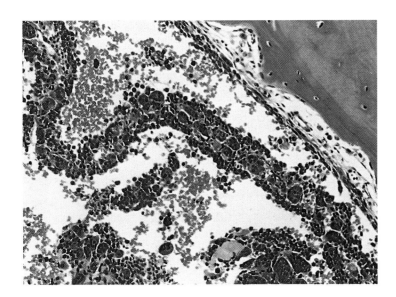

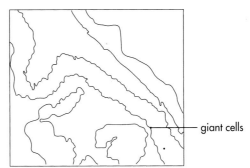

Figure 19.22 Higher power photomicrograph demonstrates the many giant cells lining the septa. This feature helps to distinguish the aneurysmal bone cyst lining from the fibrous lining space of a simple bone cyst (H&E, × 10 obj.).

— giant cells

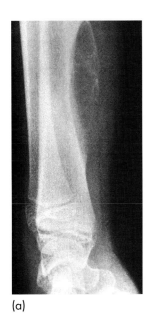

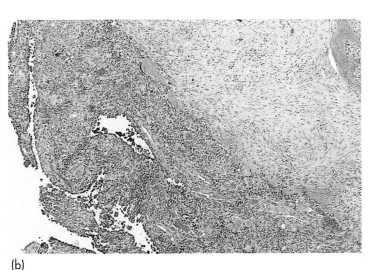

Figure 19.23 (a) Radiograph of the lower arm, showing an eccentric and expanded cystic lesion of the lower diaphysis of the distal radius. An intact shell of periosteal bone is seen over most of the lesion. In the shaft of the radius there is a poorly defined central lucency. In this case of an aneurysmal bone cyst, there was microscopic evidence of an underlying focus of fibrous dysplasia.
(b) Photomicrograph demonstrating the juxtaposition of the aneurysmal bone cyst (darker, lower left) and a focus of coexisting fibrous dysplasia (upper right) (H&E, × 10 obj.).

(a)   (b)

GIANT-CELL REPARATIVE GRANULOMA (SOLID ANEURYSMAL BONE CYST)

A giant-cell reparative granuloma is a benign, non-neoplastic, intraosseous lesion most commonly seen in the mandible or maxilla, but also reported in the small bones of the hands and feet (Fig. 19.24) as well as in other bones. Although these lesions may present at any age, most patients are in the second or third decade of life. The clinical signs are localized pain and swelling of variable duration. Radiographic examination reveals a lucent defect expanding the bone. The cortex is frequently thinned and there is little evidence of surrounding sclerosis.

On gross examination, tissue obtained from a giant-cell reparative granuloma appears grayish-brown and is often friable. Microscopic examination of the tissue may reveal varying degrees of cellularity, with predominantly unremarkable fibroblast-like spindle cells (Fig. 19.25). Histiocytes are also present.

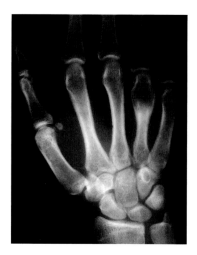

Figure 19.24 Radiograph of a giant-cell reparative granuloma of the fourth metacarpal. A lucent lesion expands the bone with thinning and expansion of the cortex. No calcification has occurred. The shaft of the bone protrudes into the expansile lesion, resembling 'a finger inside a balloon'. This radiologic finding is also common in aneurysmal bone cysts when they affect small tubular bones and is evidence of rapid growth.

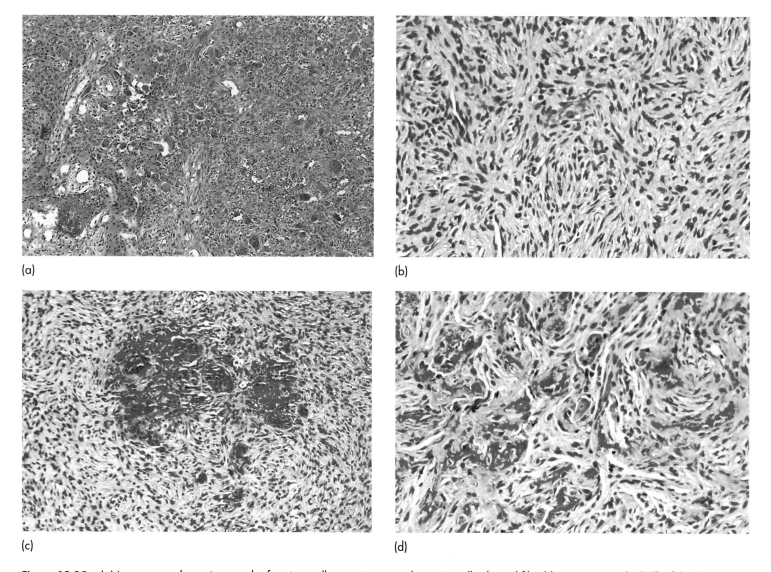

(a)

(b)

(c)

(d)

Figure 19.25 (a) Low-power photomicrograph of a giant-cell reparative granuloma. Spindle-shaped fibroblasts constitute the bulk of the lesion. Foci of giant cells can be seen, clustered in areas of extravasated blood and often accompanied by iron hemosiderin deposits (H&E, × 4 obj.). (b) A higher power shows the characteristic matted fibrous stroma (H&E, × 10 obj.). (c) Giant cells are generally found around foci of extravasated blood (H&E, × 10 obj.). (d) Areas of irregular reactive bone are frequently present (H&E, × 10 obj.). In giant-cell reparative granuloma, the differential diagnosis will therefore include a giant-cell tumor, aneurysmal bone cyst and occasionally a bone-forming neoplasm.

Characteristically, giant cells clustered in areas of recent and old hemorrhage are scattered throughout the lesion. Mitotic activity is rare. New bone formation and osteoid may be seen, again usually at sites of hemorrhage. Focal or scattered lymphocytic infiltration has been noted.

The differential diagnosis of giant-cell reparative granuloma may include the 'brown' tumor of hyperparathyroidism, conventional giant-cell tumor, and aneurysmal bone cyst. The following considerations may prove helpful in sorting through the differential diagnosis of a suspected giant-cell reparative granuloma. The clinical presentation of a solitary lesion, as well as laboratory findings of normocalcemia and normophosphatemia, mitigate against a 'brown' tumor of hyperparathyroidism. A conventional giant-cell tumor has a more homogeneous morphology, with diffuse uniform distribution of the giant cells; the stromal cells of a giant-cell tumor are more rounded and less spindle shaped, and little or no inflammation is evident. However, the differential diagnosis may be difficult in the case of an involutional giant-cell tumor. A giant-cell reparative granuloma lacks the large blood-filled channels seen in aneurysmal bone cysts. As with all bone tumors, it is important to note that the typical locations and clinical presentations of the various lesions are different.

Treatment of a giant-cell reparative granuloma consists of curettage or excision of the involved bone; however, recurrences are common in curetted lesions.

DEVELOPMENTAL OR HAMARTOMATOUS TUMORS

HEMANGIOMA OF BONE

Intraosseous hemangiomas are usually asymptomatic and solitary. These lesions typically affect the vertebral bodies or the skull though they may affect any bone. When they present clinically it is usually in patients in the middle years of life. There is no familial tendency.

Although hemangiomas are among the most frequently occurring tumors in the vertebral column, they are usually only identified as an incidental finding on a radiographic survey or after a careful autopsy study. As a clinical cause of disease they represent only about 2–3% of spinal tumors. The most common presentation is that of neurologic symptoms caused by extension of the angiomatous tissue into the epidural space.

These lesions occur most commonly in the lower thoracic vertebrae, somewhat less frequently in the lumbar spine, and infrequently in the cervical spine and the sacrum. Erosion of the horizontal trabeculae of the vertebral bodies leads to the typical radiographic appearance of accentuated, somewhat thickened vertical trabeculae (Fig. 19.26). In children, the affected bone may have a stippled or mottled appearance on radiographic examination. Cortical expansion may be seen in flat bones such as the ribs and skull (Fig. 19.27). In the skull a characteristic sunburst appearance is often present.

Gross examination of a sectioned hemangioma reveals a cystic, dark-red cavity (Fig. 19.28). The microscopic structure of this cavity consists of thin-walled cavernous blood vessels or proliferating capillaries lined with thin, flattened epithelium (Fig. 19.29).

Hemangiomas usually follow an indolent course, but they may be complicated by a fracture, extraosseous extension or hemorrhage.

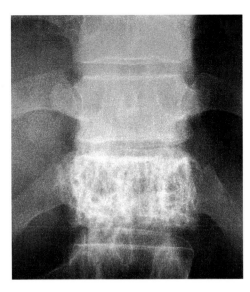

Figure 19.26 Radiograph of a hemangioma of a vertebral body demonstrates the characteristic, accentuated coarse trabecular pattern of the lesion.

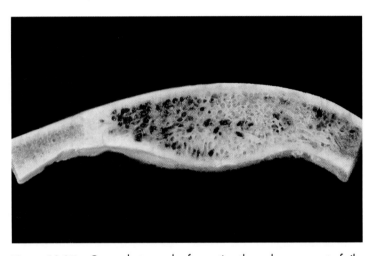

Figure 19.27 Gross photograph of a section through a segment of rib which contains an expanding hemangioma. Both in the rib and in the vault of the skull such lesions may radiographically have a 'sunburst' appearance. (Courtesy of Dr Miguel Calvo.)

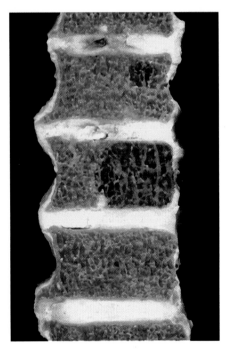

Figure 19.28 Gross photograph of hemangiomas of the vertebral bodies shows two well-demarcated, coarsely trabeculated red lesions, clearly demarcated from the normal cancellous bone.

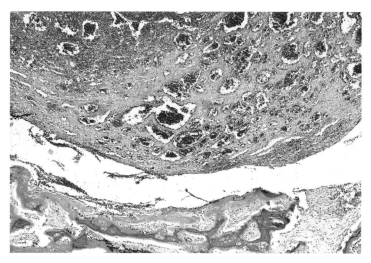

Figure 19.29   Photomicrograph of a hemangioma of bone reveals characteristic increased vascular channels of various sizes. Note in the lower part of the photograph reactive bone formation at the rim of the lesion (H&E, × 4 obj.).

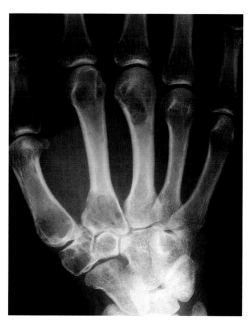

Figure 19.30 Radiograph of a hand with multiple hemangiomas. Lucent zones well demarcated from surrounding bone are evident.

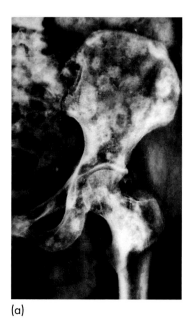

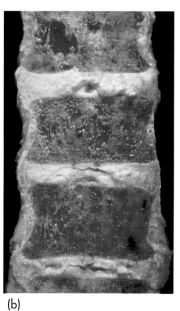

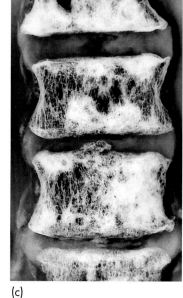

(a)   (b)   (c)

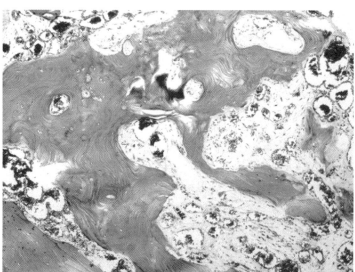

(d)

Figure 19.31   (a) Radiologically hemangiomas are characteristically lucent lesions, although the surrounding bone reaction may be sufficiently sclerotic to result in radiodensity. Sometimes this appearance is the dominant pattern, as seen in this clinical radiograph, with multiple densities throughout the skeleton mimicking a malignant bone-forming metastatic tumor. (b) Cross-section of the spine removed at autopsy from the patient with hemangiomatosis shown in (a). Note the disruption of the normal cancellous architecture of the vertebral bone. Multiple areas of dense bone, often with dark reddish centers, can be seen adjoining areas of osteopenia, in which the underlying yellow fat is readily evident. (c) Radiograph of the specimen shown in (b). Within the areas of density there are relatively lucent foci which represent the hemangioma. (d) Photomicrograph of one of the dense lesions illustrated in (b) and (c). Vascular channels of various sizes and shapes can be seen. The thickened bone appears to be immature, with increased cellularity and irregular architecture (H&E, × 4 obj.).

SKELETAL HEMANGIOMATOSIS/ LYMPHANGIOMATOSIS (CYSTIC ANGIOMATOSIS OF BONE, LYMPHANGIECTASIS OF BONE)

When systemic hemangiomatosis/lymphangiomatosis involves the skeleton the condition is usually diagnosed incidentally on radiologic examination, or as the result of complications such as pathologic fractures, soft-tissue masses (rarely), or chylous or hemorrhagic effusions. The patients are usually in the first 3 decades of life at the time of diagnosis. Hemangiomas or lymphangiomas in the skeleton are often seen in association with visceral hemangiomas and lymphangiomas, most commonly involving the spleen, pleura, and skin. There is no known familial tendency.

The radiographic features of skeletal hemangiomatosis/lymphangiomatosis are similar to those of solitary hemangiomas. The lesions usually have a fine peripheral rim of increased density (Fig. 19.30). Rare cases of hemangiomatosis with diffuse blastic skeletal lesions may mimic metastatic cancer; however, in these cases closer scrutiny reveals central lytic areas surrounded by dense sclerotic bone (Fig. 19.31).

On gross examination the lesions are generally cystic, with a reddish fluid indicative of blood or a clear yellow fluid indicating a lymphatic origin. Combinations of hemangiomas and lymphangiomas may be observed. On microscopic examination, the lesions consist of thin-walled vascular spaces lined with flattened endothelial cells and separated by collagen septa.

Laboratory findings in patients with this condition are usually unremarkable, although increases in alkaline phosphatase activity have been noted.

The prognosis for patients with this disorder is variable, depending on the degree and sites of involvement. The condition is usually self-limiting.

BENIGN TUMORS

EOSINOPHILIC GRANULOMA (LANGERHANS' GRANULOMATOSIS)

Because the clinical presentation and radiologic images in this condition very often suggest a malignancy, the discussion of eosinophilic granuloma is often included under the rubric of neoplasia. However, although the etiology is unknown, it seems more likely that this is a reactive inflammatory condition. Both the clinical course of this disease and its histopathology indicate that it is not neoplastic in nature.

Eosinophilic granuloma of bone may present as a unifocal lesion or as multifocal lesions, sometimes with systemic soft-tissue involvement. About 80% of cases of eosinophilic granuloma of bone are solitary. Classically, they present in males in the first decade of life and 75% of cases occur before the age of 20. The most commonly affected parts of the skeleton are the proximal femoral metaphysis, the skull, mandible, ribs, and vertebral column (Fig. 19.32). Patients may complain of pain or local tenderness. Laboratory tests are usually unremarkable, although the erythrocyte sedimentation rate may be elevated. Eosinophilic granuloma may also occur in soft tissue, including the skin, oral mucosa, lymph nodes, and lungs. When the lung is affected, patients may develop progressive fibrosis with impaired pulmonary function.

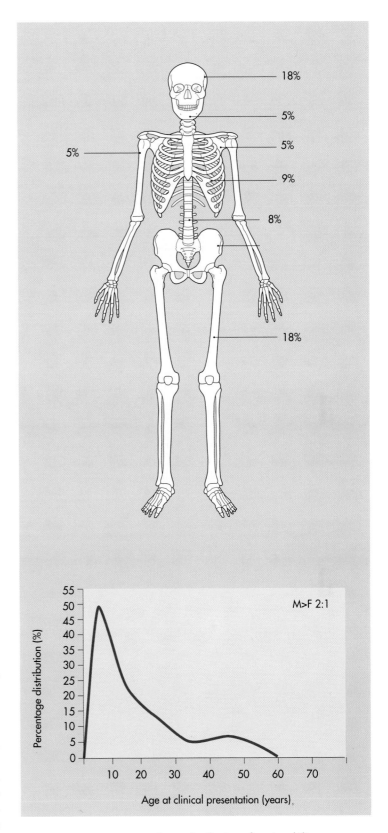

Figure 19.32   Location and age distribution of eosinophilic granuloma.

The term Hand–Schüller–Christian syndrome, which originally referred to a classic triad of skull defects, exophthalmos, and diabetes insipidus, is now used to include instances of more chronic evolution, occurring generally in children older than 3 years, with multiple cranial and other bony lesions and sometimes involvement of other systems or with one of the other classic symptoms (exophthalmos or diabetes insipidus). However, the complete triad has been rarely noted in the reported cases.

On radiologic examination, one or more circumscribed lytic defects may be evident in a bone (Fig. 19.33). These defects usually lack sclerotic margins. In the spine, collapse of a vertebral body is a common presentation (Fig. 19.34). In the long bones the lesion is usually located in the diaphysis and the cortex is often eroded. Sometimes in long bones a destructive permeative pattern with periosteal new bone formation can be seen, which may suggest malignancy (Fig. 19.35).

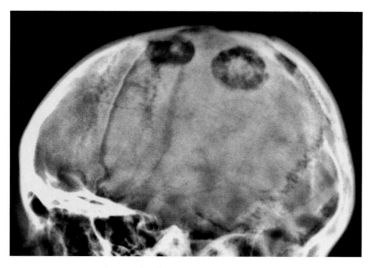

Figure 19.33   Radiograph of the skull in a child with eosinophilic granulomas. Several lytic lesions are evident; within the largest, the beveled edge that is typical of this presentation of eosinophilic granuloma can be appreciated.

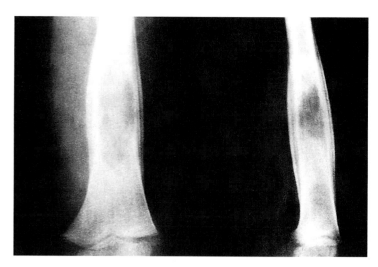

Figure 19.35   Radiograph of a child who presented with a slight fever, pain and swelling in the lower femur. Biopsy proved the lesion to be an eosinophilic granuloma. The radiologic differential diagnosis might include Ewing's sarcoma, osteomyelitis or even osteosarcoma.

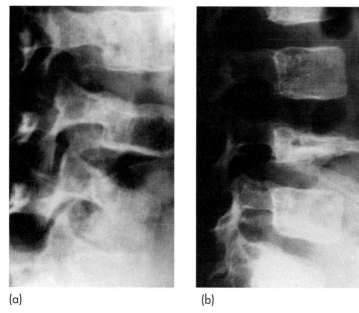

(a)   (b)

Figure 19.34   Lateral radiograph (**a**) of the lumbar spine in an 8-year-old child, showing a lytic lesion of L3, with partial collapse. A lateral radiograph (**b**) of the same patient, 1 month later, shows that the vertebral body has now collapsed down to a thin sclerotic wafer, which is somewhat increased in AP diameter. This appearance is characteristic of Calve's disease, which at one time was felt to be a form of osteochrondritis, but which is now recognized to be most often the result of eosinophilic granuloma.

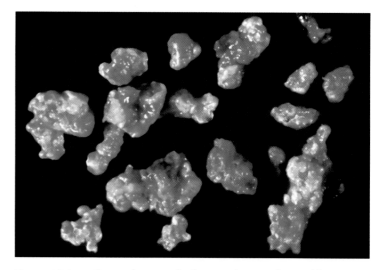

Figure 19.36   Gross photograph of curetted tissue obtained from a patient with an eosinophilic granuloma shows typically scant reddish-gray fragments of tissue flecked with dense yellow areas. These yellow areas represent loci of lipid accumulation or necrosis.

Surgical specimens submitted for pathologic examination are usually in the form of multiple curetted tissue fragments, typically consisting of glistening reddish tissue with flecks of opaque yellow material throughout (Fig. 19.36). The tissue is characterized microscopically by a mixture of eosinophils, plasma cells, histiocytes, and peculiar large mononuclear and multinucleated giant cells (Langerhans' cells) with abundant pale-staining cyto-

plasm and indented or cleaved nuclei. A variable degree of necrosis and fibrosis may be evident, as may reactive cells such as foamy macrophages. Mitotic activity is minimal (Fig. 19.37). On electron microscopy the Langerhans' cell displays characteristic 'racket-shaped' inclusion bodies in the cytoplasm (Birbeck granules) (Fig. 19.38). The Langerhans' cells show positivity for the S-100 protein and CD1A. (Because of the heterogeneity of the

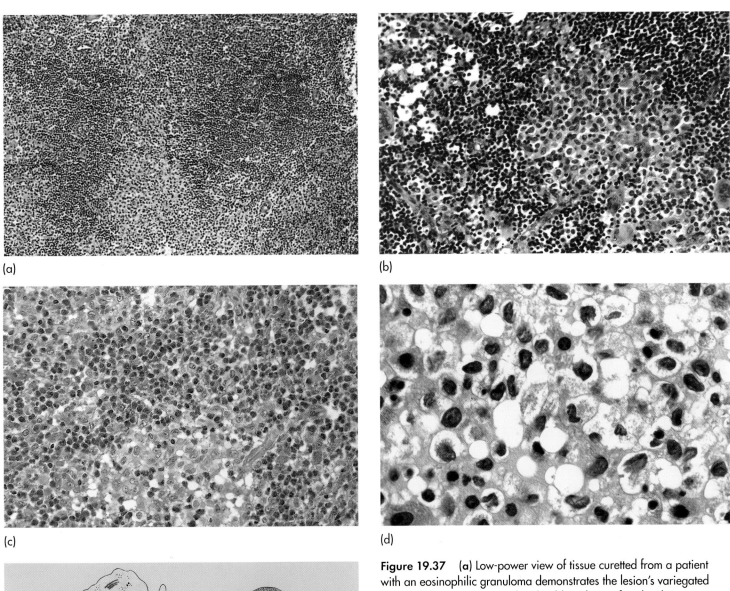

(a)

(b)

(c)

(d)

(e)

Figure 19.37   (a) Low-power view of tissue curetted from a patient with an eosinophilic granuloma demonstrates the lesion's variegated hypercellular appearance. This should not be confused with inflammatory tissue from a patient with osteomyelitis (H&E, × 4 obj.). (b) A higher power of (a) demonstrating lymphocytes, histiocytes and occasional giant cells (H&E, × 10 obj.). (c) In this photomicrograph, the mixed cellular appearance of an eosinophilic granuloma can be appreciated. In addition to plasma cells and eosinophils, large histiocytes (Langerhans' histiocytes) are present. Occasionally, especially if the tissue is scarred, confusion with Hodgkin's disease may be a problem (H&E, × 25 obj.). (d) A higher power to show the variegated appearance of the histiocytes. A few eosinophils are present (H&E, × 40 obj.). (e) Diagram of the various cells seen in eosinophilic granuloma (drawn to scale). (a) Histiocyte, (b) plasma cell showing a cartwheel nucleus, (c) eosinophil, and (d) lymphocyte.

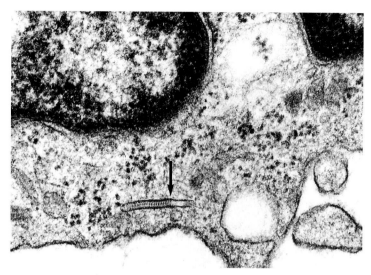

Figure 19.38 Electron micrograph of a histiocytic giant cell from a patient with eosinophilic granuloma shows a typical Birbeck granule in the cytoplasm (magnification × 100,000).

lesion, it is occasionally mistaken microscopically for Hodgkin's disease, however, it should be remembered that Hodgkin's disease is decidedly rare in people under the age of 10).

Patients with unifocal lesions may show spontaneous regression. If treatment is indicated, then curettage or small doses of radiation for inaccessible lesions is generally used. In general, the prognosis is good if a second lesion does not appear within 1 year. In patients who present with a more systemic illness characterized by fever, organomegaly, and multiple osseous lesions, the course of the disease is likely to be protracted.

Eosinophilic granulomas have been considered as one of a group of disorders known as the histiocytoses, which include (in addition to eosinophilic granuloma) Hand–Schüller–Christian disease and Letterer–Siwe disease. The former is probably better thought of as multiple eosinophilic granuloma, and Letterer–Siwe disease (a rare disease of infants with a characteristically fulminant course) is probably an unrelated neoplastic condition.

LIPID GRANULOMATOSIS OF BONE (CHESTER–ERDHEIM DISEASE)

Rare cases have been described of a granulomatous condition characterized radiographically by a diffuse symmetrical sclerosis of the metaphysis and diaphysis of major long bones. This disease usually affects multiple bones and tends to affect the metaphysis most prominently. Most of the subjects have been aged in their 40s and 50s. These patients do not in general have hypercholesterolemia. The affected individuals may have vague, localizing, aching pain but this is not always present. The first two cases of this condition were described by Chester, a pupil of the Viennese pathologist Erdheim. In one of Chester's cases there was also visceral involvement by lipid granulomatosis.

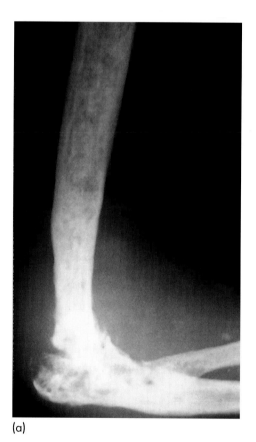

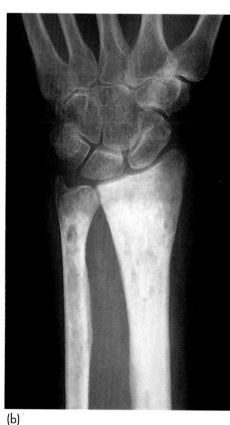

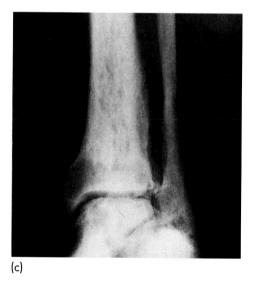

(a)

(b)

(c)

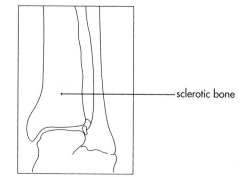

sclerotic bone

Figure 19.39 Radiographs of left elbow (a), left wrist (b), and lower leg (c) in a 50-year-old female patient with lipogranulomatosis of the bone (Chester–Erdheim disease). Note the patchy sclerosis with coarsening of the trabeculae. Unlike in Paget's disease, the cortex is generally smooth and the bone contour unaffected.

The radiographs in these cases have shown coarsening of the trabeculae, endosteal thickening and sometimes cortical rarefaction (Fig. 19.39). Unlike in Paget's disease, no change in the long bony contour is generally seen.

Microscopic examination of the bone has shown replacement of the marrow spaces by foamy histiocytes with focal fibrosis, mild chronic inflammation and new bone formation (Fig. 19.40). The microscopic appearance is not diagnostic and in the absence of radiographic and clinical correlation may be interpreted as a healed eosinophilic granuloma or nonossifying fibroma, or as a lipid storage disease (Gaucher's disease). In some cases it is possible to find groups of cleaved histiocytes which are S-100 positive. This has led some to believe that Chester–Erdheim disease is related to Langerhans' cell histiocytosis and is an indolent late stage of the disease.

SINUS HISTIOCYTOSIS WITH MASSIVE LYMPHADENOPATHY (ROSAI–DORFMAN DISEASE)

Sinus histiocytosis with massive lymphadenopathy (SHML) is distinguished by a proliferation of the distinctive lining histiocytes of the sinusoids of the lymph nodes or hematopoietic system which demonstrate numerous phagocytized lymphocytes in their cytoplasm.

This lesion may present as a primary lesion in bone and about one-third of the bone cases reported have had no evidence of lymphadenopathy. The majority of the patients are teenagers or young adults. The lesions in bone are typically osteolytic and may be confused with either eosinophilic granuloma or malignant lymphoma (Fig. 19.41). The presenting symptoms are generally

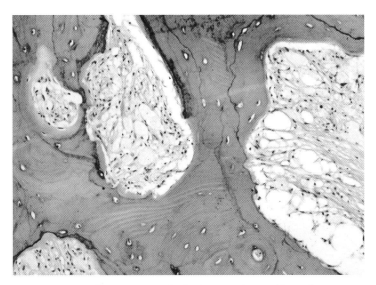

Figure 19.40   Photomicrograph of a biopsy obtained from the patient shown in Figure 19.39. In addition to thickening of the bone trabeculae, there is a replacement of the fatty marrow by foamy histiocytes, fibroblasts and occasional inflammatory cells (H&E, × 10 obj.).

fever and a general malaise. Evidence of an immune disorder is present in less than 50% of the patients.

With local disease the prognosis is good, however, it is graver in the presence of widely disseminated disease.

The typical appearance of the histiocytes in this disorder is of cells with large vesicular nuclei, occasionally prominent nucleoli,

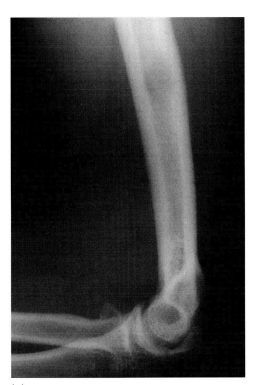

(b)

(a)

Figure 19.41   **(a)** Lateral radiograph of the arm of a 26-year-old male with localizing symptoms which on biopsy proved to be Rosai–Dorfman disease. The differential diagnosis included eosinophilic granuloma, malignant lymphoma, infection or metastasis. (Courtesy of Dr Howard Dorfman.) **(b)** A 32-year-old male with recent back pain on radiographic examination was shown to have a well-defined lytic lesion of the left ilium with a sclerotic margin, suggesting a benign process such as fibrous dysplasia, chondromyxoid fibroma or fibroxanthoma. Biopsy revealed Rosai–Dorfman disease.

and abundant eosinophilic cytoplasm with darker staining in the perinuclear area. Lymphocytophagocytosis, is one of the hallmarks of this disease. Most of the internalized lymphocytes are well preserved and located within cytoplasm vacuoles. Occasionally, plasma cells, red blood cells, and other hematolymphoid elements also can be present within the cytoplasm of the histiocytes. A foamy appearance of some of the histiocytes is an unusual secondary feature (Fig. 19.42).

The histiocytes in Rosai–Dorfman disease are S-100 protein positive and CD1 negative.

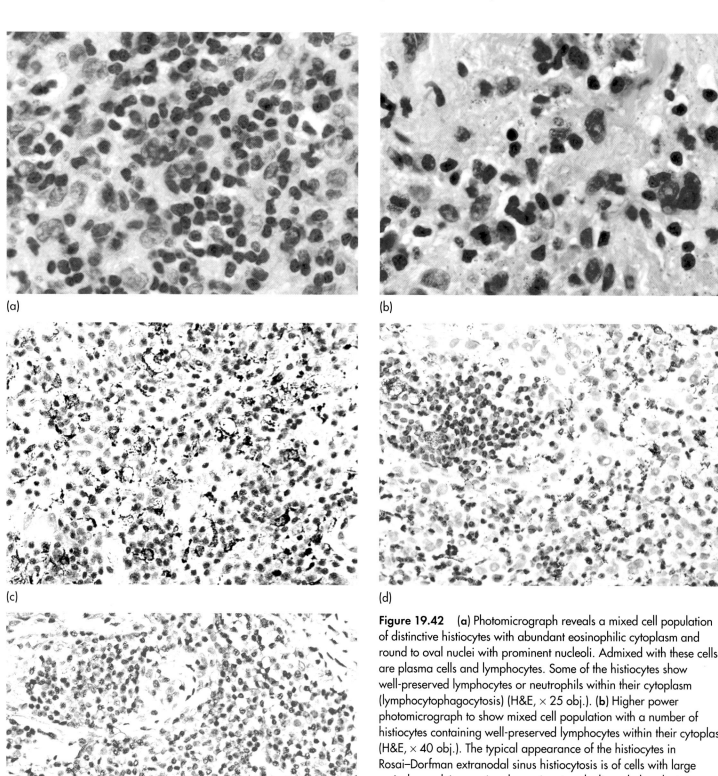

Figure 19.42 (a) Photomicrograph reveals a mixed cell population of distinctive histiocytes with abundant eosinophilic cytoplasm and round to oval nuclei with prominent nucleoli. Admixed with these cells are plasma cells and lymphocytes. Some of the histiocytes show well-preserved lymphocytes or neutrophils within their cytoplasm (lymphocytophagocytosis) (H&E, × 25 obj.). (b) Higher power photomicrograph to show mixed cell population with a number of histiocytes containing well-preserved lymphocytes within their cytoplasm (H&E, × 40 obj.). The typical appearance of the histiocytes in Rosai–Dorfman extranodal sinus histiocytosis is of cells with large vesicular nuclei, occasional prominent nucleoli, and abundant eosinophilic cytoplasm with darker staining in the perinuclear area. (c) Immunoperoxidase staining using CD68 antibody reveals positive histiocytes throughout the lesional tissue (× 10 obj.). (d) Immunoperoxidase staining using CD64 antibody confirms the presence of histiocytes (× 10 obj.). (e) Immunoperoxidase staining using S100 protein antibody confirms the presence of histiocytes (× 10 obj.).

SYSTEMIC MASTOCYTOSIS

Systemic mastocytosis is a rare condition involving the bone and other organs. Generally it is a benign indolent disease but exceptionally it may pursue an aggressive course. Usually it is characterized by osteoporosis and/or osteosclerosis, hepatosplenomegaly, lymphadenopathy, and mast cell infiltration in the skin (urticaria pigmentosa), gastrointestinal tract, heart, and lungs. This form may be accompanied by anemia, leukocytosis, leukopenia, eosinophilia, basophilia, or hypocholesterolemia.

Since mast cells secrete a variety of pharmacologically active agents, including histamine, heparin, prostaglandins, serotonin, and mucopolysaccharidases, in some individuals the clinical presentation is characterized by the pharmacologic effects following degranulation of mast cells. Among these effects are flushing, pounding headache, bronchospasm, hypotension, diarrhea, rhinorrhea, urticaria, palpitation, dyspnea, peptic ulcer, and gastrointestinal bleeding.

In patients with skeletal involvement, radiographs typically show diffuse, poorly demarcated sclerotic and lucent areas which involve predominantly the axial skeleton (Fig. 19.43). However, circumscribed lesions can occur, especially in the skull and extremities. This focal lesion may be mistaken for metastatic disease (Fig. 19.44).

Because in a child the condition may first appear as a localized permeative and occasionally sclerotic tumor, it may be mistaken for Ewing's sarcoma. In such a case, isotope bone scanning is useful, and both technetium and gallium scans may demonstrate diffuse generalized uptake; gallium in particular is taken up by the mast cells.

Microscopic examination of tissue removed from the bone of patients with mastocytosis shows diffuse or focal replacement of the bone marrow, usually with a mixture of cells including lymphocytes, eosinophils, plasma cells, fibroblasts and, of course, mast cells. The latter, however, may be easily overlooked unless a metachromatic stain is done. Occasionally the cellular infiltrate is composed predominantly of mast cells (Fig. 19.45).

In rare cases, mastocytosis may closely mimic a malignant lymphoma with leukemia, the mast cells showing cytological features of atypia.

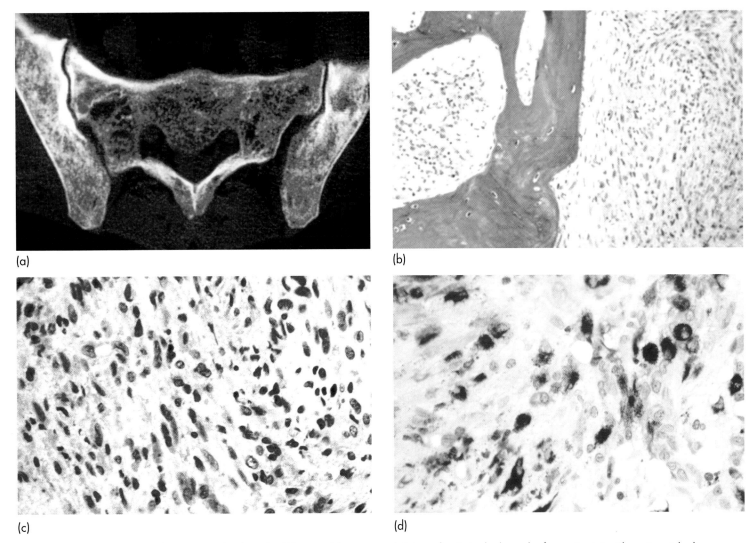

(a)

(b)

(c)

(d)

Figure 19.43 (a) CT scan of sacrum and pelvis of a 70-year-old man complaining of pain in the buttock of recent origin. There is patchy bony sclerosis with perhaps focal osteolysis. The presumptive diagnosis was metastatic carcinoma. (b) A biopsy of the item reveals a mixed fibrous and inflammatory infiltrate of the marrow space, but no evidence of tumor (H&E, × 4 obj.). (c) A higher power reveals that many of the mononuclear cells have a granular cytoplasm (H&E, × 25 obj.). (d) Giemsa stain reveals the granules within the mast cells in this case of mastocytosis (Giemsa stain, × 25 obj.).

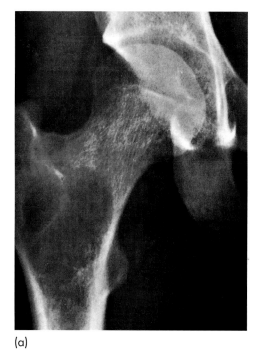

(a)

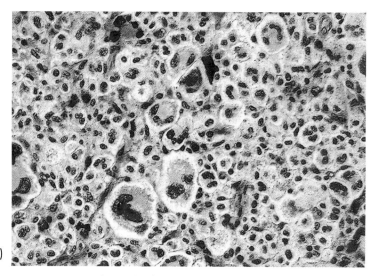

(b)

Figure 19.44   (a) Radiograph of a 14-year-old girl with a 6-month history of pain in the hip, which proved histologically to be caused by a mastocytoma. (b) Photomicrograph of tissue obtained from the case demonstrated in the radiograph in (a). The rounded bizarre cells with abundant cytoplasm and many giant cell forms suggested a malignancy, although careful searching showed no mitotic figures. Electron microscopic studies in this case confirmed the presence in the cells of typical mast cell granules (H&E, × 25 obj.). (Courtesy of Dr Ed McCarthy, Baltimore, MD.)

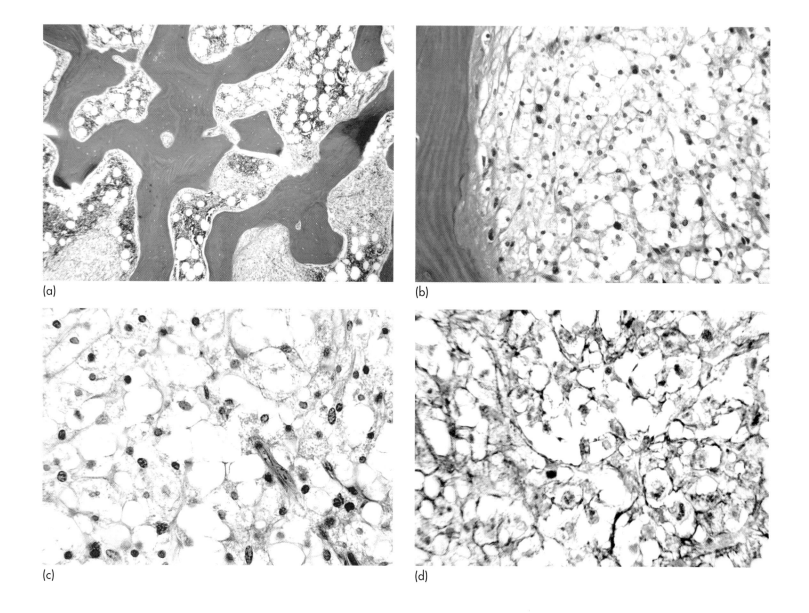

(a)

(b)

(c)

(d)

GIANT-CELL TUMOR

A conventional giant-cell tumor of bone is a locally aggressive neoplasm most commonly seen in the epiphyseal ends of long bones (usually the lower end of the femur, the upper end of the tibia, or the lower end of the radius; however, in the axial skeleton the sacrum is the most common site. In rare cases the jaw or the spine may be involved, and in such cases evidence of pre-existing Paget's disease should be sought). Giant-cell tumors most often occur in the third and fourth decades of life, and are rare in skeletally immature subjects. (However in rare cases in children, in which the growth plate is not closed, the lesions are metaphyseal in location.) Females are affected about one-and-a-half times more frequently than males. Affected individuals may complain of pain, show signs of local swelling, or have a pathologic fracture through the lesion. Multicentric lesions have been reported but are extremely rare (Fig. 19.46).

Radiographs generally reveal a well-defined defect in the metaphysis and epiphysis which is usually eccentrically located and extends to the subchondral bone end-plate of the articular surface. There is usually no evidence of sclerosis around the lesion (Figs 19.47 and 19.48). An aggressive radiographic appearance does not generally correlate with aggressive histologic features or prognosis.

Grossly the unaltered lesional tissue appears rather homogeneous, with a tan color and a moderately firm consistency (Fig. 19.49). However, foci of hemorrhage and/or necrosis may be observed in many tumors.

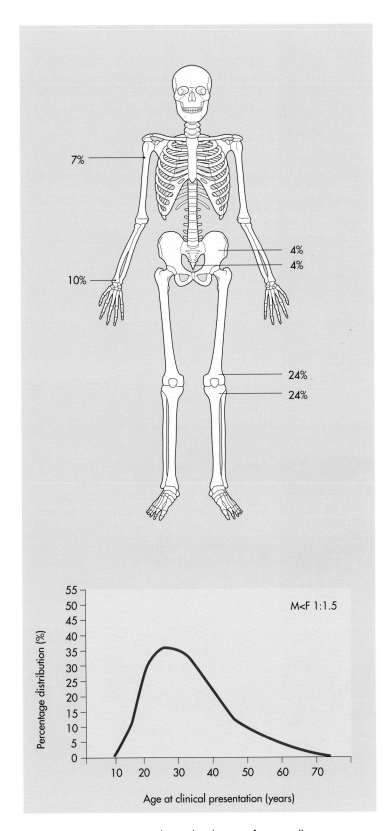

Figure 19.46   Location and age distribution of giant-cell tumor.

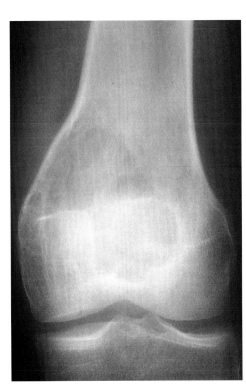

Figure 19.47
Radiograph of the distal femur and knee joint of a 30-year-old woman with complaints of pain in the knee shows a sharply demarcated lytic and eccentric lesion involving the epiphysis and metaphysis in a manner characteristic of a giant-cell tumor.

Figure 19.45   (a) Photomicrograph demonstrates sheets of pale vacuolated cells focally replacing the bone marrow. Note there is some thickening of the trabeculae which reflects the spotty diffuse sclerosis seen in clinical radiographs of patients with mast cell disease (H&E, × 4 obj.).
(b) A higher power photomicrograph shows the large foamy cells with bland nuclei and a faintly granular cytoplasm (H&E, × 10 obj.). (c) Another slightly higher power view of the cells which stained poorly with the traditional stains used to demonstrate mast cell granules (H&E, × 25 obj.).
(d) Immunoperoxidase strongly positive staining using anti-mast cell tryptase (× 25 obj.). The cells were also strongly positive when CD117 was used.

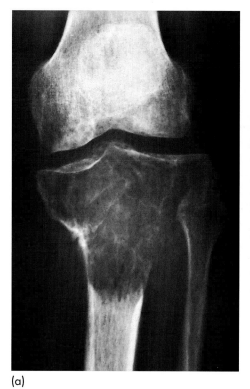

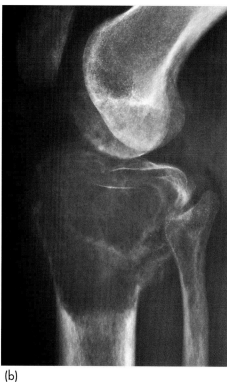

(a)   (b)

Figure 19.48   (a) Antero-posterior radiograph of a knee demonstrates a large lytic defect involving the proximal tibial epiphysis and metaphysis. Note the well-defined but nonsclerotic margin. (b) In the lateral radiograph a pathologic fracture can be seen posteriorly. (Courtesy of Dr Alex Norman.)

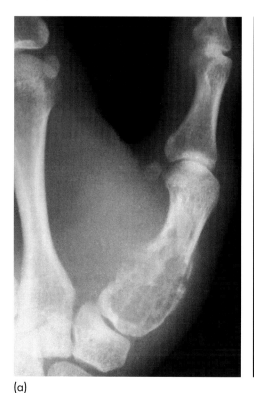

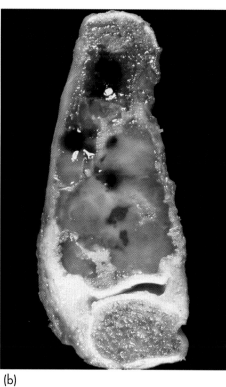

(a)   (b)

Figure 19.49   (a) Radiograph of a lytic lesion in the proximal end of the first metacarpal bone, through which there has been a pathologic fracture. On biopsy, this lesion proved to be a conventional giant-cell tumor. (b) Photograph of the transected specimen removed from (a). The pinkish-tan soft tissue seen here is typical of a giant-cell tumor.

The microscopic features of the tumor include a background of proliferating, homogeneous mononuclear cells. These have a round to ovoid shape, relatively large nuclei with inconspicuous nucleoli, and display multinucleated giant cells dispersed evenly throughout the tissue (Figs 19.50 and 19.51). Focal areas with spindle cells may be present, giving a pattern of benign fibrous histiocytoma (Fig. 19.52). In many cases, foci of reactive bone are present, particularly at the periphery of the tumor (Fig. 19.53). In other areas, involutional changes with lipid-filled histiocytes may be observed (Fig. 19.54). These infrequent patterns may give rise to occasional problems in differential diagnosis. Immunohistochemical studies show that the cells in giant-cell

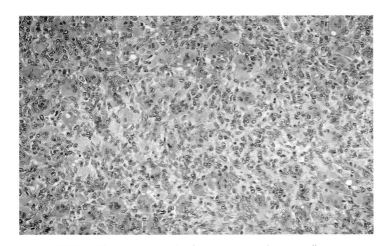

Figure 19.50 Photomicrograph of a conventional giant-cell tumor reveals the cellular nature of the lesion and the giant cells that are evenly distributed throughout. (The presence of giant cells alone does not confirm the diagnosis of a giant-cell tumor. Many lesions contain giant cells; it is the combination of mononuclear stromal cells and giant cells that is diagnostic of a giant-cell tumor) (H&E, × 25 obj.).

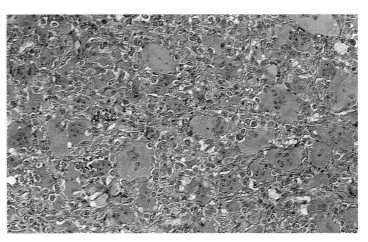

Figure 19.51 Another field of the same tumor demonstrates the homogenous, mononuclear stromal cells and the evenly distributed multinucleated giant cells. However, compared with the previous photomicrograph, some of the giant cells are much larger and appear to be phagocytosing adjacent mononuclear cells (H&E, × 25 obj.).

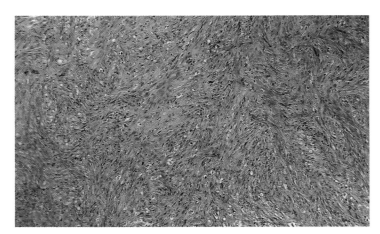

Figure 19.52 It is not unusual in giant-cell tumors to see a focal spindling out of the stromal cells which form a storiform pattern similar to that seen in a nonossifying fibroma or benign histiocytoma (H&E, × 10 obj.).

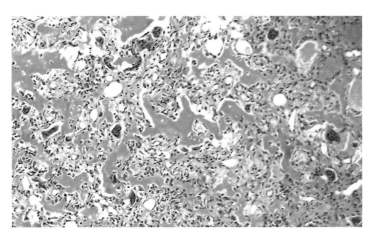

Figure 19.53 Photomicrograph demonstrating irregular and extensive bone formation in the periphery of an otherwise typical conventional giant-cell tumor. Such an appearance should not be confused with a giant cell-rich osteosarcoma (H&E, × 10 obj.).

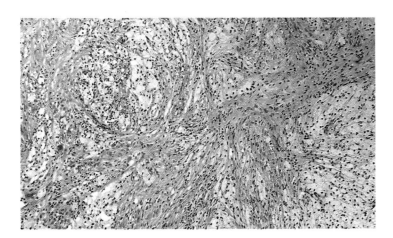

Figure 19.54 Photomicrograph of tissue obtained from a giant-cell tumor of longstanding shows foci of lipid-laden macrophages, fibrosis, and chronic inflammation. In some cases, especially following fractures, such involutional areas may be widespread (H&E, × 10 obj.).

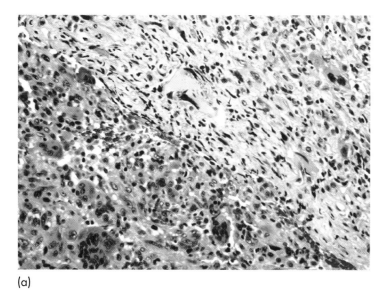

(a)

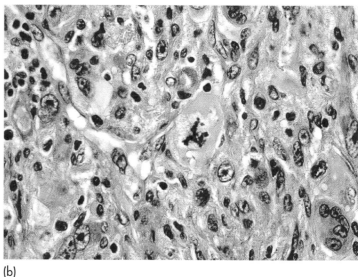

(b)

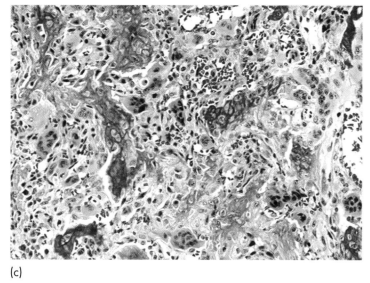

(c)

Figure 19.55 (a) Photomicrograph showing a conventional giant-cell tumor on the lower left and dedifferentiated tumor on the upper right (H&E, × 10 obj.). (b) Within the dedifferentiated tumor there is an atypical mitosis and cells with large nuclei and clumped chromatin (H&E, × 25 obj.). (c) In other areas of the dedifferentiated tumor, malignant bone matrix formation is present (H&E, × 10 obj.).

tumors have phenotypic features of both macrophages and osteo-clasts.

After curettage, conventional giant-cell tumors have a high local recurrence rate (50%). Surgical excision is therefore the treatment of choice. In conventional giant-cell tumors, lung metastases only rarely appear, and can be successfully treated by surgical excision.

Malignant dedifferentiation within a conventional giant-cell tumor has long been recognized as an occasional complication of radiation therapy. The interval between radiation and the diagnosis of malignancies has varied between 1 and 25 years, with an average interval of 8 years.

Dedifferentiation within a conventional giant-cell tumor occurring in the absence of prior radiation therapy is extremely rare.

Microscopically, malignant transformation is characterized by the presence of focal areas of anaplastic pleomorphic tumor cells and atypical mitoses; it is necessary that there are areas of identifiable giant-cell tumor present or in the case of postradiation sarcoma that the prior diagnosis of a giant-cell tumor be established (Fig. 19.55).

It is important to note that vascular invasion, soft-tissue extension and high mitotic activity do not establish malignancy.

Malignant degeneration in giant-cell tumors should be regarded as similar to the malignant degeneration/dedifferentiation described in other soft-tissue and osseous neoplasms, such as pigmented villonodular synovitis, low-grade osteogenic sarcoma, enchondroma and low-grade chondrosarcoma.

LIPOMA OF BONE

Benign fatty tumors of bone are among the rarest skeletal tumors. They have been described in patients of all ages, especially in the long bones. They may present as either subperiosteal or intramedullary lesions. In either case they are lytic, although occasionally calcification within necrotic fat may give rise to confusion with a bone infarct (Fig. 19.56). The intramedullary lesions have well-defined borders and occasionally a bubbly appearance. The periosteal lesions are also lytic and usually erode the cortex; sometimes spicules of periosteal new bone are associated with the lesion. MRI is particularly useful for localization of such lesions, because fat gives a characteristic signal.

On gross examination, the tumor is characteristically a lobulated, soft, yellow mass. Microscopic examination reveals mature fat, usually containing thin, residual cancellous bone trabeculae.

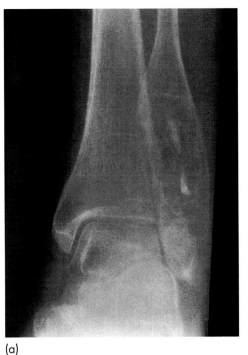

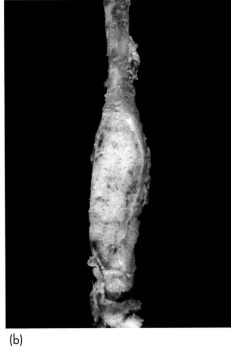

(a)   (b)

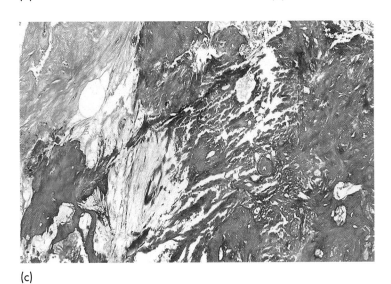

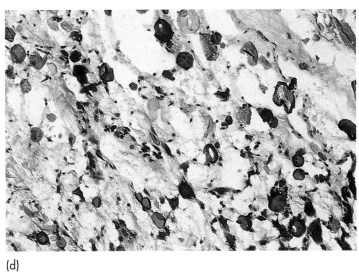

(c)   (d)

Figure 19.56   (a) Radiograph of an ankle shows fusiform swelling of the lower end of the fibula due to a lytic trabeculated intraosseous mass. In the center of the lesion there is focal dense calcification. (b) Photograph of a section through the dissected distal fibula shown in (a). The lesion is composed of an admixture of fat and fine cancellous bone. (c) Photomicrograph of tissue from the densely calcified area seen on the radiograph (a) shows heavily calcified scarring of necrotic fat within the lipoma (H&E, × 4 obj.). (d) Photomicrograph of the lesional tissue in another area of the specimen shown in (b), demonstrating punctate calcification within an area of fat necrosis (H&E, × 25 obj.). (Courtesy of Dr Leonard Kahn.)

MALIGNANT NONMATRIX-PRODUCING BONE TUMORS

This chapter will consider malignant small-cell tumors found in bone and their differential diagnosis. Also considered are vascular neoplasms and metastatic tumors.

EWING'S SARCOMA

Ewing's sarcoma is a small-cell malignant neoplasm of bone which develops in the diaphysis or metaphysis of long bones, most often the femur, tibia, and humerus, as well as in the pelvis, scapulae, ribs, and other bones. It is essentially a tumor of childhood, with most patients under 20 years of age. Males and females are about equally affected, although there is a small predominance in males. Ewing's tumors very rarely arise in the soft tissues (Fig. 20.1).

Patients usually complain of pain or tenderness in the affected bone of several weeks' or months' duration. Physical examination may reveal swelling and tenderness. Fever, anemia, leukocytosis, and elevated erythrocyte sedimentation rates often suggest a diagnosis of osteomyelitis and, because of the histologic appearance of the tumor, osteomyelitis is the most important microscopic differential diagnosis of Ewing's tumor.

Radiographic examination usually reveals a lytic, moth-eaten, mottled appearance (Figs 20.2 and 20.3), or sometimes even sclerosis; classically, laminated periosteal reactive bone is present, likened by some to an onion peel (Fig. 20.4). (However, this onion-peel appearance should not be considered diagnostic of Ewing's tumor.) The occasional finding of bone sclerosis may suggest the radiologic diagnosis of osteosarcoma.

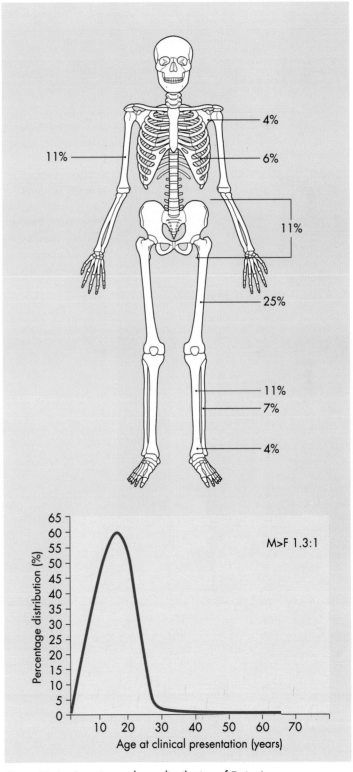

Figure 20.1   Location and age distribution of Ewing's sarcoma.

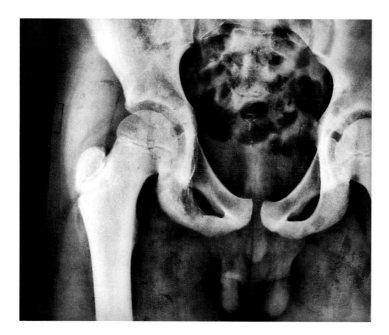

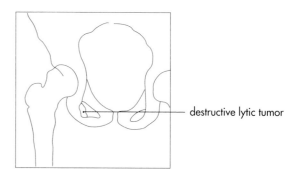

Figure 20.2   Radiograph of a 9-year-old child complaining of the pain in the hip joint shows a permeative destructive lesion of the ischium. Biopsy of this area showed a malignant round-cell tumor consistent with Ewing's sarcoma.

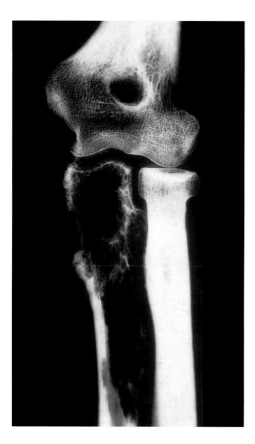

Figure 20.3
Radiograph of a resected arm with Ewing's tumor to show more clearly than is normally seen in a clinical radiograph the pattern of bone destruction.

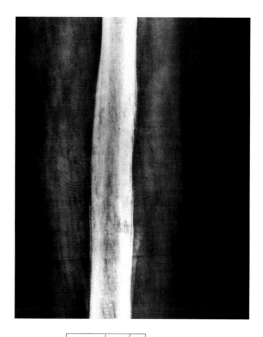

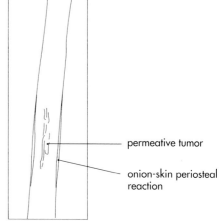

Both magnetic resonance imaging (MRI) and computerized tomography (CT) provide better pretreatment assessment of the intramedullary and soft-tissue extent of the tumor, which is often much greater than suggested on plain films. Gross examination of intact specimens reveals poorly demarcated, grayish-white tumor tissue with areas of hemorrhage, cystic degeneration, and necrosis. The actual extent of bone destruction is usually greater than that evident on radiographs, and extension of the tumor into adjacent soft tissue is common.

On microscopic examination Ewing's sarcoma consists of a homogeneous population of densely packed small cells. Nuclei are regular with finely granular nuclear chromatin and 1–2

Figure 20.4   Radiograph of the femur in a 13-year-old adolescent complaining of pain in the thigh shows an extensive permeative lesion in the midshaft of the femur, with elevation of the overlying periosteum, and periosteal new bone formation which is present in several layers, giving an 'onion-skin' appearance. Ewing's tumors are frequently located in the diaphysis, and in this respect are distinguished from osteosarcoma, the other common malignant primary tumor of bone in young people, which usually occurs in the metaphysis.

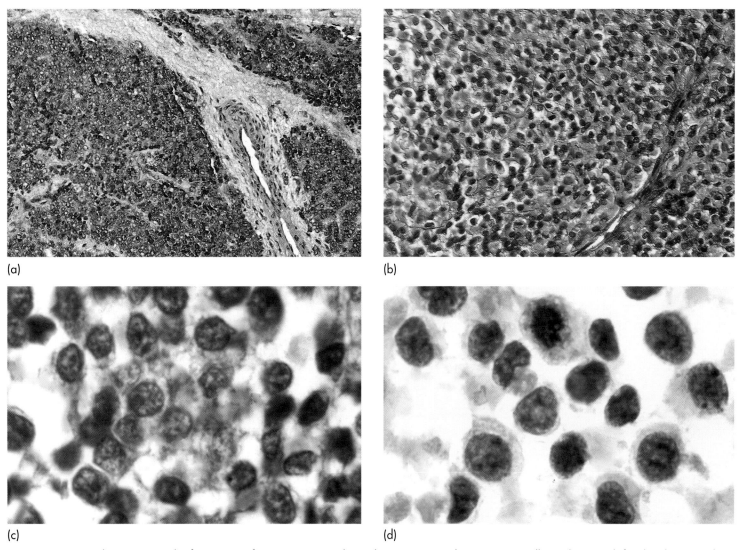

Figure 20.5 (a) Photomicrograph of a portion of a Ewing's tumor shows the monotonous, homogeneous cell population with focal, pyknotic nuclei. It is common for the lesion to show extensive necrosis or hemorrhage (H&E, × 4 obj.). (b) Intermediate power to demonstrate the characteristic uniformity of a Ewing's tumor with scattered cells having smaller and denser pyknotic nuclei (H&E, × 10 obj.). (c) High-power view of a portion of a Ewing's tumor shows the small, round cells and the indistinct lacy appearance of the cytoplasm. Note the lack of prominent nucleoli in these cells (H&E, × 40 obj.). (d) Photomicrograph of a direct imprint of fresh tumor tissue on a glass slide, subsequently stained with hematoxylin–eosin. By this technique, the cytologic detail of the cells is clearly demonstrated. A thin rim of delicate cytoplasm is seen around the vesicular nuclei, which lack any obvious nucleoli. A mitotic structure is noted in the upper part of the field (× 100 obj.).

small nucleoli. The cell wall is indistinct in histologic sections but may be visible on tissue-touch imprints. The cytoplasm is generally delicate and lace-like. Mitoses are relatively infrequent (Fig. 20.5). Reticulin fibers are sparse, but glycogen is evident after periodic acid–Schiff (PAS) staining in over 70% of cases and is usually found to be abundant on ultrastructural examination (Fig. 20.6). Areas of hemorrhage and necrosis are typically present. Scattered dark apoptotic cells as well as nests of small pyknotic cells are typically found. Although commonly referred to as a 'small-cell' tumor, Ewing's cells are actually two to three times larger than lymphocytes.

Reciprocal translocation between chromosomes 11 and 22 involving bands q24 and q12 t(11;22)(q24;q12) occurs in the majority of cases and is also present in the related small-cell peripheral neuroectodermal tumors, and Askin's tumors. These cytogenetic techniques are effective when fresh tumor tissue is available. Most Ewing's tumors will also show positivity for the CD99 antibody and vimentin is positive in the majority of cases.

Neural differentiation is present in some cases of Ewing's as well as in peripheral neuroectodermal tumor, and may be demonstrated by neuron-specific enolase, S100 protein and other neural markers. Electron microscopy may demonstrate neurosecretory granules.

The microscopic differential diagnosis of Ewing's sarcoma includes osteomyelitis, eosinophilic granuloma, and the group of small-cell tumors that includes lymphoma, leukemia, and metastatic neuroblastoma (and, in the case of soft-tissue Ewing's sarcoma, embryonal rhabdomyosarcoma). However, with molecular probes and immunohistochemical techniques, differentiation between these entities should no longer present significant problems (Fig. 20.7).

Ewing's sarcoma has a high incidence of early metastatic spread, usually to the lungs or to other bones. However, the use of adjuvant chemotherapy with radiation and surgical resection has considerably improved the outlook for patients with this tumor.

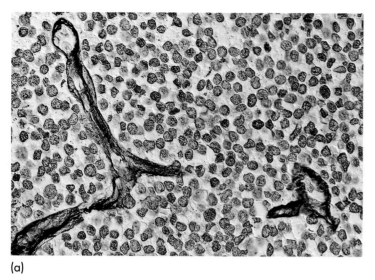

(a)

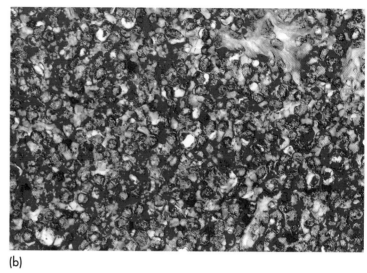

(b)

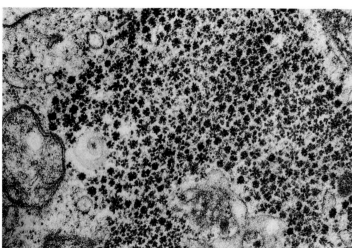

(c)

Figure 20.6   (a) Photomicrograph of a Ewing's tumor stained by the Wilder's method to demonstrate reticulin fibers. Note the lack of any reticulin network around the cells (× 25 obj.). (b) Photomicrograph of a portion of a Ewing's tumor stained by the PAS method demonstrates red-staining glycogen granules in the cytoplasm of most of the tumor cells (× 25 obj.). (c) Electron photomicrograph of a Ewing's sarcoma cell shows the packing of cytoplasm with glycogen granules (× 30,000).

Figure 20.7   Photomicrograph of a Ewing's tumor stained with antibody to *myc2* [CD99] antigen (× 40 obj.).

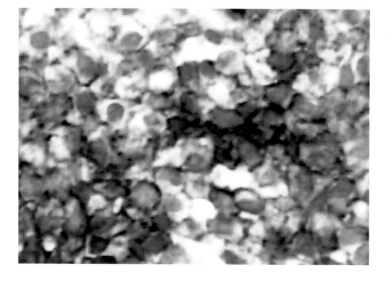

IMMUNOHEMATOPOIETIC TUMORS

In clinical cases of lymphoma, secondary involvement of the bone is present in approximately 20% of all patients and a diffuse involvement of the bone marrow is a feature of all types of leukemia. For these reasons therefore many patients with these conditions will complain of bone pain.

Primary intraosseous lymphomas are uncommon, but it is important to recognize that patients with primary bone lymphomas and no systemic involvement have a substantially better prognosis than those with disseminated disease (Fig. 20.8). Primary bone lymphoma can occur at any age but is rare in patients during the first decade of life (c.f. Ewing's sarcoma). Although local pain is usually present at the time of initial eval-

but diagnosis depends also on the identification of the immunological phenotype of the specific class of cell involved.

PRIMARY NON-HODGKIN'S LYMPHOMA

Primary non-Hodgkin's lymphomas of bone are usually large-cell lymphomas of B cell origin. They usually involve the bones of the extremities, and occur mostly in patients over 20 years of age (more than 50% of these tumors occur in patients over 40). NonHodgkin's lymphoma occurs mainly in the trunk bones including the ribs, pelvis, sternum and clavicle. However, a significant number of cases involve the long bones of the appendicular skeleton. Some cases present with multifocal lesions. The characteristic clinical picture is that of a patient in generally good health but with complaints of localized pain, swelling, or tenderness. No fever or marked weight loss is noted in the typical case. An appropriate staging procedure is required to rule out extraskeletal disease.

On radiographs, osteolysis is the predominant change observed, with the resulting appearance of a moth-eaten destructive lesion with no periosteal reaction (Fig. 20.9). MRI and CT are necessary in evaluating the extent of the lesions; especially soft-

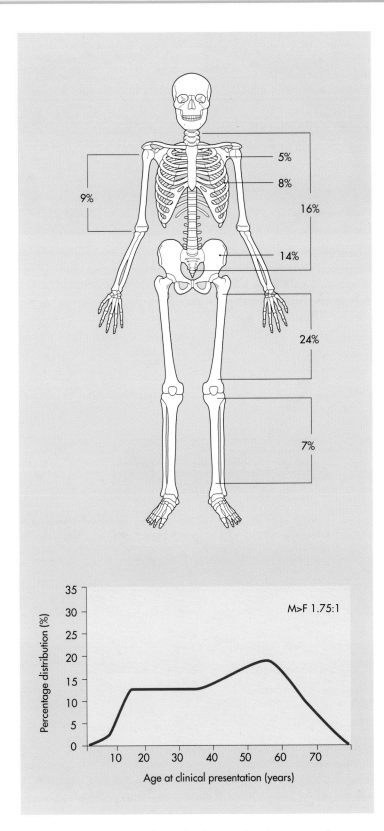

Figure 20.8 Location and age distribution of malignant lymphoma.

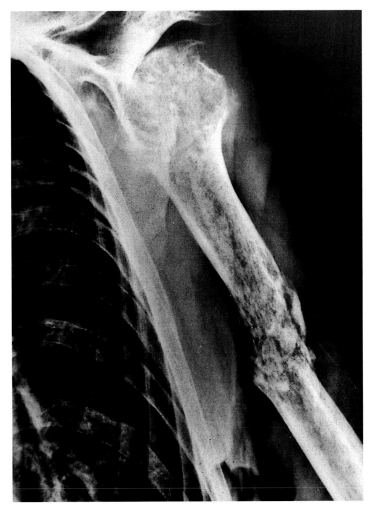

Figure 20.9 A 45-year-old man complained of sudden onset of pain in the left arm. Radiograph shows a pathologic fracture through an area of permeative destruction of both the cortical and medullary bone, which proved on biopsy to be due to lymphoma. The fracture is recent, and there is little or no periosteal reaction either to the tumor or to the complicating fracture.

uation, the overall general health of the patient is good. Early changes on radiographs include vague, mottled lucent areas. Considerable bone destruction may result from longstanding lesions. Microscopic identification depends on the presence of cells of the lymphoid series that solidly pack the marrow space, tissue extension and radioisotope studies help to document multifocal involvement. Gross examination reveals grayish-white tissue infiltrating the bone (Fig. 20.10).

Microscopically, the tumor consists of sheets of lymphoid cells with variable nuclear characteristics that depend on the type of lymphoma (Fig. 20.11). Most commonly, primary lesions are composed of a mixture of large cells with irregular cleaved nuclei, large cells with oval nuclei containing prominent nucleoli, and small cells with cleaved, hyperchromatic nuclei. Some lesions have a decidedly spindled appearance and may be difficult to recognize as lymphoma. Secondary lesions usually have a predominance of small cells, regardless of the pattern seen in the lymph nodes. The lack of glycogen (indicated by negative PAS staining) and the abundance of reticulin fibers separating each cell help to differentiate most lymphomas from Ewing's sarcoma. In addition to Ewing's tumor, the differential diagnosis includes poorly differentiated metastatic carcinoma, melanoma and, if the tissue is poorly preserved, osteomyelitis.

A panel of immunologic markers is necessary for positive identification of cell type, including leukocyte common antigen, CD20 (a pan B cell marker), CD45Ro (CD3) as a T cell marker and Ki1 for the rare large-cell Ki-lymphoma.

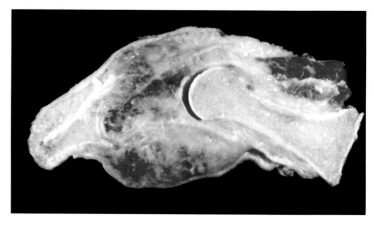

Figure 20.10 An amputated toe from a patient with a primary non-Hodgkin's lymphoma of the bone. The middle phalanx has been completely destroyed by a fleshy pink tumor which has extended both dorsally and ventrally into the soft tissue.

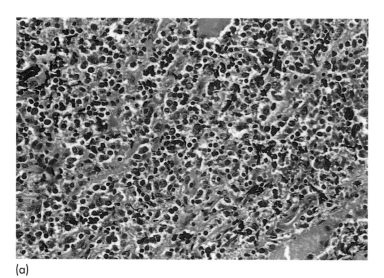

(a)

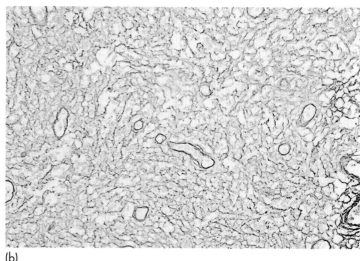

(b)

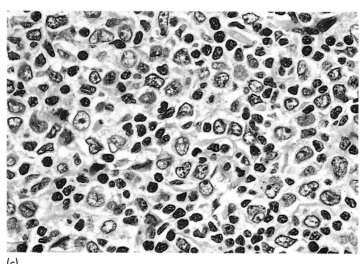

(c)

Figure 20.11 (a) Low-power photomicrograph of an area of non-Hodgkin's lymphoma shows the crowded, irregular cells. At high power these cells frequently show nuclear indentation and clefts. Compared with the cells of Ewing's tumor, these cells are larger and the cytoplasmic borders are more distinct. The cells in a non-Hodgkin's lymphoma usually lack glycogen (H&E, × 10 obj.). (b) Reticulin staining of the tumor shown in (a) reveals a fine network of reticulum separating small groups of cells as well as individual cells (× 10 obj.). (c) Photomicrograph of a primary non-Hodgkin's lymphoma in the bone. The crowded cells are larger and more irregular in outline than those seen in Ewing's sarcoma. Note the mixed cell population and the large irregular cleaved cells with prominent nucleoli (H&E, × 50 obj.).

The use of nonlymphoma markers such as keratin, desmin, and smooth-muscle actin, can help rule out other small-cell tumors.

The treatment of choice is local radiation, with or without chemotherapy, depending on the stage.

HODGKIN'S DISEASE

Hodgkin's disease is often present with bone pain and tenderness, sometimes with a palpable mass. However, primary osseous involvement is rare and may appear anywhere in the skeleton. Lesions in the ribs and sternum may result in significant swelling and extension into soft tissues. Vertebral involvement may cause neurologic disorders.

The radiographic features of Hodgkin's disease in the bone are variable; lesions may be lytic, blastic, or mixed. The radiologic finding of a dense 'ivory' vertebra is a classic presentation (Fig. 20.12). Usually multiple bones are involved, even if this is not apparent radiographically.

Microscopically, a characteristic mixed cell population can be observed, including plasma cells, lymphocytes, histiocytes, and eosinophils (Fig. 20.13). A large amount of fibrous stroma may complicate the diagnostic process. The pathognomonic and necessary finding in Hodgkin's lymphoma is the Sternberg–Reed cell. The Sternberg–Reed cell is large, with sharply delineated, abundant cytoplasm and a mirror-image double nucleus with a large, prominent, central eosinophilic nucleolus (Fig. 20.14). Conventional Sternberg–Reed cells express CD15 and CD30. Large, irregular mononuclear cells are also present, with similar nuclear features and prominent eosinophilic nucleoli. These cells are referred to as 'Hodgkin's cells'.

The differential diagnosis in Hodgkin's disease may be difficult and especially with reactive or inflammatory conditions. The positive identification of Sternberg–Reed cells is therefore essential.

LEUKEMIA

Diffuse involvement of the bone marrow is a hallmark of all types of leukemia. Skeletal pain constitutes the presenting complaint of 25% of children and 5% of adults with acute leukemia. Radiographic bone changes ultimately occur in 70–90% of leukemic patients and are described as: (1) transverse lucent metaphyseal line in children, (2) osteolytic destruction, (3) periosteal elevation, (4) generalized osteopenia, or (5) focal sclerosis.

A characteristic finding in children is a radiolucent band in the metaphysis of the long bones; similar bands may be found in the vertebral bodies just beneath the end-plates (Fig. 20.15). Perhaps the most common radiographic finding in both children and adults is diffuse demineralization of the spine with compression fractures, usually seen as anterior wedging. Epidural extension of the tumor is not uncommon in leukemia, and sometimes constitutes the presenting symptom. In addition, replacement of bone marrow by leukemic tissue may lead to ischemic necrosis of the affected bone and bone marrow (Fig. 20.16). Radiographic periosteal elevation is caused by subperiosteal leukemic masses. Sclerotic lesions are rare and are usually juxtaposed with lytic lesions. Radiographic features may mimic Ewing's sarcoma and other round-cell lesions.

The clinical diagnosis is especially difficult when a solid tumor develops significantly before the characteristic hematologic changes of leukemia. Solid leukemic tumors are found in as many as 40% of cases at autopsy, and they are the presenting feature of leukemia in up to 2% of cases.

Myelogenous leukemia can produce solid tumors called chloromas or granulocytic sarcomas. Granulocytic sarcomas are

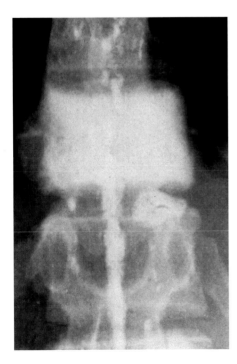

Figure 20.12 Antero-posterior radiograph of a 35-year-old male who presented with vague back pain. A single dense sclerotic vertebra is seen in the lower thoracic spine which, on biopsy, proved to be Hodgkin's disease. In the bone, Hodgkin's disease frequently exhibits considerable marrow fibrosis and reactive bone formation, which may be so severe as to obscure the lymphomatous tissue.

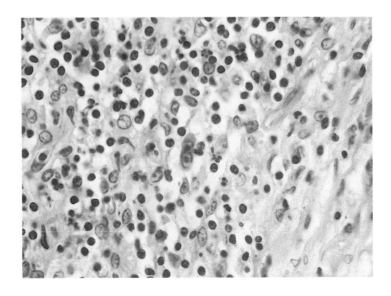

Figure 20.13 Photomicrograph of an area of Hodgkin's disease in bone shows a fibrous stroma with mixed cellular infiltrate of small, round cells and larger histiocytes (H&E, × 40 obj.).

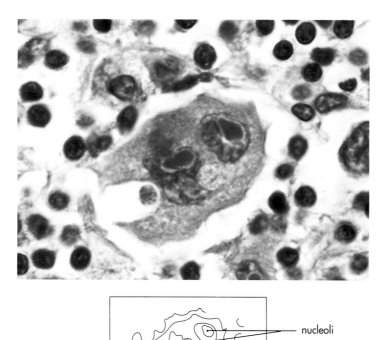

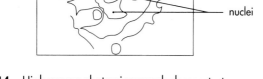

Figure 20.14   High-power photomicrograph demonstrates a binucleate Sternberg–Reed cell with prominent eosinophilic nucleoli (H&E, × 100 obj.).

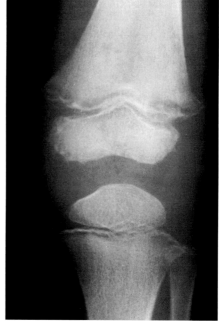

Figure 20.15   Antero-posterior radiograph of the knee in an infant with recent onset of fever, showing a radiolucent zone in the metaphysis adjacent to the growth plate, which is a classic radiologic sign of acute leukemia.

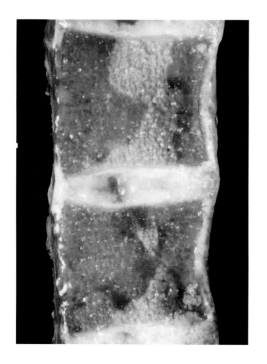

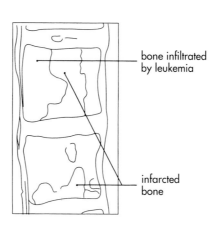

Figure 20.16   Photograph of a segment of the spine from a child who died of leukemia. Within the vertebral bodies are geographic areas of necrosis identified as yellow opacification of the bone and marrow. These are surrounded by a thin rim of hyperemic tissue. Note that the viable bone marrow has a fleshy tan color, reflecting the leukemic infiltrate.

collections of myelogenous leukemic cells outside of the bone marrow. Their 'characteristic yellow–green color' is frequently absent, so granulocytic sarcoma is a more accurate name for these leukemic tumors than is chloroma. Granulocytic sarcomas are most commonly found in the orbit and long bones, as well as in perineural spaces, lymph nodes, ovaries, and kidneys.

Wright–Giemsa and chloracetate esterase stains and electron microscopy of tissue are necessary to diagnose granulocytic sarcoma. Bone marrow examination and electron microscopy of biopsy tissue are diagnostic of leukemia and are important in all investigations of round-cell tumors of bone.

Myelofibrosis, which is often a precursor of leukemia, is discussed in Chapter 9, p. 235.

MULTIPLE MYELOMA

Multiple myeloma is the most common primary tumor of bone, with a predilection for marrow-containing bones. The spine is almost always involved, although the primary presentation may be in the skull, ribs, sternum, or pelvis. Multiple myeloma usually affects individuals over the age of 50 but is occasionally seen in patients at a younger age; men are affected almost twice as often

as women. The usual clinical picture is one in which pain predominates. Anemia is common, the ESR is usually elevated, and occasionally, especially in association with bed rest and concomitant osteoporosis, hypercalcemia is present. The most important diagnostic test involves the identification of a monoclonal protein by serum electrophoresis (Fig. 20.17). Light-chain subunits of immunoglobulins (Bence–Jones proteins) are usually found in the urine. In more than half of patients, pathologic fractures lead to an overall loss of vertebral body height, with swelling of the adjacent intervertebral discs into the affected bodies and a resulting 'fish-mouth' appearance (Fig. 20.18).

Multiple myeloma is characterized radiographically by the presence of round lytic defects in the bone, with no significant sclerotic reaction surrounding them (Fig. 20.19). Occasionally,

Serum protein electrophoresis

	%	Normal range
Albumin	32.3	56.4–71.6
Alpha-1	3.6	1.9–4.5
Alpha-2	5.3	7.3–15.0
Beta	6.8	6.2–11.5
Gamma	52.0	7.8–18.2

Quantitative immunoglobulin

	mg/dL	Normal range
IgG	275	600–1450
IgA	2964	60–340
IgM	10.4	25–200

Immunofixation electrophoresis gel

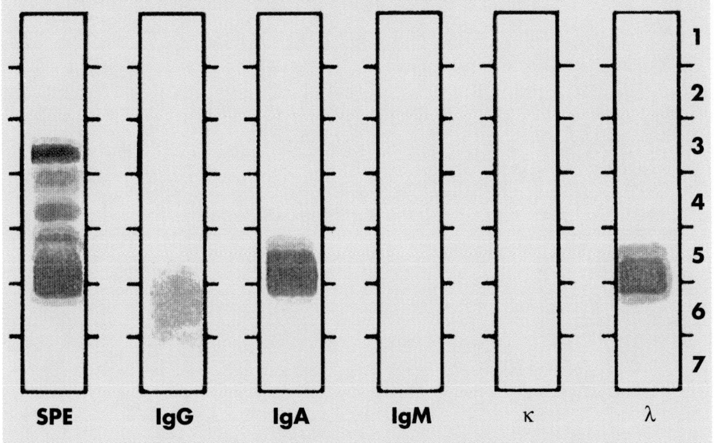

| SPE | IgG | IgA | IgM | κ | λ |

Increased IgA-lambda present

Figure 20.17 Immunoelectrophoregram of the serum from a patient with myeloma. Note that there is an excess of gammaglobulin, which is overwhelmingly IgA (λ).

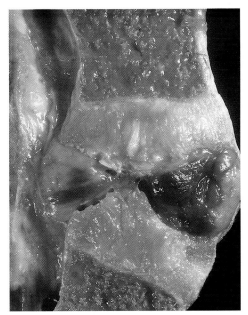

Figure 20.18
Collapse of the fifth lumbar vertebra and replacement by a gelatinous, pinkish-gray tissue is seen in this gross photograph of the lower spine removed at autopsy from a patient with multiple myeloma.

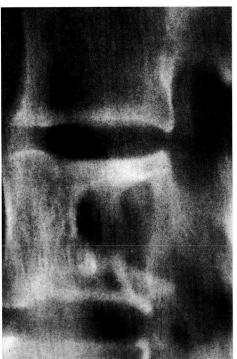

Figure 20.19
Lateral tomogram of L2, with parts of L1 and L3, in a 55-year-old male with multiple myeloma, demonstrating the well-defined lytic lesions, devoid of significant sclerosis, which are characteristic of this disease.

however, lytic defects may not be apparent and the radiographic picture suggests a diffuse osteopenia. In such cases, the differential diagnosis from osteoporosis must be made by laboratory examination.

Very rarely, multiple myeloma produces sclerotic lesions, such that the correct diagnosis may not at first be considered. (Sclerotic lesions are typical of the rare POEMS syndrome, in which *Polyneuropathy*, *Organomegaly*, *Endocrinopathy*, an *M*-component spike on electrophoresis of the serum, and *Skin* changes are characteristic.)

Gross examination of the affected bones reveals either a diffuse gelatinous red infiltration of the marrow or tan tumor nodules (Fig. 20.20). Microscopic examination reveals sheets of plasma cells, which may exhibit various degrees of differentiation; however, the atypicality of the cells (Fig. 20.21) has no prognostic significance. CD38 and plasma cell-associated antigen (PCA) are typically positive. In multiple myeloma the deposited proteins are related to the light change immunoglobulin (λ). In approximately 10% of patients with myeloma, amyloidosis occurs as a complication and amyloid deposits can be found within the bone (Fig. 20.22).

Multiple myeloma is a strikingly aggressive tumor which in the past led to early death. However, in a few cases palliative chemotherapy and bone marrow transplantation have been effective in prolonging the survival time.

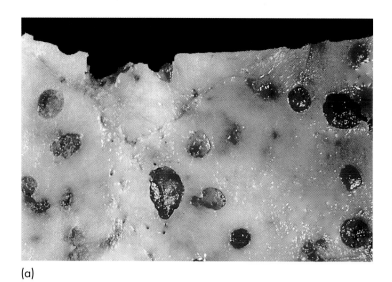

(a)

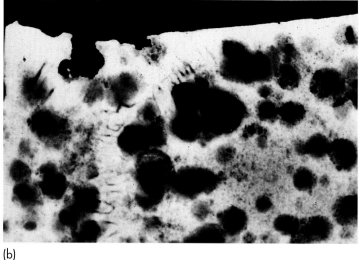

(b)

Figure 20.20 (a) Portion of the skull removed from a patient with multiple myeloma shows many round defects filled with pinkish-gray tissue. (b) Radiograph of the portion of skull shown in (a) demonstrates the clearly demarcated, lytic, punch-out lesions.

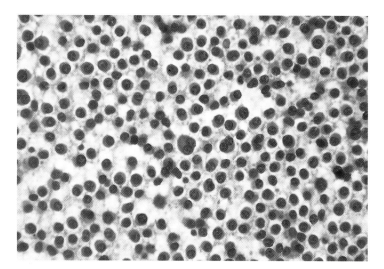

Figure 20.21 Photomicrograph of multiple myeloma shows closely packed plasma cells with some variation in shape and size, and an occasional double nucleus (H&E, × 40 obj.).

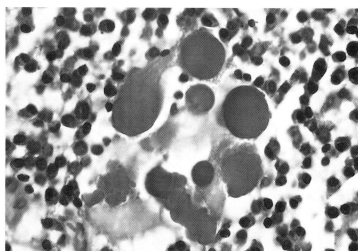

Figure 20.22 In some cases of multiple myeloma, foci of smooth, homogeneous pink material (amyloid) may be found, as shown in this photomicrograph (H&E, × 40 obj.).

SOLITARY (LOCALIZED) MYELOMA (PLASMACYTOMA)

The occurrence of a large solitary focus of plasma cell proliferation associated with radiologic evidence of bone destruction can
be considered a distinct entity from multiple myeloma if the following criteria are met: (1) there are no other radiographically
evident lesions; (2) a bone marrow biopsy from a site other than
the solitary focus reveals no malignant cells; and (3) no significant protein or immunoglobulin abnormality is discernible in the
serum and urine analyses (or, if a monoclonal spike is present on
serum electrophoresis, this disappears after treatment of the solitary lesion).

Patients who meet these criteria tend to be younger than those
with multiple myeloma and have a better prognosis. As with
multiple myeloma, men are more often affected. The site of
involvement is usually a long bone or a vertebral body (or, in
exceptional cases it is confined to the soft tissue). Long-bone
lesions may be expansile and often present with a pathologic fracture (Fig. 20.23).

In the spine, solitary myelomas are quite likely to present with
rapidly developing paraplegia and gibbous deformity as a result of
vertebral collapse (Fig. 20.24). (In fact, paraplegia is much more
frequently associated with solitary myeloma than with multiple
myeloma, probably because patients with multiple myeloma die
before paraplegia can develop.) However, paraplegia is by no
means always present and the patient may present with only
pain, as in the case illustrated in Figure 20.25.

About 70% of patients who present with an apparently solitary focus of myeloma will develop multiple myelomatosis and
will usually die within 5 years. The remaining patients may be
cured after radiation therapy or surgical en-bloc resection. A few
cases may develop generalized disease only after many years.
Microscopically, the tissue obtained in a case of solitary myeloma
may range from well differentiated to poorly differentiated plasma
cells, however, it does not seem that this variation affects the
prognosis in these patients.

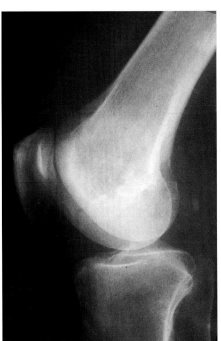

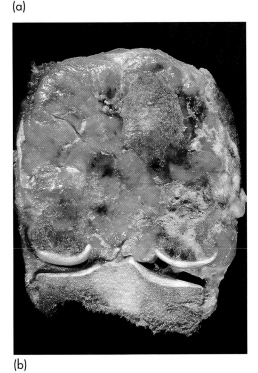

Figure 20.23   (a)
Radiograph of a 54-year-
old man who complained
of severe pain in the knee
shows a well-demarcated
lytic lesion on the femur
which, when biopsied,
was found to contain only
plasma cells. **(b)** Gross
photograph of the
specimen obtained from
the patient shown in **(a)**.
At the time of resection
no other evidence of
myeloma was present in
this patient.

(a)

(b)

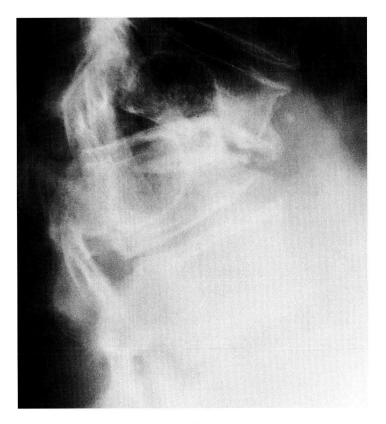

Figure 20.24   Lateral radiograph of a 45-year-old male who
presented with severe thoracolumbar pain following a fall. A fracture
dislocation of T10 and T12 is demonstrated, with virtual absence of T11.
Biopsy of the area showed myeloma. No other sites of myeloma were
demonstrated on radiographic survey. The patient received local
radiation therapy and a 10-year follow-up showed no evidence of local
or generalized disease.

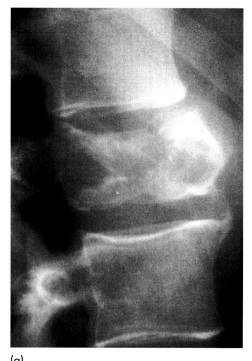
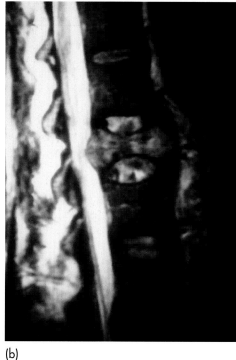

(a)   (b)

Figure 20.25   (a) Lateral radiograph of a
40-year-old male with a history of back pain
for 1 year, for which he had been treated with
physical therapy. (b) MRI shows the extent of
the plasmacytoma as well as the cord
compression.

VASCULAR NEOPLASMS

Vascular neoplasms of bone are rare. They include tumors
arising from the endothelium (hemangioendothelioma or
angiosarcoma) and tumors arising from the pericytes (hemangiopericytoma). Endothelial tumors vary from differentiated and
locally aggressive lesions (hemangioendothelioma) to highly
anaplastic, poorly differentiated metastasizing neoplasms
(angiosarcoma). The presence of multiple intraosseous lesions at
the time of initial diagnosis is common in both well-differentiated
and poorly differentiated tumors. Radiologic examination may
reveal multiple lesions either confined to a single long bone or to
the entire lower limb.

WELL-DIFFERENTIATED ENDOTHELIAL TUMORS

Hemangioendothelioma is a locally aggressive tumor which predominantly affects the long bones in adults. Complaints of pain
or swelling are common. These tumors are osteolytic and may be
poorly demarcated on radiographs (Fig. 20.26). Periosteal new
bone formation is unusual in hemangioendotheliomas.
Macroscopically, a multiloculate hemorrhagic tumor mass is typically found. The tumor is characterized microscopically by anastomosing cords of vascular channels lined with plump
endothelial cells, often with an epithelioid appearance (epithelioid
hemangioendothelioma), which lack pleomorphism or significant
mitotic activity. Solid foci of polygonal cells may also be seen (Fig.
20.27).

In some cases an inflammatory infiltrate is present in which
eosinophils may be prominent. The lining cells express factor
VIII-related antigen as well as CD31 and CD34.

Wide resection is the treatment of choice. Although these
tumors may recur they rarely, if ever, metastasize.

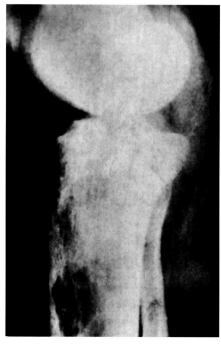

Figure 20.26
A 50-year-old man was
admitted to the hospital
complaining of pain in
the upper part of the leg.
A lateral radiograph
revealed a lytic and
permeative lesion in the
upper tibia, which on
biopsy proved to be a
well-differentiated vascular
neoplasm.

POORLY DIFFERENTIATED ENDOTHELIAL TUMORS

Angiosarcoma is a fully malignant, metastasizing neoplasm
which predilects the lower limb and affects adults of all ages,
more usually males. These tumors are characterized by rapid
growth and extensive bone destruction, with erosion of the

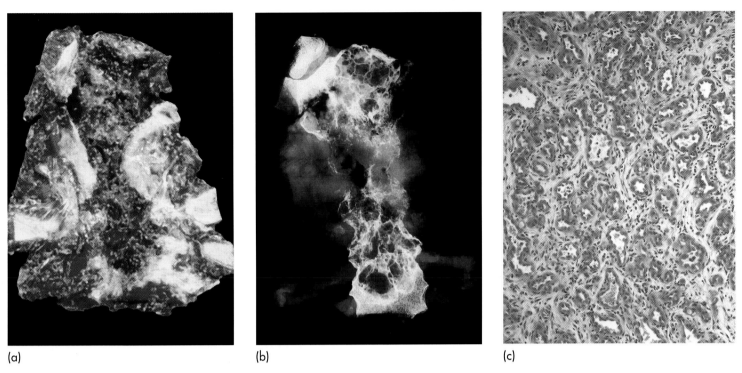

(a)   (b)   (c)

Figure 20.27   (a) Gross photograph of the sternum of a patient with a well-differentiated vascular tumor. The tumor has extensively involved the sternum and extends into the adjacent soft tissue. (b) Specimen radiograph of the tumor shown in (a). Note the lytic, destructive character of the tumor. (c) Photomicrograph of the tumor illustrated in (a) and (b) shows a fibrous stroma filled with proliferating vascular channels, lined with plump endothelial cells which lack obvious pleomorphism or significant mitotic activity (H&E, × 4 obj.).

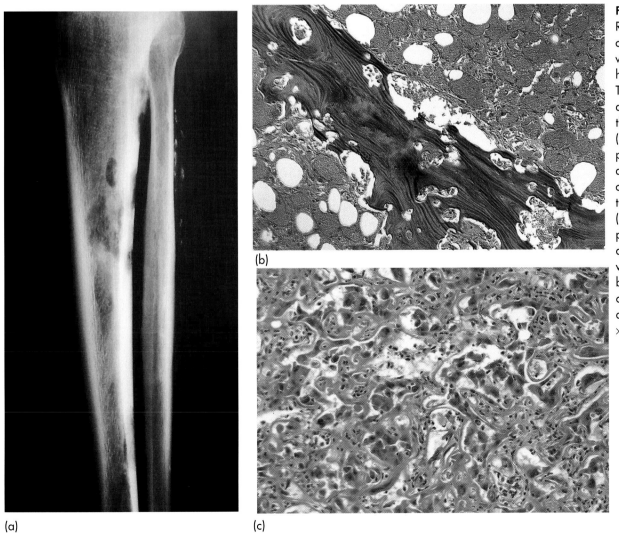

Figure 20.28   (a) Radiograph of the leg of a 70-year-old male with a few months' history of mild pain. There are several well-defined lytic lesions in the upper diaphysis. (b) Low-power photomicrograph to demonstrate the erosion of the bone by the tumor (H&E, × 4 obj.). (c) High-power photomicrograph to demonstrate numerous vascular spaces lined by large pleomorphic cells, consistent with an angiosarcoma (H&E, × 25 obj.).

(a)   (c)

cortices and extension into the soft tissues. Metastases to the lungs and other organs are common. The lesion consists of irregular, anastomosing vascular channels lined with malignant cells which exhibit prominent intravascular budding and striking cellular anaplasia with frequent mitoses (Fig. 20.28). Solid undifferentiated areas are often present and may suggest a poorly differentiated carcinoma or an anaplastic lymphoma. As with other sarcomas, foci of necrosis are common. Immunoperoxidase staining for factor VIII and other endothelial markers may be helpful in some cases.

Radical surgery is the treatment of choice.

HEMANGIOPERICYTOMA

Hemangiopericytoma is a rare, low-grade vascular tumor which occasionally occurs as a primary intraosseous lesion. Patients may present with localized pain. Radiographs are nonspecific and may reveal either lysis or focal sclerosis. Gross examination is likely to show a solid tumor.

The intervascular stroma contains typical spindle-shaped mononuclear cells believed to arise from a perivascular precursor cell (the pericyte) with the characteristics of smooth muscle. The key to the diagnosis of hemangiopericytoma is recognition that the neoplastic cells surround the vascular spaces and are not formed from the endothelial lining cells (Fig. 20.29). This finding can be confirmed by immunoperoxidase staining for factor VIII or reticulin staining. Because in some cases of mesenchymal chondrosarcoma the predominant pattern may be that of a hemangiopericytoma, it is important to look for evidence of cartilage formation when the diagnosis of hemangiopericytoma is being considered. It is also important to rule out a metastatic angioblastic meningioma.

Surgery is the treatment of choice; the prognosis is guarded, as metastases may occur.

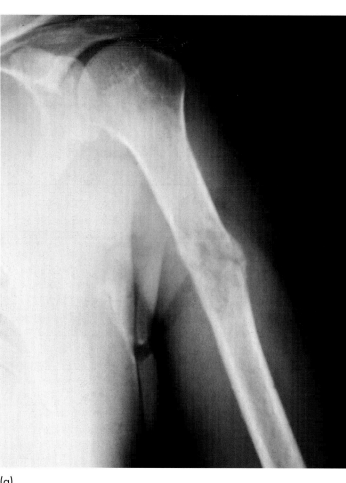

(a)

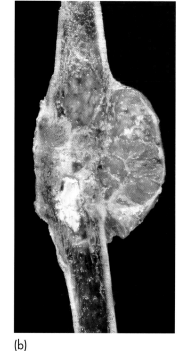

(b)

Figure 20.29 (a) Radiograph of a 30-year-old male with a 1-year history of vague pain in the left arm. A recent acute injury necessitated admission. A well-demarcated lytic lesion of the upper diaphysis is apparent. (b) Section through the resected segment of the humerus from the patient in (a) shows a fleshy tumor extending into the soft tissue from the intramedullary space. The opaque yellow infarcted area may be related to a past fracture in this area. (c) Photomicrograph of tissue obtained from the case shown in (a) and (b) shows crowded, uniform round cells surrounding vascular spaces in a pattern characteristic of hemangiopericytoma (H&E, × 25 obj.). In such a case it would be important to search for islands of cartilage since in mesenchymal chondrosarcoma identical areas of hemangiopericytoma may be found.

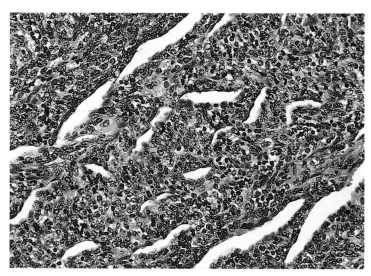

(c)

METASTATIC CANCER

Metastatic cancer is the most frequent malignant tumor found in bone and it usually causes pain. It is considerably more common than the primary bone tumor and should always be considered in the differential diagnosis, even of a solitary lesion. Reflecting the general prevalence of cancer in the population, most metastatic bone lesions are metastases from primary lesions in the breast, prostate, lung, kidney, thyroid, or colon (Figs 20.30 and 20.31). (A diagnosis of neuroblastoma, rhabdomyosarcoma, or retinoblastoma should be considered in young children.)

On radiographic studies, metastatic tumors may appear as sclerotic or lytic, solitary or multiple. Scintigraphy has greatly facilitated the identification of multiple bone metastases. In general, whereas purely blastic or sclerotic lesions are seen with prostate and breast carcinoma, kidney and thyroid metastases are destructive and frequently 'expansile.' It is not unusual for

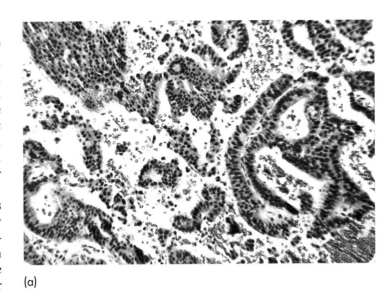

(a)

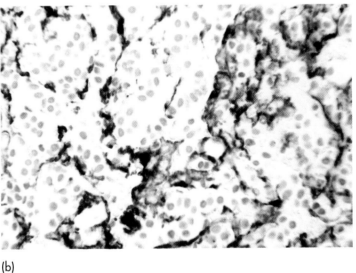

(b)

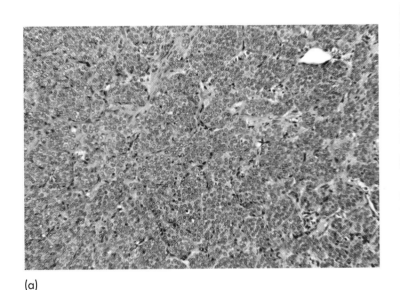

(a)

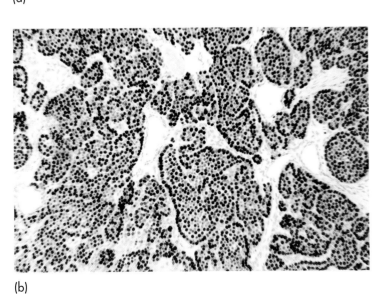

(b)

Figure 20.30   (a) Photomicrograph of metastatic lobular carcinoma of the breast (H&E, × 10 obj.). (b) Estrogen receptor marker is seen to be positive on the nuclei of this case (immunoperoxidase, × 10 obj.).

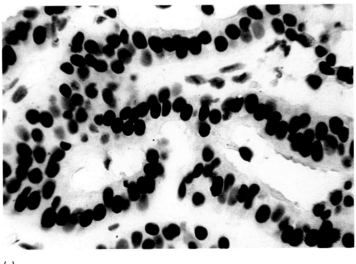

(c)

Figure 20.31   (a) Photomicrograph of metastatic adenocarcinoma which proved to be from the breast (H&E, × 10 obj.). (b) Gross cystic disease fluid protein-15 (BRST-2) is seen running in between the cords of cells (immunoperoxidase, × 25 obj.). (c) Estrogen receptor marker is positive on the nuclei (immunoperoxidase, × 25 obj.).

patients with an undiagnosed primary tumor (e.g. in the kidney) to present initially with a solitary lytic lesion in the bone, and in such a case problems of differential diagnosis may arise (Fig. 20.32).

The diagnosis of metastatic disease is often aided by fine-needle aspiration biopsy. In these circumstances, smears should be made to facilitate the interpretation of fine cytologic detail, and both core bone and blood (clot) should be processed and examined. The blood clot may exhibit evidence of cancer in many cases in which crushed tumor tissue precludes interpretation of the bone sample (Fig. 20.33).

Microscopic identification of the primary site from which the

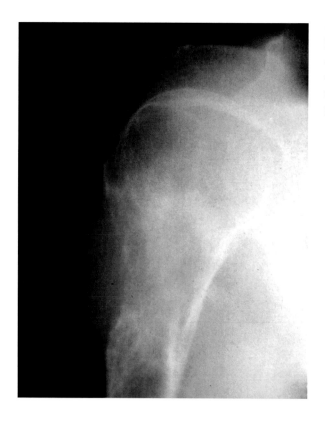

Figure 20.32   Radiograph of an aggressive lesion in the proximal humerus of a 70-year-old male who was in otherwise good health. A primary bone tumor could not be excluded radiographically. The differential would include malignant fibrous histiocytoma, solitary myeloma and chondrosarcoma. Further investigation revealed a primary carcinoma in the kidney.

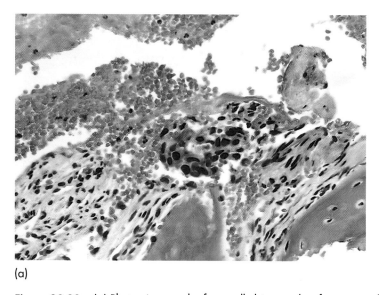

(a)

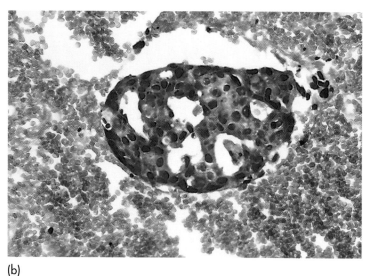

(b)

Figure 20.33   (a) Photomicrograph of a needle biopsy taken from a vertebral body with a sclerotic lesion suspected of arising from metastatic cancer. There is obviously active new bone formation as well as fibrous scarring, and a clump of atypical cells is strongly suggestive of tumor. Definitive diagnosis may be difficult on this type of tissue (H&E, × 40 obj.). (b) Within the aspirated clot there is clear evidence of adenocarcinoma. Often, in needle biopsies of bone, severe crushing artifacts preclude interpretation of the tissue sample. For this reason, the aspirated blood clot should always be submitted for examination, and will frequently give positive results when the bone tissue sample is negative or equivocal (H&E, × 40 obj.).

metastasis has originated may be difficult, especially in poorly differentiated neoplasms. Well-differentiated tumors may show squamous pearls if they are from a squamous carcinoma, and mucin-producing glands if they stem from an adenocarcinoma. (It should be noted that whereas gastrointestinal adenocarcinomas usually produce mucin, those from the lung may not, and those from the kidney rarely do.) The clear cells of renal cancer may create considerable diagnostic confusion, suggesting a clear-cell chondrosarcoma, chordoma, or even liposarcoma. Appropriate immunologic markers are often indicated.

The preferential deposition of tumor cells in bone marrow may be explained by the latter's rich vascularity and large sinusoidal channels.

In the case of osteoblastic metastases, the bone that is formed is reactive and is present as fine spicules of woven bone adherent to the residual existing bone (Fig. 20.34).

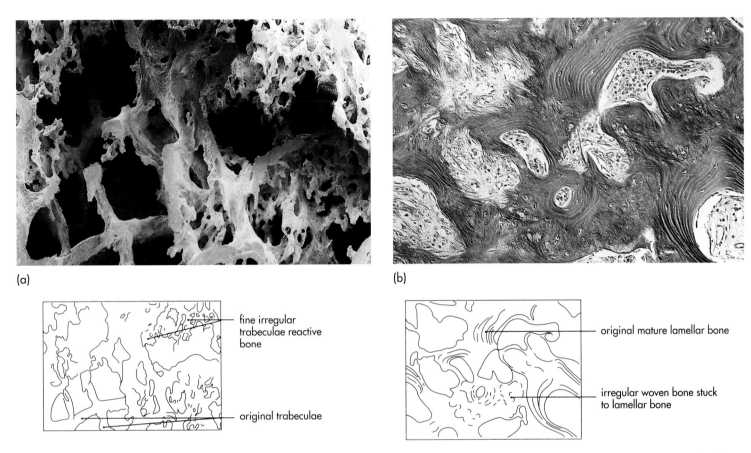

(a)　　　　　　　　　　　　　　　　　　(b)

fine irregular trabeculae reactive bone

original trabeculae

original mature lamellar bone

irregular woven bone stuck to lamellar bone

Figure 20.34 (a) Scanning electron micrograph of a portion of bone obtained from metastases from an osteoblastic prostatic carcinoma. The fine trabeculae of bone produced in response to the tumor are apparent (× 10 magnification). (b) Photomicrograph of the same specimen shows the woven character of the new bone, which is firmly adherent to the surface of the lamellar bone of the vertebral body. The spaces in between are filled with fibrous tissue and malignant cells (H&E, × 10 obj.).

SOFT-TISSUE TUMORS

BENIGN SOFT-TISSUE TUMORS

BENIGN SYNOVIAL LESIONS

SYNOVIAL HEMANGIOMA

A synovial hemangioma is usually a solitary, benign lesion, most commonly seen in the knee joints of children and adolescents.

The patient may present clinically with a swollen knee associated with mild pain or limitation of movement. Occasionally, the patient may report a history of recurrent episodes of pain and joint swelling of several years' duration.

A soft-tissue mass may be evident on radiographic examination, although magnetic resonance imaging (MRI) may be necessary to show it clearly. In severe cases, a periosteal reaction or lucent zones in the adjacent bones may also be present.

Gross examination of the resected synovial tissue reveals a soft, brown, doughy mass with overlying villous hyperplastic synovium which is frequently stained mahogany brown as a result of repeated bleeds. When the mass is viewed microscopically, arborizing vascular channels of different sizes are seen (Fig. 21.1). The overlying synovial lining is hyperplastic, and in chronic cases with repeated hemarthrosis, copious iron deposition can be observed.

Complete surgical excision may be difficult to effect, and this fact probably accounts for the occasionally reported cases of recurrence.

In Figure 21.2, a capillary hemangioma resected from a tendon sheath of a patient clinically diagnosed as de Quervain's disease, is illustrated.

HOFFA'S DISEASE (LIPOMA ARBORESCENS, VILLOUS LIPOMATOUS PROLIFERATION OF THE SYNOVIUM)

Hoffa's disease is a post-traumatic reactive condition of the synovium, clinically most often seen in the knee and characterized by enlargement of the infrapatellar fat pad on either side of the patellar tendon. However, the condition may occur in association with any joint. The patient usually complains of pain or a deep aching in the anterior compartment of the knee which is usually aggravated by physical activity. A recurrent effusion may be the consequence of repeated synovial injury. The treatment of Hoffa's disease is surgical reduction in the volume of extrasynovial fat.

When the lesion is examined macroscopically, the synovium has a marked papillary yellow fatty appearance; microscopically,

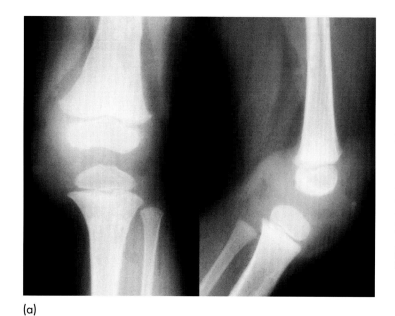

(a)

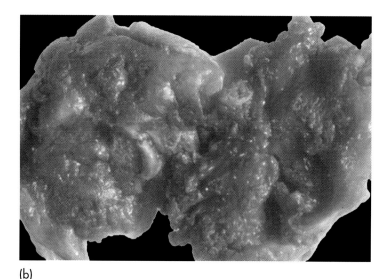

(b)

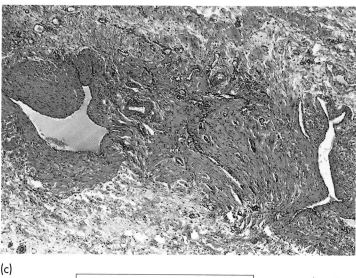

(c)

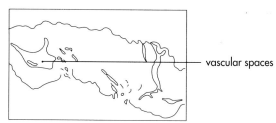

Figure 21.1   (a) Antero-posterior and lateral radiograph of the right knee of a 2-year-old who had been irritable for about 1 year, which her mother attributed to a swelling of the knee. On examination, a nontender mass was felt on the medial aspect of the knee. (b) Gross specimen removed from the knee of a patient with a history of recurrent hemorrhages into the joint. Marked hemosiderin staining of the tissues has occurred, but the synovium does not show either the villous appearance seen in association with hemophilia or the papillary appearance usually seen in patients with pigmented villonodular synovitis. (c) Photomicrograph of part of the synovial tissue shown in (b) demonstrates the vascular malformation in this patient's synovium. At the synovial surface, copious hemosiderin deposits and hyperplastic reactive tissue were evident (H&E, × 10 obj.).

there is mild hyperplasia of the synovial lining cells with abundant unremarkable fat extending to the synovial lining. Occasionally a mild to moderate chronic inflammatory infiltrate may be present (Fig. 21.3).

PRIMARY SYNOVIAL CHONDROMATOSIS (PRIMARY SYNOVIAL CHONDROMETAPLASIA)

Primary synovial chondromatosis is a rare condition characterized by the metaplastic proliferation of islands of irregularly hypercellular cartilage in the synovium of a major joint, often the knee or occasionally in a tendon sheath. These findings distinguish primary synovial chondromatosis from the much more commonly observed occurrence of articular cartilage fragments, often with associated reactive proliferative cartilage, in the syn-ovial tissues of patients with a post-traumatic osteochondral fragment, osteochondritis dissecans or osteoarthritis (OA).

Patients with primary synovial chondromatosis have been observed in their second through seventh decades of life, and males appear to be affected about twice as frequently as females. The patients usually report the gradual onset of pain, stiffness, or an enlarging mass around the affected joint. Limitation of motion is a characteristic finding on clinical examination. The knee is most commonly affected and most other cases present in the hip or elbow. Most of the remaining cases occur in the tendon sheaths of the hands or feet.

The radiologic signs of this disorder include multiple loose bodies of variable size, many of which show varying degrees of calcification and occasional ossification (Fig. 21.4). However, in a minority of cases there is no calcification and in such cases con-

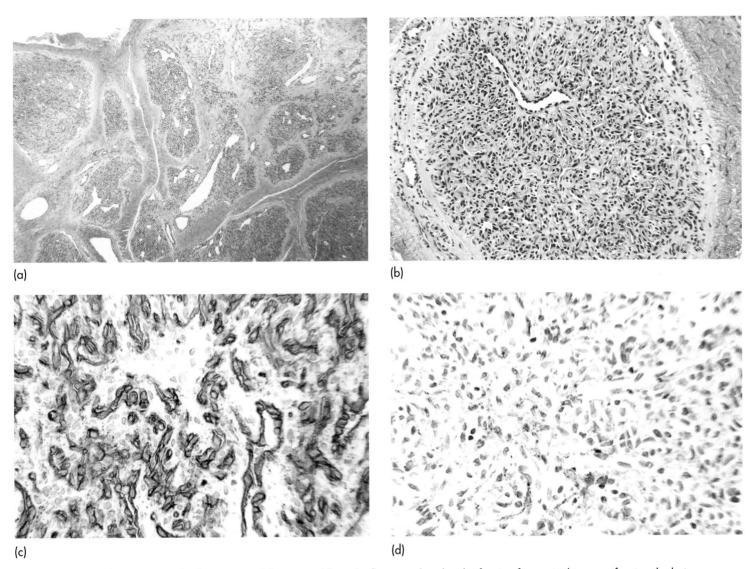

(a)

(b)

(c)

(d)

Figure 21.2   (a) Photomicrograph of a 3-mm nodule removed from the flexor tendon sheath of a ring finger. At this magnification the lesion appears to consist of vascular channels surrounded by cellular tissue, suggesting a glomus tumor (H&E, × 4 obj.). (b) At a higher power the cellular tissue is formed of closely packed capillaries (H&E, × 10 obj.), confirmed by CD34 immunoperoxidase stain (× 25 obj.) (c). (d) Smooth-muscle actin is only faintly positive (× 25 obj.).

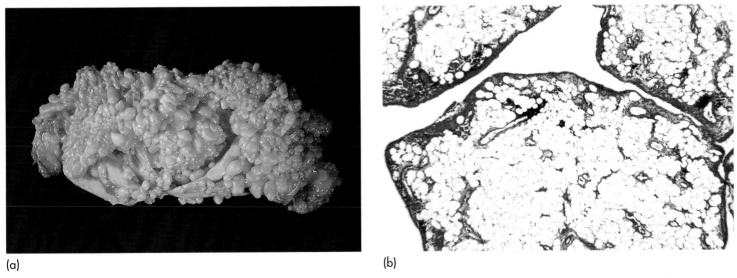

(a)

(b)

Figure 21.3   (a) Gross photograph of the synovium resected from a patient with fullness of the knee joint. Note the fatty appearance of the tissue and the papillomatous folds arising on the surface. (b) Photomicrograph of a section through the synovium shown in (a), showing fatty infiltration of the subsynovial tissue in Hoffa's disease (H&E, × 10 obj.).

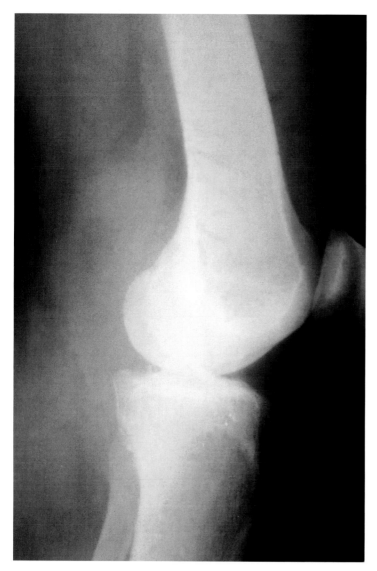

Figure 21.4   Lateral radiograph of the knee joint of a middle-aged man complaining of vague knee pain and swelling. Multiple small opacifications both in and around the joint are particularly prominent in the popliteal space. On biopsy, this proved to be due to primary synovial chondromatosis.

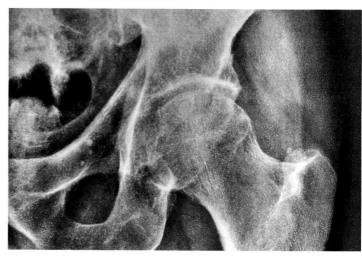

(a)

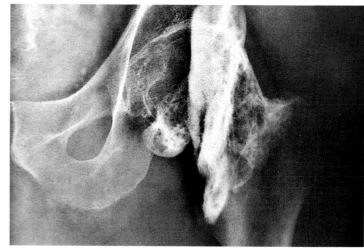

(b)

Figure 21.5   (a) Radiograph of a 65-year-old man who presented with an intermittent 20-year history of mild pain in the right hip, shows no obvious lesion in the joint. (b) Arthrogram of the patient shown in (a) demonstrates many small, round filling defects in the synovium, consistent with synovial chondromatosis. The individual nodules of cartilage were neither calcified nor ossified, and therefore failed to show up on plain radiographs. (Courtesy of Dr Alex Norman.)

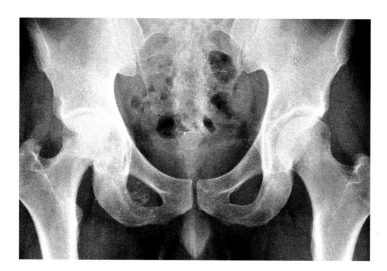

Figure 21.6   Radiograph of a young man with synovial chondromatosis which first presented as a calcified lesion in the right obturator foramen. Note that there is also distinct erosion of the medial neck of the right femur as compared with the left.

trast arthrography or MRI may be necessary to demonstrate the lesions (Fig. 21.5). In some cases of synovial chondromatosis affecting the hip joint, erosion of the bone of the neck of the femur has been observed (Fig. 21.6).

At surgery, there are usually multiple cartilaginous loose bodies, both free in the joint and attached to the synovium (Fig. 21.7). The larger cartilage loose bodies often have a multinodular surface, giving them a mulberry-like appearance. Microscopic examination reveals discrete nodules of cartilaginous tissue in the synovium, characterized by cellular crowding with cytologic atypia; many binucleate cells may be present and myxoid areas may be present such that if seen in an intramedullary lesion would be considered as chondrosarcoma (Fig. 21.8). This disordered appearance differentiates primary synovial chondromatosis

from the much more common secondary cartilaginous loose bodies, which occur in association with OA, traumatic arthritis and osteochondritis dissecans (see discussion in Chapters 10, p. 254 and 11, p. 281).

The condition frequently recurs because of the difficulty of achieving complete excision. Rare cases of malignant degeneration in synovial chondromatosis have been described.

PIGMENTED VILLONODULAR SYNOVITIS (GIANT-CELL TUMOR OF TENDON SHEATH; BENIGN SYNOVIAL HISTIOCYTOMA)

Pigmented villonodular synovitis (PVNS) is a locally aggressive synovial tumor which affects both large joints and tendon

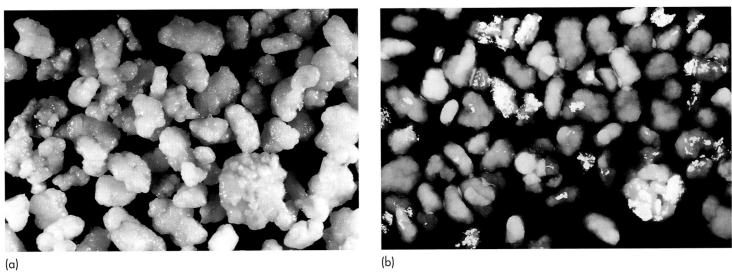

(a)   (b)

Figure 21.7   (a) Gross photograph of multiple loose bodies removed from a patient with synovial chondromatosis. (b) Radiograph of the tissue shown in (a) demonstrates that only a few of the loose bodies contain calcium.

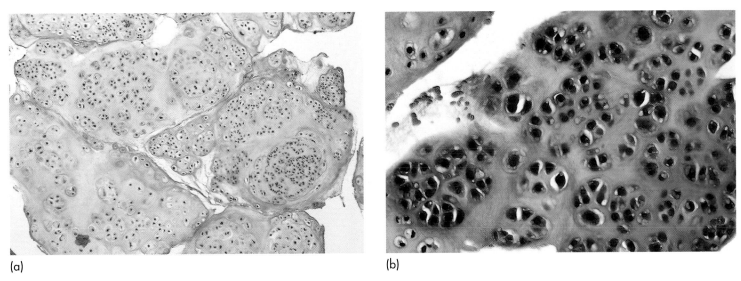

(a)   (b)

Figure 21.8   (a) Photomicrograph of the synovium removed from a patient with primary synovial chondromatosis shows nodules of hypercellular cartilage within the synovium (H&E, × 10 obj.). (b) Higher power view of primary synovial chondromatosis lesion shows atypical cells which are crowded and clumped. This histologic picture helps to distinguish primary synovial chondromatosis from the secondary chondromatosis that is frequently seen in association with osteoarthritis and trauma (compare this with Figure 10.36) (H&E, × 25 obj.).

sheaths, and which is much more frequently found as a solitary nodule and more rarely as a diffuse multinodular lesion. The most common sites involved are the knee or fingers, but this tumor sometimes occurs in the hip, ankle, foot, or wrist. The lesion is usually painless or only mildly painful; the pain appears to be more severe when the lesion is diffuse throughout a major joint. In general, the condition is confined to a single joint or tendon sheath.

The solitary lesions usually present clinically in the small joints or tendon sheaths of the hands or feet, whereas the multinodular diffuse form presents clinically in the large joints.

The radiologic signs of PVNS depend on the site of occurrence. In the finger, only soft-tissue swelling may be evident, although cortical bone erosion may occur (Fig. 21.9). In the knee, the only

consistent radiographic change is soft-tissue swelling in and around the joint, which may be massive. In the hip, joint narrowing and lytic defects in the bone may be present on both sides of the joint (Fig. 21.10). Local juxta-articular bone destruction may also be quite prominent in joints such as the wrist and ankle (Fig. 21.11).

MRI and computed tomography (CT) are useful to document the extent of the lesion and on T_1-weighted MRI the iron deposits may show up as punctate signal voids within the lesion.

On gross examination, the lesions tend to have a tan color, which is often more prominent at the periphery, and their texture may vary in firmness depending upon how much fibrous tissue they contain. In the tendon sheath of a finger the lesion is usually solitary and well circumscribed (Fig. 21.12). When it occurs

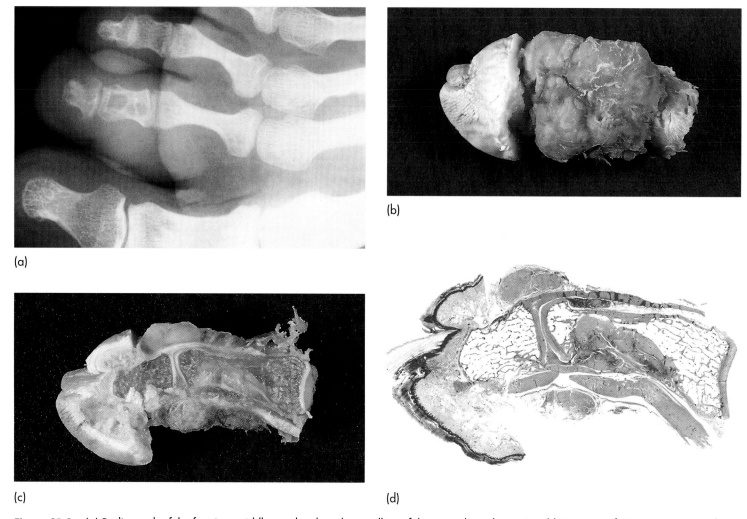

(a)

(b)

(c)

(d)

Figure 21.9 (a) Radiograph of the foot in a middle-aged male with a swelling of the second toe shows, in addition to a soft-tissue mass, several intraosseous lytic areas in the middle phalanx. (b) Lateral view of the amputated second toe in the patient shown in (a) shows a tan tumor enveloping the bone. (c) Gross photograph of a section through the specimen shown in (b). A soft-tissue tumor can be seen extending around and involving the distal interphalangeal joint. The lesion is also invading the medullary cavity of the phalanx. Focally, the tumor has a tan color. Histologically, this lesion proved to be PVNS. (d) Photomicrograph of a sagittal section through the toe shown in (c). Tumor tissue is seen both in the soft tissue and invading the bone and joint space. The pinker areas within the tumor tissue represent areas of collagenization (phloxine and tartrazine, × 1 obj.).

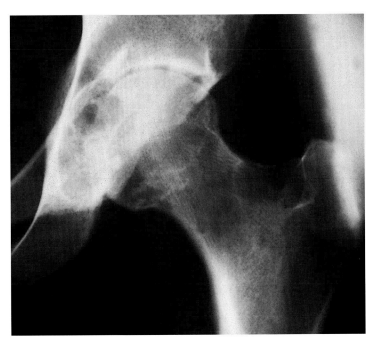

(a)

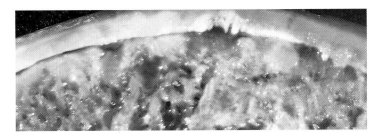

(b)

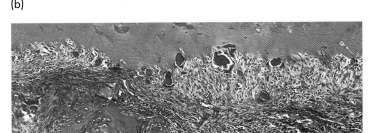

(c)

Figure 21.10   (a) Radiograph of a young woman with a history of rapid deterioration of function in the hip shows destructive changes on both sides of the joint, with marked narrowing of the joint space. Because of these radiographic findings, a diagnosis of tuberculosis was considered; however, at surgery abundant hemosiderotic synovium containing nodular fleshy areas was found. Gross section of the femoral head (b) reveals dissection of the articular cartilage, with proliferation of soft tissue between the bone and cartilage. Histologic section of this tissue (c) reveals proliferating mononuclear cells and giant cells in the subchondral bone. A diagnosis of PVNS was confirmed in this patient (H&E, × 10 obj.).

joint space narrowing and irregularity

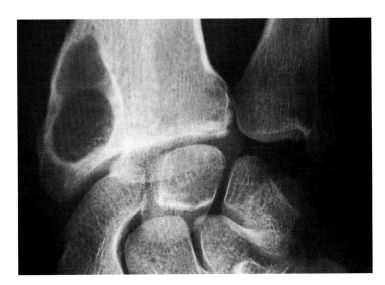

Figure 21.11   Radiograph of the wrist of a 30-year-old male who presented with swelling and pain in the joint. The lytic defect in the lower radius was due to erosion of the bone by PVNS.

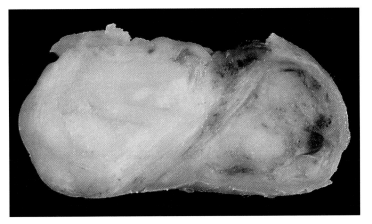

Figure 21.12   Photograph of a transected nodule removed from a finger. The nodule is firm and on cut section is found to be formed mostly of white tissue with focal areas of yellow tissue which correspond to xanthomatous areas microscopically. Pigmentation seems to be confined to the periphery of the lesion. Pigmentation is often found in lesions of PVNS and probably occurs as a result of secondary hemorrhage into the lesion following trauma.

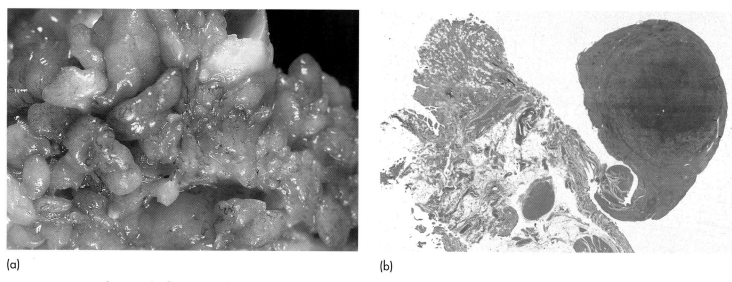

(a)   (b)

Figure 21.13   (**a**) Photograph of synovium obtained at total knee replacement from a patient with osteoarthritis. An incidental finding was the grayish nodule seen in the upper central part of the image. (**b**) Photomicrograph of the nodule seen in (**a**) proved to be a solitary area of PVNS (H&E, × 1 obj.).

in the knee joint it is most commonly as a solitary incidental finding (Fig. 21.13). In obvious clinical cases of PVNS in a large joint, the lesion commonly consists of multiple nodules, often with dramatic associated hyperplastic villous changes and extensive hemosiderin deposition in the adjacent unaffected synovium (Fig. 21.14).

On microscopic examination, the lesion is composed of proliferating, collagen-producing polyhedral cells, often with scattered, multinucleated giant cells (Fig. 21.15). Iron deposits and aggregates of foam cells may be present, but these are usually seen in the periphery of the lesion and are most consistent with secondary changes following hemorrhage into the lesion. Abundant production of collagen may be evident in patients with long-standing disease (Fig. 21.16). Occasionally, the cellularity of the lesion, especially when associated with a trabecular pattern of the intercellular matrix, may give a pseudosarcomatous appearance (Fig. 21.17).

The lesional tissue is localized below the lining cells of the synovial membrane (Fig. 21.18). The lesion is usually noninflammatory or contains only a sparse scattering of mononuclear cells, lymphocytes, and plasma cells. The differential diagnosis of PVNS includes hemosiderotic synovitis, which is seen in patients with chronic intra-articular bleeding (e.g. in hemophilia) as well as in foreign body giant cell reaction following total joint replacement (see Chapter 14, p. 342). Although a lesion of hemosiderotic synovitis contains a significant amount of pigment, it lacks the distinct submembranous mononuclear and giant-cell nodular cell proliferation that characterizes PVNS. In some cases of rheumatoid arthritis, extensive hemorrhage may lead to hemosiderin deposition and suggest PVNS at surgery (Fig. 21.19).

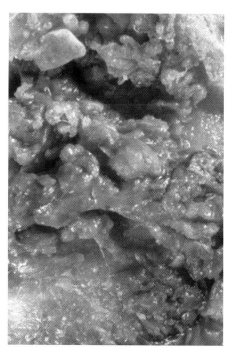

Figure 21.14   Gross photograph of synovium resected from the knee of a patient with PVNS. Note the reddish-brown staining due to hemosiderin deposition, as well as the plump papillary projections which result from cell proliferation. This appearance often causes diagnostic confusion with hemosiderotic synovitis.

The treatment of PVNS is excision; however, because complete surgical removal is often difficult, in diffuse cases clinical recurrence is fairly frequent. Very rare cases of malignant transformation have been reported.

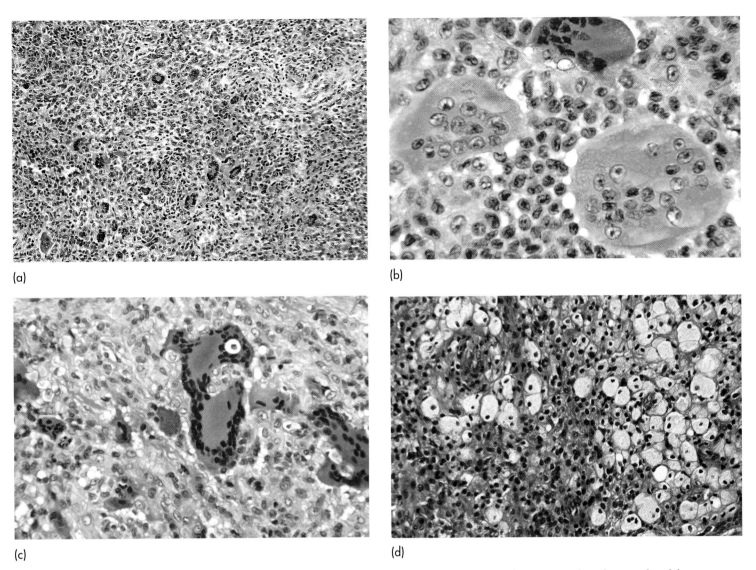

(a)

(b)

(c)

(d)

Figure 21.15   **(a)** Low-power photomicrograph of a typical area of pigmented villonodular synovitis demonstrates the subsynovial nodular accumulation of mononuclear cells with interspersed giant cells, which frequently have peripherally arranged giant cells (H&E, × 4 obj.). **(b)** Higher power shows the typical large stromal histiocytes (H&E, × 25 obj.). **(c)** In many areas of the lesion it is common to find spindle cells with collagen production as illustrated here (H&E, × 10 obj.). **(d)** Accumulation of xanthoma cells may on occasion be extensive (H&E, × 10 obj.).

Figure 21.16   Photomicrograph to demonstrate collagen production in PVNS (H&E, × 25 obj.).

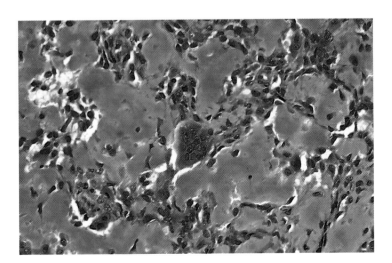

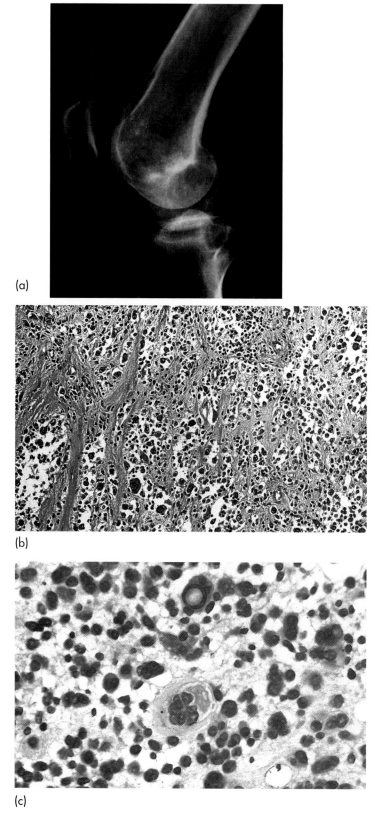

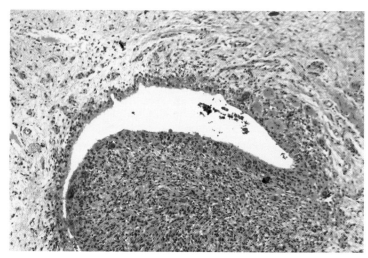

Figure 21.18 Photomicrograph illustrates a focus of PVNS with adjacent uninvolved proliferative synovium (H&E, × 4 obj.).

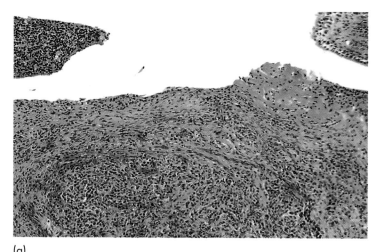

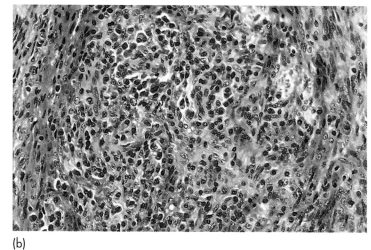

Figure 21.17 (a) Lateral radiograph of the right knee of a young man complaining of knee pain attributed clinically to a meniscal tear. The radiograph shows posterior lytic lesions on both the tibial and femoral side of the joint, suggestive of an arthritic rather than a neoplastic process. (b) Photomicrograph of this case of PVNS in which the collagen is seen in a trabeculated pattern with loose pseudoalveolar spaces between. This pattern, together with the heterogeneity of the cells, gives a pseudosarcomatous appearance to the tissue (H&E, × 10 obj.). (c) A higher power view to demonstrate the pseudosarcomatous appearance which can be seen in some cases of PVNS (H&E, × 25 obj.).

Figure 21.19 (a) Photomicrograph of synovial tissue obtained from a case of RA. There is considerable hemosiderin deposition in the deep parts of the synovium (H&E, × 10 obj.). (b) Higher power shows the hemosiderin as well as fibrous scarring. A chronic inflammatory infiltrate of lymphocytes and plasma cells is present. Nevertheless, a superficial resemblance to PVNS caused diagnostic problems in this case (H&E, × 25 obj.).

BENIGN FIBROUS LESIONS

Fibrous tumors and tumor-like lesions are common in the soft tissues and tend to be complicated. Some, such as the desmoid tumor, look at first sight to be histologically perfectly bland yet are infiltrative lesions which are poorly circumscribed and therefore tend to recur repeatedly following excision and may ultimately be lethal depending upon their location.

Others such as nodular fasciitis, proliferative fasciitis and proliferative myositis grow rapidly, are cellular, disorganized and have a high mitotic rate; they look like sarcomas and yet are readily cured by excision.

FIBROMA OF TENDON SHEATH

This is a distinct entity most commonly seen in the hands and feet. It usually presents clinically as a small mass, slowly growing, which may have been present for many years. Men are more commonly affected and most are adults between the ages of 20 and 50.

Grossly the lesions generally measure < 2 cm in diameter, have a very circumscribed lobular appearance and on cut section they are firm and appear gray–white (Fig. 21.20). Microscopically they are made up of collagen-producing fibroblastic cells with characteristic elongated vascular cleft-like spaces throughout the lesion. Myxoid areas are common. Occasionally cellular areas with some pleomorphism are present and in these areas there may be a storiform pattern (Fig. 21.21).

FIBROMATOSIS

Under the generic term of the fibromatoses are grouped a number of conditions that are characterized by fibroblastic tissue which, by its cellularity and capacity to infiltrate surrounding tissue, mimic a low-grade fibrosarcoma. However, these lesions do not metastasize. They may arise in many parts of the body and are known by a variety of names (e.g. desmoid tumor, Peyronie's disease, etc.). Of particular interest to the orthopaedic surgeon are palmar fibromatosis (Dupuytren's contracture), which is very common, and its plantar equivalent, which is decidedly rare.

Extra-abdominal fibromatosis (aggressive fibromatosis; desmoid tumor)

This is a relatively common tumor seen in young to middle aged adults. The tumor arises in the connective tissues of the muscles and aponeurosis, most commonly of the shoulder, pelvic girdle, and thigh. Because of its deceptively harmless microscopic appearance, it is unfortunately often mismanaged clinically.

The patient usually presents with a deep-seated, fixed, firm mass which has been evident to the patient for a few weeks at the time of presentation. Depending on location it may be painful (Fig. 21.22).

Characteristically these tumors are poorly circumscribed and infiltrate the surrounding tissue. It cannot be sufficiently emphasized that a wide surgical excision is necessary for successful management of the condition.

Microscopically the lesion is composed of uniform, elongated spindle cells separated by abundant collagen. Atypia and mitoses are not a feature of the lesion. These lesions are not encapsulated and at their periphery will be found to be invasive into the surrounding muscle and fat.

Because of inadequate marginal excisions the rate of regrowth is very high and at subsequent re-operation it may be difficult both for the surgeon and the pathologist to distinguish recurrent tumor from scar tissue.

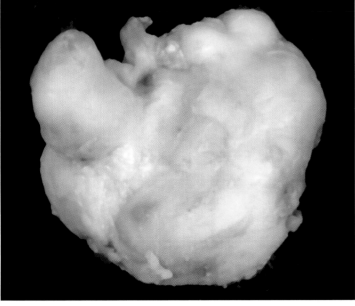

(a)

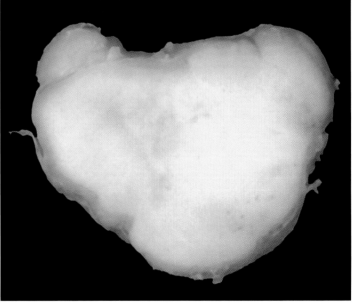

(b)

Figure 21.20 (a) This fairly well-defined, lobulated nodule measuring 2.8 cm was removed from the index finger of a 41-year-old male. (b) The cut surface reveals a firm, fibrous mass.

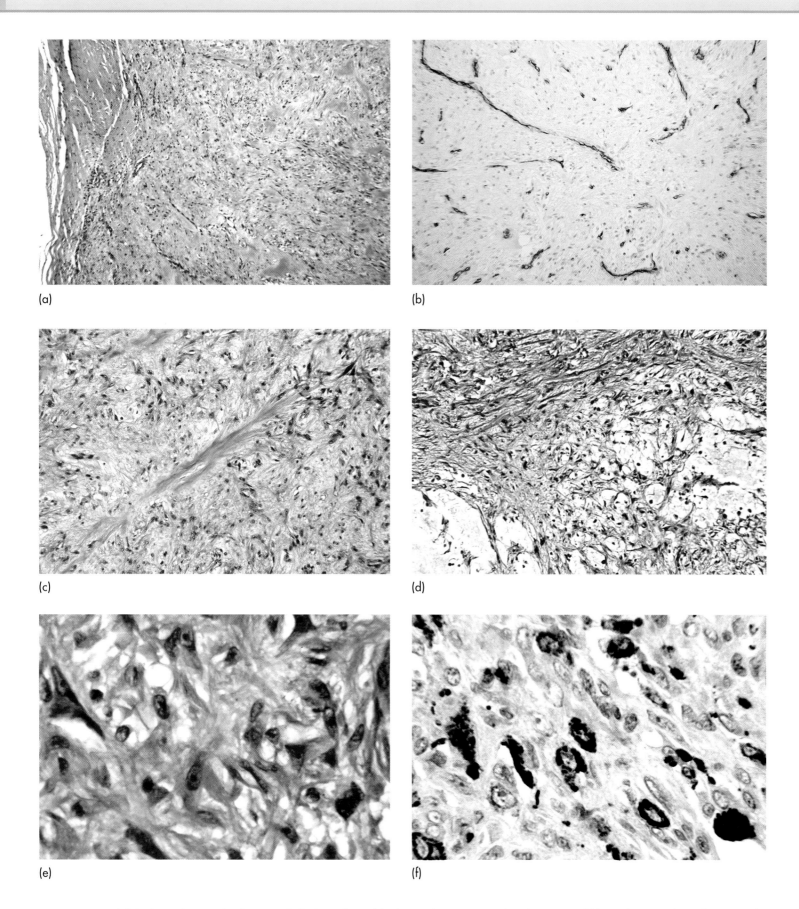

Figure 21.21   (a) A photomicrograph taken to include the surface of the lesion shows a somewhat disorganized fibrous lesion with patchy areas of hyalinized collagen and compressed vascular channels which are highlighted in (b). [(a) H&E, × 4 obj.; (b) CD31, × 4 obj.]. (c) Collagenous bundles can be seen coursing through the lesion and there are focal myxoid areas (d). [(c and d), H&E, × 4 obj.]. (e) Foci of atypical cells may be present (H&E, × 40 obj.). (f) Staining for macrophages (CD68) shows focal positivity (immunoperoxidase, × 25 obj.).

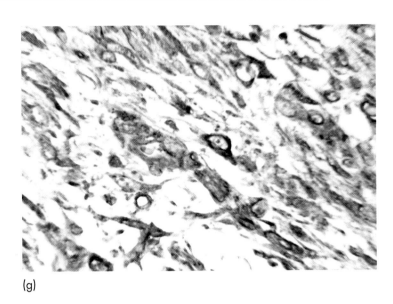

Figure 21.21   (*contd*) (**g**) Staining for smooth-muscle actin also shows focal positivity (immunoperoxidase, × 25 obj.).

(g)

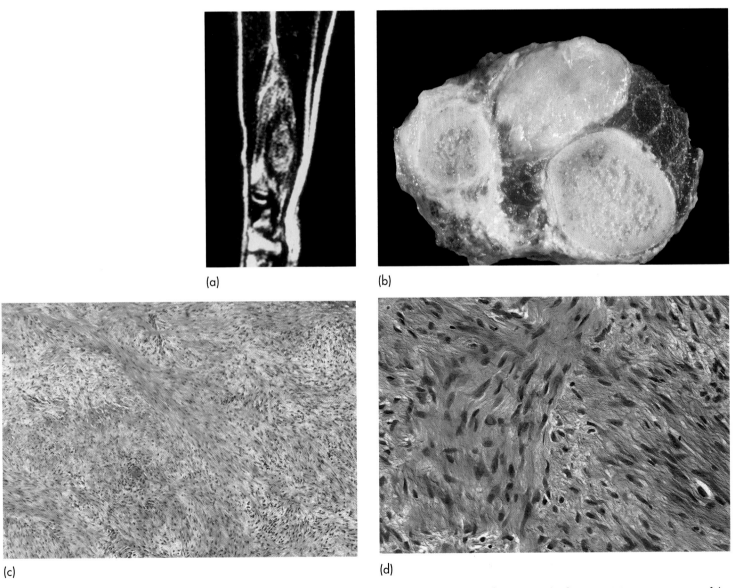

(a)

(b)

(c)

(d)

Figure 21.22   (**a**) An MR image of the right forearm of an 18-year-old male with a recent history of a mass in the forearm. (**b**) A cross-section of the amputated forearm showing the relationship of the mass to the radius and ulna. (**c**) A low-power photomicrograph to show the typical appearance of an extra-abdominal desmoid tumor. Interdigitating bundles of fibroblasts with abundant intercellular collagen matrix (H&E, × 10 obj.). (**d**) A higher power photomicrograph to show the bland appearance of the fibroblasts (H&E, × 25 obj.).

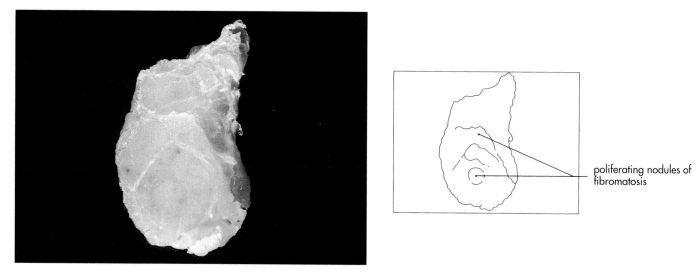

Figure 21.23 Cross-section of thickened palmar fascia removed from a patient with Dupuytren's contracture. The aponeurotic tissue has a grayish-white, glistening appearance, and within this tissue can be seen thickened nodular areas having a more opaque, white–orange appearance. These areas represent foci of proliferating fibromatosis. In longstanding Dupuytren's contracture, the entire aponeurosis may be scarred, and the proliferating nodules are no longer evident.

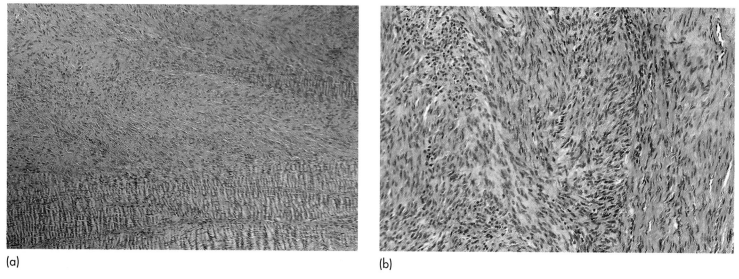

(a)   (b)

Figure 21.24 (a) Photomicrograph (partially polarized) to show part of the palmar fascia (refractile) with an adjacent nodule of cellular fibrous tissue in a case of Dupuytren's contracture (H&E, × 4 obj.). (b) Higher power view to show the packed, cellular, interdigitating fibrous bundles in early Dupuytren's contracture (H&E, × 10 obj.).

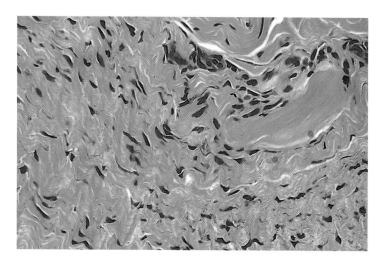

Figure 21.25 Photomicrograph of a section through a nodule from a case of longstanding Dupuytren's contracture shows heavily collagenized stroma without the obvious cellular proliferation characteristic of early lesions (H&E, × 25 obj.).

Dupuytren's contracture

Palmar fibromatosis usually occurs in older adults and has an incidence of 10–20% in the general population. It is three to four times more common in men than in women and is frequently bilateral. It may be familial. In some instances it is associated with diabetes mellitus as well as epilepsy and alcoholic cirrhosis of the liver. Patients present with nodular thickening of the palmar fascia (Fig. 21.23) and flexion contracture of the fingers (usually the third, fourth, and fifth). On histologic examination, the lesions vary in cellularity; some are very cellular and others are heavily collagenized (Figs 21.24 and 21.25). The cellular lesions are in all probability the more recent, whereas the collagenized lesions have been present for a longer period of time.

The cellular lesions are made up of plump, crowded fibroblasts with a variable number of mitoses and this may suggest to the microscopist a fibrosarcoma. However, this diagnosis is extremely unlikely in the setting of a typical clinical presentation of Dupuytren's contracture. Foci of mild chronic inflammation and hemosiderin deposition may be present.

Cytogenetic abnormalities, including trisomy of chromosomes 7 and 8 and loss of the Y chromosome, have been reported.

Plantar fibromatosis

Plantar fibromatosis is very rare in comparison with Dupuytren's. The incidence of plantar fibromatosis increases with age, however unlike Dupuytren's contracture it also occurs in younger patients, and may present with larger nodules than is usually the case in patients with palmar fibromatosis (Fig. 21.26). However, plantar fibromatosis is not associated with the formation of contractures.

Surgical excision is the treatment of choice; however, because

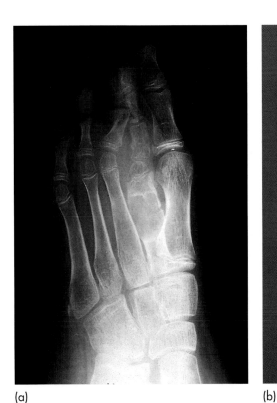

(a)

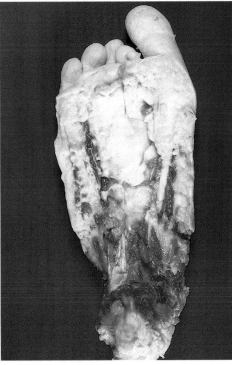

(b)

Figure 21.26 (a) Radiograph of a 13-year-old girl with a history of two excisions of plantar fibromatosis who was admitted to the hospital because of recurrence with bone involvement. Both soft-tissue swelling and invasion of the second metatarsal bone can be appreciated. (b) This amputated specimen from the patient in (a) with plantar skin removed, clearly shows the extent of the tumor. (c) Cross-section of the foot shown in (b) demonstrates the extent of tumor infiltration and involvement of the second metatarsal bone. (d) Low-power photomicrograph of the tumor illustrated in (a–c) demonstrates the bland appearance of the plantar fibromatous tissue (H&E, × 10 obj.).

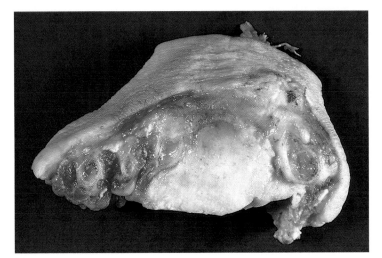

(c)

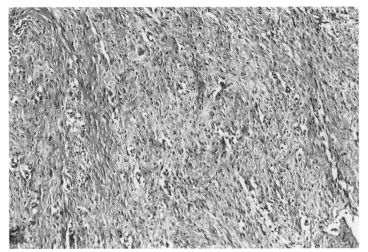

(d)

of the infiltrative nature of the lesion local recurrence is common.

The microscopic features are similar to those seen in palmar fibromatosis. Since the lesions in the foot tend to be operated on earlier than those in the hand, they appear relatively more cellular; this and the rarity of the condition means that problems in differential diagnosis are more likely to occur in the foot lesions than with Dupuytren's contracture.

Calcifying aponeurotic fibroma (juvenile aponeurotic fibromatosis, Keasbey tumor)

Calcifying aponeurotic fibroma usually presents as a slowly growing, painless mass commonly in the hands or, less frequently, in the feet of children or young adults. Occasionally, adults may be affected. The mass has usually been present for several months or even years at the time of presentation. Radiographically, calcific stippling may be apparent. Grossly, the lesion is usually an ill-

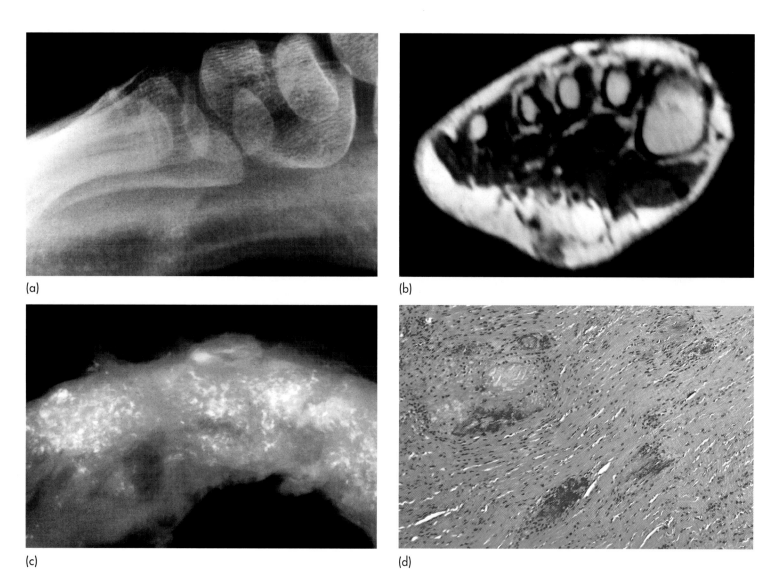

(a)

(b)

(c)

(d)

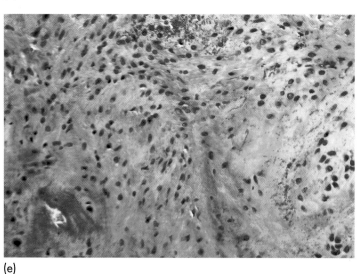

(e)

Figure 21.27 (a) A 4-year-old boy presented with a mass in the sole of the foot. A radiograph shows a focus of irregular calcification in the subcutaneous tissue below the base of the metatarsals. (b) The location is better demonstrated in an MR image. (c) Fine-grain radiograph of the resected specimen shows fine stippled calcification throughout the specimen (magnification, × 10). (d) Low-power photomicrograph shows that the lesion is composed of fibrocartilaginous tissue with irregular areas of calcification (H&E, × 4 obj.). (e) Higher power demonstrates the irregularly arranged fibrocartilaginous cells together with stippled calcification (H&E, × 10 obj.).

defined, firm, white–gray nodular mass < 3 cm in diameter. Because of calcification it may have a gritty consistency when sectioned. Microscopic examination shows foci of plump cellular fibroblasts separated by more densely collagenized tissue. Mitotic figures are rare. Foci of calcification are generally present within the lesion and are usually associated with areas of cartilaginous metaplasia (Fig. 21.27). However, in very young children calcification may not be evident, making the differentiation from infantile fibromatosis difficult. In such cases, the location in the fingers or the palm of the hand should suggest the diagnosis.

In older patients the lesion may suggest soft-tissue chondroma (Fig. 21.28). However, in calcifying aponeurotic fibroma the calcification is more focal and does not have the diffuse pattern of calcification seen in soft-tissue chondroma. Conservative surgical management is generally recommended.

NODULAR FASCIITIS

Nodular fasciitis is a relatively common pseudosarcomatous proliferation of fibroblasts which because of its rapid growth, atypia, cellularity and mitotic rate can be mistaken for a malignant condition.

It occurs most frequently in patients between the ages of 10 and 40 and is seen most often on the volar surface of the forearm. Less commonly it may occur in the head and neck region, the trunk and on the lower extremity.

In most cases when the patient is first seen the lesion has been present for 1–2 weeks, and it is usually less than 2 cm in diameter and well circumscribed.

Microscopically the lesional tissue is composed of plump immature fibroblasts, having pale nuclei and prominent nucleoli, which in general do not vary from each other. Although mitoses may be frequent, no atypical mitoses are seen. The fibroblasts are generally arranged in short irregular interlacing bundles and in addition to a scant collagen matrix there is generally a focally mucoid matrix. Scattered through the lesion there are often focal mild inflammatory infiltrates (Fig. 21.29). Generally an attachment to the fascia can be found.

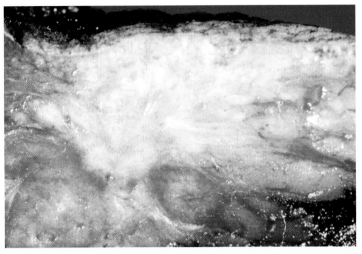

(a)

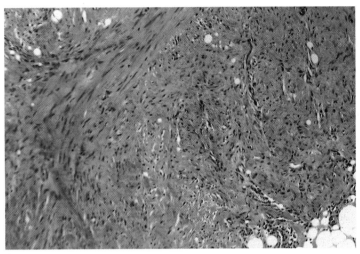

(b)

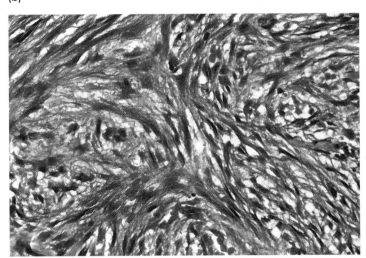

(c)

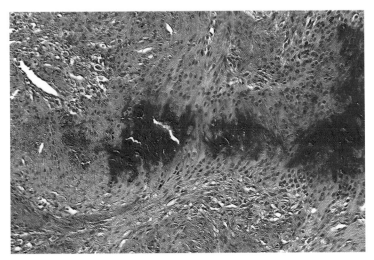

Figure 21.28   Photomicrograph to show the interdigitating bundles of fibrocartilage together with irregular foci of calcification in a young person with a calcifying aponeurotic fibroma (H&E, × 10 obj.).

Figure 21.29   (a) Photograph of a subcutaneous nodule resected from the forearm. The tumor is not well demarcated and appears to be infiltrating the surrounding tissue. (b) Photomicrograph of the lesion shows a cellular tumor which seems to be intimately associated with a fascial plane seen in the upper left quadrant of the photograph (H&E, × 4 obj.). (c) High-power view to demonstrate the matted arrangement of the fibroblasts. Generally, collagen production is slight in such cases of nodular fasciitis and there is often a loose mucoid appearance to the intercellular matrix (H&E, × 25 obj.).

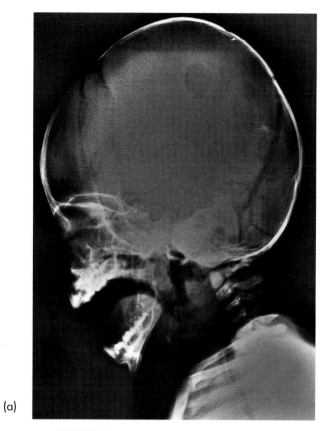

(a)

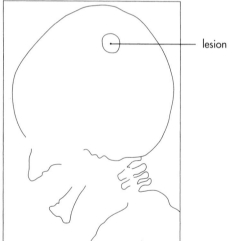

lesion

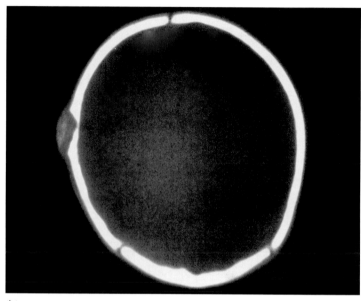

(b)

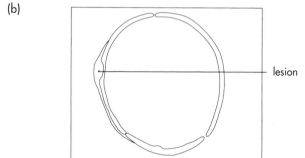

lesion

Figure 21.30 (a) Radiograph of a 5-month-old infant with a slowly growing mass on the head present since shortly after birth. The radiograph suggests a differential diagnosis including epidermoid inclusion cyst, eosinophilic granuloma, or cranial fasciitis. (b) The CT scan shows that the lesion is extraosseous and involves the bone by secondary erosion. (c) Photomicrograph of the tissue removed from the case illustrated in (a and b). The lesional tissue has a fibrous appearance (H&E, × 1 obj.). (d) Photomicrograph of a portion of the tumor removed from the patient illustrated in (a–c) shows the typical loose, swirling pattern of fasciitis, with immature fibroblastic cells producing an extracellular matrix rich in proteoglycan (foci of basophilic staining) and sparse collagen. Scattered chronic inflammatory cells are present (H&E, × 10 obj.).

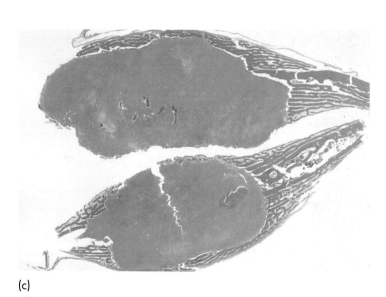

(c)

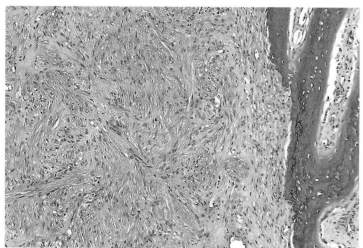

(d)

Proliferative fasciitis and proliferative myositis are related conditions which tend to occur in an older population than in nodular fasciitis, as well as in somewhat different locations; most of the former occur in the extremities whilst most of the latter occur on the trunk, especially around the chest and shoulder.

The histologic features are similar to those seen in nodular fasciitis and like that condition it would appear that proliferative fasciitis and myositis are reactive conditions and self-limiting.

Cranial fasciitis

Cranial fasciitis is a rare condition which is seen exclusively in the cranium of infants and small children.

Radiologic examination usually reveals a defect in the outer table of the skull, which results from pressure erosion consequent upon a soft-tissue mass. Gross examination of the resected tumor reveals a firm, rubbery mass which may be a few centimeters in diameter and on cut section has a glistening appearance. Microscopic examination reveals a proliferation of plump fibroblasts in a mucoid matrix. Some mitotic activity is usually present (Fig. 21.30).

Because of its rarity, rapid growth, and pseudosarcomatous appearance, the lesion may be misdiagnosed as fibrosarcoma. However, the lesion is entirely benign and self-limited.

ELASTOFIBROMA

Elastofibroma is an uncommon, self-limited lesion found in older adults. With rare exceptions, the lesion occurs in the soft tissue between the rib fascia and the inferior portion of the scapula. On gross examination the tumor is firm and rubbery in consistency and, although circumscribed, is not encapsulated but rather merges with the surrounding tissue.

On microscopic examination the lesion is formed of dense collagen and fat, interspersed with eosinophilic globules and fibers. Histochemically and ultrastructurally, these fibers and globules consist of elastin (a fibrous protein) and elastin precursors (Fig. 21.31).

It is generally agreed that the lesion is the result of trauma. Treatment is usually by surgical excision.

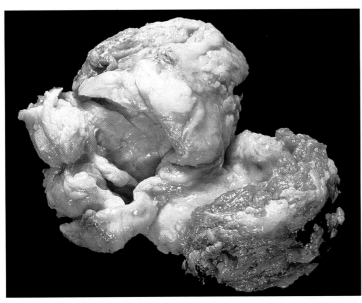

(a)

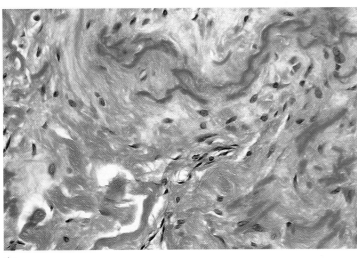

(b)

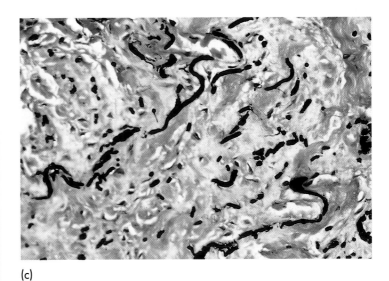

(c)

Figure 21.31   (a) Photograph of a mass excised from the soft tissues overlying the scapula. The lump had been present clinically for several years. (b) Photomicrograph of a portion of the mass illustrated in (a) to demonstrate the disorderly collagenous matrix and bland cellular appearance of the lesional tissue (H&E, × 25 obj.). (c) The same tissue as shown in (b), stained with an elastic tissue stain. Note the abundant fragmented elastic fibers in the tissue typical of an elastofibroma (Verhoeff–Van Gieson, × 25 obj.).

▌ PERIPHERAL NERVE LESIONS

TRAUMATIC (AMPUTATION) NEUROMA

Traumatic neuroma is an exuberant but non-neoplastic proliferation of nerve tissue resulting from a lacerating injury (often surgery). Clinically it presents as a firm nodule that is occasionally tender or painful.

Grossly the lesions are circumscribed, white–gray nodules located in continuity with the proximal end of the injured or transected nerve. Microscopically they consist of a haphazard proliferation of interdigitating nerve fascicles within scar tissue (Fig. 21.32).

Rarely these lesions may be difficult for the microscopist to differentiate from neurofibromas, especially if there is myxoid degeneration.

MORTON'S NEUROMA

Morton's neuroma is a distinct clinico-pathologic entity characterized by thickening and degeneration of one of the interdigital nerves of the foot, most commonly that between the third and fourth metatarsal heads. The patient, usually a woman, experiences sharp shooting pains that are worse when standing. These pains characteristically begin in the sole of the foot and radiate to the exterior surface. At surgery, a fusiform swelling proximal to the bifurcation of the plantar interdigital nerve is usually seen. When dissected, the resected specimen usually includes the neurovascular bundle (Fig. 21.33).

Histologic sections generally show three characteristic microscopic features: endarterial thickening of the digital artery, often with thrombosis and occlusion of the lumen; extensive fibrosis both around and within the nerve, giving rise to demyelinization and a marked depletion of axons within the digital nerve; and evidence of Schwann cell and fibroblast proliferation (Figs 21.34 and 21.35). The histologic findings are most consistent with recurrent nerve trauma, probably caused by the wearing of poorly fitting shoes.

Morton's neuroma should be differentiated from amputation (traumatic) neuroma, which may also occur in the interdigital nerves of the feet, although very much more rarely.

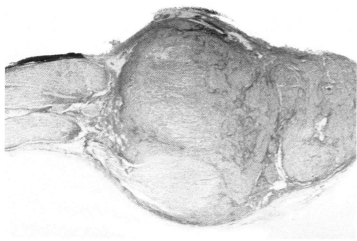

(a)

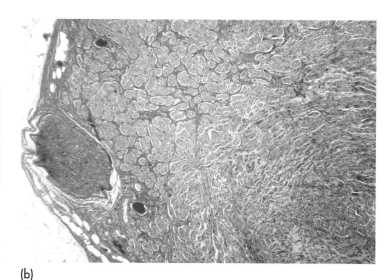

(b)

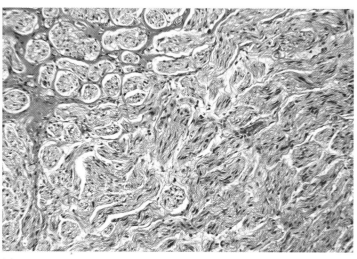

(c)

Figure 21.32 (a) Low-power histologic section of an amputation neuroma stained with Masson trichrome shows the increased fibrous scar tissue (blue staining). The proximal nerve stump is seen at left (× 1 obj.). (b) Higher power view of a traumatic neuroma showing the characteristic interdigitating bundles of proliferating nerve fascicles which characterize this condition and at the left-hand margin a portion of the nerve trunk (H&E, × 4 obj.). (c) Higher power shows a detailed view of the interdigitating bundles (H&E, × 25 obj.).

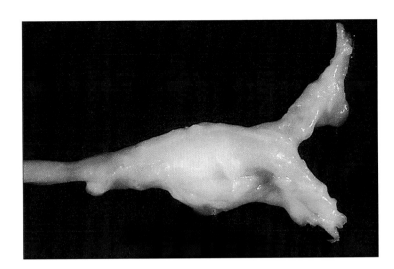

Figure 21.33   Gross photograph of a segment of the plantar interdigital nerve resected from the space between the third and fourth metatarsal heads in a patient with Morton's neuroma shows fusiform swelling of the neurovascular bundle just proximal to the bifurcation.

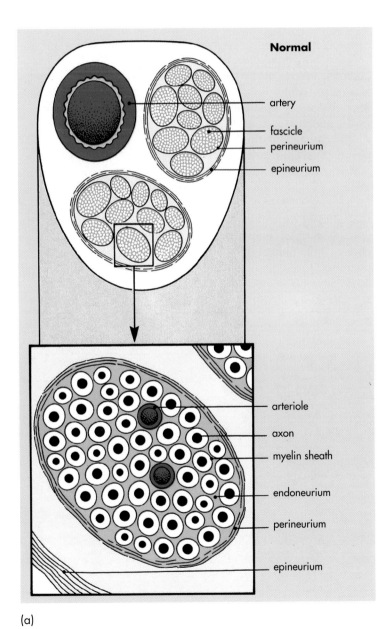

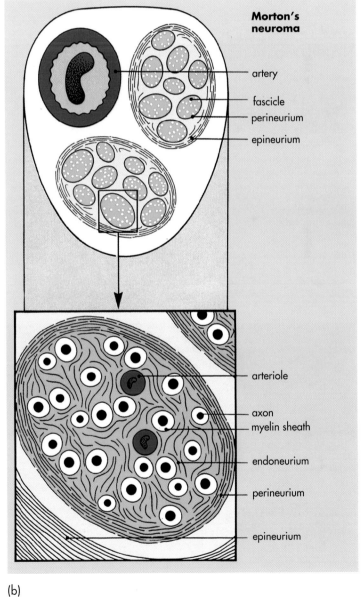

(a)   (b)

Figure 21.34   (a) Schematic diagram of a normal neurovascular bundle illustrating the relationship of the digital nerves and artery. (b) Schematic diagram of the neurovascular bundle from a patient with a Morton's neuroma. Note the increased fibrosis in the epineurium, perineurium, and endoneurium. In addition, there is marked endothelial thickening of the artery, with narrowing of the lumen.

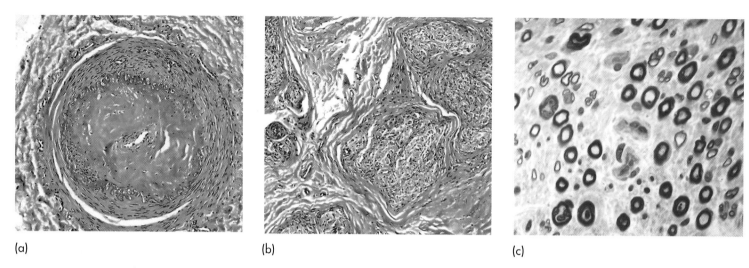

(a)   (b)   (c)

Figure 21.35 (a) Histologic section of a narrowed and occluded vessel from a patient with Morton's neuroma (H&E, × 4 obj.). (b) Morton's neuroma. The increased fibrosis of the nerve can be appreciated in this histologic section (H&E, × 10 obj.). (c) High-power photomicrograph of a single nerve fascicle shows the loss of myelinated nerve fibers together with increased endoneural fibrosis (H&E, × 100 obj.).

NEURILEMOMA (BENIGN SCHWANNOMA)

Neurilemoma is an encapsulated nerve sheath tumor which consists histologically of two components: a highly ordered cellular component (Antoni A area) and a loose myxoid component (Antoni B area).

Neurilemomas occur at all ages but are relatively common in persons of both sexes between the ages of 20 and 50 years. They have a predilection for the head, neck, and flexor surfaces of the upper and lower extremities. They almost always occur as solitary lesions. They grow slowly and usually have been present several years before diagnosis is made.

Grossly these are encapsulated tumors which in small nerves may have fusiform shape, and in larger nerves may present as eccentric masses over which the nerve fibers are splayed. On cut section the tumor is soft and has a pink, white, or yellow appearance. It usually measures < 5 cm and occasionally has foci of cystification and/or calcification (Fig. 21.36).

Microscopically, the hallmark of a neurilemoma is the pattern of alternating Antoni A and B areas of varying amounts. Antoni A areas are composed of compact spindle cells that are arranged in short bundles with nuclear palisading or interlacing fascicles of whorling cells. Antoni B areas are far less cellular; the spindled or oval cells are arranged haphazardly within the loosely textured matrix, which is punctuated by microcystic change, inflammatory cells, and delicate collagen fibers. Intense immunostaining for the S100 protein is seen in the cells (Fig. 21.37).

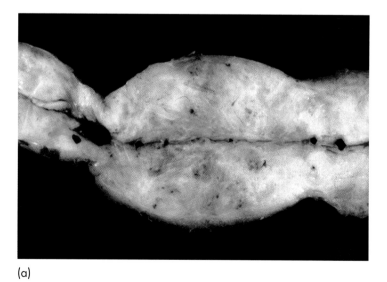

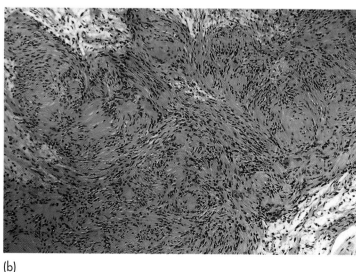

(a)   (b)

Figure 21.36 (a) Photograph of a resected neurilemoma which has been sliced longitudinally. The variegated fibrous and myxoid appearance has been likened to that of 'watered silk'. (b) Photomicrograph of the tumor showing mainly the Antoni A pattern with spindle cells in a whirling pattern and focal palisaded nuclei. At the margins of the picture is loose myxoid tissue consistent with Antoni B pattern (H&E, × 4 obj.).

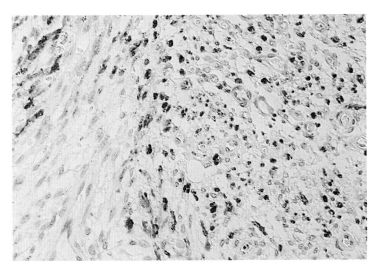

Figure 21.37 Photomicrograph of the Antoni B area of a neurilemoma stained with antibody to S100 protein (immunoperoxidase stain, × 10 obj.).

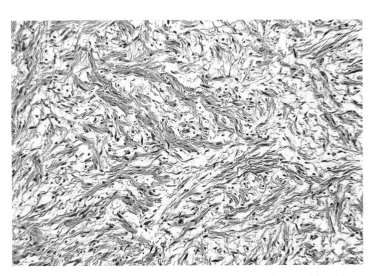

Figure 21.38 Photomicrograph of a neurofibroma shows a bland but disorderly collagen-rich, fibroblastic tumor (H&E, × 10 obj.).

SOLITARY NEUROFIBROMA

The vast majority of neurofibromas are solitary lesions. Multiple neurofibromas (neurofibromatosis or von Recklinghausen's disease) are decidedly less common. Neurofibroma differs from neurilemoma in that it is not encapsulated, though it generally appears to be a circumscribed lesion.

Clinically most present in patients aged between 20 and 30 years, these are superficial painless lesions seen in the dermis over any part of the body surface. Grossly they are firm white–gray tumors.

Microscopically the neurofibroma varies, depending on its content of cells, mucin, and collagen. Most commonly it shows interlacing bundles of elongated cells with wavy, dark-staining nuclei with intercellular wire like strands of collagen, and small to moderate amounts of mucoid material that separate the cells

and collagen. The stroma of the tumor is dotted with occasional mast cells and lymphocytes (Fig. 21.38).

Generally the S100 stain is much less intense than in neurilemoma.

MISCELLANEOUS LESIONS

LIPOMA

Benign fatty tumors are the commonest soft-tissue tumors and come in a wide variety of forms and locations. The fatty tissue may be admixed with vascular tissue (angiolipoma), muscle tissue (myolipoma), cartilage tissue (chondrolipoma) or be a mixture of any of these elements (Fig. 21.39). Occasionally,

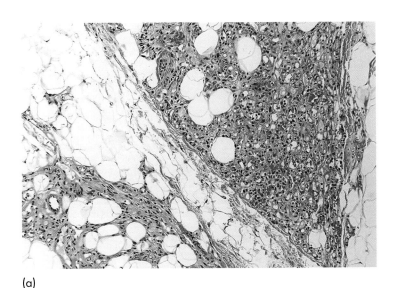

(a)

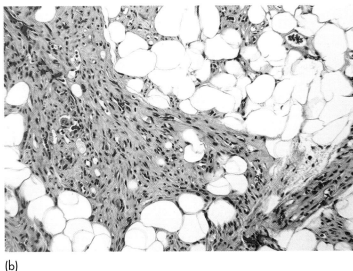

(b)

Figure 21.39 (a) Photomicrograph of an angiolipoma in which the fat is admixed with nodules of packed capillaries (H&E, × 4 obj.). (b) Higher power to show the compressed capillaries (H&E, × 10 obj.).

calcification or ossification may be seen in a lipoma. A subcutaneus location is the commonest but lipomas may also appear in muscles, tendon sheaths, nerves and joints. Neural lipomas may be associated with a fibrolipomatosis hamartoma and macrodactyly (Fig. 21.40). This lesion usually presents in childhood. In its extreme form – Proteus syndrome – fibrolipomatous hamartoma is responsible for causing the deformities seen in the 'Elephant man'.

Lipomas are rarely seen in young people and clinically usually present in patients over 40. They appear to be somewhat more common in men and are occasionally multiple. Most lipomas are superficial in location and present on the trunk and the proximal portions of the extremities. Deep lipomas are decidedly rarer and therefore often present more of a problem in diagnosis.

Grossly, soft-tissue lipomas are generally well-circumscribed, soft, yellow tumors measuring between 4–10 cm in diameter (Fig. 21.41). Microscopically, they normally do not significantly differ from the surrounding fat, though they are usually lobulated and may have admixed fibrous, myxoid or other connective-tissue elements. Secondary changes such as hemorrhage, infarction and calcification are not unusual and rests of foamy macrophages are common.

Occasionally, atypical cells may result in confusion with liposarcoma.

HEMANGIOMA

Hemangiomas are the commonest tumors seen in infancy and childhood and are usually superficial lesions with a predilection for the head and neck region. The majority have a capillary pattern, small nodules of capillary-sized vessels lined by flattened to plump endothelium, the nodules being clumped in a lobular pattern (Fig. 21.42). In some cases the vascular nature of the lesion may be obscured by the plumpness of the endothelial cells,

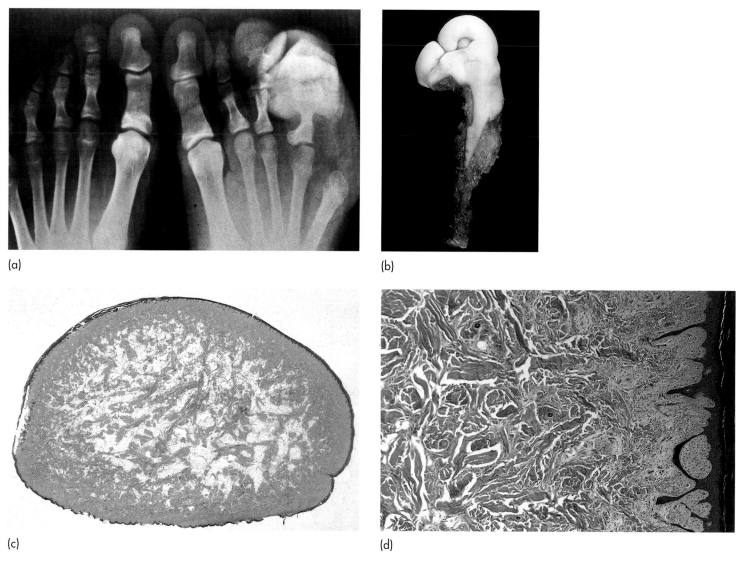

(a)

(b)

(c)

(d)

Figure 21.40 (a) A radiograph showing localized gigantism involving the third, fourth, and fifth rays of the right foot. (b) Photograph of a giant deformed toe in a case of macrodactyly lipomatosis. (c) Low-power photomicrograph of a section across the toe demonstrated in (b) shows the disorderly fat and fibrous tissue. Note the absence of skin appendages (H&E, × 1 obj.). (d) Photomicrograph of the skin and subcutaneous tissue of the toe, demonstrating macrodactyly illustrated in (a and b). There is an overabundance of interdigitating bundles of collagen-rich fibroblasts (H&E, × 4 obj.).

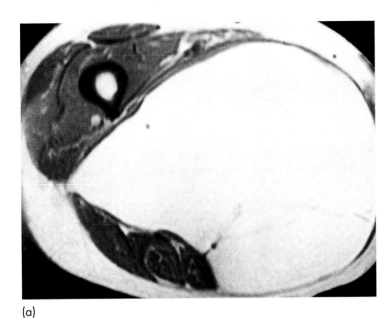

(a)

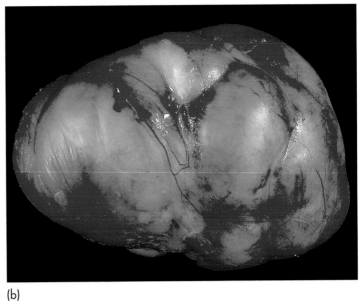

(b)

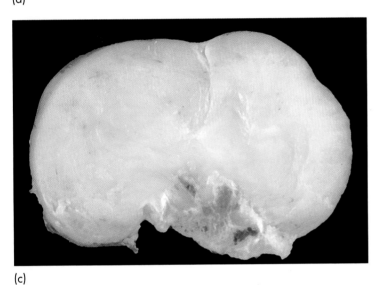

(c)

Figure 21.41 (a) Lipoma. An MRI showing sections through the thigh. There is a large mass in the posterior compartment of the thigh, producing compression of the adjacent muscles. (From: Beltran J. *MRI: Musculoskeletal System*. London: Gower Medical Publishing, 1990.) (b) Photograph of a resected lipoma showing an intact delicate fibrous capsule. (c) Photograph of the sectioned tumor shown in (b) reveals the yellow, fatty, lobulated nature of the lesion.

giving a solid appearance to the tumor. In these instances immunohistochemistry using vascular markers such as CD31 or Factor VIII can be most helpful.

Cavernous hemangiomas are less common, are usually larger in size than capillary hemangiomas and frequently involve deep structures such as muscles (Fig. 21.43). On radiographs it is sometimes possible to visualize calcified thrombi with a long curvilineal pattern, or more typically with a nodular pattern (phleboliths).

Sometimes multiple hemangiomas are seen in association with multiple enchondromatosis (Maffucci's syndrome, see Chapter 17, p. 405) (Fig. 21.44).

Epithelioid hemangioma is a rare but distinctive variety of hemangioma characterized by inflammatory cells, particularly eosinophils, but in addition plasma cells, mast cells and lymphocytes. The cells lining the vessels have an epithelioid appearance with eosinophilic cytoplasm and frequently appear as a line of 'tombstones' (Fig. 21.45).

MYOSITIS OSSIFICANS

The diagnostic term myositis ossificans includes two entirely different clinical diseases: myositis ossificans circumscripta and fibrodysplasia (myositis) ossificans progressiva.

Fibrodysplasia (myositis) ossificans progressiva

Fibrodysplasia ossificans progressiva is a rare progressive disease in which groups of muscles, tendons, and ligaments (usually the muscles of the back and those around major joints of the upper limb) become progressively fibrosed, calcified and ossified, thereby producing severe functional disability (Fig. 21.46). Symptoms of the disease usually begin in childhood, generally before the age of 10. In some cases the condition is inherited, and several members of a family may be affected. In most instances, however, it is probably the result of a spontaneous mutation.

The disorder is often associated with symmetrical malformation or absence of the digits of the hands and feet. The sexes are equally affected and there is no racial predilection.

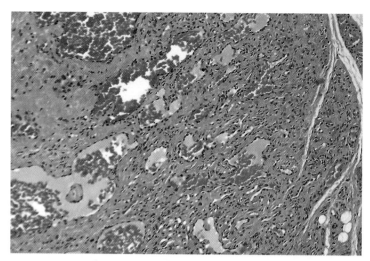

Figure 21.42   Photomicrograph to demonstrate a hemangioma. In this example, the packed vascular channels vary in size, have an irregular branching pattern and the endothelial lining is unremarkable (H&E, × 4 obj.).

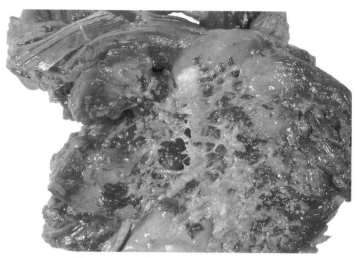

Figure 21.43   Photograph of a resected intramuscular hemangioma. Note the spongy and fibrous nature of the angiomatous component.

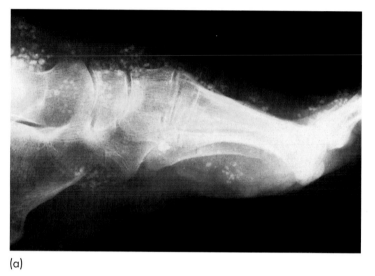

(a)

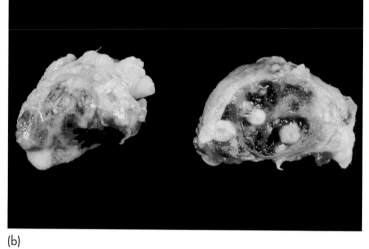

(b)

Figure 21.44   (a) Lateral radiograph of a foot. There are many calcified nodules of approximately the same size in the soft tissues which represent calcified phleboliths in an extensive soft-tissue hemangioma in a patient with Maffucci's syndrome. (b) Photograph of a resected hemangioma to demonstrate in situ phleboliths.

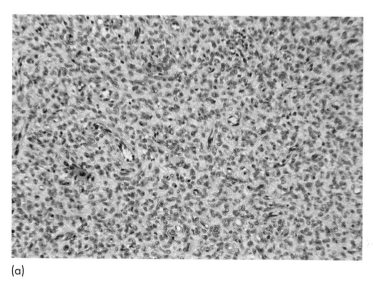

(a)

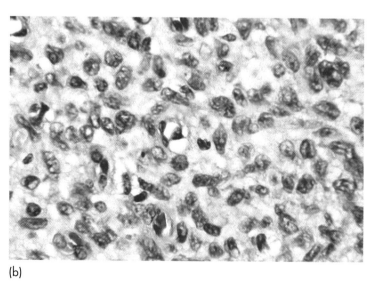

(b)

Figure 21.45   (a) Photomicrograph of an epithelioid hemangioma to demonstrate the packed and solid appearance of the tumor due to the compression of the vascular spaces (H&E, × 4 obj.). (b) At a higher power some of the vascular space can be discerned (H&E, × 25 obj.).

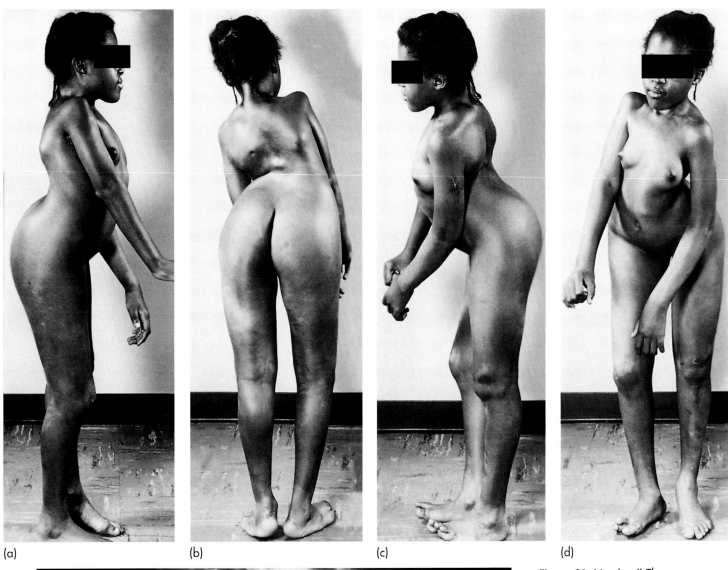

(a) (b) (c) (d)

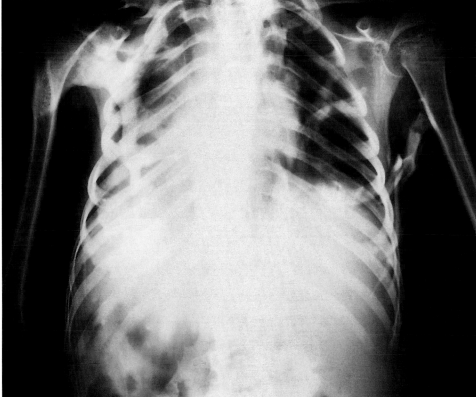

(e)

Figure 21.46 **(a–d)** These photographs demonstrate severe deformities of the limbs, spine, and neck, resulting from myositis ossificans progressiva. **(e)** Clinical radiograph of the patient in **(a–d)** shows ossification around both shoulder joints as well as in the paravertebral area.

It is thought that the underlying biochemical defect in this condition is an overexpression of bone morphogenetic protein-4 (BMP4).

Microscopic examination of the early lesions, which consist of nodular swellings in the muscles and subcutis, reveal a loose proliferation of fibroblasts and interstitial edema which may be confused with a desmoid tumor.

Microscopic examination of advanced lesions reveals poorly organized bone (both lamellar and woven), dense, fibrous scar tissue, and islands of poorly formed cartilage (Fig. 21.47). This disorder is usually fatal because of progressive functional disability, including impairment of pulmonary function.

Myositis ossificans circumscripta

Myositis ossificans circumscripta is a solitary, nonprogressive, benign ossifying lesion of soft tissues. The patient is usually an athletic adolescent or young adult who presents with a lump in a muscle which has been evident for some weeks and may have been somewhat painful. A history of trauma can usually be elicited, but these traumatic incidents are, more often than not, trivial in nature. A radiograph taken soon after the onset of symptoms may not reveal any calcification, but within 1 week or 2 a poorly defined area of opacification will appear. Over the following weeks the periphery of this shadow becomes increasingly well delineated from the surrounding soft tissue (Fig. 21.48). Diagnostic problems in such cases occur when the lesion is biopsied in the early phase before peripheral maturation has occurred.

Gross examination of a focus of myositis ossificans circumscripta that has been present for 1 month or 2 reveals a shell of bony tissue with a soft reddish-brown central area. The lesion is usually 2–5 cm in diameter and is adherent to the surrounding muscle.

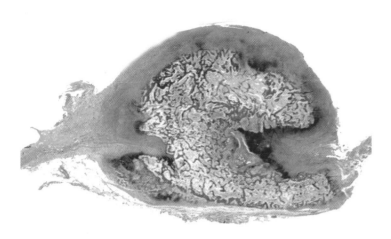

(a)

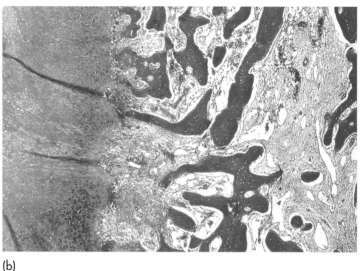

(b)

Figure 21.47   (a) Photomicrograph of a portion of ossified soft tissue taken from the hip joint of a patient with myositis ossificans progressiva demonstrates both immature bone and cartilage formation, with areas of dense fibrous connective tissue also in evidence (H&E, × 1 obj.). (b) Higher power photomicrograph of the tissue in (a) shows bone and cartilage formation within the soft tissue (H&E, × 10 obj.).

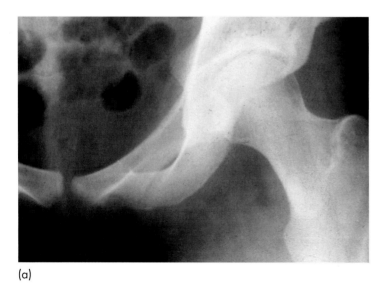

(a)

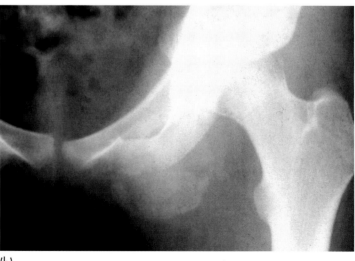

(b)

Figure 21.48   (a) Clinical radiograph of a young woman who developed pain in the region of the pubis after childbirth reveals no obvious abnormality. (b) This radiograph of the patient in (a) taken 1 month later, demonstrates a well-defined ossifying mass in the soft tissue adjacent to the pubis.

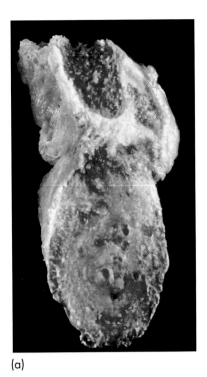

(a)

Figure 21.49   (a) Gross photograph of the specimen removed from the patient in Figure 21.48. In the upper part can be seen a segment of normal bone pubic ramus, and immediately underlying this segment is a well-circumscribed ossified mass which though attached to the periosteum did not arise from the bone tissue. (b) Photomicrograph of a section through an intact specimen of myositis ossificans circumscripta clearly shows the fibrous cellular center and the limiting outer layer of more mature bone (H&E, × 1 obj.). (c) High-power photomicrograph of tissue taken from the center of the mass shown in (a) demonstrates a spindle-cell lesion. The cells have a disorderly arrangement and are producing collagen (H&E, × 40 obj.). (d) Photomicrograph of an area adjacent to the tissue seen in (c) demonstrates immature bone matrix formation. The cellularity of this tissue might cause concern and lead to an erroneous diagnosis of sarcoma (H&E, × 25 obj.). (e) Histologic section taken from the periphery of the lesion demonstrated in the previous figures shows mature bone formation, characteristic of myositis ossificans circumscripta (H&E, × 10 obj.).

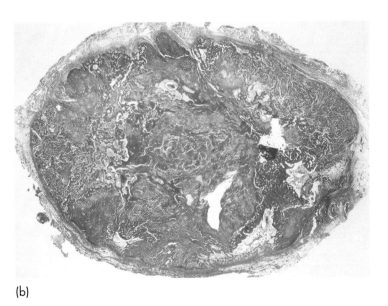

(b)

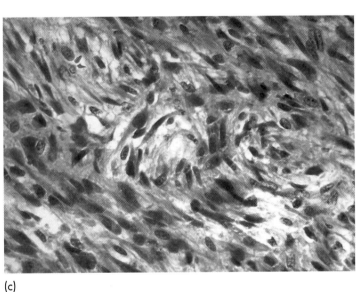

(c)

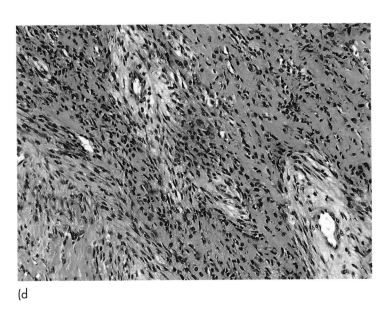

(d)

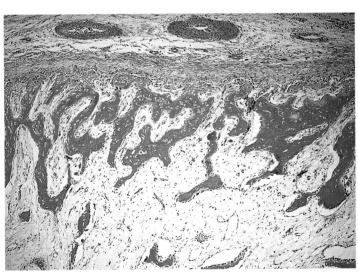

(e)

Microscopic examination of myositis ossificans circumscripta reveals an irregular mass of active, immature fibroblastic cells in the center of the lesion, with foci of interstitial microhemorrhages that are rarely extensive. At some distance from the center of the lesion, depending on the age of the entity in question, small foci of osteoid production can be seen. The resulting tissue may be disorganized and hypercellular. Near the periphery, more and more clearly defined trabeculae are evident. The bone is usually of the immature woven type, with large, round, and crowded osteocytes; however, in longstanding lesions the bone may be mature and have a lamellar pattern and a fatty/hematopoietic marrow (Fig. 21.49).

Especially in its acute stage, it may be difficult on the basis of histologic evidence alone to differentiate a focus of myositis, from a sarcoma. Careful correlation of the clinical and radiologic findings is therefore essential. An important distinction to be emphasized is that whereas myositis ossificans is most mature at its periphery and least mature at its center, the opposite is true of a malignant tumor (see discussion of soft-tissue osteosarcoma in Chapter 22, p. 534). Treatment of myositis ossificans is usually conservative, with the option of excision of the mass.

[Three conditions which appear to be related to myositis ossificans circumscripta – subungual exostosis, reactive periostitis, and bizarre parosteal osteochondromatous proliferation (BPOP) – have already been discussed in Chapter 16, p. 365.]

SOFT-TISSUE CHONDROMA

Cartilaginous lesions in the soft tissues are rare. Most soft-tissue chondromas have been described in the hands or feet of patients 30–60 years of age. In general, the lesions measure between 1 and 2 cm in diameter and about one-third of the lesions are densely calcified on radiographic examination.

Grossly, the lesions are usually firmly adhered to adjacent structures, tendons, tendon sheaths or joint capsules, and have a hard, often gritty, consistency. Microscopic examination shows

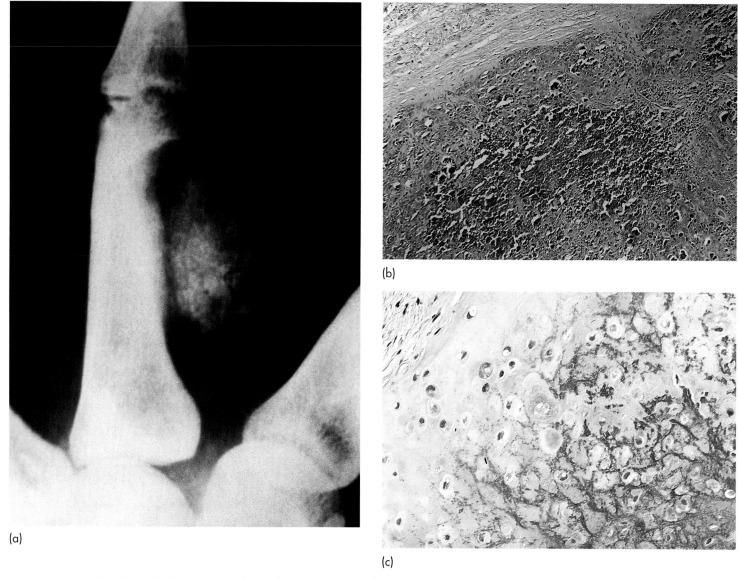

(a)

(b)

(c)

Figure 21.50 (a) Radiograph showing a heavily calcified tumor on the volar aspect of a proximal phalanx. Note the punctate appearance of the calcification. (b) Photomicrograph of a portion of the periphery of the lesion illustrated in (a) shows heavily calcified cartilage with only a few viable chondrocytes at the periphery, consistent with soft-tissue chondroma (H&E, × 10 obj.). (c) Photomicrograph of a peripheral field of the tumor to demonstrate viable cartilage and a delicate lace-like pattern of calcification around some of the cells (H&E, × 25 obj.).

considerable variation. Some consist of mature hyaline cartilage arranged in a lobular pattern. Others show, in addition to the cartilage, areas of fibrosis, myxoid change or hemorrhage. About one-third reveal heavy granular calcification which may obscure the chondrocytes and suggest the diagnosis of tumoral calcinosis (Fig. 21.50). In many of these latter cases foci of reactive epithelioid histiocytes and multinucleated giant cells further complicate the histologic presentation. Because of the variable and sometimes bizarre appearance these lesions may be occasionally mistaken for chondrosarcoma, especially if they have a myxoid stroma. The differential diagnosis should also include primary synovial chondromatosis and tophaceous pseudogout.

SOFT-TISSUE GIANT-CELL TUMOR

These rare lesions seem to most commonly occur in the superficial or deep soft tissue of the hand or arm (Fig. 21.51). Microscopically they are similar to giant-cell tumor of bone and have a similar immunophenotypic profile.

They should be readily distinguishable from nodular tenosynovitis (giant-cell tumor of the tendon sheath) not only by their different location but also by the lack of heterogeneity, which is the hallmark of nodular tenosynovitis. Metaplastic bone may be present usually at the periphery of the lesion.

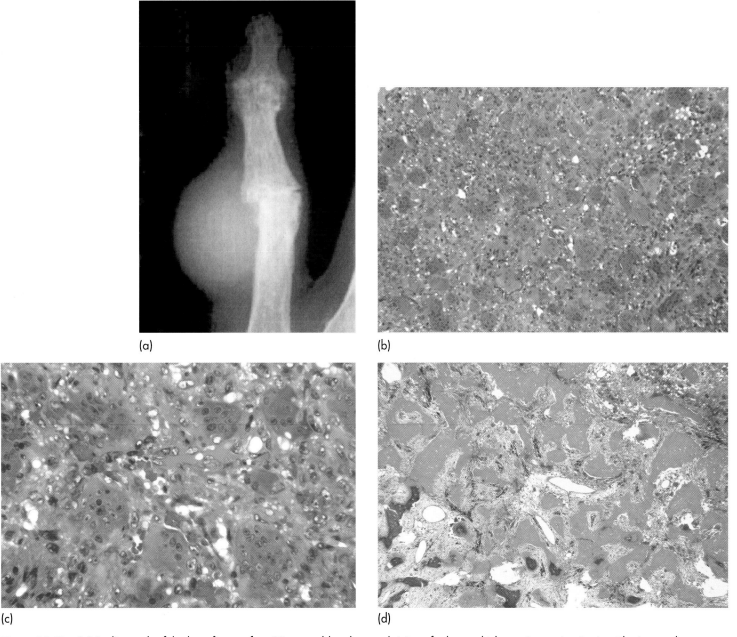

(a)

(b)

(c)

(d)

Figure 21.51 (a) Radiograph of the long finger of an 83-year-old male complaining of a lump which was increasing in size. The image shows destructive changes in the proximal and distal interphalangeal joints, and a large soft-tissue mass adjacent to the proximal joint. (b) Photomicrograph of tissue obtained from the resected soft-tissue mass shows a tumor composed of closely packed giant cells separated by mononuclear stromal cells and indistinguishable from a giant-cell tumor of bone (H&E, × 4 obj.). (c) Higher power view (H&E, × 25 obj.). (d) At the periphery of the lesion there is reactive bone formation (H&E, × 4 obj.).

GANGLION

A ganglion is a fibrous-walled cyst filled with clear mucinous fluid and usually lacking a recognizable lining of differentiated cells (Fig. 21.52). Ganglia occur in the soft tissues, usually dissecting between tendon planes. They are often seen in the hands and feet, particularly on the extensor surfaces near joints. (The most common location is around the wrist joint.)

Ganglia may arise either as herniations of the synovium or from cystification of foci of myxoid degeneration within dense fibrous connective tissue, possibly secondary to trauma. Rarely, a communication with the joint cavity can be demonstrated. On occasion, these lesions may erode the adjacent bone and subsequently become totally intraosseous. The most common site for such an intraosseous ganglion is the medial malleolus of the tibia (see Chapter 19, p. 446). Ganglia are often seen in the parameniscal tissue of the knee joint, usually in proximity to the lateral meniscus (Figs 21.53 and 21.54). Synovial cysts may also

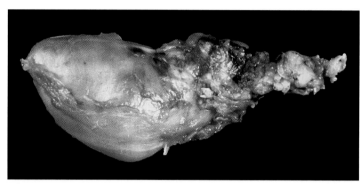

(a)

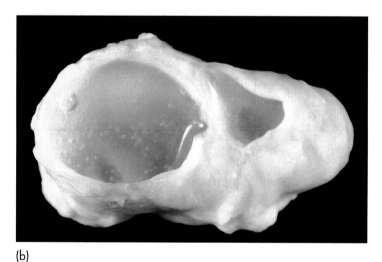

(b)

(c)

Figure 21.52 (a) Gross photograph of an intact, excised ganglion cyst. Note the smooth fibrous wall and the translucent appearance. (b) Gross photograph of a bisected ganglion shows a multiloculated cyst filled with clear glairy fluid. (c) Photomicrograph of a ganglion shows the dense fibrous multiloculated connective-tissue wall, with a thin layer of flattened cells lining the cyst (H&E, × 10 obj.).

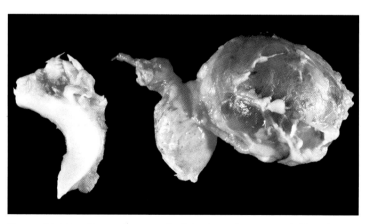

Figure 21.53 Gross photograph of the lateral meniscus (left) and a parameniscal cyst (right). As is apparent here, cysts of the lateral meniscus may occasionally grow to a very large size.

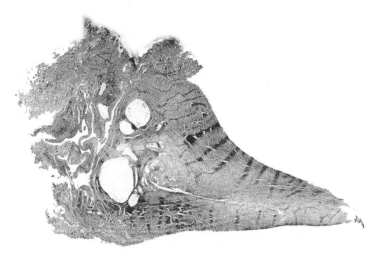

Figure 21.54 Photomicrograph of a cross-section of the lateral meniscus shows focal cystic degeneration in the outer third of the meniscus. Microscopic foci of myxoid degeneration and cystification are common findings in histologic sections of the meniscus (H&E, × 4 obj.).

develop in the vertebral column, where they may result in pressure on the nerve root, or on the spinal canal contents (Fig. 21.55).

On microscopic examination, the wall of a ganglion cyst is formed of dense, collagenized fibrous tissue, often with foci of myxoid tissue (Fig. 21.56). Chronic inflammatory cells may be observed, especially if the cyst has been previously ruptured.

If clinically troublesome, surgical excision of the cyst is the treatment of choice.

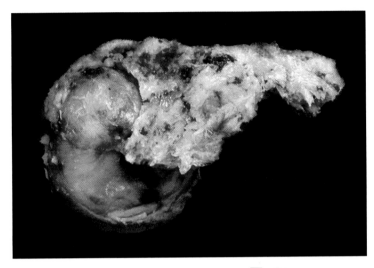

Figure 21.55 Photograph of a ganglion cyst with a portion of the lamina bone taken from the lumbar spine of a patient with symptoms of nerve root compression.

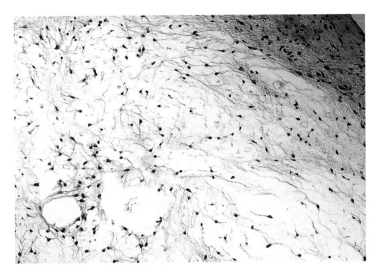

Figure 21.56 Photomicrograph of a portion of the wall of a ganglion, showing extensive myxoid change (H&E, × 10 obj.).

MALIGNANT SOFT-TISSUE TUMORS

Malignant tumors arising in the soft connective tissues are about three times commoner than those arising in the skeletal tissues, but to put things in perspective, they are 20 times less common than lung cancer.

The commonest soft-tissue sarcomas are malignant fibrous histiocytoma, liposarcoma, rhabdomyosarcoma and synovial sarcoma.

(Soft-tissue sarcomas tend to show considerable variation in their histologic patterns and can be very difficult to diagnose accurately. In these cases it is often wise to seek a second opinion from some authority in the subject.)

MALIGNANT FIBROUS HISTIOCYTOMA

The commonest form of malignant fibrous histiocytoma (MFH) is a pleomorphic high-grade tumor which is characterized by a storiform, matted or pinwheel pattern and is generally seen in older adults. The microscopic diagnosis is one of exclusion and should not be made until a panel of immunohistochemical stains has been performed to exclude a rhabdomyosarcoma, leiomyosarcoma, liposarcoma, tumors of peripheral nerve origin, and poorly differentiated melanoma or carcinoma.

The term MFH was first introduced in 1963 and before that time most of these cases would have been diagnosed as pleomorphic rhabdomyosarcoma or fibrosarcoma.

Most of the patients are in the fifth to seventh decades of life and two-thirds are males. The tumor is most often seen in the lower extremity, particularly the thigh and at the initial presentation has usually been present for several months or even a year or two. Most of the lesions are intramuscular. Occasionally an MFH may arise in a previously irradiated area.

Grossly the tumor is generally a lobulated, fleshy gray–white mass, between 5 and 10 cm in diameter, which appears circumscribed, even though microscopically it may have infiltrated into the surrounding tissue and along fascial planes (Fig. 22.1). Occasionally there may be evidence of extensive necrosis and/or hemorrhage. About 20% of these tumors have a decidedly myxoid appearance which may grossly suggest a myxoid liposarcoma.

Microscopically these tumors are quite variable. Most of them have a storiform pleomorphic pattern and the rest show either a myxoid, a predominantly giant-cell pattern, or an inflammatory infiltration both of acute and chronic inflammatory cells which tends to obscure the underlying tumor.

In the classic storiform-pleomorphic pattern, plump spindle cells are arranged in a matted pattern of short fascicles. Focally there are large pleomorphic cells, many of them multinucleate giant cells, together with many mitotic figures both typical and atypical (Fig. 22.2).

As already stated, the diagnosis depends on careful exclusion of other entities by the use of immunohistochemistry.

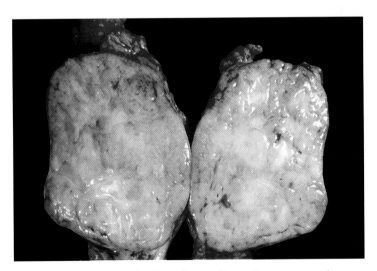

Figure 22.1 Photograph of a malignant fibrous histiocytoma. These tumors, though they appear well circumscribed, usually show microscopic extension into the surrounding tissue. The excision shown here was inadequate.

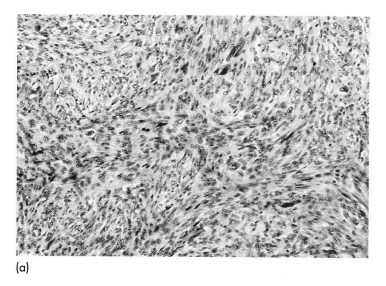

(a)

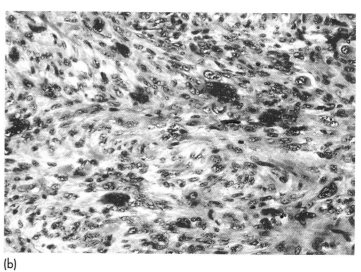

(b)

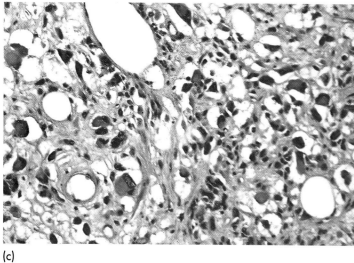

(c)

Figure 22.2 (**a**) Photomicrograph to demonstrate a storiform pattern in an MFH (H&E, × 10 obj.). (**b**) Higher power view to demonstrate giant cells amongst the spindle cells (H&E, × 25 obj.). (**c**) Another high-power field to demonstrate the variability seen in these tumors (H&E, × 25 obj.).

▌LIPOSARCOMA

Liposarcomas most often present in the deep soft tissue of the lower extremity, particularly the thigh, or in the retroperitoneum. They tend to occur in older adults and are frequently large at the time of clinical presentation.

There are five subtypes of liposarcoma which can be conveniently grouped into three. The subtypes are distinct from each other histologically, biologically and cytogenetically (Table 22.1).

Well-differentiated liposarcomas are large multilobular yellow tumors with varying amounts of fibrous tissue coursing through them (Fig. 22.3). Microscopically the well-differentiated liposar-

Table 22.1 Types and outcomes of liposarcoma

Groups (freq.)	Subtypes	Age	Cytogenetics	Recurrence and mets
1 (40%)	Well-differentiated liposarcoma	50–70	Giant and ring chromosomes	Recurrence is more common in retroperitoneal tissue
	Well-differentiated liposarcoma with dedifferentiation			41% local recurrence 17% metastasize
2 (50%)	Myxoid liposarcoma	25–45	Reciprocal translocation between chromosomes 12 and 16	Predominantly myxoid tumors 23% metastasizes
	Round cell liposarcoma			When round cells exceed 25% of the tumor, 58% metastasize
3 (10%)	Pleomorphic liposarcoma	50–70		Increased rate of fatality with this pattern

comas are formed predominantly of mature fat with varying numbers of atypical spindle cells with hypochromatic nuclei and vacuolated lipoblasts; varying degrees of fibrosis and chronic inflammation may be present (Fig. 22.4).

Dedifferentiation occurs in around 6% of the extremity lesions but is somewhat more commonly seen in retroperitoneal lesions. The dedifferentiated areas most often have the pattern of an MFH or high-grade fibrosarcoma. Dedifferentiation of a well-differentiated liposarcoma needs to be distinguished from an ab initio pleomorphic liposarcoma (Fig. 22.5).

Myxoid/round-cell liposarcomas are also large multilobular tumors but with a grayish myxoid gross appearance with more solid areas depending on the proportion of the tumor having a round-cell pattern (Fig. 22.6). Microscopically myxoid liposarcomas are multinodular with each nodule generally paucicellular

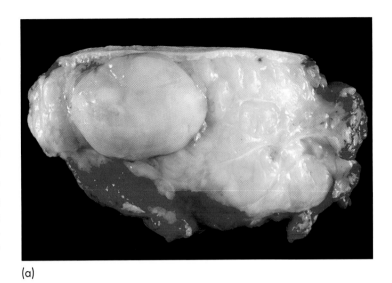

(a)

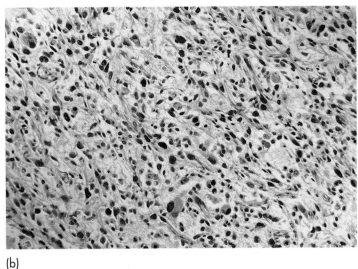

(b)

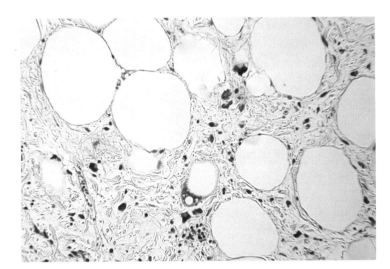

Figure 22.3 Photograph of a resected liposarcoma to show the well-encapsulated appearance which most of these tumors have.

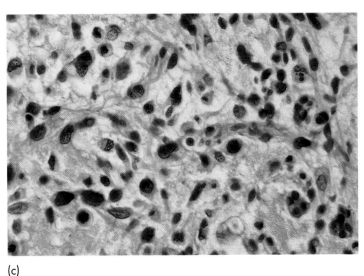

(c)

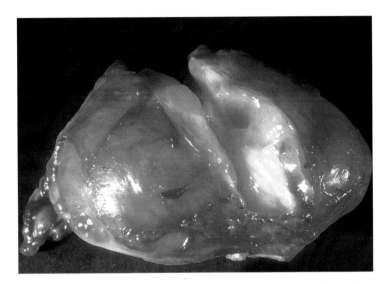

Figure 22.4 In low-grade well-differentiated liposarcomas, much of the tissue may be indistinguishable from lipoma. However, some fibrosis and chronic inflammation may be present and careful searching will show large atypical lipoblasts as seen in this photomicrograph (H&E, × 10 obj.).

Figure 22.5 (a) Photograph of a pleomorphic liposarcoma in section. The tumor is surrounded by subcutaneous fat and lies just below the skin. Note how well the tumor is demarcated from the surrounding tissue. (b) Photomicrograph to demonstrate the pattern in a pleomorphic liposarcoma (H&E, × 4 obj.). (c) Higher power view to demonstrate the pleomorphism of the cells. Occasionally, very bizarre and giant lipoblasts are seen in this form of tumor (H&E, × 25 obj.).

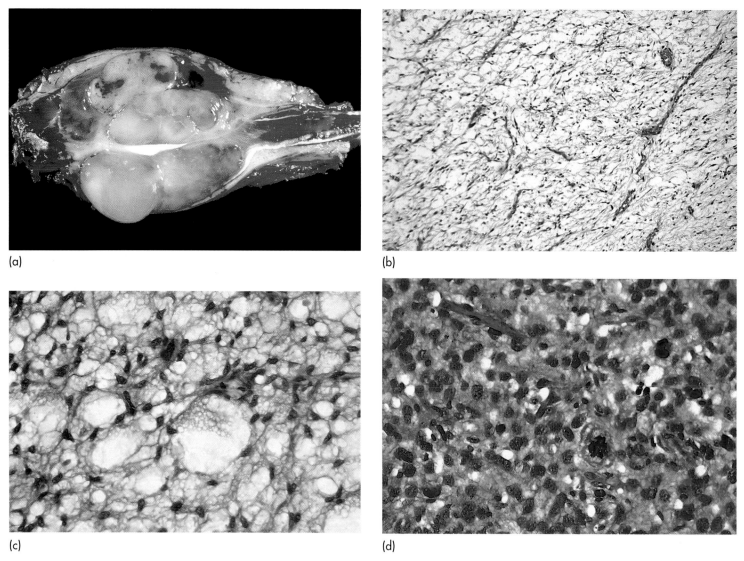

Figure 22.6   (a) Photograph of the cut surface of a myxoid liposarcoma to show the typical mucoid appearance of these tumors.
(b) Photomicrograph of a myxoid liposarcoma shows the typical loose myxoid cellular arrangement of the tumor which is characterized by a network of fine branching capillaries (H&E, × 4 obj.). (c) Higher power view of myxoid liposarcoma (H&E, × 25 obj.). (d) Photomicrograph of a liposarcoma with a closely packed round-cell pattern (H&E, × 25 obj.).

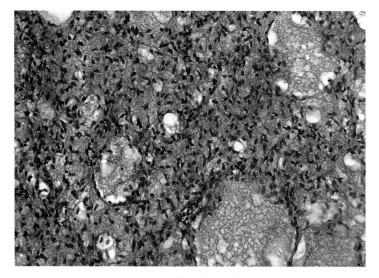

Figure 22.7   Photomicrograph of a myxoid liposarcoma containing pools of mucus which in areas resulted in a lace-like pattern (H&E, × 10 obj.).

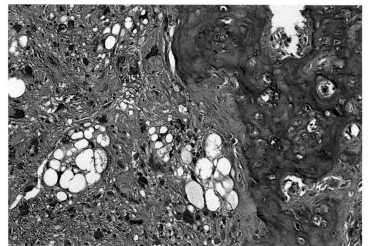

Figure 22.8   Photomicrograph to demonstrate bone formation in a liposarcoma (H&E, × 10 obj.).

in the central area and more cellular at the periphery. The cells are bland fusiform or round cells in a myxoid matrix of hyaluronic acid. Usually lipoblasts can be readily recognized (Fig. 22.7). Characteristically there is a delicate plexiform capillary network coursing through the tumor. Occasionally, as in other forms of liposarcoma, immunohistochemical stains will demonstrate occasional myoblastic cells as well as keratin-positive cells.

As with lipomas, on occasion foci of cartilage or bone may be present within a liposarcoma (Fig. 22.8).

RHABDOMYOSARCOMA

Rhabdomyosarcoma is a malignant tumor arising from skeletal muscle and is the most common soft-tissue sarcoma of children and to a lesser extent young adults. It is rare in people over the age of 40 (Fig. 22.9).

Rhabdomyosarcomas have considerable histologic heterogeneity depending on cellularity, pattern of growth and cellular differentiation. Generally they are classified as embryonal (botryoid or spindle-cell variants of embryonal), alveolar, or pleomorphic. Those with botryoid and spindle-cell variants of embryonal rhabdomyosarcoma have the best prognosis; those with conventional embryonal rhabdomyosarcoma have an intermediate prognosis and those with alveolar rhabdomyosarcoma and undifferentiated sarcoma have a poor prognosis.

Embryonal rhabdomyosarcoma with its botryoid and spindle-cell subtypes affects mainly children between birth and 15 years of age. Alveolar rhabdomyosarcoma affects a somewhat older age group between the ages of 10 and 25. Pleomorphic sarcomas are rare and seen in patients over 45 years of age. Most embryonal tumors occur in the head and neck or trunk, commonly around the orbit or the paratesticular region. Many of the alveolar and rare pleomorphic types occur in the extremities.

Embryonal rhabdomyosarcoma resembles microscopically the various stages of muscle development from poorly differentiated monotonous round-cell tumors to well-differentiated tumor cells with cross-striations resembling rhabdomyoblasts (Fig. 22.10).

Alveolar rhabdomyosarcoma resembles a poorly differentiated embryonal rhabdomyosarcoma but with poorly defined cellular aggregates separated by vascularized dense fibrous septae. Frequently the cells in the center of these aggregates show loss of cohesion, resulting in an 'alveolar' pattern.

In the case of poorly differentiated embryonal tumors, it may be difficult without immunohistochemical staining to distinguish between Ewing's tumor, neuroblastoma, melanoma or rhabdomyosarcoma.

The most useful immunohistochemical stains for the diagnosis of the rhabdomyosarcoma are desmin, muscle-specific actin and myoglobin.

Metastases are very common and are often found at the time of initial presentation.

Cytogenetic abnormalities of embryonal and alveolar rhabdomyosarcoma are distinct.

Embryonal sarcomas are characterized by a consistent loss of heterozygosity for multiple closely linked loci at chromosome 11p15.5. Trisomy 8 has also been reported.

Most alveolar rhabdomyosarcomas have t(2;13)(q35:14) translocation.

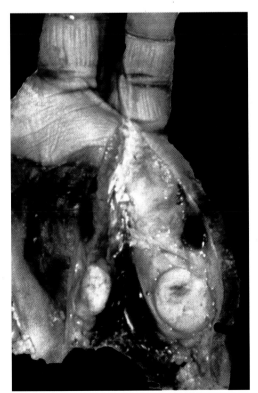

Figure 22.9 Photograph of a rhabdomyosarcoma which presented in the hypothenar eminence.

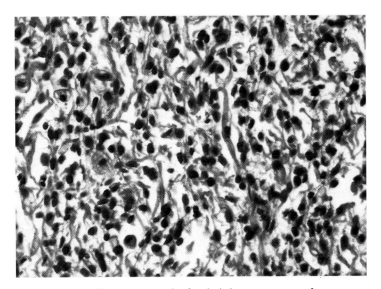

Figure 22.10 Photomicrograph of a rhabdomyosarcoma of embryonal type shows immature cells with elongated eosinophilic cytoplasm (H&E, × 25 obj.).

SYNOVIAL SARCOMA (MALIGNANT SYNOVIOMA)

Synovial sarcomas are rare malignant neoplasms of unknown histogenesis, affecting the extremities, most commonly the lower. Most involve soft tissue in the vicinity of joints, especially the knee. Although the name implies an origin from synovial lining cells, true intra-articular synovial sarcomas are decidedly rare. Usually sharply circumscribed, these tumors may extend along fascial planes and/or invade bone.

Both biphasic and monophasic types of synovial sarcoma are recognized. The classic type has both a spindle-cell and an epithelial component. A monophasic spindle-cell tumor, requires positive immunohistochemical or cytogenetic identification.

Patients with synovial sarcoma usually present between the ages of 15 and 40 with pain and/or with a slow-growing mass. The tumor is decidedly rare in children. A lobulated soft-tissue shadow may be seen on radiographs, and irregular, spotty calcification is evident in about 20% of affected individuals (Figs 22.11 and 22.12). Although the lesion may grossly appear to be encapsulated, on microscopic examination it usually exhibits diffuse infiltration of the surrounding tissues. On gross examination the tumor has a rubbery consistency and may contain evidence of hemorrhage, cysts and calcification (Fig. 22.13).

On histologic examination, classic synovial sarcoma has a biphasic pattern of plump uniform spindle cells and well-differentiated cuboidal to columnar cells forming gland-like spaces, in which cytokeratin and epithelial membrane antigen can be demonstrated (Fig. 22.14). The glandular zones contain mucus-like material which stains positively with PAS, alcian blue and mucicarmine. Microscopic calcifications are usually found; foci of hyalinization and bone formation may also be present (Fig. 22.15). Mast cells are a typical feature, usually being more numerous in the spindle-cell component.

Monophasic synoviomas are as frequently diagnosed as the classic biphasic variety. These tumors are characterized by a monotonous, small spindle-cell population lacking the gland-forming components typically seen in classic synovial sarcoma (Fig. 22.16). In these cases positive identification depends on the demonstration of epithelial antigens by immunohistochemistry. Usually it is only a few cells which will be positive for cytokeratin but rarely it may be the majority (Fig. 22.17).

Consistent specific translocation t(x:18)(p11.2q:11.2) is found in 90% of synovial sarcomas.

Synovial sarcoma has a high rate of local recurrence, as well as metastasis (Fig. 22.18). Some clinicians report a poorer prognosis for patients with the so-called monophasic variant of synovial sarcoma.

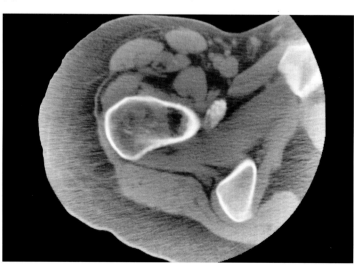

Figure 22.11 (a) Radiograph of a young male with discomfort in the hip shows a calcified mass on the medial side of the femoral neck which, as can be seen in the CT (**b**), is not attached to the bone. This proved to be a synovioma.

(a)

(b)

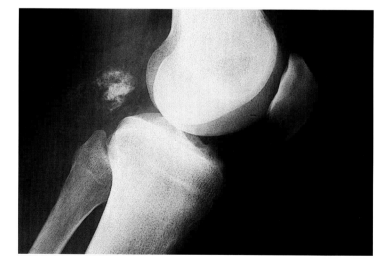

Figure 22.12 Radiograph of a calcified soft-tissue mass in the popliteal space. Although many cases of synovioma will not have radiologic evidence of calcification, around 50% will show some microscopic evidence.

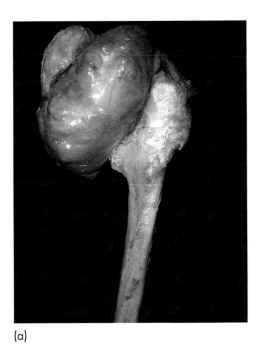
(a)

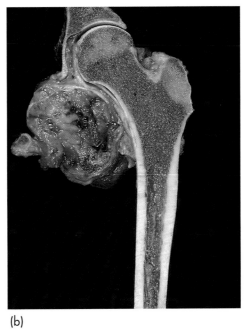
(b)

Figure 22.13 (a) Photograph of a synovioma which is closely applied to the femoral neck in a 19-year-old female. (b) Transected gross specimen of the upper end of the femur and acetabulum shows the tumor abutting against the neck of the femur. (Typically, synoviomas do not involve the joint space.)

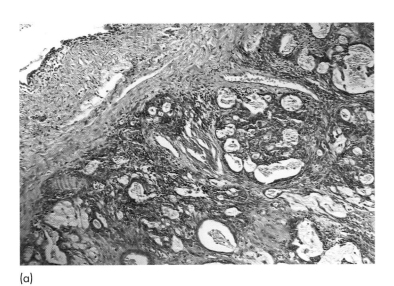
(a)

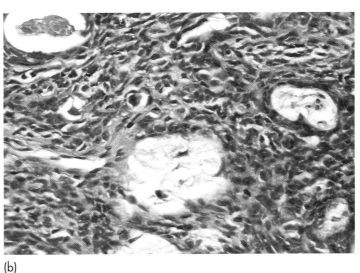
(b)

Figure 22.14 (a) Photomicrograph of a malignant synovioma demonstrates the biphasic appearance of such lesions. Gland-like spaces lined with columnar epithelial cells are seen, as well as a fibrosarcomatous stroma. The ratio of these two components may vary considerably (H&E, × 10 obj.). (b) A higher power view to better show the spindle-cell stroma (H&E, × 25 ob.j).

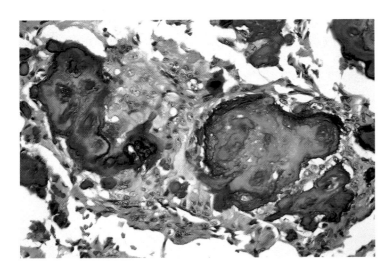

Figure 22.15 Photomicrograph to demonstrate a foci of calcification within a synovial sarcoma. Calcification is more usual at the margins of the tumor (H&E, × 25 obj.).

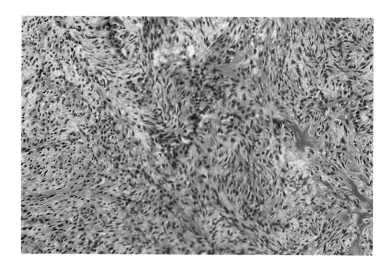

Figure 22.16 Photomicrograph of a monophasic synovioma. Cytokeratin stains in such a case will show occasional positive epithelioid cells. Note the foci of hyalinized intercellular matrix which is occasionally present (H&E, × 10 obj.).

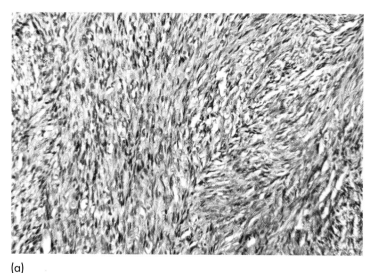

(a)

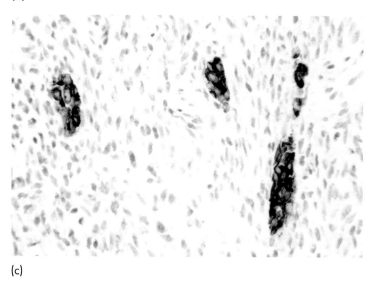

(c)

(b)

Figure 22.17 The photomicrograph is of tissue removed from the elbow joint of a 27-year-old male who presented clinically with pain and limitation of motion. The clinical diagnosis was loose bodies and synovitis. The microscopic finding was of a spindle-cell neoplasm (a) which stained diffusely positive with vimentin antibody (b), and focally positive with cytokeratin antibody (AE-1/AE-3) (c). [(a) H&E, × 4 obj.; (b) immunoperoxidase, × 4 obj.; (c) immunoperoxidase, × 25 obj.]. Malignant synovioma is only very rarely seen in the joint space.

FIBROSARCOMA

Fibrosarcoma is a malignant tumor of fibroblasts, i.e. collagen-producing cells, which shows no other evidence of differentiation i.e. the production of bone matrix or cartilage matrix.

At one time this was the most commonly diagnosed malignant connective-tissue tumor. However, with the increasing use of immunohistochemistry, the segregation of desmoid tumors and benign reactive processes such as fasciitis, the diagnosis of fibrosarcoma has become a diagnosis of exclusion and is much less commonly made.

Most patients are in their 30s to 50s and most of the tumors are seen on the extremities, more frequently the lower extremity. Generally these individuals have slowly growing tumors and in most cases the tumor has been present 2 years or more when they have been seen clinically. The tumor generally arises in the deep structures, either intramuscularly or in the intermuscular septae. Grossly the excised tumors are firm and gray–white in color (Fig. 22.19) and measure < 10 cm in diameter.

Microscopically the lesions consist of uniform spindle cells with scanty cytoplasm which are organized into rather uniform fascicles. Mitoses are generally present but vary in number. Occasionally myxoid changes are seen in the matrix. The lesions are generally regarded as either well or poorly differentiated. In a well-differentiated fibrosarcoma, there is generally a very distinct 'herring-bone' pattern with a variable degree of collagenization (Fig. 22.20). In the less well-differentiated tumors there is generally more cellular crowding, more mitoses, a less distinct pattern and foci of necrosis. Differentiation from monophasic synovioma or peripheral nerve sheath tumors requires immunohistochemical stains for accuracy.

With wide marginal excision the 5-year survival rate for well-differentiated tumors is about 60%, whereas for poorly differentiated tumors it is about 30%.

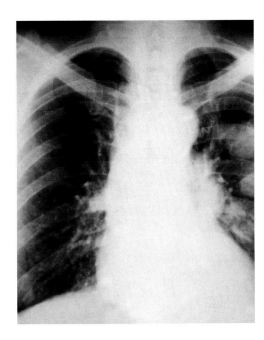

Figure 22.18 Radiograph to demonstrate lung metastases in a case of synovioma.

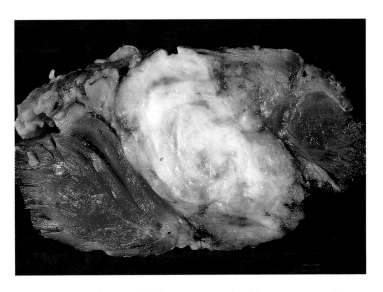

Figure 22.19 Photograph of an intramuscular fibrosarcoma to show the cut surface.

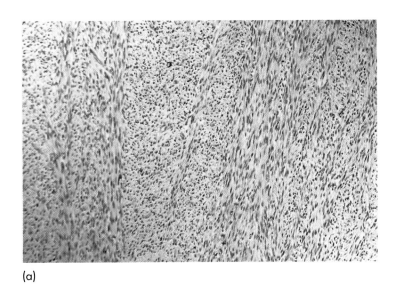

(a)

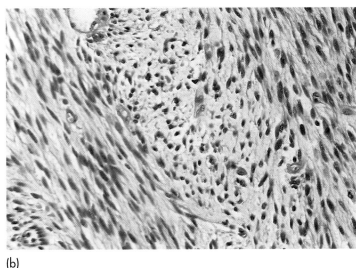

(b)

Figure 22.20 (a) Photomicrograph of a fibrosarcoma to show the packed spindle-cell pattern (H&E, × 4 obj.). (b) A higher power shows the 'herring-bone' pattern (H&E, × 10 obj.).

MALIGNANT PERIPHERAL NERVE SHEATH TUMORS (MALIGNANT NEURILEMOMA)

A malignant peripheral nerve sheath tumor (MPNST) is a spindle-cell sarcoma which arises from a nerve or from a neurofibroma, or has histologic features felt to be characteristic of a nerve sheath. This tumor accounts for about 10% of all soft-tissue sarcomas and up to half of the cases occur in association with neurofibromatosis. In patients with neurofibromatosis, the development of a painful mass should alert the clinician to the possibility of an MPNST. Most patients with MPNSTs are between the ages of 25 and 40 at the time of presentation.

Most cases are seen in relationship to major nerves of either the brachial or sciatic plexus and hence in the proximal upper or lower extremity.

Microscopically most MPNSTs resemble fibrosarcomas in their pattern. However, unlike the symmetrical nuclei of fibroblasts, the nuclei in cases of MPNST are often wavy in outline; there may be nuclei palisading and the lesion may demonstrate a nodular or plexiform arrangement (Fig. 22.21). Occasional cases of MPNST demonstrate myoblastic differentiation (Triton tumor) whilst others show vascular or epithelial differentiation. Mature islands of cartilage or bone may be present.

The differential diagnosis of MPNST from fibrosarcoma, monophasic synovioma or leiomyosarcoma may be difficult. It depends on the microscopic morphology in addition to a careful evaluation of a panel of immunohistochemical stains. The most useful stain for nerve sheath differentiation is the S100 protein. However, there are no specific markers and the careful evaluation of a panel of antigens is necessary to arriving at a correct diagnosis. The rates of recurrence and metastases in MPNST are around 50%.

It may be especially difficult to differentiate a cellular neurilemoma from an MPNST and impossible with a small biopsy. However, generally the S100 protein is more diffusely distributed in a neurilemoma and generally typical morphologic features of neurilemoma can be found such as the Antoni A and B pattern.

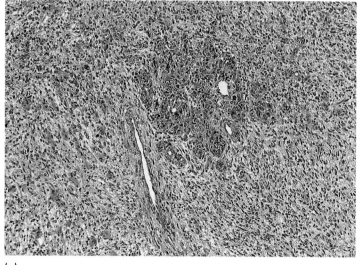

(a)

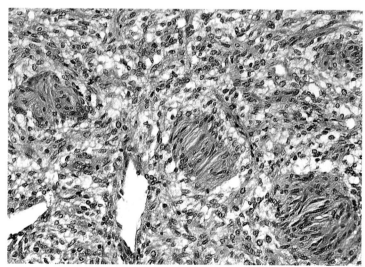

(b)

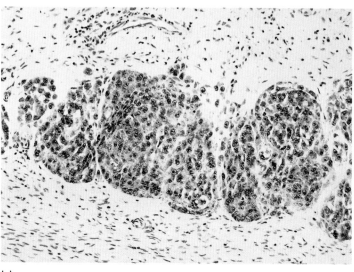

(c)

Figure 22.21 (a) Photomicrograph of a malignant peripheral nerve sheath tumor. At low power, there is a cellular spindle-cell lesion with a nondescript pattern (H&E, × 4 obj.). (b) At a higher power, there are distinct foci of nuclear palisading in this field (H&E, × 10 obj.). (c) Another field stained for S100 protein (× 10 obj.).

EPITHELIOID SARCOMA

Epithelioid sarcoma is a fully malignant, painless soft-tissue sarcoma which when it first presents is likely to be mistaken for granulation tissue, ulcerated squamous-cell carcinoma, or a synovial sarcoma. The patients are generally young adults (aged 10–35) and males appear to be more frequently affected. These lesions most often present in the superficial subcutis or deep tendon sheaths of the hand, wrist, or fingers, but may also extend to involve the skin and ulcerate. The lesions vary considerably in size from a few millimeters in diameter to several centimeters. The smaller lesions in particular will tend to be underdiagnosed both clinically and pathologically. The histo-genesis of this neoplasm remains obscure, but a synovial origin has been suggested.

On microscopic examination, epithelioid sarcoma is a nodular growth composed of a densely eosinophilic polyhedral cell population with prominent nucleoli and an epithelial appearance, however occasionally the cells are spindled (Fig. 22.22). Pleomorphism is variable, and central necrosis may be evident. Immunohistochemical stains are generally positive with both vimentin and epithelial markers (Fig. 22.23). These tumors have a tendency to recur and may disseminate via the lymphatic and vascular systems, eventually leading to both lymph node and lung metastases. The prognosis is poor.

The treatment of choice is wide excision.

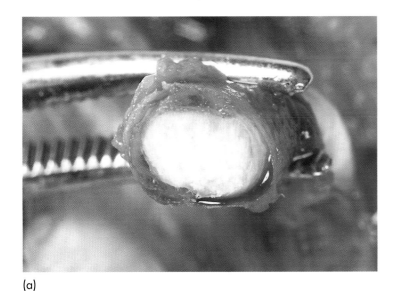

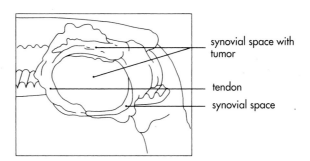

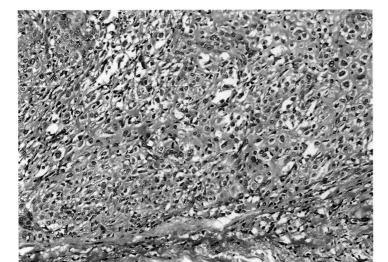

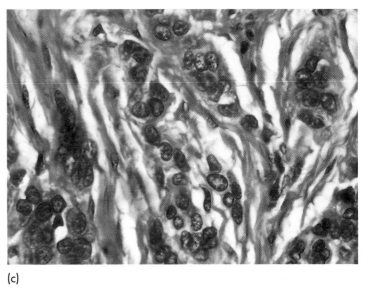

Figure 22.22   (a) In this patient with an epithelioid sarcoma, the tumor initially arose in the distal portion of the tendon sheath of the extensor pollicis longus. At amputation, as demonstrated in this photograph, the tumor was found to be in the subsynovial space, wrapping around the tendon. (b) Photomicrograph of an epithelioid sarcoma shows plump, oval to polyhedral cells which have a dense eosinophilic cytoplasm. The predominant pattern here is epithelial, but in other areas a spindle fibrosarcomatous appearance can be expected (H&E, × 10 obj.). (c) Higher power view of nests of epithelioid cells (H&E, × 40 obj.).

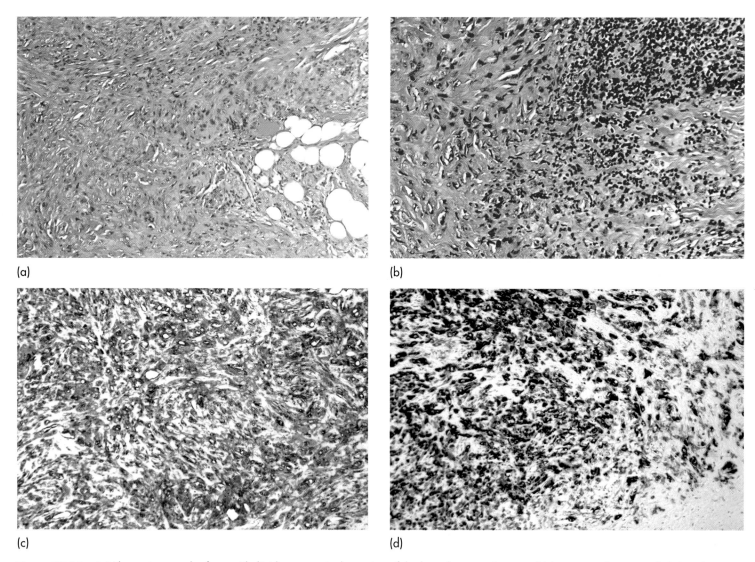

(a)   (b)

(c)   (d)

Figure 22.23   (a) Photomicrograph of an epithelioid sarcoma in the region of the hypothenar eminence which presented as a small, irritated nodule. There is a nodular pattern of swollen cells with smaller spindle cells running between them. It seems in the lower right to be invading fat (H&E, × 10 obj.). (b) In another area of the tumor there are admixed chronic inflammatory cells (H&E, × 10 obj.). It is perhaps not difficult to see that such an appearance may be confused with reparative tissue. (c) Nearly all the cells stain for vimentin (immunoperoxidase, × 10 obj.). (d) The larger swollen cells, but not the smaller spindle cells, also stain for cytokeratin (CAM5.2) (immunoperoxidase, × 10 obj.).

SOFT-TISSUE (EXTRASKELETAL) OSTEOSARCOMA

Rare cases of bone-forming mesenchymal tumors have been described in the soft tissues, usually intramuscularly and most commonly in the thigh. These are usually round to ovoid lesions which exhibit radiographically trabeculated bone formation throughout. They occur in older individuals with a mean age of around 50. The duration of symptoms at the time of presentation is usually only a few months. In some cases the lesion has been associated with prior radiotherapy.

Grossly the excised tumors are soft to firm, gritty and have a variegated hemorrhage and necrotic appearance. They may appear to be well circumscribed or infiltrative. Microscopically they may be fibroblastic or extremely cellular, usually with fine lace-like osteoid and mineralized bone (Fig. 22.24).

Since metaplastic bone is found in a variety of other mesenchymal tumors including synovial sarcoma, malignant fibrous histiocytoma and liposarcoma, differential diagnosis may on occasion be very difficult. In general the prognosis is poor with early metastases.

EXTRASKELETAL MYXOID CHONDROSARCOMA (CHORDOID TUMOR)

Extraskeletal myxoid chondrosarcoma is a rare tumor which usually presents in the deep soft tissue of an extremity, most often the thigh or popliteal fossa. Generally it is a slow-growing tumor and metastasizes late. Most of the patients are middle-aged or older and males are more commonly affected.

Grossly the tumor is generally well circumscribed with a soft to firm consistency. On sectioning it characteristically has a nodular gelatinous appearance and there may be focal hemorrhage. From the gross appearance the lesion is most likely to be initially diagnosed as a myxoid liposarcoma.

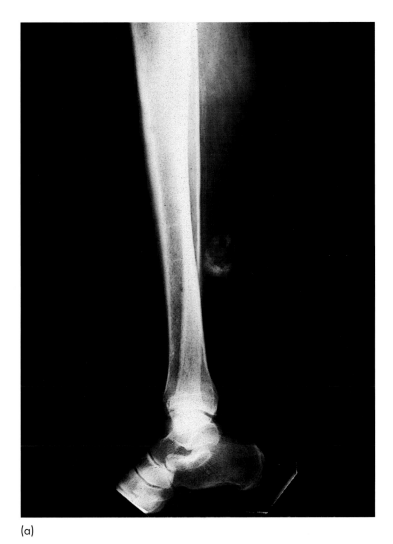

(a)

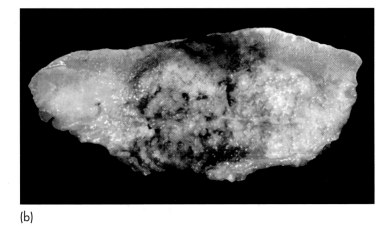

(b)

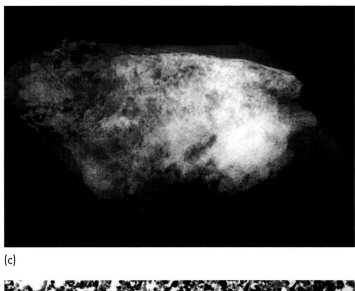

(c)

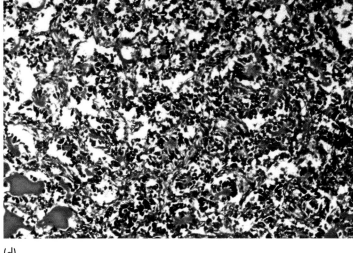

(d)

Figure 22.24 (a) Radiograph of a 50-year-old man who presented with a small, painful mass in the calf region. A well-defined ossified lesion is evident in the soft tissue. (b) Gross lesion resected from the patient in (a). (c) Radiograph of the specimen shows the formation of mineralized tissue throughout the lesion. There is no evidence of maturation of the bone toward the periphery, a finding in contrast to that found in myositis ossificans, a lesion that can be mistaken for a soft-tissue osteosarcoma. (d) Photomicrograph of a portion of the tumor demonstrates the hypercellular anaplastic nature of the lesion and the microscopic foci of osteoid that are being formed by the tumor cells. This is in marked contrast to the histologic picture found in cases of myositis ossificans circumscripta (see Figure 21.49) (H&E, × 10 obj.).

Microscopically the cells have small hyperchromatic nuclei with a thin rim of eosinophilic cytoplasm. Frequently the cells are arranged in short anastomosing strands with abundant extracellular mucoid matrix; they stain with alcian blue and colloidal iron and are resistant to hyaluronidase digestion. PAS stains will usually demonstrate intracellular glycogen. Differentiated chondrocytes are rare but can usually be found after careful searching. Mitotic figures are generally rare (Fig. 22.25).

Immunohistochemical staining shows diffuse S100 staining in maybe 50% of cases; however, since most of the lesions in the dif-ferential diagnosis are S100 positive, this is not very helpful. Epithelial markers will be negative, which differentiates this lesion from chordoma and mixed tumors of salivary gland or sweat gland origin.

Extraskeletal myxoid chondrosarcoma is characterized by a balanced translocation t(9:22)(q22;q12).

Mesenchymal chondrosarcoma, which has already been discussed in Chapter 17, p. 420 may also occur in the soft tissues in almost 25% of cases, mostly around the head and neck region or in the thigh.

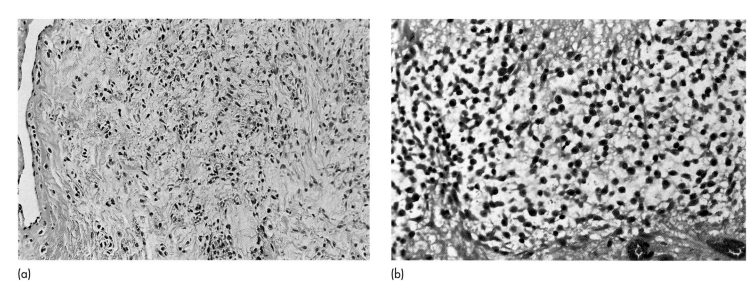

(a)   (b)

Figure 22.25   (a) A photomicrograph of a popliteal mass in a 30-year-old male, which proved to be a myxoid chondrosarcoma. The tumor is composed of small cells in a loose myxoid matrix (H&E, × 4 obj.). (b) A higher power shows small hyperchromatic nuclei with scant eosinophilic cytoplasm in a myxoid stroma (H&E, × 10 obj.).

FURTHER READING

GENERAL

BONE AND JOINTS

Bilezikian JP, Raisz LG, Rodan GA. *Principles of bone biology*, 2 edn. San Diego, CA: Academic Press, 2002.

Brookes M, Revell WJ. *Blood supply of bone: scientific aspects*. London: Springer, 1998.

Burstein AH, Wright TM. *Fundamentals of orthopedic biomechanics*. Baltimore: Williams & Wilkins, 1994.

Crock HV. *Atlas of vascular anatomy of the skeleton and spinal cord*. London: Martin Dunitz, 1996.

Crock HV, Crock C. *The blood supply of the lower limb bones in man*. Edinburgh: Livingstone, 1967.

Crock HV, Yoshizawa H. *The blood supply of the vertebral column and spinal cord in man*. New York: Springer-Verlag, 1977.

Enlow DH. *Principles of bone remodeling*. Springfield, IL: Charles C Thomas, 1963.

Hall BK. *Bone*, Vol. 7. Caldwell, NJ: Telford Press, 1990.

Malluche HH, Faugere MC. *Atlas of mineralized bone histology*. New York: Karger, 1986.

Martin L, Boyde A, Trine F et al. *Scanning microscopy of vertebrate mineralized tissues*. Chicago, IL: AMF O'Hare, 1988.

Mow VC, Hayes WC. *Basic orthopaedic biomechanics*, 2 edn. Philadelphia: Lippincott-Raven, 1997.

Murray PDF. *Bones: a study of the development and structure of the vertebrate skeleton*. Cambridge: Cambridge University Press, 1985.

Nordin M, Frankel VH. *Basic biomechanics of the musculoskeletal system*. Philadelphia: Lippincott Williams & Wilkins, 2001.

Ortner D, Putshar W. *Identification of pathological conditions in human skeletal remain. Smithsonian Contribution to Anthropology, No 28*. Washington, D.C.: Smithsonian Institution Press, 1981.

Thompson DW. *On growth and form, abridged ed. by Bonner, JT*. London: Cambridge University Press, 1961.

Trueta J. *Development and decay of the human frame*. London: Heinemann, 1968.

Wolff J. *The law of bone remodeling, translated by Maquet P, Furlong R*. New York: Springer-Verlag, 1986.

ORTHOPEDICS AND RHEUMATOLOGY

Buckwalter JA, Einhorn TA, Simon SR. *Orthopaedic basic science: biology and biomechanics of the musculoskeletal system*, 2 edn. Rosemont, IL: American Academy of Orthopaedic Surgeons, 2000.

Bullough PG, Boachie-Adjei O. *Atlas of spinal diseases*. New York: Gower Medical Publishing, 1988.

Coe FL, Favus MJ. *Disorders of bone and mineral metabolism*, 2 edn. Philadelphia: Lippincott Williams & Wilkins, 2002.

Doherty M. *Color atlas and text of osteoarthritis*. London: Wolfe, 1994.

Favus MJ. *Primer on the metabolic bone diseases and disorders of mineral metabolism*, 4 edn. Philadelphia: Lippincott Williams & Wilkins, 1999.

Hirohata K, Morimoto K, Kimura H. *Ultrastructure of bone and joint diseases*, 2 edn. Tokyo: Igaku-Shoin, 1981.

Jaffe HL. *Metabolic, degenerative, and inflammatory diseases of bones and joints*. Philadelphia: Lea & Febiger, 1972.

Klippel JH, Dieppe P. *Rheumatology*, 2 edn. London: Mosby, 1998.

Klippel JH, Weyand CM, Crofford LJ et al. *Primer on the rheumatic diseases*, 12 edn. Atlanta, GA: Arthritis Foundation, 2001.

Milgram JH. *Radiologic and histologic pathology of nontumorous diseases of bones and joints*. Northbrook, IL: Northbrook Publishing, 1990.

Peltier LF. *Orthopaedics: a history and iconography*. San Francisco: Norman Publishing, 1993.

Rang M. *The story of orthopaedics*. Philadelphia: W.B. Saunders, 2000.

Resnick D. *Diagnosis of bone and joint disorders*, 4 edn. Philadelphia: Saunders, 2002.

Schmorl G, Junghanns H. *The human spine in health and disease*, 2 Am. edn. New York: Grune & Stratton, 1971.

Sissons HA, Murray RO, Kemp HBS. *Orthopaedic diagnosis: clinical, radiological, and pathological coordinates*. Berlin: Springer-Verlag, 1984.

TUMORS

Dorfman HD, Czerniak B. *Bone tumors*. St. Louis: Mosby, 1998.

Fechner RE, Mills SE. *Tumors of the bones and joints*. Washington, D.C.: Armed Forces Institute of Pathology, 1993.

Fletcher CDM, McKee PH. *Pathobiology of soft tissue tumours*. Edinburgh: Churchill Livingstone, 1990.

Fletcher CDM, Unni KK, Mertens F. *World Health Organization classification of tumours: pathology and genetics of tumours of soft tissue and bone*. Lyon: International Agency for Research on Cancer (IARC) Press, 2002.

Forest M, Tomeno G, Vanel D. *Orthopaedic surgical pathology: diagnosis of tumors and pseudotumoral lesions of bone and joints*. Edinburgh: Churchill Livingstone, 1998.

Greenspan A, Remagen W. *Differential diagnosis of tumors and tumor-like lesions of bones and joints*. Philadelphia: Lippincott-Raven, 1997.

Jaffe HL. *Tumors and tumorous conditions of the bones and joints*. Philadelphia: Lea & Febiger, 1958.

Kempson RL. *Tumors of the soft tissues*. Washington, D.C.: Armed Forces Institute of Pathology, 2001.

Kilpatrick SE, Renner JB. *Diagnostic musculoskeletal surgical pathology: clinicoradiologic and cytologic correlations*, 1 edn. Philadelphia: W.B. Saunders, 2004.

Mirra JM, Picci P, Gold RH. *Bone tumors: clinical, radiologic, and pathologic correlations*. Philadelphia: Lea & Febiger, 1989.

Schajowicz F. *Tumors and tumorlike lesions of bone: pathology, radiology, and treatment*, 2 edn. New York: Springer-Verlag, 1994.

Sciubba JJ, Fantasia JE, Kahn LB. *Tumors and cysts of the jaws*. Washington, D.C.: Armed Forces Institute of Pathology, 2001.

Unni KK. *Dahlin's bone tumors: general aspects and data on 11,087 cases*, 5 edn. Philadelphia: Lippincott-Raven, 1996.

Weiss SW, Goldblum JR. *Enzinger and Weiss's Soft tissue tumors*, 4 edn. St. Louis, MO: Mosby, 2001.

SECTION I – NORMAL

1. NORMAL BONE STRUCTURE AND DEVELOPMENT

Bones

Anderson HC. Mechanism of mineral formation in bone. *Lab Invest* 1989; **60**: 320–30.

Bertram JE, Swartz SM. The 'law of bone transformation': a case of crying Wolff? *Biol Rev Camb Philos Soc* 1991; **66**: 245–73.

Bianco P. Immunohistology of bone proteins, bone quality, and bone turnover. *Clin Rheumatol* 1994; **13 Suppl 1**: 69–74.

Boskey AL. Pathogenesis of cartilage calcification: mechanisms of crystal deposition in cartilage. *Curr Rheumatol Rep* 2002; **4**: 245–51.

Carando S, Portigliatti Barbos M, Ascenzi A et al. Orientation of collagen in human tibial and fibular shaft and possible correlation with mechanical properties. *Bone* 1989; **10**: 139–42.

Ghokaley JA, Robey PG, Boskey AL. The biochemistry of bone. In: *Osteoporosis* (Marcus R, Feldman D, Kelsey J, eds), 2 edn. San Diego: Academic Press, 2001: 107–88.

Hanna SL, Fletcher BD, Fairclough DL et al. Magnetic resonance imaging of disseminated bone marrow disease in patients treated for malignancy. *Skeletal Radiol* 1991; **20**: 79–84.

Iwasaki M, Le AX, Helms JA. Expression of indian hedgehog, bone morphogenetic protein 6 and gli during skeletal morphogenesis. *Mech Dev* 1997; **69**: 197–202.

Marks SC, Jr., Popoff SN. Bone cell biology: the regulation of development, structure, and function in the skeleton. *Am J Anat* 1988; **183**: 1–44.

Martin TJ, Ng KW, Suda T. Bone cell physiology. *Endocrinol Metab Clin North Am* 1989; **18**: 833–58.

McDonald JA. Extracellular matrix assembly. *Annu Rev Cell Biol* 1988; **4**: 183–207.

Miller A. Collagen: the organic matrix of bone. *Philos Trans R Soc Lond B Biol Sci* 1984; **304**: 455–77.

Mitchell DG, Rao VM, Dalinka M et al. Hematopoietic and fatty bone marrow distribution in the normal and ischemic hip: new observations with 1.5-T MR imaging. *Radiology* 1986; **161**: 199–202.

Ruoslahti E. Structure and biology of proteoglycans. *Annu Rev Cell Biol* 1988; **4**: 229–55.

Schneider RA, Hu D, Helms JA. From head to toe: conservation of molecular signals regulating limb and craniofacial morphogenesis. *Cell Tissue Res* 1999; **296**: 103–9.

Tonna EA, Cronkite EP. The periosteum. Autoradiographic studies on cellular proliferation and transformation utilizing tritiated thymidine. *Clin Orthop* 1963; **30**: 218–33.

Woodard HQ. The composition of human cortical bone: effect of age and of some abnormalities. *Clin Orthop* 1964; **37**: 187–93.

Wozney JM, Rosen V, Celeste AJ et al. Novel regulators of bone formation: molecular clones and activities. *Science* 1988; **242**: 1528–34.

Joints

Bullough P, Goodfellow J. The significance of the fine structure of articular cartilage. *J Bone Joint Surg Br* 1968; **50**: 852–7.

Bullough PG, Jagannath A. The morphology of the calcification front in articular cartilage. Its significance in joint function. *J Bone Joint Surg Br* 1983; **65**: 72–8.

Cooper RR, Misol S. Tendon and ligament insertion. A light and electron microscopic study. *J Bone Joint Surg Am* 1970; **52**: 1–20.

Frank CB, Woo SL-Y, Andriacchi T. Normal ligament: structure, function and composition. In: *Injury and repair of the musculoskeletal soft tissues* (Woo SL-Y, Buckwalter JA, eds). Park Ridge, IL: American Academy of Orthopaedic Surgeons, 1988: 45–101.

Goodfellow J, O'Connor JJ. The design of synovial joints. In: *Scientific foundations of orthopaedics and traumatology* (Owen R, Goodfellow J, Bullough P, eds). London: Heinemann, 1980.

Henderson B. The synovial lining cell and synovitis. *Scand J Rheumatol Suppl* 1988; **76**: 33–8.

MacConaill MA. The movements of bones and joints. *J Bone Joint Surg Br* 1950; **32**: 244.

Ogston A. On articular cartilage. *J Anat* 1876; **10**: 49–74.

Schenk RK, Eggli PS, Hunziker EB. Articular cartilage morphology. In: *Articular cartilage biochemistry* (Kuettner KE, Schleyerbach R, Hascall VC, eds). New York: Raven Press, 1986.

Bone growth and development

Hunter SJ, Caplan AI. Control of cartilage differentiation. In: *Cartilage* (Hall BK, ed). New York: Academic Press, 1983.

Ogden JA. Changing patterns of proximal femoral vascularity. *J Bone Joint Surg Am* 1974; **56**: 941–50.

2. METHODS OF EXAMINATION

Gross examination

Anderson C. *Manual for the examination of bone.* Boca Raton, FL: CRC Press, 1982.

Cutignola L, Bullough PG. Photographic reproduction of anatomic specimens using ultraviolet illumination. *Am J Surg Pathol* 1991; **15**: 1096–9.

Dickson G. *Methods of calcified tissue preparation.* New York: Elsevier, 1984.

Microscopic examination

Bullough PG, Bansal M, DiCarlo EF. The tissue diagnosis of metabolic bone disease. Role of histomorphometry. *Orthop Clin North Am* 1990; **21**: 65–79.

Clark G, Bartholomew JW. *Staining procedures,* 4 edn. Baltimore: Williams & Wilkins, 1981.

Eriksen EF, Axelrod DW, Melsen F. *Bone histomorphometry.* New York: Raven Press, 1994.

Frost HM. Relation between bone tissue and cell population dynamics, histology and tetracycline labeling. *Clin Orthop* 1966; **49**: 65–75.

Keen CE, Crocker PR, Brady K et al. Intraosseous secondary calcium salt crystal deposition: an artefact of acid decalcification. *Histopathology* 1995; **27**: 181–5.

Milch R, Rall D, Tobie J. Fluorescence of tetracycline antibiotics in bone. *J Bone Joint Surg Am* 1958; **40**: 897–910.

Recker RR. *Bone histomorphometry, techniques and interpretation.* Boca Raton, FL: CRC Press, 1983.

3. IMAGING TECHNIQUES, INTERPRETATION AND STRATEGIES

Bohndorf K, Imhof H, Pope TL. *Musculoskeletal imaging: a concise multimodality approach.* New York: Thieme, 2001.

Collier D, Fogelman I, Rosenthal L. *Skeletal nuclear medicine.* St. Louis: Mosby, 1996.

Greenspan A. *Orthopedic radiology: a practical approach,* 3 edn. Philadelphia: Lippincott Williams & Wilkins, 2000.

Helms CA. *Fundamentals of skeletal radiology,* 2 edn. Philadelphia: W.B. Saunders, 1995.

Kaplan P. *Musculoskeletal MRI.* Philadelphia: Saunders, 2001.

Manaster BJ. *Musculoskeletal imaging: the requisites,* 2 edn. St. Louis: Mosby, 2002.

Resnick D. *Diagnosis of bone and joint disorders,* 4 edn. Philadelphia: Saunders, 2002.

Stoller DW. *Magnetic resonance imaging in orthopaedics & sports medicine,* 2 edn. Philadelphia: Lippincott-Raven, 1997.

Vahlensieck M. *MRI of the musculoskeletal system.* New York: Thieme, 2000.

Van Holsbeeck M, Introcaso JH. *Musculoskeletal ultrasound,* 2 edn. St. Louis: Mosby, 2001.

SECTION II – RESPONSE TO INJURY

4. INJURY AND REPAIR

Allbrook DB. Muscle breakdown and repair. In: *Scientific foundations of orthopaedics and traumatology* (Owen R, Goodfellow J, Bullough P, eds). Philadelphia: WB Saunders, 1980.

Byers PD, Gray JC, Mostafa A et al. The healing of bone and articular cartilage. In: *Tissue repair and regeneration. Handbook of inflammation* (Glynn LE, ed), Vol. 3. Amsterdam: Elsevier North-Holland, 1981.

Campanacci M, Nicoll EA, Pagella P. The differential diagnosis of congenital pseudarthrosis of the tibia. *Int Orthop* 1981; **4**: 283–8.

Gain P, Thuret G, Chiquet C et al. Value of two mortality assessment techniques for organ cultured corneal endothelium: trypan blue versus TUNEL technique. *Br J Ophthalmol* 2002; **86**: 306–10.

Hargens AR, Mubarak SJ. Current concepts in the pathophysiology, evaluation, and diagnosis of compartment syndrome. *Hand Clin* 1998; **14**: 371–83.

Hayda RA, Brighton CT, Esterhai JL, Jr. Pathophysiology of delayed healing. *Clin Orthop* 1998: S31–40.

Heppenstall RB. *Fracture treatment and healing.* Philadelphia: Saunders, 1980.

Hock JM, Krishnan V, Onyia JE et al. Osteoblast apoptosis and bone turnover. *J Bone Miner Res* 2001; **16**: 975–84.

Noguchi T, Oka M, Fujino M et al. Repair of osteochondral defects with grafts of cultured chondrocytes. Comparison of allografts and isografts. *Clin Orthop* 1994; **302**: 251–8.

Ogden JA. *Skeletal injury in the child,* 3 edn. New York: Springer, 2000.

Ordman LJ, Gillman T. Studies in the healing of cutaneous wounds. I. The healing of incisions through the skin of pigs. *Arch Surg* 1966; **93**: 857–82.

Peacock EE. *Wound repair,* 3 edn. Philadelphia: Saunders, 1984.

Phalen GS. The birth of a syndrome, or carpal tunnel revisited. *J Hand Surg [Am]* 1981; **6**: 109–10.

Sunderland S. The anatomic foundation of peripheral nerve repair techniques. *Orthop Clin North Am* 1981; **12**: 245–66.

Tidball JG. Inflammatory cell response to acute muscle injury. *Med Sci Sports Exerc* 1995; **27**: 1022–32.

Verdan C. *Tendon surgery of the hand,* 1 edn. Edinburgh: Churchill Livingstone, 1979.

Vortkamp A. The Indian hedgehog—PTHrP system in bone development. *Ernst Schering Res Found Workshop* 2000: 191–209.

Walter JB, Talbot IC, Israel MS. *Walter and Israel general pathology,* 7 edn. New York: Churchill Livingstone, 1996.

5. BONE AND JOINT INFECTION

Pyogenic and other nongranulomatous infections

Abel L, Casanova J. Immunogenetics of the host response to bacterial and parasites in humans. In: *Immunology of infectious diseases* (Kaufmann SHE, Sher A, Ahmed R, eds). Washington, D.C.: ASM Press, 2002: 395–406.

Anderson SE, Heini P, Sauvain MJ et al. Imaging of chronic recurrent multifocal osteomyelitis of childhood first presenting with isolated primary spinal involvement. *Skeletal Radiol* 2003; **32**: 328–36.

Ashby ME. Serratia osteomyelitis in heroin users. A report of two cases. *J Bone Joint Surg Am* 1976; **58**: 132–4.

Barnard J, Newman LS. Sarcoidosis: immunology, rheumatic involvement, and therapeutics. *Curr Opin Rheumatol* 2001; **13**: 84–91.

Broner FA, Garland DE, Zigler JE. Spinal infections in the immunocompromised host. *Orthop Clin North Am* 1996; **27**: 37–46.

Costerton JW, Stewart PS, Greenberg EP. Bacterial biofilms: a common cause of persistent infections. *Science* 1999; **284**: 1318–22.

Gifford DB, Patzakis M, Ivler D et al. Septic arthritis due to pseudomonas in heroin addicts. *J Bone Joint Surg Am* 1975; **57**: 631–5.

Green NE, Edwards K. Bone and joint infections in children. *Orthop Clin North Am* 1987; **18**: 555–76.

Greenspan A, Norman A, Steiner G. Case report 146. Squamous cell carcinoma arising in chronic, draining sinus tract secondary to osteomyelitis of right tibia. *Skeletal Radiol* 1981; **6**: 149–51.

Gustilo RB, Gruninger RP, Tsukayama DT. *Orthopaedic infection: diagnosis and treatment.* Philadelphia: Saunders, 1989.

Jarvis JG, Skipper J. Pseudomonas osteochondritis complicating puncture wounds in children. *J Pediatr Orthop* 1994; **14**: 755–9.

Mader JT, Calhoun J. Osteomyelitis. In: *Mandell, Douglas, and Bennett's principles and practice of infectious diseases* (Mandell GL, Douglas RG, Bennett JE et al., eds), 5 edn. Philadelphia: Churchill Livingstone, 2000: 1182–96.

Mascola L. The rising incidence of congenital syphilis: back to the future. *N Y State J Med* 1990; **90**: 485–6.

Nade S. Infection after joint replacement—what would Lister think? *Med J Aust* 1990; **152**: 394–7.

Ramos OM. Chronic osteomyelitis in children. *Pediatr Infect Dis J* 2002; **21**: 431–2.

Rasool MN, Govender S. The skeletal manifestations of congenital syphilis. A review of 197 cases. *J Bone Joint Surg Br* 1989; **71**: 752–5.

Resnick D. Enostosis, hyperostosis, and periostitis. In: *Bone and joint imaging* (Resnick D, ed), 2 edn. Philadelphia: W.B. Saunders, 1996: 1211–31.

Rosenberg ZS, Norman A, Solomon G. Arthritis associated with HIV infection: radiographic manifestations. *Radiology* 1989; **173**: 171–6.

Stephens MM, MacAuley P. Brodie's abscess. A long-term review. *Clin Orthop* 1988: 211–6.

Tehranzadeh J, Wong E, Wang F et al. Imaging of osteomyelitis in the mature skeleton. *Radiol Clin North Am* 2001; **39**: 223–50.

Thornburg LP. Infantile cortical hyperostosis (Caffey-Silverman syndrome). Animal model: craniomandibular osteopathy in the canine. *Am J Pathol* 1979; **95**: 575–8.

Waldvogel FA, Papageorgiou PS. Osteomyelitis: the past decade. *N Engl J Med* 1980; **303**: 360–70.

Wu PC, Khin MM, Pang SW. Salmonella osteomyelitis. An important differential diagnosis of granulomatous osteomyelitis. *Am J Surg Pathol* 1985; **9**: 531–7.

Granulomatous inflammation of bones and joints

Autzen B, Elberg JJ. Bone and joint tuberculosis in Denmark. *Acta Orthop Scand* 1988; **59**: 50–2.

Bjarnason DF, Forrester DM, Swezey RL. Destructive arthritis of the large joints. A rare manifestation of sarcoidosis. *J Bone Joint Surg Am* 1973; **55**: 618–22.

Brown BA, Wallace RJJ. Infections due to nontuberculous mycobacteria. In: *Mandell,*

Douglas, and Bennett's principles and practice of infectious diseases (Mandell GL, Douglas RG, Bennett JE et al., eds), 5 edn. Philadelphia: Churchill Livingstone, 2000: 2630–6.

Fyfe B, Amazon K, Poppiti RJ, Jr. et al. Intraosseous echinococcosis: a rare manifestation of echinococcal disease. *South Med J* 1990; **83**: 66–8.

Hooper J, McLean I. Hydatid disease of the femur. Report of a case. *J Bone Joint Surg Am* 1977; **59**: 974–6.

Lemley DE, Katz P. Granulomatous musculoskeletal disease: sarcoidosis versus tuberculosis. *J Rheumatol* 1987; **14**: 1199–201.

Lieberman J. *Sarcoidosis.* Orlando: Grune & Stratton, 1985.

Shannon FB, Moore M, Houkom JA et al. Multifocal cystic tuberculosis of bone. Report of a case. *J Bone Joint Surg Am* 1990; **72**: 1089–92.

Smith MB, Molina CP, Schnadig VJ et al. Pathologic features of Mycobacterium kansasii infection in patients with acquired immunodeficiency syndrome. *Arch Pathol Lab Med* 2003; **127**: 554–60.

Walker AN, Fechner RE. Granulomatous inflammation of bones and joints. In: *Pathology of granulomas* (Ioachim HL, ed). New York: Raven Press, 1983.

SECTION III – METABOLIC DISTURBANCES

6. DISEASES RESULTING FROM ABNORMAL SYNTHESIS OF MATRIX COMPONENTS

Disturbances in collagen synthesis

Bullough PG, Davidson DD, Lorenzo JC. The morbid anatomy of the skeleton in osteogenesis imperfecta. *Clin Orthop* 1981: 42–57.

Byers PH. Disorders of collagen biosynthesis and structure. In: *The metabolic and molecular bases of inherited disease* (Scriver CR, Beaudet AL, Sly W et al., eds), 8 edn. New York: McGraw-Hill, 2001: 5241–86.

Caffey J. Chronic poisoning due to excess of vitamin A. *Amer J Roentgenology* 1951; **65**: 12.

Fell HB, Mellanby E. The effect of hypervitaminosis A on embryonic limb bones cultured in vitro. *J Physiol* 1952; **116**: 320–49.

Grahame R. Heritable disorders of connective tissue. *Baillieres Best Pract Res Clin Rheumatol* 2000; **14**: 345–61.

Nakamura K, Kurokawa T, Nagano A et al. Familial occurrence of hyperplastic callus in osteogenesis imperfecta. *Arch Orthop Trauma Surg* 1997; **116**: 500–3.

Prockop DJ. The Gordon Wilson lecture. Mutations in type I procollagen genes. An explanation for brittle bones and a paradigm for other diseases of connective tissue. *Trans Am Clin Climatol Assoc* 1988; **100**: 70–80.

Valentic JP, Elias AN, Weinstein GD. Hypercalcemia associated with oral isotretinoin in the treatment of severe acne. *Jama* 1983; **250**: 1899–900.

Wang Q, Marini JC. Antisense oligodeoxynucleotides selectively suppress expression of the mutant alpha 2(I) collagen allele in type IV osteogenesis imperfecta fibroblasts. A molecular approach to therapeutics of dominant negative disorders. *J Clin Invest* 1996; **97**: 448–54.

Mucopolysaccharidoses

Eggli KD, Dorst JP. The mucopolysaccharidoses and related conditions. *Semin Roentgenol* 1986; **21**: 275–94.

Haskins M, Casal M, Ellinwood NM et al. Animal models for mucopolysaccharidoses and their clinical relevance. *Acta Paediatr Suppl* 2002; **91**: 88–97.

Neufeld EF, Muenzer J. The mucopolysaccharidoses. In: *The metabolic and molecular bases of inherited disease* (Scriver CR, Beaudet AL, Sly W et al., eds), 8 edn., Vol. 4. New York: McGraw-Hill, 2001: 3421–52.

Wraith JE. The mucopolysaccharidoses: a clinical review and guide to management. *Arch Dis Child* 1995; **72**: 263–7.

Disturbances in mineral formation

Courvoisier B, Baud CA, Donath A. *Fluoride and bone: Second Symposium CEMO Centre d'etude des maladies osteo-articulaires de Geneve), Nyon, Switzerland, October 9th-12th, 1977.* Bern: Huber, 1978.

Crespo-Pena M, Torrijos-Eslava A, Gijon-Banos J. Benign familial hyperphosphatasemia: a report of two families and review of the literature. *Clin Exp Rheumatol* 1997; **15**: 425–31.

Horwith M, Nunez EA, Krook L et al. Hereditary bone dysplasia with hyperphosphatasaemia: response to synthetic human calcitonin. *Clin Endocrinol (Oxf)* 1976; **5 Suppl**: 341S-52S.

Hoshino T, Kumasaka K, Kawano K et al. A case of benign familial hyperphosphatasemia of intestinal origin. *Clin Biochem* 1993; **26**: 421–5.

Lum G. Significance of low serum alkaline phosphatase activity in a predominantly adult male population. *Clin Chem* 1995; **41**: 515–8.

Silve C. Hereditary hypophosphatasia and hyperphosphatasia. *Curr Opin Rheumatol* 1994; **6**: 336–9.

Whyte MP. Hypophosphatasia and the role of alkaline phosphatase in skeletal mineralization. *Endocr Rev* 1994; **15**: 439–61.

Dwarfism (Chondro-osseous dysplasia)

Dutton RV. A practical radiologic approach to skeletal dysplasias in infancy. *Radiol Clin North Am* 1987; **25**: 1211–33.

Olsen BR. Mutations in collagen genes resulting in metaphyseal and epiphyseal dysplasias. *Bone* 1995; **17**: 45S-9S.

Wynne-Davies R, Hall CM, Apley AG. *Atlas of skeletal dysplasias.* Edinburgh: Churchill Livingstone, 1985.

7. DISEASES RESULTING FROM DISTURBANCES IN CELL LINKAGE

Osteosclerotic conditions

Altman RD. Arthritis in Paget's disease of bone. *J Bone Miner Res* 1999; **14 Suppl 2**: 85–7.

Applegate LJ, Applegate GR, Kemp SS. MR of multiple cranial neuropathies in a patient with camurati-engelmann disease: case report. *AJNR Am J Neuroradiol* 1991; **12**: 557–9.

Basle MF, Mazaud P, Malkani K et al. Isolation of osteoclasts from Pagetic bone tissue: morphometry and cytochemistry on isolated cells. *Bone* 1988; **9**: 1–6.

Bevier WC, Wiswell RA, Pyka G et al. Relationship of body composition, muscle strength, and aerobic capacity to bone mineral density in older men and women. *J Bone Miner Res* 1989; **4**: 421–32.

Bollerslev J, Andersen PE, Jr. Radiological, biochemical and hereditary evidence of two types of autosomal dominant osteopetrosis. *Bone* 1988; **9**: 7–13.

Johnston CC, Melton LJI, Lindsay R. Clinical indication for bone mass measurement. *J Bone Miner Res* 1989; **4**: 1–28.

Lieschke GJ, Stanley E, Grail D et al. Mice lacking both macrophage- and granulocyte-macrophage colony-stimulating factor have macrophages and coexistent osteopetrosis and severe lung disease. *Blood* 1994; **84**: 27–35.

Mankin HJ, Mankin CJ. Metabolic bone disease: an update. *Instr Course Lect* 2003; **52**: 769–84.

Marks SC, Jr. Osteopetrosis—multiple pathways for the interception of osteoclast function. *Appl Pathol* 1987; **5**: 172–83.

McAfee JG. Radionuclide imaging in metabolic and systemic skeletal diseases. *Semin Nucl Med* 1987; **17**: 334–49.

Monson DK, Finn HA, Dawson PJ et al. Pseudosarcoma in Paget disease of bone. A case report. *J Bone Joint Surg Am* 1989; **71**: 453–5.

Nuovo MA, Nuovo GJ, MacConnell P et al. In situ analysis of Paget's disease of bone for measles-specific PCR-amplified cDNA. *Diagn Mol Pathol* 1992; **1**: 256–65.

Paget J. On a form of chronic inflammation of bones (osteitis deformans). *Med Chir Trans* 1877; **60**: 37–63.

Rebel A, Basle M, Pouplard A et al. Bone tissue in Paget's disease of bone. Ultrastructure and Immunocytology. *Arthritis Rheum* 1980; **23**: 1104–14.

Reddy SV, Kurihara N, Menaa C et al. Paget's disease of bone: a disease of the osteoclast. *Rev Endocr Metab Disord* 2001; **2**: 195–201.

Resnick D. Paget disease of bone: current status and a look back to 1943 and earlier. *AJR Am J Roentgenol* 1988; **150**: 249–56.

Shapiro F. Osteopetrosis. Current clinical considerations. *Clin Orthop* 1993: 34–44.

Singer FR. *Paget's disease of bone*. New York: Plenum Medical Book Co., 1977.

Sparkes RS, Graham CB. Camurati-Engelmann disease. Genetics and clinical manifestations with a review of the literature. *J Med Genet* 1972; **9**: 73–85.

Van Buchem FS. The pathogenesis of hyperostosis corticalis generalisata and calcitonin. *Proc K Ned Akad Wet C* 1970; **73**: 243–53.

Vanhoenacker FM, De Beuckeleer LH, Van Hul W et al. Sclerosing bone dysplasias: genetic and radioclinical features. *Eur Radiol* 2000; **10**: 1423–33.

Vuillemin-Bodaghi V, Parlier-Cuau C, Cywiner-Golenzer C et al. Multifocal osteogenic sarcoma in Paget's disease. *Skeletal Radiol* 2000; **29**: 349–53.

Whyte MP. Sclerosing bone disorders. In: *Primer on the metabolic bone diseases and disorders of mineral metabolism* (Favus MJ, ed). Philadelphia: Lippincott William & Wilkins, 1999: 367–83.

Osteopenic conditions

Bullough PG. Massive osteolysis. *N Y State J Med* 1971; **71**: 2267–78.

Burr DB, Martin RB. Errors in bone remodeling: toward a unified theory of metabolic bone disease. *Am J Anat* 1989; **186**: 186–216.

Dickson GR, Hamilton A, Hayes D et al. An investigation of vanishing bone disease. *Bone* 1990; **11**: 205–10.

Lakhanpal S, Ginsburg WW, Luthra HS et al. Transient regional osteoporosis. A study of 56 cases and review of the literature. *Ann Intern Med* 1987; **106**: 444–50.

Riggs BL, Melton LJ. *Osteoporosis: etiology, diagnosis, and management*. Philadelphia: Lippincott-Raven Publishers, 1995.

Whedon GD. Disuse osteoporosis: physiological aspects. *Calcif Tissue Int* 1984; **36 Suppl 1**: S146–50.

8. BONE DISEASE RESULTING FROM DISTURBANCES IN MINERAL HOMEOSTASIS

Calcium and phosphorus homeostasis

Elder G. Pathophysiology and recent advances in the management of renal osteodystrophy. *J Bone Miner Res* 2002; **17**: 2094–105.

Freemont AJ. The pathology of dialysis. *Semin Dial* 2002; **15**: 227–31.

Glorieux FH. Hypophosphatemic vitamin D-resistant rickets. In: *Primer on the metabolic bone diseases and disorders of mineral metabolism* (Favus MJ, ed), 4 edn. Philadelphia: Lippincott Williams & Wilkins, 1999: 328–30.

Grech P. *Diagnosis of metabolic bone disease*. London: Chapman and Hall Medical, 1985.

Kleerekoper M, Siris ES, McClung M. *The bone and mineral manual: a practical guide*. San Diego: Academic Press, 1999.

Malluche H, Faugere MC. Renal bone disease 1990: an unmet challenge for the nephrologist. *Kidney Int* 1990; **38**: 193–211.

Parfitt AM. Parathyroid hormone and periosteal bone expansion. *J Bone Miner Res* 2002; **17**: 1741–3.

Rasmussen H. The calcium messenger system (1). *N Engl J Med* 1986; **314**: 1094–101.

Rasmussen H. The calcium messenger system (2). *N Engl J Med* 1986; **314**: 1164–70.

Stern PH. Vitamin D and bone. *Kidney Int Suppl* 1990; **29**: S17–21.

Whyte MP. Hypophosphatasia. In: *Primer on the metabolic bone diseases and disorders of mineral metabolism* (Favus MJ, ed), 4 edn. Philadelphia: Lippincott Williams & Wilkins, 1999: 337–9.

Hypercalcemia

Bassler T, Wong ET, Brynes RK. Osteitis fibrosa cystica simulating metastatic tumor. An almost-forgotten relationship. *Am J Clin Pathol* 1993; **100**: 697–700.

Burtis WJ, Wu TL, Insogna KL et al. Humoral hypercalcemia of malignancy. *Ann Intern Med* 1988; **108**: 454–7.

Genant HK, Baron JM, Straus FH et al. Osteosclerosis in primary hyperparathyroidism. *Am J Med* 1975; **59**: 104–13.

Heath H, 3rd, Hodgson SF, Kennedy MA. Primary hyperparathyroidism. Incidence, morbidity, and potential economic impact in a community. *N Engl J Med* 1980; **302**: 189–93.

Hypocalcemia

Sherrard DJ, Andress DL. Aluminum-related osteodystrophy. *Adv Intern Med* 1989; **34**: 307–23.

Hahn TJ. Drug-induced disorders of vitamin D and mineral metabolism. *Clin Endocrinol Metab* 1980; **9**: 107–27.

Roth KS, Foreman JW, Segal S. The Fanconi syndrome and mechanisms of tubular transport dysfunction. *Kidney Int* 1981; **20**: 705–16.

Boyce BF, Smith L, Fogelman I et al. Focal osteomalacia due to low-dose diphosphonate therapy in Paget's disease. *Lancet* 1984; **1**: 821–4.

Mundy GR, Guise TA. Hypercalcemia of malignancy. *Am J Med* 1997; **103**: 134–45.

McMurtry CT, Godschalk M, Malluche HH et al. Oncogenic osteomalacia associated with metastatic prostate carcinoma: case report and review of the literature. *J Am Geriatr Soc* 1993; **41**: 983–5.

Parfitt AM. Osteomalacia and related disorders. In: *Metabolic bone disease and clinically related disorders* (Avioli LM, S.M. K, eds), 3 edn. San Diego: Academic Press, 1998.

Sherrard DJ. Renal osteodystrophy. In: *Principles and practice of dialysis* (Heinrich WL, ed). Baltimore: Williams & Wilkins, 1994: 234–45.

Nuovo MA, Dorfman HD, Sun CC et al. Tumor-induced osteomalacia and rickets. *Am J Surg Pathol* 1989; **13**: 588–99.

Soft-tissue calcification

Anderson HC. Calcific diseases. A concept. *Arch Pathol Lab Med* 1983; **107**: 341–8.

Boskey AL, Vigorita VJ, Spencer O et al. Chemical, microscopic, and ultrastructural characterization of the mineral deposits in tumoral calcinosis. *Clin Orthop* 1983: 258–69.

Connor JM. *Soft tissue calcification*. New York: Springer-Verlag, 1983.

Hodge JC, Schneider R, Freiberger RH et al. Calcific tendinitis in the proximal thigh. *Arthritis Rheum* 1993; **36**: 1476–82.

Martinez S. Tumoral calcinosis: 12 years later. *Semin Musculoskelet Radiol* 2002; **6**: 331–39.

Russell RGG, Kanis JA. Ectopic calcification and ossification. In: *Metabolic bone and stone disease* (Nordin BEC, ed), 2 edn. Edinburgh: Churchill Livingstone, 1984: 344–65.

Slavin RE, Wen J, Kumar D et al. Familial tumoral calcinosis. A clinical, histopathologic, and ultrastructural study with an analysis of its calcifying process and pathogenesis. *Am J Surg Pathol* 1993; **17**: 788–802.

9. ACCUMULATION OF ABNORMAL METABOLIC PRODUCTS AND VARIOUS HEMATOLOGIC DISORDERS

Deposition and storage disease

Benhamou CL, Pierre D, Geslin N et al. Primary bone oxalosis: the roles of oxalate deposits and renal osteodystrophy. *Bone* 1987; **8**: 59–64.

Brayton C. Amyloidosis, hemochromatosis, and atherosclerosis in a roseate flamingo (Phoenicopterus ruber). *Ann N Y Acad Sci* 1992; **653**: 184–90.

Chapman RH, Cotter F. The carpal tunnel syndrome and amyloidosis. A case report. *Clin Orthop* 1982: 159–62.

Devouassoux G, Lantuejoul S, Chatelain P et al. Erdheim-Chester disease: a primary macrophage cell disorder. *Am J Respir Crit Care Med* 1998; **157**: 650–3.

Goldblatt J, Sacks S, Beighton P. The orthopedic aspects of Gaucher disease. *Clin Orthop* 1978: 208–14.

Julian BA, Faugere MC, Malluche HH. Oxalosis in bone causing a radiographical mimicry of renal osteodystrophy. *Am J Kidney Dis* 1987; **9**: 436–40.

Kalimo H, Sourander P, Jarvi O et al. Vascular changes and blood–brain barrier damage in the pathogenesis of polycystic lipomembranous osteodysplasia with sclerosing leukoencephalopathy (membranous lipodystrophy). *Acta Neurol Scand* 1994; **89**: 353–61.

Kay J, Bardin T. Osteoarticular disorders of renal origin: disease-related and iatrogenic. *Baillieres Best Pract Res Clin Rheumatol* 2000; **14**: 285–305.

Kenan S, Abdelwahab IF, Klein MJ et al. Case report 754: Xanthoma of the Achilles tendon. *Skeletal Radiol* 1992; **21**: 471–3.

Kim NR, Ko YH, Choe YH et al. Erdheim-Chester disease with extensive marrow necrosis: a case report and literature review. *Int J Surg Pathol* 2001; **9**: 73–9.

Machinami R. Degenerative change of adipose tissue; the so-called membranous lipodystrophy. *Virchows Arch A Pathol Anat Histopathol* 1990; **416**: 373–4.

Rousselin B, Helenon O, Zingraff J et al. Pseudotumor of the craniocervical junction during long-term hemodialysis. *Arthritis Rheum* 1990; **33**: 1567–73.

Springfield DS, Landried M, Mankin HJ. Gaucher hemorrhagic cyst of bone. A case report. *J Bone Joint Surg Am* 1989; **71**: 141–4.

Stubgen JP, Lotz BP. Membranous lipodystrophy. Clinical and electrophysiological observations in the first South African case. *S Afr Med J* 1992; **81**: 620–2.

Tagliabue JR, Stull MA, Lack EE et al. Case report 610: Amyloid arthropathy of the left ankle. *Skeletal Radiol* 1990; **19**: 448–52.

Vogelgesang SA, Klipple GL. The many guises of amyloidosis. Clinical presentations and disease associations. *Postgrad Med* 1994; **96**: 119–22, 26–7.

Yamaguchi K, Grant J, Noble-Jamieson G et al. Hypercalcaemia in primary oxalosis: role of increased bone resorption and effects of treatment with pamidronate. *Bone* 1995; **16**: 61–7.

Skeletal manifestations of hematological diseases

Bennett OM, Namnyak SS. Bone and joint manifestations of sickle cell anaemia. *J Bone Joint Surg Br* 1990; **72**: 494–9.

Gratwick GM, Bullough PG, Bohne WH et al. Thalassemic osteoarthropathy. *Ann Intern Med* 1978; **88**: 494–501.

Mundy GR. Myeloma bone disease. *Eur J Cancer* 1998; **34**: 246–51.

Schumacher HR, Straka PC, Krikker MA et al. The arthropathy of hemochromatosis. Recent studies. *Ann N Y Acad Sci* 1988; **526**: 224–33.

Visani G, Finelli C, Castelli U et al. Myelofibrosis with myeloid metaplasia: clinical and haematological parameters predicting survival in a series of 133 patients. *Br J Haematol* 1990; **75**: 4–9.

SECTION IV – ARTHRITIS

10. THE DYSFUNCTIONAL JOINT

Function and anatomy

Deutsch AL, Mink JH, Shellock FG. Magnetic resonance imaging of injuries to bone and articular cartilage. Emphasis on radiographically occult abnormalities. *Orthop Rev* 1990; **19**: 66–75.

Bullough PG, Jagannath A. The morphology of the calcification front in articular cartilage. Its significance in joint function. *J Bone Joint Surg Br* 1983; **65**: 72–8.

Hunter W. Of the structure and diseases of articulating cartilages. *Phil Trans* 1743: 267–71.

Ettinger L, Doljanski F. On the generation of form by the continuous interactions between cells and their extracellular matrix. *Biol Rev Camb Philos Soc* 1992; **67**: 459–89.

Goodfellow JW, Bullough PG. The pattern of ageing of the articular cartilage of the elbow joint. *J Bone Joint Surg Br* 1967; **49**: 175–81.

Bullough P, Goodfellow J. The significance of the fine structure of articular cartilage. *J Bone Joint Surg Br* 1968; **50**: 852–7.

Normal joint physiology

Bullough PG, Yawitz PS, Tafra L et al. Topographical variations in the morphology and biochemistry of adult canine tibial plateau articular cartilage. *J Orthop Res* 1985; **3**: 1–16.

Hascall VC, Kuettner KE. *The many faces of osteoarthritis*. Basel: Birkhauser Verlag, 2002.

MacConaill MA. The movements of bones and joints. *J Bone Joint Surg Br* 1950; **32**: 244.

Mainil-Varlet P, Aigner T, Brittberg M et al. Histological assessment of cartilage repair: a report by the Histology Endpoint Committee of the International Cartilage Repair Society (ICRS). *J Bone Joint Surg Am* 2003; **85–A Suppl 2**: 45–57.

McCarthy J, Noble P, Aluisio FV et al. Anatomy, pathologic features, and treatment of acetabular labral tears. *Clin Orthop* 2003: 38–47.

Wormsley T. The articular mechanism of the diarthroses. *J Bone Joint Surg Am* 1928; **10**: 40.

Arthritic joint

Brandt KD. Response of joint structures to inactivity and to reloading after immobilization. *Arthritis Rheum* 2003; **49**: 267–71.

Curwin SL. Tendon injuries: pathophysiology and treatment. In: *Athletic injuries and rehabilitation* (Zachazewski JE, Magee DJ, Quillen WS, eds). Philadelphia: Saunders, 1996: 27–54.

Fernandes JC, Martel-Pelletier J, Pelletier JP. The role of cytokines in osteoarthritis pathophysiology. *Biorheology* 2002; **39**: 237–46.

Frank CB. Ligament injuries: pathophysiology and healing. In: *Athletic injuries and rehabilitation* (Zachazewski JE, Magee DJ, Quillen WS, eds). Philadelphia: Saunders, 1996: 9–26.

Freemont A, Denton J. The cytology of synovial fluid. In: *Diagnostic cytopathology* (Gray W, ed), pp. 887–98. Edinburgh: Churchill Livingstone, 1995.

Poole AR. Can serum biomarker assays measure the progression of cartilage degeneration in osteoarthritis? *Arthritis Rheum* 2002; **46**: 2549–52.

Schumacher HR, Reginato AJ. *Atlas of synovial fluid analysis and crystal identification*. Philadelphia: Lea & Febiger, 1991.

Swan A, Amer H, Dieppe P. The value of synovial fluid assays in the diagnosis of joint disease: a literature survey. *Ann Rheum Dis* 2002; **61**: 493–8.

11. NONINFLAMMATORY ARTHRITIS

Osteoarthritis (Degenerative joint disease)

Bennett GA, Waine H, Bauer KW. *Changes in the knee joint at various ages with particular reference to the nature and development of degenerative joint disease*. New York: The Commonwealth Fund, 1942.

Brown MF. Cartilage changes in osteoarthritis and rheumatoid arthritis. In: *Sciences basic to orthopaedics* (Hughes SPF, McCarthy ID, eds). London: W.B. Saunders, 1998: 156–67.

Buckwalter JA. Were the Hunter brothers wrong? Can surgical treatment repair articular cartilage? *Iowa Orthop J* 1997; **17**: 1–13.

Bullough P, Goodfellow J, O'Conner J. The relationship between degenerative changes and load-bearing in the human hip. *J Bone Joint Surg Br* 1973; **55**: 746–58.

Eichenholtz SN. *Charcot joints*. Springfield, IL: Charles C. Thomas, 1966.

Harris WH. Etiology of osteoarthritis of the hip. *Clin Orthop* 1986: 20–33.

Heine J. Uber die Arthritis deformans. *Virchows Arch* 1926; **260**: 521–663.

Hunziker EB. Articular cartilage repair: basic science and clinical progress. A review of the current status and prospects. *Osteoarthritis Cartilage* 2002; **10**: 432–63.

Johanson NA. Endocrine arthropathies. *Clin Rheum Dis* 1985; **11**: 297–323.

Kellgren JH, Lawrence JS. Radiological assessment of osteoarthrosis. *Ann Rheum Dis* 1957; **16**: 494.

Macys JR, Bullough PG, Wilson PD, Jr. Coxarthrosis: a study of the natural history based on a correlation of clinical, radiographic, and pathologic findings. *Semin Arthritis Rheum* 1980; **10**: 66–80.

Moskowitz RW. *Osteoarthritis: diagnosis and medical/surgical management*, 3 edn. Philadelphia: Saunders, 2001.

Peyron JG. Is osteoarthritis a preventable disease? *J Rheumatol Suppl* 1991; **27**: 2–3.

Ochronosis

Gaines JJ, Jr. The pathology of alkaptonuric ochronosis. *Hum Pathol* 1989; **20**: 40–6.

Schumacher HR, Holdsworth DE. Ochronotic arthropathy. I. Clinicopathologic studies. *Semin Arthritis Rheum* 1977; **6**: 207–46.

Arthritis secondary to subchondral insufficiency fracture

Yamamoto T, Bullough PG. Subchondral insufficiency fracture of the femoral head: a differential diagnosis in acute onset of coxarthrosis in the elderly. *Arthritis Rheum* 1999; **42**: 2719–23.

Yamamoto T, Bullough PG. The role of subchondral insufficiency fracture in rapid destruction of the hip joint: a preliminary report. *Arthritis Rheum* 2000; **43**: 2423–7.

Yamamoto T, Schneider R, Bullough PG. Subchondral insufficiency fracture of the femoral head: histopathologic correlation with MRI. *Skeletal Radiol* 2001; **30**: 247–54.

Osteochondritis dissecans

Barrie HJ. Osteochondritis dissecans 1887–1987. A centennial look at Konig's memorable phrase. *J Bone Joint Surg Br* 1987; **69**: 693–5.

Slipped capital femoral epiphysis (Adolescent coxa vara)

Boyer DW, Mickelson MR, Ponseti IV. Slipped capital femoral epiphysis. Long-term follow-up study of one hundred and twenty-one patients. *J Bone Joint Surg Am* 1981; **63**: 85–95.

Rattey T, Piehl F, Wright JG. Acute slipped capital femoral epiphysis. Review of outcomes and rates of avascular necrosis. *J Bone Joint Surg Am* 1996; **78**: 398–402.

Congenital dislocation of the hip

Leck I. Congenital dislocation of the hip. In: *Antenatal and neonatal screening* (Wald N, Leck I, eds), 2 edn. Oxford: Oxford University Press, 2000: 398–424.

Lee J, Jarvis J, Uhthoff HK et al. The fetal acetabulum. A histomorphometric study of acetabular anteversion and femoral head coverage. *Clin Orthop* 1992: 48–55.

12. INFLAMMATORY ARTHRITIDES

Inflammatory arthritis associated with diffuse connective-tissue disease

Cassidy JT, Martel W. Juvenile rheumatoid arthritis: clinicoradiologic correlations. *Arthritis Rheum* 1977; **20**: 207–11.

Cassidy JT, Hillman LS. Abnormalities in skeletal growth in children with juvenile rheumatoid arthritis. *Rheum Dis Clin North Am* 1997; **23**: 499–522.

Imal Y, Yamakawa M. Morphology, function and pathology of follicular dendritic cells. *Pathol Int* 1996; **46**: 807–33.

Naides SJ. Viral arthritis including HIV. *Curr Opin Rheumatol* 1995; **7**: 337–42.

Rodriguez-Merchan EC. Pathogenesis, early diagnosis, and prophylaxis for chronic hemophilic synovitis. *Clin Orthop* 1997: 6–11.

Soren A. *Histodiagnosis and clinical correlation of rheumatoid and other synovitis.* Philadelphia: Lippincott, 1978.

Verschure PJ, Van Noorden CJ, Van Marle J et al. Articular cartilage destruction in experimental inflammatory arthritis: insulin-like growth factor-1 regulation of proteoglycan metabolism in chondrocytes. *Histochem J* 1996; **28**: 835–57.

Diseases resulting from deposition of metabolic products in joint tissues

Boss GR, Seegmiller JE. Hyperuricemia and gout. Classification, complications and management. *N Engl J Med* 1979; **300**: 1459–68.

Fam AG. What is new about crystals other than monosodium urate? *Curr Opin Rheumatol* 2000; **12**: 228–34.

Hough AJ, Banfield WG, Sokoloff L. Cartilage in hemophilic arthropathy. Ultrastructural and microanalytical studies. *Arch Pathol Lab Med* 1976; **100**: 91–6.

Ishida T, Dorfman HD, Bullough PG. Tophaceous pseudogout (tumoral calcium pyrophosphate dihydrate crystal deposition disease). *Hum Pathol* 1995; **26**: 587–93.

Resnick D, Niwayama G, Goergen TG et al. Clinical, radiographic and pathologic abnormalities in calcium pyrophosphate dihydrate deposition disease (CPPD): pseudogout. *Radiology* 1977; **122**: 1–15.

Sissons HA, Steiner GC, Bonar F et al. Tumoral calcium pyrophosphate deposition disease. *Skeletal Radiol* 1989; **18**: 79–87.

Zaharopoulos P, Wong JY. Identification of crystals in joint fluids. *Acta Cytol* 1980; **24**: 197–202.

13. SPINAL ARTHRITIS AND DEGENERATIVE DISC DISEASE

Displacement of disc tissue

Adams MA, Dolan P, Hutton WC. The stages of disc degeneration as revealed by discograms. *J Bone Joint Surg Br* 1986; **68**: 36–41.

Fraser RD, Sandhu A, Gogan WJ. Magnetic resonance imaging findings 10 years after treatment for lumbar disc herniation. *Spine* 1995; **20**: 710–4.

Golub BS, Rovit RL, Mankin HJ. Cervical and lumbar disc disease: a review. *Bull Rheum Dis* 1971; **21**: 635–42.

Hilton RC, Ball J, Benn RT. Vertebral end-plate lesions (Schmorl's nodes) in the dorsolumbar spine. *Ann Rheum Dis* 1976; **35**: 127–32.

Kirkaldy-Willis WH, Wedge JH, Yong-Hing K et al. Pathology and pathogenesis of lumbar spondylosis and stenosis. *Spine* 1978; **3**: 319–28.

Milgram JW. Osteoarthritic changes at the severely degenerative disc in humans. *Spine* 1982; **7**: 498–505.

Resnick D, Niwayama G. Intravertebral disk herniations: cartilaginous (Schmorl's) nodes. *Radiology* 1978; **126**: 57–65.

Inflammatory spondylitis

Ball J. New knowledge of intervertebral disc disease. *J Clin Pathol Suppl (R Coll Pathol)* 1978; **12**: 200–4.

Bywaters EG. Rheumatoid and other diseases of the cervical interspinous bursae, and changes in the spinous processes. *Ann Rheum Dis* 1982; **41**: 360–70.

Cruickshank B. Lesions of cartilaginous joints in ankylosing spondylitis. *J Pathol Bacteriol* 1956; **71**: 73.

Jacobs JC. Spondyloarthritis and enthesopathy. Current concepts in rheumatology. *Arch Intern Med* 1983; **143**: 103–7.

Little H, Swinson DR, Cruickshank B. Upward subluxation of the axis in ankylosing spondylitis. A clinical pathologic report. *Am J Med* 1976; **60**: 279–85.

Resnick D, Shapiro RF, Wiesner KB et al. Diffuse idiopathic skeletal hyperostosis (DISH) [ankylosing hyperostosis of Forestier and Rotes-Querol]. *Semin Arthritis Rheum* 1978; **7**: 153–87.

14. TISSUE RESPONSE TO IMPLANTED PROSTHESES

Usual tissue response to clinically nonfailed articular implants

Johanson NA, Bullough PG, Wilson PD, Jr. et al. The microscopic anatomy of the bone-cement interface in failed total hip arthroplasties. *Clin Orthop* 1987: 123–35.

Joshi AB, Porter ML, Trail IA et al. Long-term results of Charnley low-friction arthroplasty in young patients. *J Bone Joint Surg Br* 1993; **75**: 616–23.

Mears DC. *Materials and orthopaedic surgery.* Baltimore: Williams & Wilkins Co., 1979.

Morbidity associated with total joint replacements

Brien WW, Salvati EA, Healey JH et al. Osteogenic sarcoma arising in the area of a total hip replacement. A case report. *J Bone Joint Surg Am* 1990; **72**: 1097–9.

Keel SB, Jaffe KA, Petur Nielsen G et al. Orthopaedic implant-related sarcoma: a study of twelve cases. *Mod Pathol* 2001; **14**: 969–77.

Kim KC, Ritter MA. Hypotension associated with methyl methacrylate in total hip arthroplasties. *Clin Orthop* 1972; **88**: 154–60.

Lalor PA, Revell PA, Gray AB et al. Sensitivity to titanium. A cause of implant failure? *J Bone Joint Surg Br* 1991; **73**: 25–8.

Santavirta S, Hoikka V, Eskola A et al. Aggressive granulomatous lesions in cementless total hip arthroplasty. *J Bone Joint Surg Br* 1990; **72**: 980–4.

Widmer AF. New developments in diagnosis and treatment of infection in orthopedic implants. *Clin Infect Dis* 2001; **33 Suppl 2**: S94–106.

Willert HG, Bertram H, Buchhorn GH. Osteolysis in alloarthroplasty of the hip. The role of bone cement fragmentation. *Clin Orthop* 1990: 108–21.

Wroblewski BM, Siney PD, Fleming PA. Fatal pulmonary embolism and mortality after revision of failed total hip arthroplasties. *J Arthroplasty* 2000; **15**: 437–9.

Tissues around noninfected, clinically failed articular implants

Bansal M, Goldman AB, Bullough PG et al. Case report 706: Silicone-induced reactive synovitis. *Skeletal Radiol* 1992; **21**: 49–51.

Black J, Sherk H, Bonini J et al. Metallosis associated with a stable titanium-alloy femoral component in total hip replacement. A case report. *J Bone Joint Surg Am* 1990; **72**: 126–30.

Bullough PG. Metallosis. *J Bone Joint Surg Br* 1994; **76**: 687–8.

Christiansen K, Holmes K, Zilko PJ. Metal sensitivity causing loosened joint prostheses. *Ann Rheum Dis* 1980; **39**: 476–80.

DiCarlo EF, Bullough PG. The biologic responses to orthopedic implants and their wear debris. *Clin Mater* 1992; **9**: 235–60.

Gordon M, Bullough PG. Synovial and osseous inflammation in failed silicone-rubber prostheses. *J Bone Joint Surg Am* 1982; **64**: 574–80.

Howie DW, Haynes DR, Rogers SD et al. The response to particulate debris. *Orthop Clin North Am* 1993; **24**: 571–81.

Lee JM, Salvati EA, Betts F et al. Size of metallic and polyethylene debris particles in failed cemented total hip replacements. *J Bone Joint Surg Br* 1992; **74**: 380–4.

Masri BA, Salvati EA, Duncan CP. Polyethylene properties and their role in osteolysis after total joint arthroplasty. In: *Advances in osteoarthritis* (Tanaka S, Hamanishi C, eds). Tokyo: Springer, 1999: 271–85.

Rae T. The biological response to titanium and titanium-aluminium-vanadium alloy particles. II. Long-term animal studies. *Biomaterials* 1986; **7**: 37–40.

15. OSTEONECROSIS AND BONE INFARCTION

Osteonecrosis of the femoral head

Bullough PG, DiCarlo EF. Subchondral avascular necrosis: a common cause of arthritis. *Ann Rheum Dis* 1990; **49**: 412–20.

Franchi A, Bullough PG. Secondary avascular necrosis in coxarthrosis: a morphologic study. *J Rheumatol* 1992; **19**: 1263–8.

Glickstein MF, Burk DL, Jr., Schiebler ML et al. Avascular necrosis versus other diseases of the hip: sensitivity of MR imaging. *Radiology* 1988; **169**: 213–5.

McCarthy EF. Aseptic necrosis of bone. An historic perspective. *Clin Orthop* 1982: 216–21.

Mitchell DG, Steinberg ME, Dalinka MK et al. Magnetic resonance imaging of the ischemic hip. Alterations within the osteonecrotic, viable, and reactive zones. *Clin Orthop* 1989: 60–77.

Sissons HA, Nuovo MA, Steiner GC. Pathology of osteonecrosis of the femoral head. A review of experience at the Hospital for Joint Diseases, New York. *Skeletal Radiol* 1992; **21**: 229–38.

Necrosis following fracture

Catto M. A histological study of avascular necrosis of the femoral head after transcervical fracture. *J Bone Joint Surg Br* 1965; **47**: 749–76.

Catto M. The histological appearances of late segmental collapse of the femoral head after transcervical fracture. *J Bone Joint Surg Br* 1965; **47**: 777–91.

Legg-Calve-Perthes disease

Burwell RG. Perthes' disease: growth and aetiology. *Arch Dis Child* 1988; **63**: 1408–12.

Landin LA, Danielsson LG, Wattsgard C. Transient synovitis of the hip. Its incidence, epidemiology and relation to Perthes' disease. *J Bone Joint Surg Br* 1987; **69**: 238–42.

Thompson GH, Salter RB. Legg-Calve-Perthes disease. Current concepts and controversies. *Orthop Clin North Am* 1987; **18**: 617–35.

Idiopathic, nontraumatic or primary osteonecrosis of the femoral head

Bradway JK, Morrey BF. The natural history of the silent hip in bilateral atraumatic osteonecrosis. *J Arthroplasty* 1993; **8**: 383–7.

Bone infarctions not associated with caisson disease

Bullough PG, Kambolis CP, Marcove RC et al. Bone infarctions not associated with caisson disease. *J Bone Joint Surg Am* 1965; **47**: 477–91.

SECTION V – BONE TUMORS

16. BONE-FORMING TUMORS AND TUMOR-LIKE CONDITIONS

Reactive or post-traumatic lesions

Campanacci DA, Guarracino R, Franchi A et al. Bizarre parosteal osteochondromatous proliferation (Nora's lesion). Description of six cases and a review of the literature. *Chir Organi Mov* 1999; **84**: 65–71.

Kahn LB, Wood FW, Ackerman LV. Fracture callus associated with benign and malignant bone lesions and mimicking osteosarcoma. *Am J Clin Pathol* 1969; **52**: 14–24.

Meneses MF, Unni KK, Swee RG. Bizarre parosteal osteochondromatous proliferation of bone (Nora's lesion). *Am J Surg Pathol* 1993; **17**: 691–7.

Miller-Breslow A, Dorfman HD. Dupuytren's (subungual) exostosis. *Am J Surg Pathol* 1988; **12**: 368–78.

Oviedo A, Simmons T, Benya E et al. Bizarre parosteal osteochondromatous proliferation: case report and review of the literature. *Pediatr Dev Pathol* 2001; **4**: 496–500.

Pavlov H, Torg JS. *The running athlete : roentgenograms and remedies*. Chicago: Year Book Medical Publishers, 1987.

Spjut HJ, Dorfman HD. Florid reactive periostitis of the tubular bones of the hands and feet. A benign lesion which may simulate osteosarcoma. *Am J Surg Pathol* 1981; **5**: 423–33.

Developmental of hamartomatous tumors

Buch B, Noffke C, de Kock S. Gardner's syndrome— the importance of early diagnosis: a case report and a review. *Sadj* 2001; **56**: 242–5.

Greenspan A, Steiner G, Sotelo D et al. Mixed sclerosing bone dysplasia coexisting with dysplasia epiphysealis hemimelica (Trevor-Fairbank disease). *Skeletal Radiol* 1986; **15**: 452–4.

Greenspan A, Steiner G, Knutzon R. Bone island (enostosis): clinical significance and radiologic and pathologic correlations. *Skeletal Radiol* 1991; **20**: 85–90.

Greenspan A, Azouz EM. Bone dysplasia series. Melorheostosis: review and update. *Can Assoc Radiol J* 1999; **50**: 324–30.

Benign tumors

Bullough PG. Ivory exostosis of the skull. *Postgrad Med* 1965; **41**: 277–81.

Dorfman HD, Weiss SW. Borderline osteoblastic tumors: problems in the differential diagnosis of aggressive osteoblastoma and low-grade osteosarcoma. *Semin Diagn Pathol* 1984; **1**: 215–34.

Freiberger RH, Loitman BS, et al. Osteoid osteoma. A report on 80 cases. *AJR* 1959; **82**: 194.

Greenspan A, Elguezabel A, Bryk D. Multifocal osteoid osteoma. A case report and review of the literature. *Am J Roentgenol Radium Ther Nucl Med* 1974; **121**: 103–6.

Greenspan A. Benign bone-forming lesions: osteoma, osteoid osteoma, and osteoblastoma. Clinical, imaging, pathologic, and differential considerations. *Skeletal Radiol* 1993; **22**: 485–500.

Keim HA, Reina EG. Osteoid-osteoma as a cause of scoliosis. *J Bone Joint Surg Am* 1975; **57**: 159–63.

Marsh BW, Bonfiglio M, Brady LP et al. Benign osteoblastoma: range of manifestations. *J Bone Joint Surg Am* 1975; **57**: 1–9.

Mirra JM, Cove K, Theros E et al. A case of osteoblastoma associated with severe systemic toxicity. *Am J Surg Pathol* 1979; **3**: 463–71.

Worland RL, Ryder CT, Johnston AD. Recurrent osteoid-osteoma. Report of a case. *J Bone Joint Surg Am* 1975; **57**: 277–8.

Malignant tumors

Anderson RB, McAlister JA, Jr., Wrenn RN. Case report 585: Intracortical osteosarcoma of tibia. *Skeletal Radiol* 1989; **18**: 627–30.

Ayala AG, Raymond AK, Jaffe N. The pathologist's role in the diagnosis and treatment of osteosarcoma in children. *Hum Pathol* 1984; **15**: 258–66.

Ayala AG, Ro JY, Papadopoulos NK et al. Small cell osteosarcoma. *Cancer Treat Res* 1993; **62**: 139–49.

Bane BL, Evans HL, Ro JY et al. Extraskeletal osteosarcoma. A clinicopathologic review of 26 cases. *Cancer* 1990; **65**: 2762–70.

el-Khoury JM, Haddad SN, Atallah NG. Osteosarcomatosis with Rothmund-Thomson syndrome. *Br J Radiol* 1997; **70**: 215–8.

Greenspan A, Steiner G, Norman A et al. Case report 436: Osteosarcoma of the soft tissues of the distal end of the thigh. *Skeletal Radiol* 1987; **16**: 489–92.

Hansen MF. Molecular genetic considerations in osteosarcoma. *Clin Orthop* 1991: 237–46.

Hermann G, Abdelwahab IF, Kenan S et al. Case report 795. High-grade surface osteosarcoma of the radius. *Skeletal Radiol* 1993; **22**: 383–5.

Jundt G, Schulz A, Berghauser KH et al. Immunocytochemical identification of osteogenic bone tumors by osteonectin antibodies. *Virchows Arch A Pathol Anat Histopathol* 1989; **414**: 345–53.

Kilpatrick SE, Abdul-Karim FW, Renner JB et al. Interobserver variability among expert orthopedic pathologists for diagnosis, histologic grade, and determination of the necessity for chemotherapy in osteosarcoma. *Pediatr Patholo Mol Med* 2000; **19**: 337–58.

Klein MJ, Kenan S, Lewis MM. Osteosarcoma. Clinical and pathological considerations. *Orthop Clin North Am* 1989; **20**: 327–45.

Kurt AM, Unni KK, McLeod RA et al. Low-grade intraosseous osteosarcoma. *Cancer* 1990; **65**: 1418–28.

Parham DM, Pratt CB, Parvey LS et al. Childhood multifocal osteosarcoma. Clinicopathologic and radiologic correlates. *Cancer* 1985; **55**: 2653–8.

Picci P, Campanacci M, Bacci G et al. Medullary involvement in parosteal osteosarcoma. A case report. *J Bone Joint Surg Am* 1987; **69**: 131–6.

Rayne J, Bullough P. A case of Gardner's syndrome. *Br J Surg* 1966; **53**: 824–6.

Schajowicz F, McGuire MH, Santini Araujo E et al. Osteosarcomas arising on the surfaces of long bones. *J Bone Joint Surg Am* 1988; **70**: 555–64.

Sim FH, Unni KK, Beabout JW et al. Osteosarcoma with small cells simulating Ewing's tumor. *J Bone Joint Surg Am* 1979; **61**: 207–15.

Smith J, Botet JF, Yeh SD. Bone sarcomas in Paget disease: a study of 85 patients. *Radiology* 1984; **152**: 583–90.

Steiner G. Post-radiation sarcoma of bone. *Cancer* 1965; **18**: 603–12.

Tsuneyoshi M, Dorfman HD. Epiphyseal osteosarcoma: distinguishing features from clear cell chondrosarcoma, chondroblastoma, and epiphyseal enchondroma. *Hum Pathol* 1987; **18**: 644–51.

Unni KK, Dahlin DC, Beabout JW. Periosteal osteogenic sarcoma. *Cancer* 1976; **37**: 2476–85.

17. CARTILAGE-FORMING TUMORS AND TUMOR-LIKE CONDITIONS

Reactive or post-traumatic lesions

D'Ambrosia R, Ferguson AB, Jr. The formation of osteochondroma by epiphyseal cartilage transplantation. *Clin Orthop* 1968; **61**: 103–15.

Developmental or hamartomatous tumors

Kettelkamp DB, Campbell CJ, Bonfiglio M. Dysplasia epiphysealis hemimelica. *J Bone Joint Surg Am* 1966; **48**: 746.

Liu J, Hudkins PG, Swee RG et al. Bone sarcomas associated with Ollier's disease. *Cancer* 1987; **59**: 1376–85.

Mendez AA, Keret D, MacEwen GD. Isolated dysplasia epiphysealis hemimelica of the hip joint. A case report. *J Bone Joint Surg Am* 1988; **70**: 921–5.

Peterson HA. Multiple hereditary osteochondromata. *Clin Orthop* 1989: 222–30.

Shapiro F. Ollier's Disease. An assessment of angular deformity, shortening, and pathological fracture in twenty-one patients. *J Bone Joint Surg Am* 1982; **64**: 95–103.

Trevor D. Tarso-epiphysial aclasis: a congenital error of epiphysial development. *J Bone Joint Surg Br* 1950; **32**: 204–13.

Voegeli E, Laissue J, Kaiser A et al. Case report 143. Multiple hereditary osteocartilaginous exostoses affecting right femur with an overlying giant cystic bursa (exostosis bursata). *Skeletal Radiol* 1981; **6**: 134–7.

Benign tumors

Bauer TW, Dorfman HD, Latham JT, Jr. Periosteal chondroma. A clinicopathologic study of 23 cases. *Am J Surg Pathol* 1982; **6**: 631–7.

Green P, Whittaker RP. Benign chondroblastoma. Case report with pulmonary metastasis. *J Bone Joint Surg Am* 1975; **57**: 418–20.

Lewis MM, Kenan S, Yabut SM et al. Periosteal chondroma. A report of ten cases and review of the literature. *Clin Orthop* 1990: 185–92.

Marcove RC, Kambolis C, Bullough PG. Fibromyxoma of bone. *Cancer* 1961; **17**: 1209.

Schajowicz F, Gallardo H. Epiphysial chondroblastoma of bone. A clinico-pathological study of sixty-nine cases. *J Bone Joint Surg Br* 1970; **52**: 205–26.

Takigawa K. Chondroma of the bones of the hand. A review of 110 cases. *J Bone Joint Surg Am* 1971; **53**: 1591–600.

Turcotte RE, Kurt AM, Sim FH et al. Chondroblastoma. *Hum Pathol* 1993; **24**: 944–9.

Zillmer DA, Dorfman HD. Chondromyxoid fibroma of bone: thirty-six cases with clinicopathologic correlation. *Hum Pathol* 1989; **20**: 952–64.

Malignant tumors

Barnes R, Catto M. Chondrosarcoma of bone. *J Bone Joint Surg Br* 1966; **48**: 729–64.

Coughlan B, Feliz A, Ishida T et al. p53 expression and DNA ploidy of cartilage lesions. *Hum Pathol* 1995; **26**: 620–4.

Culver JE, Jr., Sweet DE, McCue FC. Chondrosarcoma of the hand arising from a pre-existent benign solitary enchondroma. *Clin Orthop* 1975: 128–31.

Harwood AR, Krajbich JI, Fornasier VL. Mesenchymal chondrosarcoma: a report of 17 cases. *Clin Orthop* 1981: 144–8.

Ishida T, Kuwada Y, Motoi N et al. Dedifferentiated chondrosarcoma of the rib with a malignant mesenchymomatous component: an autopsy case report. *Pathol Int* 1997; **47**: 397–403.

Johnson S, Tetu B, Ayala AG et al. Chondrosarcoma with additional mesenchymal component (dedifferentiated chondrosarcoma). I. A clinicopathologic study of 26 cases. *Cancer* 1986; **58**: 278–86.

Mankin HJ, Cantley KP, Schiller AL et al. The biology of human chondrosarcoma. II. Variation in chemical composition among types and subtypes of benign and malignant cartilage tumors. *J Bone Joint Surg Am* 1980; **62**: 176–88.

Mankin HJ, Cantley KP, Lippiello L et al. The biology of human chondrosarcoma. I. Description of the cases, grading, and biochemical analyses. *J Bone Joint Surg Am* 1980; **62**: 160–76.

McCarthy EF, Dorfman HD. Chondrosarcoma of bone with dedifferentiation: a study of eighteen cases. *Hum Pathol* 1982; **13**: 36–40.

Miettinen M. Chordoma. Antibodies to epithelial membrane antigen and carcinoembryonic antigen in differential diagnosis. *Arch Pathol Lab Med* 1984; **108**: 891–2.

Nakashima Y, Unni KK, Shives TC et al. Mesenchymal chondrosarcoma of bone and soft tissue. A review of 111 cases. *Cancer* 1986; **57**: 2444–53.

Naumann S, Krallman PA, Unni KK et al. Translocation der(13;21)(q10;q10) in skeletal and extraskeletal mesenchymal chondrosarcoma. *Mod Pathol* 2002; **15**: 572–6.

O'Malley DP, Opheim KE, Barry TS et al. Chromosomal changes in a dedifferentiated chondrosarcoma: a case report and review of the literature. *Cancer Genet Cytogenet* 2001; **124**: 105–11.

Sanerkin NG, Gallagher P. A review of the behaviour of chondrosarcoma of bone. *J Bone Joint Surg Br* 1979; **61–B**: 395–400.

Swanson PE. Clear cell tumors of bone. *Semin Diagn Pathol* 1997; **14**: 281–91.

Ulich TR, Mirra JM. Ecchordosis physaliphora vertebralis. *Clin Orthop* 1982; **163**: 282–9.

Unni KK, Dahlin DC, Beabout JW et al. Chondrosarcoma: clear-cell variant. A report of sixteen cases. *J Bone Joint Surg Am* 1976; **58**: 676–83.

Valderrama E, Kahn LB, Lipper S et al. Chondroid chordoma. Electron-microscopic study of two cases. *Am J Surg Pathol* 1983; **7**: 625–32.

Volpe R, Mazabraud A. A clinicopathologic review of 25 cases of chordoma (a pleomorphic and metastasizing neoplasm). *Am J Surg Pathol* 1983; **7**: 161–70.

18. FIBER-FORMING TUMORS AND TUMOR-LIKE CONDITIONS

Reactive or post-traumatic lesions

Kimmelstiel P, Rapp I. Cortical defect due to periosteal desmoids. *Bull Hosp Jt Dis* 1951; **12**: 286.

Developmental or hamartomatous tumors

Bertoni F, Calderoni P, Bacchini P et al. Benign fibrous histiocytoma of bone. *J Bone Joint Surg Am* 1986; **68**: 1225–30.

Harris WH, Dudley HJ, Barry RJ. The natural history of fibrous dysplasia. *J Bone Joint Surg Am* 1962; **44**: 207.

Henry A. Monostotic fibrous dysplasia. *J Bone Joint Surg Br* 1969; **51**: 300–6.

Logel RJ. Recurrent intramuscular myxoma associated with Albright's syndrome. *J Bone Joint Surg Am* 1976; **58**: 565–8.

Marks KE, Bauer TW. Fibrous tumors of bone. *Orthop Clin North Am* 1989; **20**: 377–93.

Yabut SM, Jr., Kenan S, Sissons HA et al. Malignant transformation of fibrous dysplasia. A case report and review of the literature. *Clin Orthop* 1988: 281–9.

Benign tumors

Campanacci M, Laus M. Osteofibrous dysplasia of the tibia and fibula. *J Bone Joint Surg Am* 1981; **63**: 367–75.

Gebhardt MC, Campbell CJ, Schiller AL et al. Desmoplastic fibroma of bone. A report of eight cases and review of the literature. *J Bone Joint Surg Am* 1985; **67**: 732–47.

Ishida T, Dorfman HD. Massive chondroid differentiation in fibrous dysplasia of bone (fibrocartilaginous dysplasia). *Am J Surg Pathol* 1993; **17**: 924–30.

Sissons HA, Steiner GC, Dorfman HD. Calcified spherules in fibro-osseous lesions of bone. *Arch Pathol Lab Med* 1993; **117**: 284–90.

Malignant tumors

Campanacci M, Giunti A, Bertoni F et al. Adamantinoma of the long bones. The experience at the Istituto Ortopedico Rizzoli. *Am J Surg Pathol* 1981; **5**: 533–42.

Czerniak B, Rojas-Corona RR, Dorfman HD. Morphologic diversity of long bone adamantinoma. The concept of differentiated (regressing) adamantinoma and its relationship to osteofibrous dysplasia. *Cancer* 1989; **64**: 2319–34.

Enzinger FM. Malignant fibrous histiocytoma 20 years after Stout. *Am J Surg Pathol* 1986; **10 Suppl 1**: 43–53.

Fechner RE, Mills SE. Malignant fibrous histiocytoma. In: *Tumors of the bones and joints* (Fechner RE, Mills SE, eds), 3 edn. Washington, D.C.: Armed Forces Institute of Pathology, 1993: 163–8, 71.

Fletcher CD. Pleomorphic malignant fibrous histiocytoma: fact or fiction? A critical reappraisal based on 159 tumors diagnosed as pleomorphic sarcoma. *Am J Surg Pathol* 1992; **16**: 213–28.

Huvos AG, Higinbotham NL. Primary fibrosarcoma of bone. A clinicopathologic study of 130 patients. *Cancer* 1975; **35**: 837–47.

Kahn LB. Adamantinoma, osteofibrous dysplasia and differentiated adamantinoma. *Skeletal Radiol* 2003; **32**: 245–58.

Schajowicz F, Santini-Araujo E. Adamantinoma of the tibia masked by fibrous dysplasia. Report of three cases. *Clin Orthop* 1989: 294–301.

Weiss SW, Dorfman HD. Adamantinoma of long bone. An analysis of nine new cases with emphasis on metastasizing lesions and fibrous dysplasia-like changes. *Hum Pathol* 1977; **8**: 141–53.

19. BENIGN NONMATRIX-PRODUCING BONE TUMORS

Reactive or post-traumatic lesions

Bauer TW, Dorfman HD. Intraosseous ganglion: a clinicopathologic study of 11 cases. *Am J Surg Pathol* 1982; **6**: 207–13.

Dorfman HD, Steiner GC, Jaffe HL. Vascular tumors of bone. *Hum Pathol* 1971; **2**: 349–76.

Frassica FJ, Amadio PC, Wold LE et al. Aneurysmal bone cyst: clinicopathologic features and treatment of ten cases involving the hand. *J Hand Surg [Am]* 1988; **13**: 676–83.

Kambolis C, Bullough PG, Jaffe HI. Ganglionic cystic defects of bone. *J Bone Joint Surg Am* 1973; **55**: 496–505.

Makley JT, Joyce MJ. Unicameral bone cyst (simple bone cyst). *Orthop Clin North Am* 1989; **20**: 407–15.

Martinez V, Sissons HA. Aneurysmal bone cyst. A review of 123 cases including primary lesions and those secondary to other bone pathology. *Cancer* 1988; **61**: 2291–304.

Nuovo MA, Grimes MM, Knowles DM. Glomus tumors: clinicopathologic and immunohistochemical analysis of forty cases. *Surg Pathol* 1990; **3**: 31.

Ratner V, Dorfman HD. Giant-cell reparative granuloma of the hand and foot bones. *Clin Orthop* 1990: 251–8.

Roth SI. Squamous cysts involving the skull and distal phalanges. *J Bone Joint Surg Am* 1964; **46**: 1442.

Rozmaryn LM, Sadler AH, Dorfman HD. Intraosseous glomus tumor in the ulna. A case report. *Clin Orthop* 1987: 126–9.

Sanerkin NG, Mott MG, Roylance J. An unusual intraosseous lesion with fibroblastic, osteoclastic, osteoblastic, aneurysmal and fibromyxoid elements. "Solid" variant of aneurysmal bone cyst. *Cancer* 1983; **51**: 2278–86.

Schajowicz F, Aiello CL, Francone MV et al. Cystic angiomatosis (hamartous haemolymphagiomatosis) of bone. A clinicopathological study of three cases. *J Bone Joint Surg Br* 1978; **60**: 100–6.

Sugiura I. Intra-osseous glomus tumour: a case report. *J Bone Joint Surg Br* 1976; **58**: 245–7.

Developmental or hamartomatous tumors

Ishida T, Dorfman HD, Steiner GC et al. Cystic angiomatosis of bone with sclerotic changes mimicking osteoblastic metastases. *Skeletal Radiol* 1994; **23**: 247–52.

Kenan S, Abdelwahab IF, Klein MJ et al. Hemangiomas of the long tubular bone. *Clin Orthop* 1992: 256–60.

Moon NF. Synovial hemangioma of the knee joint. A review of previously reported cases and inclusion of two new cases. *Clin Orthop* 1973; **90**: 183–90.

Wenger DE, Wold LE. Benign vascular lesions of bone: radiologic and pathologic features. *Skeletal Radiol* 2000; **29**: 63–74.

Benign tumors

Beltran J, Aparisi F, Bonmati LM et al. Eosinophilic granuloma: MRI manifestations. *Skeletal Radiol* 1993; **22**: 157–61.

Bertoni F, Bacchini P, Staals EL. Malignancy in giant cell tumor of bone. *Cancer* 2003; **97**: 2520–9.

Bertoni F, Bacchini P, Staals EL. Malignancy in giant cell tumor. *Skeletal Radiol* 2003; **32**: 143–6.

Campanacci M, Baldini N, Boriani S et al. Giant-cell tumor of bone. *J Bone Joint Surg Am* 1987; **69**: 106–14.

Chow LT, Lee KC. Intraosseous lipoma. A clinicopathologic study of nine cases. *Am J Surg Pathol* 1992; **16**: 401–10.

Compere EL, Johnson WE, Coventry MB. Vertebra plana (Calve's disease) due to eosinophilic granuloma. *J Bone Joint Surg Am* 1954; **36**: 969.

Cook JV, Chandy J. Systemic mastocytosis affecting the skeletal system. *J Bone Joint Surg Br* 1989; **71**: 536.

Dehner LP. Juvenile xanthogranulomas in the first two decades of life: a clinicopathologic study of 174 cases with cutaneous and extracutaneous manifestations. *Am J Surg Pathol* 2003; **27**: 579–93.

Fallon MD, Whyte MP, Teitelbaum SL. Systemic mastocytosis associated with generalized osteopenia. Histopathological characterization of the skeletal lesion using undecalcified bone from two patients. *Hum Pathol* 1981; **12**: 813–20.

Foucar E, Rosai J, Dorfman R. Sinus histiocytosis with massive lymphadenopathy (Rosai-Dorfman disease): review of the entity. *Semin Diagn Pathol* 1990; **7**: 19–73.

Jacobs TP, Michelsen J, Polay JS et al. Giant cell tumor in Paget's disease of bone: familial and geographic clustering. *Cancer* 1979; **44**: 742–7.

Kenin A, Levine J, Spinner M. Parosteal lipoma. *J Bone Joint Surg Am* 1959; **41**: 1122.

Lantz B, Lange TA, Heiner J et al. Erdheim-Chester disease. A report of three cases. *J Bone Joint Surg Am* 1989; **71**: 456–64.

Lieberman PH, Jones CR, Steinman RM et al. Langerhans cell (eosinophilic) granulomatosis. A clinicopathologic study encompassing 50 years. *Am J Surg Pathol* 1996; **20**: 519–52.

Milgram JW. Intraosseous lipomas. A clinicopathologic study of 66 cases. *Clin Orthop* 1988: 277–302.

Sim FH, Dahlin DC, Beabout JW. Multicentric giant-cell tumor of bone. *J Bone Joint Surg Am* 1977; **59**: 1052–60.

Sung HW, Kuo DP, Shu WP et al. Giant-cell tumor of bone: analysis of two hundred and eight cases in Chinese patients. *J Bone Joint Surg Am* 1982; **64**: 755–61.

Weinfeld GD, Yu GV, Good JJ. Intraosseous lipoma of the calcaneus: a review and report of four cases. *J Foot Ankle Surg* 2002; **41**: 398–411.

20. MALIGNANT NONMATRIX-PRODUCING BONE TUMORS

Ewing's sarcoma

Burchill SA. Ewing's sarcoma: diagnostic, prognostic, and therapeutic implications of molecular abnormalities. *J Clin Pathol* 2003; **56**: 96–102.

Dagher R, Pham TA, Sorbara L et al. Molecular confirmation of Ewing sarcoma. *J Pediatr Hematol Oncol* 2001; **23**: 221–4.

Fellinger EJ, Garin-Chesa P, Triche TJ et al. Immunohistochemical analysis of Ewing's sarcoma cell surface antigen p30/32MIC2. *Am J Pathol* 1991; **139**: 317–25.

Jaffe R, Santamaria M, Yunis EJ et al. The neuroectodermal tumor of bone. *Am J Surg Pathol* 1984; **8**: 885–98.

Toolan BC, Steiner GC, Kenan S. Round cell tumors. In: *Orthopedics: a study guide* (Spivak JM, et al, eds). New York: McGraw Hill, 1999: 267–72.

Immunohematopoietic tumors

Epstein BS. Vertebral changes in childhood leukemia. *Radiology* 1957; **68**: 65.

Ishida T, Dorfman HD. Plasma cell myeloma in unusually young patients: a report of two cases and review of the literature. *Skeletal Radiol* 1995; **24**: 47–51.

Kyle RA. Multiple myeloma: review of 869 cases. *Mayo Clin Proc* 1975; **50**: 29–40.

Ostrowski ML, Inwards CY, Strickler JG et al. Osseous Hodgkin disease. *Cancer* 1999; **85**: 1166–78.

Sweet DL, Mass DP, Simon MA et al. Histiocytic lymphoma (reticulum-cell sarcoma) of bone. Current strategy for orthopaedic surgeons. *J Bone Joint Surg Am* 1981; **63**: 79–84.

Triche TJ. Diagnosis of small round cell tumors of childhood. *Bull Cancer* 1988; **75**: 297–310.

Valderrama JA, Bullough PG. Solitary myeloma of the spine. *J Bone Joint Surg Br* 1968; **50**: 82–90.

Vascular neoplasms

Dorfman HD, Steiner GC, Jaffe HL. Vascular tumors of bone. *Hum Pathol* 1971; **2**: 349–76.

Gutierrez RM, Spjut HJ. Skeletal angiomatosis: report of three cases and review of the literature. *Clin Orthop* 1972; **85**: 82–97.

Perkins P, Weiss SW. Spindle cell hemangioendothelioma. An analysis of 78 cases with reassessment of its pathogenesis and biologic behavior. *Am J Surg Pathol* 1996; **20**: 1196–204.

Tang JS, Gold RH, Mirra JM et al. Hemangiopericytoma of bone. *Cancer* 1988; **62**: 848–59.

Tsuneyoshi M, Dorfman HD, Bauer TW. Epithelioid hemangioendothelioma of bone. A clinicopathologic, ultrastructural, and immunohistochemical study. *Am J Surg Pathol* 1986; **10**: 754–64.

Wenger DE, Wold LE. Malignant vascular lesions of bone: radiologic and pathologic features. *Skeletal Radiol* 2000; **29**: 619–31.

Metastatic cancer

Boland PJ, Lane JM, Sundaresan N. Metastatic disease of the spine. *Clin Orthop* 1982: 95–102.

Mir R, Phillips SL, Schwartz G et al. Metastatic neuroblastoma after 52 years of dormancy. *Cancer* 1987; **60**: 2510–4.

Mohla S, Weilbacher KN, Cher ML et al. Third North American Symposium on Skeletal Complications of Malignancy: summary of the scientific sessions. *Cancer* 2003; **97**: 719–25.

Sherry HS, Levy RN, Siffert RS. Metastatic disease of bone in orthopedic surgery. *Clin Orthop* 1982: 44–52.

SECTION VI – SOFT-TISSUE TUMORS

21. BENIGN SOFT-TISSUE TUMORS

Benign synovial lesions

Arthaud JB. Pigmented nodular synovitis: report of 11 lesions in non-articular locations. *Am J Clin Pathol* 1972; **58**: 511–7.

Bullough PG. Pigmented villonodular synovitis and synovial cysts of the spine [comment]. *AJNR Am J Neuroradiol* 1992; **13**: 167–8.

Eisig S, Dorfman HD, Cusamano RJ et al. Pigmented villonodular synovitis of the temporomandibular joint. Case report and review of the literature. *Oral Surg Oral Med Oral Pathol* 1992; **73**: 328–33.

Hallam P, Ashwood N, Cobb J et al. Malignant transformation in synovial chondromatosis of the knee? *Knee* 2001; **8**: 239–42.

Hallel T, Lew S, Bansal M. Villous lipomatous proliferation of the synovial membrane (lipoma arborescens). *J Bone Joint Surg Am* 1988; **70**: 264–70.

Hermann G, Klein MJ, Abdelwahab IF et al. Synovial chondrosarcoma arising in synovial chondromatosis of the right hip. *Skeletal Radiol* 1997; **26**: 366–9.

Kahn LB. Malignant giant cell tumor of the tendon sheath. Ultrastructural study and review of the literature. *Arch Pathol* 1973; **95**: 203–8.

Martinez D, Millner PA, Coral A et al. Case report 745: Synovial lipoma arborescens. *Skeletal Radiol* 1992; **21**: 393–5.

Norman A, Steiner GC. Bone erosion in synovial chondromatosis. *Radiology* 1986; **161**: 749–52.

Schwartz HS, Unni KK, Pritchard DJ. Pigmented villonodular synovitis. A retrospective review of affected large joints. *Clin Orthop* 1989: 243–55.

Steiner GC, Meushar N, Norman A et al.

Intracapsular and paraarticular chondromas. *Clin Orthop* 1994: 231–6.

Villacin AB, Brigham LN, Bullough PG. Primary and secondary synovial chondrometaplasia: histopathologic and clinicoradiologic differences. *Hum Pathol* 1979; **10**: 439–51.

Wendt RG, Wolfe F, McQueen D et al. Polyarticular pigmented villonodular synovitis in children: evidence for a genetic contribution. *J Rheumatol* 1986; **13**: 921–6.

Benign fibrous lesions

Hoffman JK, Klein MH, McInerney VK. Bilateral elastofibroma: a case report and review of the literature. *Clin Orthop* 1996: 245–50.

Lauer DH, Enzinger FM. Cranial fasciitis of childhood. *Cancer* 1980; **45**: 401–6.

Renshaw TS, Simon MA. Elastofibroma. *J Bone Joint Surg Am* 1973; **55**: 409–12.

Weiss S. Fibromatoses. In: *Enzinger and Weiss's soft tissue tumors* (Weiss S, Goldblum JR, eds), 4 edn. St. Louis: Mosby, 2001: 309–46.

Peripheral nerve lesions

Lassmann G. Morton's toe: clinical, light and electron microscopic investigations in 133 cases. *Clin Orthop* 1979: 73–84.

Woodruff JM. Pathology of the major peripheral nerve sheath neoplasms. *Monogr Pathol* 1996; **38**: 129–61.

Miscellaneous lesions

Adeyemi-Doro HO, Olude O. Juvenile aponeurotic fibroma. *J Hand Surg [Br]* 1985; **10**: 127–8.

Allen RA, Woolner LB, Ghormley RK. Soft tissue tumors of the sole: with special reference to plantar fibromatosis. *J Bone Joint Surg Am* 1955; **37**: 14.

Arafa M, Noble J, Royle SG et al. Dupuytren's and epilepsy revisited. *J Hand Surg [Br]* 1992; **17**: 221–4.

Burk DL, Jr., Dalinka MK, Kanal E et al. Meniscal and ganglion cysts of the knee: MR evaluation. *AJR Am J Roentgenol* 1988; **150**: 331–6.

Chung EB, Enzinger FM. Chondroma of soft parts. *Cancer* 1978; **41**: 1414–24.

Cobey MC. Hemangioma of joints. *Arch Surg* 1943; **46**: 465.

Cohen RB, Hahn GV, Tabas JA et al. The natural history of heterotopic ossification in patients who have fibrodysplasia ossificans progressiva. A study of forty-four patients. *J Bone Joint Surg Am* 1993; **75**: 215–9.

DelSignore JL, Torre BA, Miller RJ. Extraskeletal chondroma of the hand. Case report and review of the literature. *Clin Orthop* 1990: 147–52.

Desai P, Steiner GC. Pathology of macrodactyly. *Bull Hosp Jt Dis Orthop Inst* 1990; **50**: 116–25.

Dionne GP, Seemayer TA. Infiltrating lipomas and angiolipomas revisited. *Cancer* 1974; **33**: 732–8.

Jones WA, Ghorbal MS. Benign tendon sheath chondroma. *J Hand Surg [Br]* 1986; **11**: 276–8.

Lagier R, Cox JN. Pseudomalignant myositis ossificans. A pathological study of eight cases. *Hum Pathol* 1975; **6**: 653–65.

Lantz B, Singer KM. Meniscal cysts. *Clin Sports Med* 1990; **9**: 707–25.

Lopez R, Kemalyan N, Moseley HS et al. Problems in diagnosis and management of desmoid tumors. *Am J Surg* 1990; **159**: 450–3.

Misawa A, Okada K, Hirano Y et al. Fibroma of tendon sheath arising from the radio-ulnar joint. *Pathol Int* 1999; **49**: 1089–92.

Norman A, Dorfman HD. Juxtacortical circumscribed myositis ossificans: evolution and radiographic features. *Radiology* 1970; **96**: 301–6.

Nuovo MA, Norman A, Chumas J et al. Myositis ossificans with atypical clinical, radiographic, or pathologic findings: a review of 23 cases. *Skeletal Radiol* 1992; **21**: 87–101.

Smith R. Fibrodysplasia (myositis) ossificans progressiva. Clinical lessons from a rare disease. *Clin Orthop* 1998; **346**: 7–14.

22. MALIGNANT SOFT-TISSUE TUMORS

Abramovici LC, Steiner GC, Bonar F. Myxoid chondrosarcoma of soft tissue and bone: a retrospective study of 11 cases. *Hum Pathol* 1995; **26**: 1215–20.

Bane BL, Evans HL, Ro JY et al. Extraskeletal osteosarcoma. A clinicopathologic review of 26 cases. *Cancer* 1990; **65**: 2762–70.

Barbashina V, Benevenia J, Aviv H et al. Oncoproteins and proliferation markers in synovial sarcomas: a clinicopathologic study of 19 cases. *J Cancer Res Clin Oncol* 2002; **128**: 610–6.

Bliss BO, Reed RJ. Large cell sarcomas of tendon sheath. Malignant giant cell tumors of tendon sheath. *Am J Clin Pathol* 1968; **49**: 776–81.

Fletcher CD. Pleomorphic malignant fibrous histiocytoma: fact or fiction? A critical reappraisal based on 159 tumors diagnosed as pleomorphic sarcoma. *Am J Surg Pathol* 1992; **16**: 213–28.

Halling AC, Wollan PC, Pritchard DJ et al. Epithelioid sarcoma: a clinicopathologic review of 55 cases. *Mayo Clin Proc* 1996; **71**: 636–42.

Kawaguchi S, Wada T, Nagoya S et al. Extraskeletal myxoid chondrosarcoma: a Multi-Institutional Study of 42 Cases in Japan. *Cancer* 2003; **97**: 1285–92.

Krall RA, Kostianovsky M, Patchefsky AS. Synovial sarcoma: a clinical, pathological, and ultrastructural study of 26 cases supporting the recognition of a monophasic variant. *Am J Surg Pathol* 1981; **5**: 137–51.

Mackenzie DH. The myxoid tumors of somatic soft tissues. *Am J Surg Pathol* 1981; **5**: 443–58.

Matsushita Y, Ahmed AR, Kawaguchi N et al. Epithelioid sarcoma of the extremities: a dismal long-term outcome. *J Orthop Sci* 2002; **7**: 462–6.

McKinney CD, Mills SE, Fechner RE. Intraarticular synovial sarcoma. *Am J Surg Pathol* 1992; **16**: 1017–20.

Milchgrub S, Ghandur-Mnaymneh L, Dorfman HD et al. Synovial sarcoma with extensive osteoid and bone formation. *Am J Surg Pathol* 1993; **17**: 357–63.

Miller TT, Hermann G, Abdelwahab IF et al. MRI of malignant fibrous histiocytoma of soft tissue: analysis of 13 cases with pathologic correlation. *Skeletal Radiol* 1994; **23**: 271–5.

Pelmus M, Guillou L, Hostein I et al. Monophasic fibrous and poorly differentiated synovial sarcoma: immunohistochemical reassessment of 60 t(X;18)(SYT-SSX)-positive cases. *Am J Surg Pathol* 2002; **26**: 1434–40.

Prat J, Woodruff JM, Marcove RC. Epithelioid sarcoma: an analysis of 22 cases indicating the prognostic significance of vascular invasion and regional lymph node metastasis. *Cancer* 1978; **41**: 1472–87.

Reitan JB, Kaalhus O, Brennhovd IO et al. Prognostic factors in liposarcoma. *Cancer* 1985; **55**: 2482–90.

Saleh G, Evans HL, Ro JY et al. Extraskeletal myxoid chondrosarcoma. A clinicopathologic study of ten patients with long-term follow-up. *Cancer* 1992; **70**: 2827–30.

Scott SM, Reiman HM, Pritchard DJ et al. Soft tissue fibrosarcoma. A clinicopathologic study of 132 cases. *Cancer* 1989; **64**: 925–31.

Tang JS, Gold RH, Mirra JM et al. Hemangiopericytoma of bone. *Cancer* 1988; **62**: 848–59.

Wright PH, Sim FH, Soule EH et al. Synovial sarcoma. *J Bone Joint Surg Am* 1982; **64**: 112–22.

Wu KK, Collon DJ, Guise ER. Extra-osseous chondrosarcoma. Report of five cases and review of the literature. *J Bone Joint Surg Am* 1980; **62**: 189–94.

INDEX

Notes:
Page numbers in **bold** refer to information in figures or tables only.